MELLONI'S ILLUSTRATED DICTIONARY OF

OBSTETRICS AND GYNECOLOGY

**FOR
REFERENCE ONLY**

MELLONI'S ILLUSTRATED DICTIONARY OF

OBSTETRICS AND GYNECOLOGY

I. G. Dox, PhD, J. L. Melloni, PhD,
and H. H. Sheld, MD

The Parthenon Publishing Group
International Publishers in Medicine, Science & Technology

NEW YORK   LONDON

Published in the USA by
The Parthenon Publishing Group Inc.
One Bluc Hill Plaza, PO Box 1564
Pearl River, New York 10965, USA

Published in the UK by
The Parthenon Publishing Group Limited
Casterton Hall
Carnforth, Lancs LA6 2LA, UK

Library of Congress Cataloging-in-Publication Data
Melloni's illustrated dictionary of obstetrics and gynecology / I. G. Dox,
    J. L. Melloni, and H. H. Sheld.
        p.; cm.
    ISBN 1-85070-710-3 (alk. paper)
    1. Gynecology – Dictionaries. 2. Obstetrics – Dictionaries. I. Title: Illustrated dictionary
    of obstetrics and gynecology. II. Dox, Ida. III. Melloni, June L. IV. Sheld, Harrison H.
    [DNLM: 1. Gynecology – Dictionary – English. 2. Obstetrics – Dictionary – English. WP
    13 M527 1999]
    RG45 .M45 1999
    618'.03 – dc21

                                                                                    99-056573

British Library Cataloguing in Publication Data
Melloni's illustrated dictionary of obstetrics and gynecology
    1. Obstetrics – Dictionaries 2. Gynecology – Dictionaries
    I. Dox, Ida II. Melloni, June L. III. Sheld, Harrison H.
    IV. Illustrated dictionary of obstetrics and gynecology
    618'.03
    ISBN 1850707103

Printed and bound by The Bath Press, Bath, UK

Preface

The aim of this dictionary is to place in one volume the terminology generally used in the study and practice of obstetrics and gynecology. The book contains a profusion of original, single-concept illustrations, which include a substantial number of anatomic renderings depicting the female reproductive system. Each illustration is placed in close proximity to its corresponding definition to act as a 'road map' for extended comprehension of the defined term. Color is used to highlight the point being made. In essence, the visual impact of each illustration ensures comprehension of the definition and promotes longer retention of the meaning of the word.

In addition to the distinctive language of obstetrics and gynecology, the defined entries also include relevant terms from disciplines that are linked to female health, such as oncology, genetics, endocrinology, immunology and embryology as well as the newer terms of the evolving infertility and imaging technologies. As a further aid to the reader, abbreviations frequently encountered in the literature of obstetrics and gynecology have been listed in the last 15 pages of the book.

Whenever possible, the definitions are written in everyday language. Many definitions are expanded to better serve the needs of the intended reader. Regarding eponyms, the time-honored use of the possessive form for entries containing the name of a person is currently decreasing, but this traditional form still predominates. This dictionary reflects that trend.

This dictionary was designed as a standard reference for obstetric and gynecologic terms. The prolific use of illustrations combined with definitions accurately written in everyday English, offers a proven understanding of these terms to anyone involved or interested in the many aspects of women's health and health care – to residents in obstetrics and gynecology, as well as other practicing physicians, to medical students and to those in the allied health sciences.

Suggestions to enhance the usefulness of this dictionary are welcomed and should be directed to Ida G. Dox, PhD, 9308 Renshaw Drive, Bethesda, Maryland 20817, USA.

The Authors

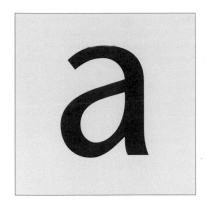

a

abandonment (ă-ban'don-ment) The unilateral termination of the doctor–patient relationship by the physician without cause or proper timely patient notification, or when alternative sources of medical care are unavailable.

abdomen (ab'dŏ-men, ab-do'men) The part of the body between the chest and the pelvis, containing the largest cavity of the body; generally divided into nine regions by hypothetical planes to identify the location of structures contained within. Abdominal contents include nerves, blood and lymph vessels, lymph nodes, and several organs (lowest part of esophagus, stomach, intestines, liver, gallbladder, pancreas, and spleen). Also called belly, and (incorrectly) stomach. See also abdominal regions, under region; abdominal cavity, under cavity.

abdomen

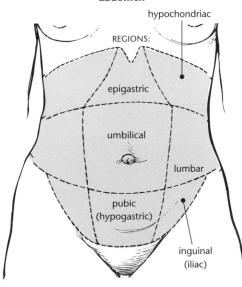

REGIONS:
- hypochondriac
- epigastric
- umbilical
- lumbar
- pubic (hypogastric)
- inguinal (iliac)

acute a. General term denoting any intra-abdominal condition that usually requires surgical treatment; common findings include tenderness, muscle guarding, abnormal or absent bowel sounds, and pain felt when pressure applied to the abdomen is released (rebound tenderness); gynecologic causes include ectopic pregnancy, a bleeding ovarian cyst, and inflammation of a fallopian (uterine) tube. Also called surgical abdomen.

   burst a. See evisceration (3).

   surgical a. See acute abdomen.

abdominal (ab-dom'ĭ-nal) Relating to the abdomen.

abdomino-, abdomin- Combining forms meaning abdomen.

abdominocentesis (ab-dom-ĭ-no-sen-te'sis) See peritoneocentesis.

abdominocystic (ab-dom-ĭ-no-sis'tik) **1.** Relating to the gallbladder. **2.** See abdominovesical.

abdominoperineal (ab-dom-ĭ-no-per-ĭ-ne'al) Relating to the abdomen and perineum, applied especially to surgical procedures involving those areas.

abdominovaginal (ab-dom-ĭ-no-vag'ĭ-nal) Relating to the abdomen and vagina.

abdominovesical (ab-dom-ĭ-no-ves'ĭ-kl) Relating to the abdomen and bladder. Also called abdominocystic.

abembryonic (ab-em-bre-on'ik) Away from the region where the embryo is located.

aberration (ab-er-a'shun) Abnormality; deviation; imperfection.

   chromosomal a. Any irregularity in the number of chromosomes or structure of a chromosome that is discernible by microscopy. Also called chromosomal anomaly.

ablatio placentae (ab-la'shio) See abruptio placentae.

ablation (ab-la'shun) **1.** Detachment. **2.** Eradication or removal of tissues by surgery, laser, or freezing radiotherapy.

   hormonal a. Ablation of a particular tissue to arrest its hormonal production (e.g., removal of the ovaries for the treatment of advanced breast cancer).

abnormal (ab-nor'mal) Not normal; differing substantially from the usual.

abnormality (ab-nor-mal'ĭ-te) **1.** The state of being abnormal. **2.** An anomaly or dysfunction.

ABO blood group International classification of human blood types according to their compatibility in transfusion, typed as A, B, AB, or O.

abort (ă-bort') **1.** To expel or to remove the products of conception before the fetus reaches the age of viability. **2.** To arrest the usual course of a disease. **3.** To cause cessation of development.

abortient (ă-bor'shent) See abortifacient.

abortifacient (ă-bor-tĭ-fa'shent) **1.** Producing an abortion. Also called abortient; abortigenic; abortive. **2.** An agent, such as a drug, that brings about an abortion.

abortigenic (ă-bor-tĭ-gen'ik) See abortifacient.

abortion (ă-bor'shun) **1.** Expulsion or extraction of all or any part of the products of conception (placenta, membranes, and embryo or fetus) before the end of 20 completed weeks (139 days) of gestation calculated from the first day of the last normal menstrual period, or at a fetal weight of less than 500 g. **2.** The arrest of any process.

> **accidental a.** Abortion resulting from injury.

> **ampullar a.** Abortion resulting from implantation of the fertilized egg within the ampulla of the fallopian (uterine) tube.

> **atraumatic a.** See menstrual aspiration, under aspiration.

> **complete a.** Abortion that includes the fetus (or embryo), placenta, and membranes, ending with cessation of both pain and copious bleeding.

> **early a.** Spontaneous abortion occurring before completion of 12 weeks of gestation; thought to be caused mainly by a chromosomal abnormality of the embryo.

> **elective a.** Induced abortion performed at the request of the pregnant woman, but not due to impaired maternal health or fetal disease and before fetal viability is reached. Also called voluntary abortion.

> **eugenic a.** See therapeutic abortion.

> **habitual a.** Three or more spontaneous abortions occurring consecutively, before 20 weeks of gestation, with the fetus weighing less than 500 g. Causes may be due to fetal or maternal factors and usually include: genetic error, hormonal abnormalities, anatomic anomalies of the reproductive tract, infection, systemic disease, and immunologic factors. Sometimes causes are unknown. Also called recurrent abortion; recurrent spontaneous abortion.

> **incomplete a.** Abortion in which some of the products of conception (usually a portion of the placenta) remain within the uterus, causing profuse uterine bleeding.

> **induced a.** Abortion deliberately carried out by means of drugs or mechanical devices or instruments, ensuring that the embryo or fetus will not survive. It may be therapeutic or nontherapeutic. See also elective abortion; therapeutic abortion.

> **inevitable a.** Bleeding of intrauterine origin occurring before 20 completed weeks of gestation with continuous and progressive dilatation of the cervix, but without expulsion of the products of conception.

> **infected a.** Abortion accompanied by fever, generalized pelvic discomfort, purulent discharge, or elevated white blood cell count; caused by infection of the genital organs with pathogenic microorganisms. Distinguished from septic abortion.

> **justifiable a.** See therapeutic abortion.

> **late a.** Spontaneous abortion occurring between 12 and 20 weeks of gestation; considered to be mainly due to maternal factors.

> **missed a.** Death of an embryo or fetus before completion of the 20th week of gestation, with retention of all the products of conception within the uterus for several weeks; manifested by absence of a fetal heartbeat, regression of breast changes, decrease of uterine size, and weight loss; may be accompanied by a bloody or brownish discharge.

> **natural a.** See spontaneous abortion.

> **nontherapeutic a.** Abortion induced without a medical reason.

> **recidive a.** The occurrence of two consecutive spontaneous abortions before 20 weeks of gestation, with the fetus weighing less than 500 g.

> **recurrent a.** See habitual abortion.

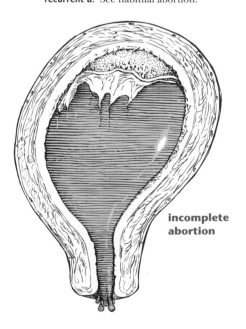

incomplete abortion

recurrent spontaneous a. See habitual abortion.

partial-birth a. (PBA) Popular term for a late pregnancy termination. Labor is induced by conventional methods and delivery is effected in the usual way, except if there is a breech presentation. In that case, the delivery may be expedited by evacuating the cranial contents with a suction catheter and then decompressing the calvaria. Also called dilatation and evacuation (D & E).

saline-induced a. Abortion performed, usually during the second trimester, by injecting a 20–25% saline solution into the amniotic sac; because the procedure has resulted in serious complications, including disseminated coagulation (DIC) and death, it has been replaced by dilatation and evacuation (D & E).

septic a. Infected abortion accompanied by life-threatening dissemination of microorganisms and toxic substances throughout the maternal blood circulation; marked by a malodorous discharge, pelvic and abdominal pain, suprapubic tenderness, and peritonitis. Distinguished from infected abortion.

spontaneous a. Expulsion of the products of conception due to natural causes, without deliberate mechanical or medicinal interference, and occurring before the fetus can survive outside the uterus. Also called fetal loss; miscarriage; natural abortion.

subclinical spontaneous a. See undiagnosed spontaneous abortion.

therapeutic a. Abortion performed before the time of fetal viability to safeguard the physical or mental health of the pregnant woman. Also called justifiable abortion; eugenic abortion.

threatened a. Slight or heavier bloody vaginal discharge, occurring during the first 20 weeks of pregnancy, with or without cramplike pain and low backache, without expulsion of the products of conception, and without dilatation of the cervix.

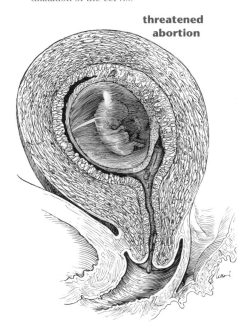

threatened abortion

tubal a. The spontaneous termination of a tubal pregnancy; commonly, the embryo separates from its implantation site within the fallopian (uterine) tube and is expelled into the peritoneal cavity through the end of the tube; less frequently, it may pass into the peritoneal cavity through a rupture of the tube's wall at the implantation site (usually at the tubal isthmus).

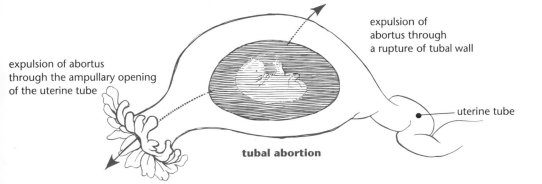

expulsion of abortus through a rupture of tubal wall

expulsion of abortus through the ampullary opening of the uterine tube

uterine tube

tubal abortion

undiagnosed spontaneous a. A pregnancy that is aborted or reabsorbed before it is recognized. Also called subclinical spontaneous abortion.

voluntary a. See elective abortion.

abortionist (ă-bor'shun-ist) One who induces abortion, especially illegally.

abortive (ă-bor'tiv) **1.** Cutting short progress (e.g., of a disease). **2.** Incompletely developed or formed; rudimentary. **3.** See abortifacient.

abortus (ă-bor'tus) A fetus or embryo aborted during the first half of gestation with all or part of its accompanying tissues and weighing less than 500 g, or measuring less than 25 cm from crown to heel.

abrachia (ă-bra'ke-ă) Congenital absence of the arms; may be unilateral or bilateral. Bones of the shoulder may be absent or reduced in size.

abruption (ab-rup'shun) A detachment or tearing away.

placental a. See abruptio placentae.

abruptio placentae (ab-rup'she-o plă-sen'te) Premature detachment of the placenta from the uterine wall. Also called ablatio placentae; placental abruption; accidental hemorrhage; premature separation of normally implanted placenta.

absence (ab'sens) Abrupt, brief loss of consciousness without loss of postural tone or autonomic function, usually without convulsions. Also called absentia epileptica; petit mal; petit mal epilepsy; absence seizure.

abscess (ab'ses) Localized accumulation of pus associated with tissue destruction; usually caused by a bacterial infection.

acute a. Abscess of short duration accompanied by fever, inflammation, and throbbing pain. Also called hot abscess.

anal a. Abscess occurring along the anal canal; may be superficial or deep and usually originates from the folds of the anorectal junction (anal crypts); caused by bacterial infection, usually resulting from infiltration of normal rectal flora (*Bacillus coli, Bacillus proteus, Bacillus subtilis*, staphylococci, and streptococci).

appendiceal a. Abscess occurring near the vermiform appendix; generally formed after perforation of an inflamed appendix. Also called periappendiceal abscess; appendicular abscess.

appendicular a. See appendiceal abscess.

Bartholin's a. Abscess in a greater vestibular (Bartholin's) gland or its duct. Sometimes, but not always, a complication of a gonorrheal infection.

breast a. See mammary abscess.

canalicular a. Abscess connected to a milk (lactiferous) duct within a breast, causing a purulent discharge from the nipple.

abruptio placentae

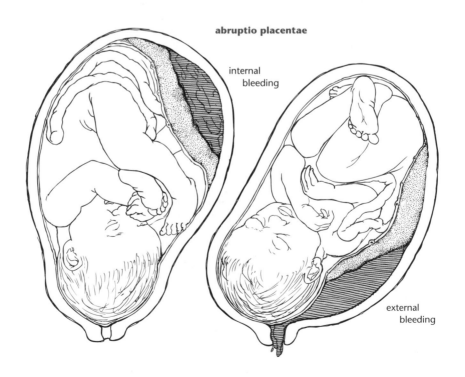

internal bleeding

external bleeding

chronic a. A long-standing, slow-developing abscess occurring without inflammation. Also called cold abscess.

cold a. See chronic abscess.

diffuse a. An abscess that is not enclosed in a capsule.

dry a. The remains of an abscess after the pus is resorbed.

gas a. Abscess containing gas due to the presence of gas-forming bacteria such as *Enterobacter aerogenes, Clostridium perfringens,* and *Escherichia coli.*

gravitation a. See perforating abscess.

gummatous a. Abscess formed subsequent to the softening and breaking down of a gumma, the characteristic tumor of tertiary syphilis. Also called syphilitic abscess.

hot a. See acute abscess.

hypostatic a. See perforating abscess.

iliac a. See psoas abscess.

mammary a. Single or multiple abscesses of the breast substance, affecting usually one breast; most commonly caused by *Staphylococcus aureus*, or occasionally by streptococci. Organisms gain entry through cracks on the nipple, most frequently during lactation, or in skin conditions such as eczema. Destroyed breast tissue may be replaced by fibrous tissue with resulting nipple retraction, which may be mistaken for a tumor. Also called breast abscess.

metastatic a. A secondary abscess caused by microorganisms carried in the bloodstream from a primary abscess.

migrating a. See perforating abscess.

pelvic a. Abscess in the retrouterine pouch occurring as a complication of abdominal or pelvic inflammatory disease.

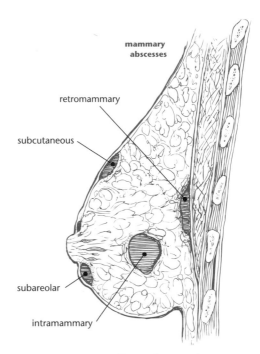

mammary abscesses

retromammary

subcutaneous

subareolar

intramammary

perforating a. Abscess that spreads to adjacent areas through a point of least resistance. Also called gravitation abscess; hypostatic abscess; migrating abscess; wandering abscess.

periappendiceal a. See appendiceal abscess.

periurethral a. Abscess involving the tissues of the urethra, causing strained, painful urination; associated with gonorrhea or other pyogenic infection.

psoas a. Abscess located along the sheath of the psoas muscle occurring as an extension of infection from a tuberculous lower spine, or

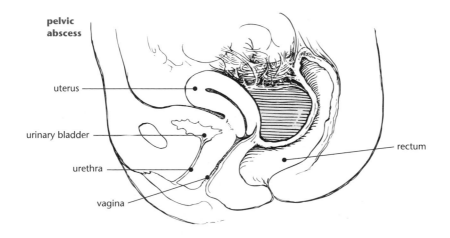

pelvic abscess

uterus

urinary bladder

urethra

vagina

rectum

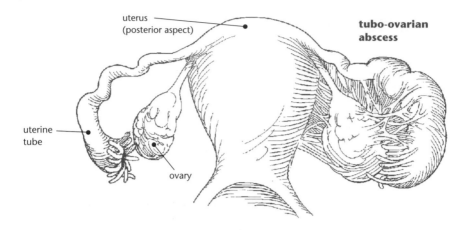

uterus
(posterior aspect)

tubo-ovarian abscess

uterine tube

ovary

from regional inflammation of the intestines. Also called iliac abscess.

    stitch a. A small abscess around a suture.

    syphilitic a. See gummatous abscess.

    tubo-ovarian a. Abscess involving both a fallopian (uterine) tube and its corresponding ovary, usually associated with inflammation of the tube; generally seen in patients with a history of pelvic infection; symptoms include an extremely tender pelvic mass, abdominal and pelvic pain, fever, nausea, and vomiting.

    wandering a. See perforating abscess.

absorptiometry (ab-sorp-she-om'ě-tre) **1.** Any procedure for measuring absorption of waves or particles. **2.** In radiology, measurement of the amount of radiation, emitted by a radioisotope, that is completely dispersed throughout a tissue.

    dual-photon a. A method of quantitating bone mineral content by comparing the transmission of two photoelectric energy peaks emitted by gandolinium 153 through bone and soft tissues; used to measure bone density of the spine and hip for diagnosis of osteoporosis and in following therapy response.

absorption (ab-sorp'shun) **1.** The process of taking up and incorporating a substance or energy (gas, liquid, light, heat). **2.** In radiology, the uptake of radiant energy by the medium through which the radiation passes.

abstinence (ab'stĭ-nens) Voluntary refraining, especially from indulging in a craving for certain foods, alcohol, or drugs, or sexual activity.

    periodic a. See rhythm method, under method.

abuse (a-bus') **1.** Habitual and excessive use. **2.** Maltreatment; injurious or offensive treatment.

    a. of children See child abuse.

    alcohol a. See alcoholism.

    child a. An act or omission, which is not accidental, committed by a parent, caregiver, or other adult, that harms, or threatens to harm, a child's physical or mental health or welfare. It may occur in the following forms: *Emotional child a.*: acts or omissions usually on the part of parents or other caregivers that cause serious behavioral, cognitive, emotional, or mental disorders in the child; may involve rejecting the child's needs, isolating the child from normal social experiences, terrorizing the child by constant verbal harassment and denigration, ignoring the child's emotional and developmental growth, and corrupting the child by engagement in antisocial behavior. Emotional abuse usually accompanies other forms of abuse and neglect. Also called psychological abuse. *Physical child a.*: abuse that results in physical injury, usually perpetrated in the name of discipline or punishment and ranging from slaps to the use of belts, kitchen utensils, lit cigarettes, etc. *Psychological child a.*: see emotional child abuse. *Sexual child a.*: any sexual activity perpetrated by an adult or older child with or upon a child, or the sexual exploitation of a child for the gratification or profit of the other. It may be assaultive, which produces physical injury and severe emotional trauma, or nonassaultive, which causes little or no physical injury.

    drug a. See substance abuse.

    polydrug a. Simultaneous abuse of several substances, usually including alcohol.

    sexual child a. See child abuse.

    substance a. The excessive and persistent use (generally self-administered) of any drug, most commonly an agent that acts on the central nervous system, without due regard for accepted medical practice. Abused substances include alcohol, tobacco, marijuana, amphetamines, cocaine, heroine, methadone, LSD (lysergic acid diethylamide), PCP (phencyclidine), and 'T's and blues'. The maternal and embryofetal damage caused by these substances when taken by a pregnant woman are numerous, ranging from spontaneous abortion to growth or mental retardation, congenital anomalies, and perinatal death. Also called drug abuse.

acanthosis nigrans (ak-an-tho'sis ni'grans) A benign hyperpigmented skin lesion characterized by papillomatous hypertrophy, associated with a variety of disorders of the endocrine system, including pituitary Cushing's syndrome, pituitary tumors, acromegaly, Addison disease, and polycystic ovarian disease. Most often there is an underlying insulin resistance.

acardia (a-kar'de-ă) Absence of the heart; a rare condition sometimes occurring in one member of conjoined twins.

accelerant (ak-sel'er-ant) See accelerator.

accelerator (ak-sel'er-a-tor) Any device, drug, nerve, or muscle that increases speed of action or function. Also called accelerant.

    linear a. In radiation therapy, a machine that creates high-energy radiation using electricity to form a stream of fast-moving subatomic particles; used in cancer treatment. Also called megavoltage (MeV) linear accelerator; linac.

    megavoltage (MeV) linear a. See linear accelerator.

accouchement (ah-koosh-maw') French for childbirth; labor.

accoucheur (ah-koo-sher') French for midwife.

acentric (ă-sen'trik) Without a center; in genetics, applied to a chromosome without a centromere.

acephaly (ă-sef'ă-le) Congenital absence of the head.

acetaminophen (ă-set-am'ĭ-no-fen) A non-prescription drug used to relieve pain and fever. It lacks anti-inflammatory properties and has been known to have harmful effects on the liver.

acetone (as'ĕ-tōn) Dimethyl ketone; one of the ketone bodies found in the blood and urine of persons with poorly controlled diabetes. See also ketone bodies, under body; ketoacidosis.

acetonemia (as-ĕ-to-ne'me-ă) Condition marked by increased concentration of acetone in the blood, as occurs when there is incomplete breakdown of large amounts of fat; seen in poorly controlled diabetes, high-fat diets, and starvation states.

acetonuria (as-ĕ-to-nu're-ă) The presence of acetone in the urine, occurs in poorly controlled diabetes mellitus and in starvation states from incomplete oxidation of fats.

acetylcholinesterase (as'ĕ-tēl-ko-lĭ-nes'tĕ-rās) An enzyme, present throughout body tissues, which promotes the hydrolysis of acetylcholine; it removes acetylcholine discharged at the neuromuscular junction, thus preventing it from re-exciting the muscle. Also called cholinesterase.

    amniotic fluid a. Acetylcholinesterase not normally present in amniotic fluid; it may be present in cases of multifactorial fetal abnormalities, such as open neural tube defects, omphalocele, cystic hygroma, and certain mendelian conditions.

acetylcysteine (as-ĕ-tēl-sis'te-ēn) The N-acetyl derivative of L-cysteine; a compound that reduces the viscosity of mucus; used to remove excessive mucus produced in certain bronchopulmonary disorders and in cases of infertility due to viscous cervical mucus; also used for the treatment of acetaminophen overdosage.

achalasia (ak-ă-la'ze-ă) Failure to relax; refers especially to a disorder of the motor innervation of the esophagus, causing impairment of coordinated muscular action (peristalsis) of the lower portion of the esophagus and failure of the esophageal sphincter to relax. Also called cardiospasm, esophageal aperistalsis.

acheilia (ă-ki'le-ă), pl. achilia Absence of one or both lips, a developmental defect. Also spelled achilia.

acheilous (ă-ki'lus) Relating to acheilia. Also spelled achilous.

acheiria (ă-ki're-ă) Absence of one or both hands; a developmental defect. Also spelled achiria.

acheiropodia, acheiropody (ă-ki-ro-po'de-ă, ă-ki-rop'o-de) Absence of one or both hands and feet; a developmental defect. Also spelled achiropodia; achiropody.

acheirous (ă-ki'rus) Relating to acheiria. Also spelled achirous.

achilia (ă-ki'le-ă) See acheilia.

achilous (ă-ki'lus) See acheilous.

achiria (ă-ki're-ă) See acheiria.

achirous (ă-ki'rus) See acheirous.

achondrogenesis (ă-kon-dro-jen'ĕ-sis) A type of hereditary dwarfism characterized by underdevelopment of bone of the four limbs, resulting in markedly short arms and legs relative to the trunk and head, which are normal in size; an autosomal recessive inheritance.

achondroplasia (ă-kon-dro-pla'ze-ă) A defect in the conversion process of cartilage into bone, resulting in dwarfism and other skeletal deformities; an autosomal dominant inheritance. Also called achondroplasty; osteosclerosis congenita.

achondroplastic (ă-kon-dro-plas'tik) Relating to achondroplasia.

achondroplasty (ă-kon'dro-plas-te) See achondroplasia.

achordia (ă-kor'de-ă) Absence of the umbilical cord.

achoresis (ak-o-re'sis) A reduction in the capacity of a hollow organ (e.g., of the bladder or stomach) resulting from a persistent contraction.

acid (as'id) A compound that can donate a hydrogen ion (proton) to a base and combine to form a salt; any substance that turns litmus indicators red. For individual acids, see specific names.

    amino a.'s Organic compounds containing an amino group (NH_2) and a carboxyl group (COOH) and forming the basic structural units of all proteins. Individual amino acid molecules are linked by chemical bonds between the amino and carboxyl groups to form chains of molecules (polypeptides). Polypeptides, in turn, join to form a protein molecule. Amino acids that cannot be made by the body and must be obtained from the diet to maintain health are called *essential amino a.'s*; those that can be made by the body from other amino acids are termed *nonessential amino acids.*

    bile a.'s Steroid acids important in digestion and absorption of fats.

    fatty a.'s A large group of organic acids, especially those present in fat, made up of molecules containing a carboxyl group (COOH) at the end of a long hydrocarbon chain; the number of carbon atoms ranges from 2 to 34. Usually classified as *saturated fatty a.'s* (those containing the maximum amount of hydrogen), *unsaturated fatty a.'s* (those whose carbon atoms contain some sites unoccupied by hydrogen), *monounsaturated fatty acids* (those whose carbon atoms contain one unoccupied site), and *polyunsaturated fatty acids* (those whose carbon atoms contain many unoccupied sites).

acidemia (as-ĭ-de'me-a) An increase in the hydrogen ion concentration of the blood; a fall below the normal pH (7.42) of the blood. See also acidosis.

acidity (ă-sid'ĭ-te) 1. The quality of being acid. 2. The acid content of a fluid.

    gastric a. The acid content of stomach fluids.

acidosis (as-ĭ-do'sis) A process tending to produce an increase in hydrogen ion concentration in body fluids; if uncompensated, it produces a lowering of the pH. Commonly used synonymously with acidemia.

    carbon dioxide a. See respiratory acidosis.

    compensated a. Condition in which the pH of blood is kept within the normal range through respiratory or renal mechanisms, although the blood bicarbonate level may be out of the usual range.

    lactic a. A metabolic acidosis in which lactic acid accumulates in the body, causing decreased bicarbonate concentration.

    metabolic a. Acidosis occurring in individuals afflicted with metabolic disorders in which acid (excluding carbonic acid) accumulates in, or bicarbonate is lost from, extracellular fluids.

    renal tubular a. (RTA) Acidosis secondary to kidney disorders in which there is defective elimination of acid or excessive loss of bicarbonate by the kidneys; characterized by elevated plasma chloride and lowered concentration of plasma bicarbonate.

    respiratory a. Acidosis caused by failure to adequately eliminate carbon dioxide (CO_2) from the blood circulation; the retained CO_2 in the blood yields carbonic acid (H_2CO_3) and its dissociation increases the hydrogen ion concentration; seen in advanced pulmonary disease. Also called carbon dioxide acidosis.

acidotic (as-ĭ-dot'ik) Relating to acidosis.

aciduria (as-ĭ-du're-ă) The presence of an abnormal amount of acids in the urine.

acro- Combining form meaning extremity; tip; an extreme.

acrocentric (ak-ro-sen'trik) Denoting a chromosome with its centromere located away from the center, close to one end.

acrocephalic (ak-ro-sĕ-fal'ik) See oxycephalic.

acrocephalopolysyndactyly (ak-ro-sef'ă-lo-pol-e-sin-dak'tĭ-le) (ACPS) General term for any of four types of inherited syndromes characterized by premature closure of the space between cranial bones (craniosynostosis), webbed fingers or toes (syndactyly), and extra digits (polydactyly). Each type has specific additional features.

acrocephalosyndactyly (ak-ro-sef-ă-lo-sin-dak'tĭ-le) Any of a group of inherited conditions occurring in varying degrees of congenital malformations of the skull and digits; characterized mainly by a high-domed or peaked head due to premature closure of the space between cranial bones (craniosynostosis), and a partial or complete webbing of fingers or toes (syndactyly); an autosomal dominant inheritance.

acrocephaly (ak-ro-sef'ă-le) See oxycephaly.

acrochordon (ak-ro-kor'don) See skin tag, under tag.

acrocyanosis (ak-ro-si-ă-no'sis) A chronic circulatory disorder marked by persistently cold and profusely sweating hands and feet, with mottled blue and red skin; the condition is intensified by cold or emotion.

acrodysesthesis (ak-ro-dis-es-the'sis) Abnormal sensations (e.g., numbness, tingling) occurring in the hands or feet.

acromioclavicular (ă-kro-me-o-klă-vik'u-lar) Denoting a relationship to the acromion and the clavicle (bones of the shoulder joint).

acromiocoracoid (ă-kro-me-o-kor'ă-koid) See coracoacromial.

acromion (ă-kro'me-on) The flattened process extending laterally from the spine of the shoulder blade (scapula); it articulates with the collarbone (clavicle), forms the most prominent point of the shoulder, and provides attachment to muscles and ligaments of the shoulder joint.

acromphalus (ă-krom'fă-lus) Abnormal protrusion of the umbilicus.

acrosome (ak'ro-sōm) The dense caplike, membrane-bound structure covering the anterior tip of a spermatozoon; it contains enzymes that facilitate penetration of the egg by the sperm during fertilization. Also called acrosomal cap.

actino- Combining form denoting a relation to a form of radiation.

Actinomyces (ak-tĭ-no-mi'sēz) A genus of filamentous bacteria that are nonmotile and nonacid-fast (family Actinomycetaceae). Some species are responsible for pathologic infections in humans and animals.

    A. israelii An anaerobic species that is the causative agent of human actinomycosis; also associated with unilateral tubo-ovarian abscess in a patient wearing an intrauterine device (IUD).

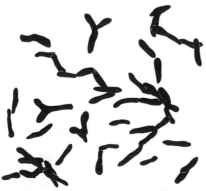

3μm Actinomyces israelii

actinomycin (ak-tĭ-no-mi'sin) Any of a group of antibiotic substances, obtained from various species of *Streptomyces*, which are active against bacteria and fungi. Some, such as actinomycin D (dactinomycin), act against the cells of certain tumors.

actinomycosis (ak-tĭ-no-mi-ko'sis) A contagious disease characterized by multiple, painful swellings that progress to form abscesses and suppurating openings in the skin of the jaw and neck and, less frequently, the vulvar skin; caused by *Actinomyces israelii*. The microorganisms may inhabit the mouth, clinging to the gums, teeth and tonsils without causing disease until they gain entrance to the tissues (e.g., through a decayed tooth or a tooth extraction). If untreated, infection may extend via the bloodstream to the lungs and intestinal tract. Also called lumpy jaw.

activator (ak'tĭ-va-tor) Any substance that stimulates, accelerates, or increases the activity of another substance, especially one that combines with an enzyme to enhance its catalytic activity.

    tissue plasminogen a. (tPA) A genetically engineered enzyme that is capable of dissolving thrombi, such as those obstructing coronary arteries; used in the treatment of myocardial infarction. Also called tissue-type plasminogen activator.

    tissue-type plasminogen a. (tPA) See tissue plasminogen activator.

activin (ak'tĭ-vin) A peptide derived from granulosa cells of the ovary; present also in the pituitary and in many other tissues (e.g., bone marrow); it stimulates secretion of follicle-stimulating hormone (FSH); in the embryo, activin is involved in mesoderm formation.

acyanotic (ă-si-ă-not'ik) Not marked by cyanosis.

acycloguanocin (a-si-klo-guan'o-sin) See acyclovir.

acyclovir (a-si'klo-vir) An antiviral compound used chiefly in the treatment of herpesvirus infections, especially genital herpes and shingles (herpes zoster).

acystia (ă-sis'te-ă) Congenital absence of the bladder.

ad- Prefix meaning to or toward; adherence; increase.

-ad Suffix used in anatomic nomenclature meaning toward the direction of (e.g., cephalad).

adactylous (a-dak'tĭ-lus) Lacking fingers or toes.

adactyly (a-dak'tĭ-le) Congenital anomaly marked by the absence of digits.

adeno-, aden- Combining forms denoting a relationship to a gland.

adenoacanthoma (ad-ĕ-no-ak-an-tho′mă) An aggressive cancerous tumor, most commonly of the uterus, that is made up of malignant glandular tissue, but most of the cells exhibit benign squamous differentiation. Also called adenosquamous carcinoma.

adenoblast (ad′ĕ-no-blast) Embryonic cell that gives origin to glandular tissue.

adenocarcinoma (ad-ĕ-no-kar-sĭ-no′mă) Glandular cancer in which the malignant tissue is derived from epithelial cells, or arranged in a glandlike pattern. It is the most common type of endometrial cancer. Also called glandular cancer.

    clear cell a. of vagina An uncommon type of vaginal cancer occurring in young females, between the ages of 10 and 35 years, whose mothers were treated with diethylstilbestrol (DES) during pregnancy for the treatment of threatened abortion.

    renal a. The most common form of cancer of the kidney, especially among people over 60 years of age; may be detected by the presence of blood in the urine; often found incidentally when a sonogram of the abdomen is obtained; may spread via the bloodstream to the lungs, bone, liver, and brain. Also called clear cell carcinoma of kidney; hypernephroma, Grawitz' tumor; renal cell carcinoma.

    secretory a. An uncommon type of endometrial cancer, occurring as a well-differentiated tumor with progestational changes and causing abnormal uterine bleeding.

    villoglandular papillary a. A generally circumscribed endocervical adenocarcinoma occurring usually at a young age (average 33 years); characterized basically by a surface papillary component of variable thickness; typically, the papillae have a fibromatous stroma; the invasive portion of the tumor is composed of elongated branching glands separated by fibromatous stroma; invasion by lymphatic or blood circulation occurs only rarely.

adenofibrosis (ad-ĕ-no-fi-bro′sis) See sclerosing adenosis, under adenosis.

adenohypophyseal, adenohypophysial (ad-ĕ-no-hi-po-fiz′e-al) Relating to the anterior, glandular portion of the pituitary (hypophysis).

adenohypophysis (ad-ĕ-no-hi-pof′ĭ-sis) The anterior, glandular portion of the pituitary (hypophysis); it synthesizes and secretes several important hormones, including thyroid-stimulating hormone (TSH), adrenocorticotropic hormone (ACTH), follicle-stimulating hormone (FSH), growth hormone, and luteinizing hormone (LH). Also called anterior lobe of pituitary, glandular lobe of pituitary. See also hypophysis; neurohypophysis.

adenoma (ad-ĕ-no′mă) Benign tumor arising from epithelial cells of glands or having a glandlike structure.

    chromophobe a., chromophobic a. See null-cell adenomas.

    growth hormone-secreting a. Pituitary adenoma composed of cells that secrete excessive growth hormone, which may cause gigantism in children and acromegaly in adults.

    gonadotroph a. Any benign, gonadotropin-secreting tumor arising from the anterior portion of the pituitary; so named because it secretes hormones targeted to the gonads (the ovaries and testes).

    hepatocellular a. A soft, pale yellow tumor in the liver that is strongly associated with the use of oral contraceptives and anabolic steroids; also seen in pregnancy; has a tendency to rupture through the liver capsule, especially during pregnancy, causing sudden pain and intraperitoneal hemorrhage. Also called liver cell adenoma.

    liver cell a. See hepatocellular adenoma.

    null-cell a.'s Pituitary adenomas composed of cells that give negative results on tests for hormone secretion; some tumors may contain functioning cells and may be associated with hyperpituitary conditions.

    ovarian tubular a. See arrhenoblastoma.

    pituitary a. Any adenoma of the anterior lobe of the pituitary occurring most frequently in the age group between 20 and 50 years; they are typically enveloped by a thin fibrous membrane and composed mostly of one

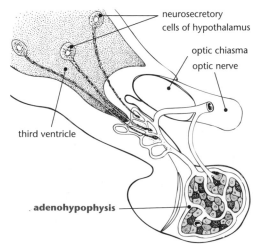

neurosecretory cells of hypothalamus

optic chiasma

optic nerve

third ventricle

adenohypophysis

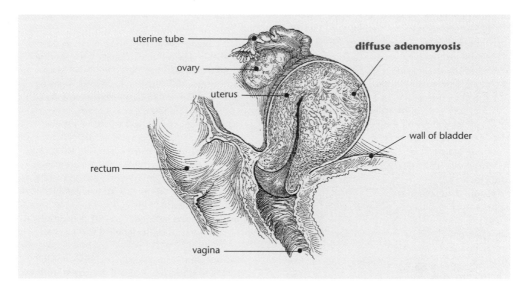

uterine tube

diffuse adenomyosis

ovary

uterus

wall of bladder

rectum

vagina

morphologic cell type which, depending on the type, may cause overproduction of specific hormones and consequent disorders (e.g., Cushing's syndrome and acromegaly).

    tubular a. A benign, usually pedunculated polyp commonly occurring on the inner lining of the colon; risk of its becoming cancerous correlates with size.

    villous a. A potentially cancerous adenoma of the inner lining of the large intestine.

adenomatoid (ăd-ĕ-no′mă-toid) Resembling an adenoma.

adenomatous (ad-ĕ-nom′ă-tus) Relating to an adenoma or to glandular overgrowth.

adenomyoma (ad-ĕ-no-mi-o′mă) See focal adenomyosis, under adenomyosis.

adenomyosis (ad-ĕ-no-mi-o′sis) The abnormal, but benign, ingrowth of the endometrium into the uterine musculature. Also called endometriosis interna.

    diffuse a. Adenomyosis involving much or all of the uterus.

    focal a. Adenomyosis concentrating in one area, forming a nodular mass that resembles a fibroid. Also called adenomyoma.

adenosarcoma (ad-ĕ-no-sar-ko′mă) A cancerous tumor containing glandular tissue.

adenosis (ad-ĕ-no′sis) **1.** Any disease of glands, especially one involving the lymph nodes. **2.** Abnormal development of glandular tissue.

    sclerosing a. A benign condition of the breast most commonly affecting young women; characterized by the formation of relatively hard nodules of glandular tissue that, occasionally, may be difficult to distinguish

from cancer. Also called adenofibrosis.

    vaginal a. Abnormal development of glandular tissue in the vagina resulting from *in utero* exposure to diethylstilbestrol (DES), causing vaginal bleeding and discharge. Abnormal tissue may occur, (1) as replacement of the normal squamous cell lining of the vagina, (2) beneath the intact normal lining, or (3) mixed with the squamous cells of the lining.

S-adenosyl-L-methionine (ă-den-o-sĭl-me-thi′o-nēn) A product of the reaction of ATP and the amino acid methionine, serving as a methyl donor in transmethylation reactions. It has been used to treat disorders that arrest or suppress bile flow (cholestasis) but its use in pregnancy is not recommended.

adhesion (ad-he′zhun) **1.** The sticking together of two surfaces that are normally separate (e.g., in inflammatory processes). **2.** One of the fibrous bands abnormally holding two surfaces together. **3.** The attraction of two surfaces in contact, such as that of blood platelets sticking to each other or to a blood vessel wall.

    abdominal a.'s Adhesions formed in the abdominal cavity, usually involving the intestines; may occur as a complication of surgery or as a result of peritonitis (i.e., inflammation of the serous membrane lining the abdominal cavity).

    labial a. Abnormal fusion of the labia majora, most commonly seen in prepubertal girls; thought to be due to age-related low levels of estrogens. The skin covering the labia becomes extremely thin; when irritated, the labia become denuded, causing them to stick together at the midline with subsequent re-epithelialization.

> **posttraumatic uterine a.'s** Formation of adhesions within the uterine cavity, usually caused by scraping off of the inner uterine lining (curettage), resulting in reduced or absent menstrual flow and, frequently, infertility. Also called Asherman's syndrome.

> **primary a.** See healing by first intention, under healing.

> **secondary a.** See healing by second intention, under healing.

adhesiotomy (ad-he-ze-ot'o-me) The surgical division of adhesions.

adip-, adipo- Combining forms meaning fat. See also lip-; lipo-.

adiponecrosis (ad-ĭ-po-ne-kro'sis) See fat necrosis, under necrosis.

adiposis (ad-ĭ-po'sis) Accumulation of fat in a body area.

adiposity (ad-ĭ-pos'ĭ-te) Obesity; excessive accumulation of fat in the body.

adjuvant (aj-ĕ-vant, ă-joo'vant) 1. Assisting, aiding (e.g., an auxiliary therapy). 2. A substance that enhances the action of another, such as a substance that, when added to a vaccine, increases the production of antibodies by the immune system, thereby enhancing the vaccine's efficacy in producing immunity.

> **a. chemotherapy** The use of anticancer drugs following removal of a tumor.

> **Freund's complete a.** A mixture of mineral oil, plant waxes, and killed tubercle bacilli; added to antigen to increase antibody production.

> **Freund's incomplete a.** Freund's complete antigen without the tubercle bacilli.

adnexa (ad-nek'să) Appendages; accessory parts.

adnexal (ad-nek'sal) Relating to accessory parts, especially the ovaries, Fallopian (uterine) tubes, and ligaments of the uterus.

adolescence (ad-o-les'ens) General term meaning the period between childhood and adulthood. It overlaps puberty. See also puberty.

adolescent (ad-o-les'ent) 1. Relating to adolescence. 2. A person in that stage of development.

adren-, adreno- Combining forms denoting a relationship to the adrenal (suprarenal) gland.

adrenal (ă-dre'nal) Term originally meaning near the kidney; now used in relation to the adrenal (suprarenal) glands.

adrenaline (ă-dren'ă-lēn) See epinephrine.

adrenarche (ad-ren-ar'ke) The normal physiologic change in which the activity of the adrenal cortex is increased; it occurs at the age of approximately 9 years.

> **premature a.** Early puberty induced by hyperactivity of the adrenal cortex; it occurs most frequently in girls.

adrenergic (ad-ren-er'jik) 1. Relating to nerve fibers of the autonomic nervous system that, upon stimulation, release norepinephrine at their endings to transmit the nerve impulse. 2. A compound that mimics such action.

adrenocortical (ad-re-no-kor'te-kal) Relating to the cortex of the adrenal (suprarenal) glands.

adrenocorticotropin (ad-re-no-kor-te-ko-trop'in) See adrenocorticotropic hormone (ACTH), under hormone.

adrenosterone (ad-re-no'ster-on) A male sex hormone (androgen) found in the adrenal cortex.

adriamycin (ă-dre-ă-mi'sin) See doxorubicin.

advanced directive A signed document (either a living will or a durable power of attorney for health care) stating a person's wishes regarding medical care in the event of becoming unable to make decisions. The document does not have to be written, reviewed, or signed by an attorney but it must be signed by two witnesses. In many American states the witnesses cannot be the patient's relatives, heirs, or physicians.

aer-, aero- Combining forms meaning air; gas.

aerobe (air'ōb) A microorganism that can live in the presence of air.

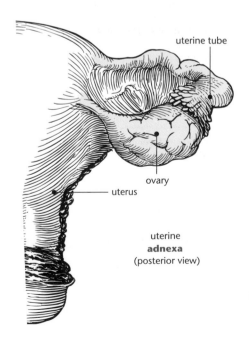

uterine tube

ovary

uterus

uterine
adnexa
(posterior view)

afibrinogenemia (ă-fi-brin-o-jĕ-ne'me-ă) Marked deficiency of fibrinogen, a blood-clotting factor in the blood

afterbirth (af'ter-berth) The placenta and fetal membranes expelled from the uterus after birth of the child. Also called secundines.

afterpains (af'ter-pānz) The normal cramps experienced after childbirth, due to contractions of the uterus while returning to its nonpregnant size.

agalactia (ă-gă-lak'she-ă) Absence of milk in the breasts after childbirth.

agalactorrhea (ă-gă-lak-to-re'ă) Absence or arrest of the milk flow.

age (āj) The time during which an individual exists.

advanced maternal a. The age of a pregnant woman, aged 35 years or older.

chronologic a. Age expressed in calendar units (days, weeks, months, years) since birth. Also called calendar age.

calendar a. See chronologic age.

a. of consent In legal medicine, the chronologic age of an individual at which she or he is regarded as legally capable to assent to sexual intercourse or marriage; depending on localities, it ranges from 14 to 18 years. See also statutory rape, under rape.

conceptional a. Age of an embryo or fetus determined (most commonly) by measuring the crown–rump length, or the crown–heel length; considered by some authorities to be an inaccurate method.

gestational a. The age of an embryo or a fetus, timed in weeks beginning with the first day of the mother's last menstruation. Also called menstrual age. See also pregnancy.

menstrual a. See gestational age.

ovulational a. Age of an embryo or fetus calculated from the date of ovulation and timed in days or weeks.

-age Combining form meaning a collection of (e.g., dosage); a result or degree of (e.g., shrinkage).

agenesis (ă-jen'ĕ-sis) Absence of an organ resulting from failure of development of the primitive cells that give rise to that organ during formation of the embryo.

bilateral renal a. Congenital absence of the kidneys, which eventually results in marked deficiency of amniotic fluid; usually associated with enlargement of the adrenal (suprarenal) glands, which may be mistaken for kidneys when observed in a sonogram. Death usually occurs *in utero*, or shortly after birth.

vaginal a. Congenital absence of the vagina; may be complete or partial.

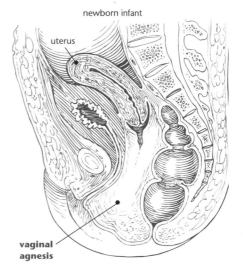

newborn infant
uterus
vaginal agnesis

agenosomia (ă-jen-o-so'me-ă) Congenital absence, or abnormal development, of the genitals; usually accompanied by protrusion of the abdominal organs through an incomplete abdominal wall.

agent (a'jent) **1.** Any substance or force capable of producing a biologic, chemical, or physical effect upon an organism. **2.** Any microorganism, chemical substance, or form of radiation whose presence, excessive presence, or (in deficiency states) relative absence is essential for the occurrence of a disorder; a causative agent.

adrenergic blocking a. Drug that slows the stimulating effects of sympathetic nerves, epinephrine, norepinephrine, and other adrenergic amines by blocking receptor sites of cells.

alkylating a.'s Highly reactive chemicals that inhibit cell division by binding to DNA, causing cross-linking of DNA strands; some are used as antineoplastics.

alpha-adrenergic blocking a. An agent that blocks the alpha receptors at nerve endings. Also called alpha-blocker.

anticancer a. A drug that destroys malignant cells or inhibits their proliferation; its selectivity is only moderate since it also harms host cells, such as those that normally undergo rapid division. Some anticancer agents (e.g., cyclophosphamide and aminotropterin) cause embryofetal malformations when taken by a pregnant woman. Also called antineoplastic agent.

antimicrobial a. A drug that acts by *(a)* disrupting bacterial wall synthesis and activating those enzymes that destroy the cell wall (e.g., penicillin, bacitracin, cephalosporin), *(b)* interfering with bacterial protein synthesis (e.g., tetracycline, erythromycin, streptomycin), *(c)* inhibiting nucleic acid synthesis (e.g., sulfonamides, para-aminosalicylic acid), or *(d)* increasing cell membrane permeability (e.g., polymixin B).

antineoplastic a. See anticancer agent.

beta-adrenergic blocking a. An agent that blocks the beta receptors at nerve endings.

blocking a. A drug that selectively interferes with the function of the autonomic nervous system by preventing transmission of the impulse at a receptor site on a cell surface, a synapse, or a neuromuscular junction. Commonly called blocker.

calcium channel-blocking a. Drug that slows muscle contraction by blocking passage of calcium across the membrane of muscle cells; also slows nerve impulses through heart muscle. Commonly called calcium channel blocker.

delta a. See hepatitis delta virus, under virus.

Eaton a. See *Mycoplasma pneumoniae,* under *Mycoplasma.*

fetotoxic a. Any agent that causes injurious alteration of fetal developmental processes through maternal exposure to that agent during pregnancy (e.g., viral, bacterial, and protozoal infections, radiation, gases, and drugs). Deleterious results include malformations, intrauterine growth retardation, and fetal death.

hepatitis B-associated delta a. See hepatitis delta virus, under virus.

hyperosmotic a. Any pharmaceutical compound that produces abnormally rapid osmosis in tissues and organs.

progestational a. See progestin.

prophylactic a. Any antibiotic, usually a broad-spectrum antibiotic, administered before and shortly after a surgical operation to prevent bacterial infections.

uterotonic a. An agent that enhances uterine contractions, e.g., one administered after delivery of the placenta to control excessive bleeding caused by undue relaxation (atony) of the uterus. Examples include oxytocin, methylergonovine, and prostaglandin $F_{2\alpha}$.

-agogue Combining form meaning inducing, promoting (e.g., lymphagogue).

agonadism (a-go′na-diz-m) Congenital absence of the gonads (testes or ovaries), which may have developed initially but degenerated shortly afterwards. Distinguished from agenesis.

ovarian a. Agonadism of the ovaries.

agonist (ag′o-nist) **1.** Denoting a muscle that initiates and maintains a particular movement, against another muscle (antagonist) that opposes such action. **2.** Denoting a chemical that interacts with specific receptors on the cell membrane, thereby initiating a cellular reaction.

gonadotropin-releasing hormone a. (GnRHa) A substance related to the 10-amino acid peptide hormone GnRH which stimulates the release of pituitary gonadotropins; used in the treatment of endometriosis, hirsutism, precocious puberty, and breast cancer. Also called gonadotropin-releasing hormone analog.

AIDS (acquired immune deficiency syndrome) The clinical state caused by a strain of the human immunodeficiency virus (cuurrently HIV1 or HIV2). The HIV infection, acquired by sexual contact or from contaminated blood products or body parts, progresses as follows. *Acute stage:* viruses enter lymphocytes (helper T cells) and, from this point on, the infected person can transmit the disease to others. About 3 to 5 weeks later, symptoms may develop (fever, muscle and joint pain, rash, hives, diarrhea), lasting 2 to 3 weeks before disappearing. T cells produce antibodies to kill the virus from the beginning, but they cannot be detected in blood tests until 5 to 6 months later. *Asymptomatic stage:* the infected person may have no symptoms for several years, but the virus population increases and destroys T cells, slowly at first, rapidly later; the immune system becomes compromised. A helper T cell (T-4) population of less than 500 cells/mm³ is a bad prognostic sign. Defenses begin to fail and symptoms, formerly called AIDS-related complex or ARC, begin to appear (weight loss, fatigue, fever, diarrhea, swollen lymph nodes). *Full-blown AIDS:* final stage of the disease; immune defenses break down completely and secondary (opportunistic) diseases attack the body (*Pneumocystis carinii* pneumonia; Kaposi's sarcoma; nervous system diseases; and fungal, bacterial, and parasitic infections). Death usually follows a few years later. Those at greatest risk for contracting AIDS are homosexual and bisexual men and intravenous drug users who share needles. Others include infants born to HIV-infected women and those who receive blood (in transfusion) or body parts (in transplants).

airway (ār′wa) **1.** The anatomic structures

through which air passes into and out of the lungs. **2.** A tube (e.g., an endotracheal tube or a tracheotomy tube) performing the function of a natural passageway to prevent loss of aeration during periods of unconsciousness or in case of an obstruction in the airflow.

albuginea (al-bu-jin'e-ă) A thick connective tissue capsule surrounding an organ, especially the testes and ovaries.

albumin (al-bu'min) A simple protein made in the liver and abundantly present in the body. It regulates movement of water between tissues and the bloodstream and helps retain substances in the circulation.

albuminuria (al-bu-mĭ-nu're-ă) Excretion of albumin in the urine in excess of the normal daily amount. See also proteinuria.

albuterol (al-bu'ter-ol) A bronchodilator used in the treatment of asthma; may cause fetal tachycardia and hypoglycemia in the newborn when taken during pregnancy. It has been known to decrease incidence of neonatal respiratory distress syndrome.

alcoholism (al'ko-hol-ism) Pathologic condition marked by a pattern of alcohol consumption accompanied by physical and psychological dependence. Regardless of the amount of alcohol consumed, alcoholism can be recognized: when it causes impairment of social or occupational functioning; by the need to increase amounts of alcohol intake to achieve desired effects (tolerance); and by severe physical (withdrawal) symptoms when alcohol intake is stopped or reduced. Also called alcohol abuse; alcohol dependence.

> **paroxysmal a.** See periodic drinking bouts, under bout.

aldosterone (al-dos'ter-ōn) A steroid hormone secreted by the outer layer (cortex) of the adrenal gland; its main function is to regulate sodium and potassium concentration in the body; it causes retention of sodium by enhancing sodium reabsorption in the kidney, the intestinal tract, and the sweat and salivary glands; sodium reabsorption is usually accompanied by increased excretion of potassium.

aldosteronism (al-dos'ter-on-izm) Condition caused by excessive production of aldosterone by the adrenal gland, usually resulting in lowered levels of potassium in the blood, muscular weakness, and hypertension.

> **primary a.** Excessive and inappropriate aldosterone production usually secondary to a unilateral adrenal adenoma, rarely in association with adrenal carcinoma. Also called Conn's syndrome.

alge-, algesi-, algio-, algo- Combining forms meaning pain.

-algia Suffix meaning pain (e.g., ostealgia).

alimentation (al-e-men-ta'shun) Providing nourishment.

> **total parenteral a.** See total parenteral nutrition, under nutrition.

alkaloid (al'kă-loid) Any of a group of nitrogenous substances (e.g., morphine, reserpine, quinine, cocaine, caffeine, nicotine) that are present in certain plants and produce strong physiologic effects.

> **vinca a.'s** Alkaloids with cytotoxic properties obtained from *Vinca rosea*, the periwinkle plant; they arrest cell division in metaphase by binding to microtubular protein in the mitotic spindle. Several vinca alkaloids (e.g., vinblastine and vincristine) have been used in combination with other drugs to treat cancer, including gynecologic cancers. Some cause congenital defects.

allantoic (al-an-to'ik) Relating to the allantois, an embryonic sac.

allantois (ă-lan'to-is) In the early embryo, an elongated outpouching from the caudal wall of the yolk sac connected with the embryonic bladder (urogenital sinus); as the bladder enlarges, the allantois involutes to form the urachus.

allel (ă-lel') See allele.

allele (ă-lēl') Any one of two or more genes that occupy the same location on homologous chromosomes and determine the heredity of a particular trait. Also spelled allel.

allergen (al'er-jen) Any agent that can trigger an allergic reaction.

allergy (al'er-je) A state of abnormal hypersensitivity to a normally harmless agent (allergen), acquired by previous exposure to that particular agent. See also allergic reaction, under reaction; anaphylaxis.

> **drug a.** Unusual sensitivity to a drug or chemical.

allo- Combining form meaning other.

alochia (ă-lo'ke-ă) Absence of vaginal discharges (lochia) after childbirth.

alopecia (al-o-pe'she-ă) Baldness; partial or complete loss of hair; may be temporary or permanent and result from genetic factors, aging, stress, physical trauma, trauma caused by local or systemic disease, or an adverse reaction to pharmaceutical drugs.

alpha-blocker (al'fă blok'er) See alpha-adrenergic blocking agent, under agent.

alpha-fetoprotein (al'fă fe-to-pro'tēn) (AFP) A plasma protein produced in the fetal liver and the yolk sac (until this structure degenerates normally at about 12 weeks of gestation). AFP reaches peak levels in fetal blood at the end of the first trimester (about 13 weeks of gestation); then levels decrease, gradually at first and rapidly after 32 weeks; the concentration of AFP is 150 times higher in fetal serum than in maternal serum. It is used as a diagnostic measure in obstetrics; considerably raised levels of AFP in the amniotic fluid and maternal serum after 14 weeks of gestation may indicate developmental defects, especially of the neural tube (e.g., spina bifida); moderately elevated levels may represent false-positive test results. In adults, AFP is produced in certain abnormal tissues, such as liver cancer (hepatoma), endodermal sinus tumors of the ovary, and testicular cancer. Used also to monitor response to antitumor therapy.

alphaprodine (al-fă-pro'dēn) A narcotic analgesic that has been used to relieve pain during labor. It may produce significant respiratory depression in the newborn because it rapidly crosses the placenta.

alprazolam (al-pra'zo-lam) A minor tranquilizer; a member of the class of benzodiazepine drugs used for management of anxiety, panic attack, and phobias; abuse may lead to addiction.

alveolus (al-ve'o-lus), pl. alveoli In anatomy, a small cavity or saclike dilatation.

   pulmonary a. One of the minute, balloonlike air sacs at the end of a bronchiole in the lungs. Exchange of the gases or respiration takes place through the alveolar walls.

amastia (ă-mas'te-ă) Congenital absence of the breasts.

ambi- Prefix meaning both.

ambisexual (am-bĭ-seks'u-al) 1. Relating to both sexes. 2. See bisexual.

ambo- Prefix meaning both.

ambulation (am-bu-la'shun) The act of walking.

ambulatory, ambulant (am'bu-lā-to-re, am'bu-lant) 1. Capable of walking; applied to patients who are not bedridden. 2. Relating to ambulation.

amenorrhea (ă-men-o-re'ă) Absence of menstruation.

   hypoestrogenic hypothalamic a. Hypothalamic amenorrhea associated with low estrogen levels.

   hypothalamic a. Amenorrhea caused by functional disturbances in the central regulation of ovulatory function.

   lactational a. Absence of menstruation associated with breast-feeding, believed to be due to elevated levels of prolactin which inhibit the pulsatile secretion of gonadotropin-releasing hormone (GnRH), subsequently affecting the cyclicity of pituitary gonadotropin secretion.

   physiologic a. Absence of menses associated with pregnancy, lactation, and menopause.

   primary a. Failure of menstruation to begin by the age of 16 years.

   secondary a. Cessation of menstruation for at least 3 months in a woman who has menstruated in the past.

   stress a. Amenorrhea resulting from excessive physical activity and loss of body weight, usually about 22% below average; seen particularly in women engaged in competitive sports, demanding activities such as ballet and modern dance, and strenuous recreational exercises.

amenorrheal (ă-men-o-re'al) Relating to amenorrhea.

amethopterin (am-eth-op'tĕ-rin) See methotrexate.

ametria (ă-me'tre-ă) Congenital absence of the uterus.

aminoaciduria (am-ĭ-no-as-ĭ-du're-ă) Excretion of excessive amounts of amino acids in the urine; seen in lead poisoning, damaged kidney tubules, and in other disorders.

aminoglutethimide (ă-me-no-gloo-teth'ĭ-mīd) A pharmaceutical drug that inhibits activity of the adrenal cortex; used in the treatment of Cushing's syndrome and some advanced cases of breast cancer.

aminoglycoside (am-ĭ-no-gli-ko'sīd) Any of a class of antibiotics effective against Gram-positive and Gram-negative bacteria by blocking protein synthesis in bacterial ribosomes; examples include streptomycin, amikacin, and gentamicin. High dosages, especially in the presence of kidney dysfunction, may cause muscle weakness; some have deleterious effects on the fetus.

aminopterin (am-ĭ-nop'ter-in) A folic acid antagonist used as a cancer chemotherapeutic agent; it causes fetal malformations if taken during the first trimester of pregnancy, or when taken unsuccessfully to induce abortion.

amiodarone (ă-me'o-dă-rōn) A potassium channel-blocker administered orally to treat atrial fibrillation and ventricular tachycardia; may cause fetal or neonatal hypothyroidism if taken during pregnancy and breast-feeding.

amitriptyline hydrochloride (am-ĭ-trip'tĭ-lēn hi-dro-klo'rīd) An antidepressant drug with sedative properties. If taken by a pregnant woman, it may cause developmental malformations, neonatal withdrawal symptoms, or neonatal urinary retention.

amniocentesis

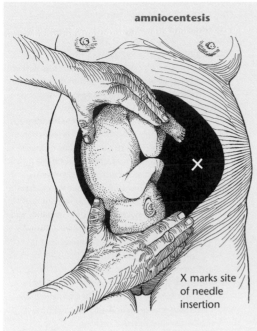

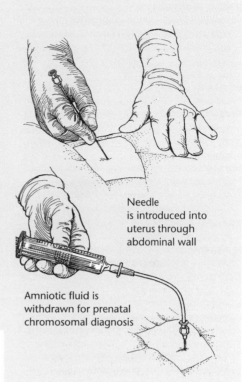

X marks site of needle insertion

Needle is introduced into uterus through abdominal wall

Amniotic fluid is withdrawn for prenatal chromosomal diagnosis

ammonia (ă-mo′ne-a) A volatile, water-soluble present in small amounts in blood plasma; ra levels occur in certain conditions (liver disease, Reye's syndrome, severe congestive heart failure, gastrointestinal hemorrhage, and erythroblastosis fetalis).

amnio- Combining form meaning amnion.

amniocentesis (am-ne-o-sen-te′sis) Diagnostic procedure in which a few milliliters of the amniotic fluid surrounding the fetus are withdrawn with a needle and syringe through the woman's abdominal wall. The fluid and fetal cells contained in the fluid can be analyzed to detect the presence of infection, fetal abnormalities, and genetic diseases.

amniochorion (am-ne-o-ko′re-on) The amnion and chorion considered together; after the third month of gestation, they remain in close contact, forming an avascular sac that contains the fetus and amniotic fluid. Commonly called the bag of waters.

amniography (am-ne-og′ră-fe) Radiography of the pregnant uterus after injection of a radiopaque solution into the amniotic fluid.

amnioinfusion (am-ne-o-in-fu′shun) The procedure of introducing saline solution at room temperature into the amniotic sac; useful in the treatment of patients with deficient amniotic fluid (oligohydramnios) where umbilical cord compression and subsequent fetal compromise can be prevented by reconstituting sufficient intrauterine fluid volume.

amnion (am′ne-on) The thin, tough, innermost layer of the membranous sac that surrounds the embryo and fills with amniotic fluid as the pregnancy advances. It covers the chorionic blood vessels (branches of the umbilical vessels) spreading throughout the chorion. See also amniochorion.

amnion

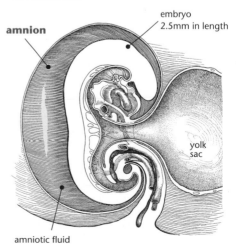

embryo 2.5mm in length

yolk sac

amniotic fluid

amnion nodosum (am'ne-on no-do'sum) Small nodules (5 mm or less) usually found on the fetal surface of the amniotic membrane; associated with deficient amniotic fluid and with underlying anomalies of the fetal genitourinary system. Also called amniotic caruncles.

amnionitis (am-ne-o-ni'tis) Inflammation of the amnion.

amniorrhea (am-ne-o-re'ă) Premature escape of amniotic fluid.

amniorrhexis (am-ne-o-rek'sis) Rupture of the amniotic membrane.

amnioscopy (am-ne-os'kŏ-pe) Direct inspection of the fetus and amniotic fluid with a specially designed viewing instrument (amnioscope) introduced through the cervical canal.

amniotic, amnionic (am-ne-ot'ik, am-ne-on'ic) Relating to the amnion.

amniotome (am'ne-o-tōm) Instrument used to puncture the fetal membranes.

amniotomy (am-ne-ot'o-me) Surgical rupture of the fetal membranes.

amobarbital sodium (am-o-bar'bĭ-tal so'de-um) An intermediate-acting barbiturate with sedative and hypnotic properties, used intravenously to treat seizure disorders. An increased incidence of congenital defects has been reported when administered during pregnancy to treat status epilepticus.

amphetamine (am-fet'a-min) Any of a group of synthetic drugs that have a strong stimulant effect on the central nervous system; pharmacologically, amphetamines are classified as sympathomimetic amines; some are appetite suppressants and have been used to treat patients who are overweight. Abuse of the drug leads to tolerance and dependence; adverse reactions to continued high doses include anxiety, hallucinations, intense fatigue after the stimulation phase, and prolonged depression with possible suicide. Amphetamine abuse during pregnancy causes a host of adverse effects, including increased incidence of preterm labor, placental abruption, intrauterine growth retardation, fetal distress, and postpartum hemorrhage.

amphi- Prefix meaning on both sides; around.

amphimixis (am-fĭ-mik'sis) The union of paternal and maternal nuclear elements following fertilization of the ovum.

ampho- Combining form meaning on both sides.

amputation (am-pu-ta'shun) The cutting off of a limb or other part of the body.

    cervical a. Surgical removal of the uterine cervix. Also called hysterotrachelectomy.

ana-, an- Prefixes meaning upward; again.

anaerobic (an-ĕ-ro'bik) Living in the absence of oxygen.

anal (a'nal) Relating to the anus.

analgesia (an-al-je'ze-ă) Loss or modulation of pain sensation; a condition in which stimuli that normally produce pain are perceived but are not interpreted as pain; it may be induced by hypnosis, or administration of drugs (e.g., relief of pain without loss of consciousness during childbirth through the administration of certain inhalation anesthetics in concentrations lower than those required for surgical anesthesia), or it may result from disease that interrupts pain pathways in the central or peripheral nervous systems.

    caudal a. Analgesia produced by injecting an appropriate local anesthetic solution into the sacral canal through the sacral hiatus.

    epidural a. In obstetrics, relief from pain of uterine contractions and delivery achieved by injecting an appropriate local anesthetic into the epidural space (i.e., between the spinal dura mater and the walls of the vertebral canal); termed *lumbar epidural a.* if the anesthetic agent is introduced through a lumbar intervertebral space. See also caudal analgesia.

    patient-controlled a. (PCA) Reduction of acute pain by self administration of narcotic drugs within limits of dose established by the physician (e.g., in a postoperative period).

    peridural a. Epidural analgesia.

    regional a. Analgesia achieved by injecting long-lasting local anesthetics in the proximity of nerves, or into the epidural space or the intrathecal space (i.e., within the dural sac).

analgesic (an-al-je'zik) Relating to analgesia.

analog, analogue (an'ă-log) 1. An organ or part similar in function to one in another organism of a different species but different in structure or development. 2. A chemical compound similar in structure to another but dissimilar in composition.

    gonadotropin-releasing hormone a., GnRH a. A hormonal analog that effects a down-regulation of the anterior pituitary (adenohypophysis); it eventually suppresses follicle-stimulating hormone (FSH) and luteinizing hormone (LH), subsequently decreasing estrogen production by the ovary. GnRH analogs are used to treat breast cancer in premenopausal women. Sometimes called gonadotropin-releasing hormone agonist.

analysis (ă-nal'ĭ-sis), pl. analyses 1. A method of study based on the separation of the object of study into smaller units. 2. The breaking up of a chemical compound into its constituent elements. **3.** See psychoanalysis.

Northern blot a. Identification of RNA fragments that have been electrophoretically separated and transferred (blotted) onto nitrocellular or other type of paper or nylon membrane. Specific RNA fragments can then be detected by radioactive probes.

multivariate a. A statistical method of analyzing data that takes into account many dependent, as well as independent, variables; it establishes the effect of one variable and, simultaneously, evaluates repeatedly the effect of additional factors that may influence the variable being tested.

saturation a. See competitive protein-binding assay, under assay.

semen a. Examination of a semen sample to determine male fertility in an infertile marriage or relationship, or to substantiate the success of vasectomy. A fresh ejaculate is examined under the microscope to count the number of spermatozoa, check their shape and size, and note their motility.

Southern blot a. A procedure (first developed by E. M. Southern) for separating and identifying DNA sequences; DNA fragments are separated by electrophoresis and transferred (blotted) onto a special filter on which specific DNA fragments can then be detected by radioactive probes.

Western blot a. A technique for identifying antibodies to a protein of specific molecular weight; proteins are electrophoretically separated and transferred (blotted) onto nitrocellulose or nylon membrane; the blots are then detected by radiolabeled antibody probes. The procedure is a more specific test than the ELISA for AIDS.

anamnesis (an-am-ne'sis) The history of an ailment as recalled by the patient.

anamnestic (an-am-nes'tik) **1.** Relating to anamnesis. **2.** Assisting the memory; mnemonic.

anaphase (an'ă-fāz) The third stage of cell division by mitosis during which the two chromatids of each chromosome separate and migrate from the equatorial plane, along spindle fibers, toward opposite poles of the cell.

anaphylactic (an-ă-fĭ-lak'tik) Relating to anaphylaxis.

anaphylaxis (an-ă-fĭ-lak'sis) An immediate, severe hypersensitivity (allergic) reaction to a previously encountered antigen (allergen) to which the person was sensitized; the reaction requires the presence of IgE antibodies formed in response to a previous exposure to the same antigen;

characterized by the release of histamine and other pharmacologically active substances into the bloodstream, with subsequent itchiness, hives, generalized flush, respiratory distress, and vascular collapse; occasionally accompanied by seizures, vomiting, abdominal cramps, and incontinence.

anasarca (an-ă-sar'kă) Massive swelling and accumulation of fluids in subcutaneous tissues and in body cavities.

anastomosis (ă-nas-to-mo'sis), pl. anastomoses **1.** The normal channel between two tubular structures. **2.** A channel between tubular structures or hollow organs, opened either surgically or pathologically.

Hyrtl's a. In embryology, the transverse anastomosis joining the two umbilical arteries immediately before, or just after they enter, the chorionic plate on the fetal surface of the placenta.

microvascular a. Anastomosis of minute blood vessels performed under a surgical microscope.

tubocornual a. The microsurgical reconstruction and joining of a fallopian (uterine) tube to the cornual portion of the uterus after removal of a section of the tube; performed to repair the damage associated with a variety of pathologic conditions (e.g., endometriosis and infections).

tubotubal a. The operation of uniting two segments of the fallopian (uterine) tube, either to reverse a tubal ligation or to re-establish continuity after removing an occluded segment caused by endometriosis, follicular salpingitis or, most frequently, an arrested tubal pregnancy.

anatomy (ă-nat'ŏ-me) **1.** The science of the structure and organization of the body parts. **2.** Dissection.

developmental a. See embryology.

gross a. Study of body parts as seen without the aid of a microscope. Also called macroscopic anatomy.

macroscopic a. See gross anatomy.

microscopic a. See histology.

surface a. Study of the outer configuration of the body in relation to underlying and deep structures.

surgical a. Study of anatomy with a view toward applying the knowledge to surgical techniques.

topographic a. Study of the location of organs and other body parts in relation to their neighboring structures.

-ance Suffix meaning action; state; condition (e.g., brilliance).

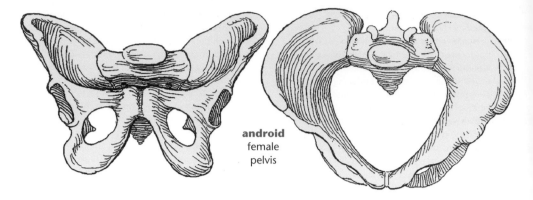

android
female
pelvis

andro- Combining form meaning male.

androblastoma (an-dro-blas-to'mă) See Sertoli-Leydig tumor, under tumor.

androgen (an'dro-jen) A hormone that stimulates development of male sex characteristics.

androgenic (an-dro-jen'ik) Relating to androgen; producing male characteristics.

androgenous (an-droj'ĕ-nus) Tending to produce mostly males.

androgynous (an-droj'ĭ-nus) Relating to female pseudohermaphroditism (i.e., a true female with male characteristics).

android (an'droid) Resembling a man; manlike (e.g., android pelvis).

andropathy (an-drop'ă-the) Any disease peculiar to males.

androstenedione (an-dro-stēn'de-ōn) An androgenic steroid produced in the testis, ovary, and adrenal cortex.

androsterone (an-dros'ter-ōn) An androgen (male sex hormone) derived from testosterone.

anechoic (an-ĕ-ko'ik) Denoting absence of echoes in an area studied with ultrasonography. Also called sonolucent.

anemia (ă-ne'me-ă) Any condition in which the concentration of blood hemoglobin decreases below normal levels for the age and sex of the person; usually there is also a decrease in the number of red blood cells per mm³ and in the number of packed red blood cells per 100 ml of blood. Anemia decreases the oxygen-carrying capacity of the blood.

    aplastic a. Anemia due to failure of bone marrow to produce the normal number of red blood cells; usually associated with decreased number of all cellular components of the blood.

    congenital hypoplastic a. Anemia occurring in infants, resulting from underdevelopment of bone marrow; minor congenital abnormalities may also occur. Also called erythrogenesis imperfecta.

    Cooley's a. See beta thalassemia major, under thalassemia.

    folic acid deficiency a. Anemia occurring during pregnancy, caused by folic acid deficiency; characterized by the presence of large embryonic red blood cells in bone marrow; it is usually mild unless associated with conditions such as systemic infection and hemolytic disease; it disappears after delivery but may recur in subsequent pregnancies.

    hemolytic a. Any of a group of diseases characterized by a shortened life span of red blood cells in the bloodstream.

    hemolytic a. of the newborn See hemolytic disease of the newborn.

    iron-deficiency a. The most common type of anemia, developed when insufficient iron is available to the bone marrow where red blood cells are formed; characterized by low concentration of hemoglobin and smaller than normal red blood cells. May be caused by dietary deficiency, increased demand for iron (e.g., in growing children, in pregnant and lactating women), malabsorption due to other conditions, or chronic blood loss (e.g., hookworm disease, peptic ulcers, colon cancer, long-term aspirin ingestion).

    physiologic a. of the newborn The normal decline of red blood cell and hemoglobin concentrations occurring in infants 2 to 3 months of age, beginning gradually after the first week of life.

    physiologic a. of pregnancy A hemodilution effect, occurring during pregnancy, from a larger increase in plasma volume than hemoglobin mass and red cell volume.

    sickle cell a. Hereditary anemia occurring almost exclusively among blacks; characterized by the presence of a large number of crescent-shaped red blood cells that contain an abnormal hemoglobin (hemoglobin S). Also called sickle-cell disease.

anencephaly (an-en-sef'ă-le) Developmental defect in which the top of the skull is absent and the brain is reduced to small masses lying at the base of the skull. The affected infant is either stillborn or does not survive beyond a few hours.

anephric (a-nef'rik) Without kidneys.

anesthesia (an-es-the'ze-ă) Total loss of sensory perception; it may include loss of consciousness; may be induced by special techniques or by administration of drugs, or it may result from a lesion of the nervous system. See also analgesia.

    balanced general a. Anesthesia achieved by a combination of drugs, each used in enough quantities to produce the maximum desired effect.

    block a. See conduction anesthesia.

    caudal a. Anesthesia produced by injecting an anesthetic solution into the sacral canal through the sacral hiatus.

    conduction a. Inhibition of nerve transmission by injecting an anesthetic solution around a nerve trunk. Also called block anesthesia.

    epidural a. Anesthesia produced by injection of an anesthetic solution into the epidural space (i.e., the space between the dura mater and the walls of the vertebral canal).

    field block a. Anesthesia produced in a local area by multiple injections of an anesthetic solution around the circumference of the operative field.

    general a. A controlled state of unconsciousness and complete loss of sensation, accompanied by partial or complete loss of protective reflexes, including the inability to independently maintain an airway or respond purposefully to verbal command; produced by administration of intravenous or inhalation anesthetic agents. Intramuscular injection and rectal instillation are rarely used in general anesthesia. Also called surgical anesthesia.

    local a. Anesthesia confined to one part of the body by injecting anesthetic into or adjacent to the site of surgery.

    monitored a. See standby anesthesia.

    nerve block a. Anesthesia produced by injecting a local anesthetic solution about peripheral nerves.

    paracervical block a. Injection of an anesthetic solution in the area along the walls of the lower uterus and the base of the broad ligament to block nerve impulse transmission

along the sensory fibers of the hypogastric plexus. Because of its possible adverse effects on the fetus, paracervical block is now considered contraindicated in obstetrics by most authorities.

    pudendal a. Anesthesia of the perineum produced by injection of an anesthetic solution into the areas near the pudendal nerves.

    rectal a. Anesthesia produced by instillation of a central nervous system depressant into the rectum.

    regional a. Any of four types of anesthesia (spinal, epidural, caudal, or nerve block) accomplished with local anesthetic techniques.

    saddle block a. Anesthesia of the buttocks, perineum, and inner thighs produced by introducing the anesthetic low in the dural sac around the spinal cord.

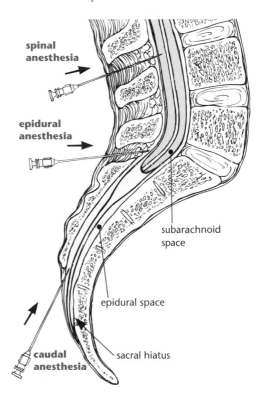

    spinal a. (1) Anesthesia of the lower part of the body produced by introducing the anesthetic solution into the subarachnoid space around a specified portion of the spinal cord. Also called subarachnoid block anesthesia. (2) Anesthesia caused by disease or injury to the spinal cord.

standby a. The use of local anesthesia by the surgeon during a surgical operation, in addition to administration of sedative-hypnotics and narcotics by the anesthesiologist. Also called monitored anesthesia.

subarachnoid block a.
See spinal anesthesia (1).

surgical a. See general anesthesia.

anesthesiologist (an-es-the-ze-ol'o-jist) A physician who specializes in anesthesiology.

anesthesiology (an-es-the-ze-ol'o-je) The study of anesthesia and its application to medical and surgical treatment.

anesthetic (an-es-thet'ik) **1.** Relating to anesthesia. **2.** An agent that produces anesthesia.

anesthetist (ă-nes'thĕ-tist) A person (physician, nurse, or technician) trained to administer anesthesia.

anesthetize (ă-nes thĕ-tīz) To produce anesthesia.

aneuploid (an'u-ploid) The state of having an abnormal number of chromosomes.

aneurysm (an'u-rizm) A localized abnormal outpouching of an arterial wall or of the heart muscle; results from pressure of the blood against a weakened or thinned area of the vessel wall or of the heart muscle. The weakening may be caused by disease, injury, or congenital defect. See also microaneurysm.

berry a. A small berry-like sacculation of a cerebral artery, occurring at the bifurcation of arteries forming the arterial circle (circle of Willis) at the base of the brain. In pregnancy, rupture of the aneurysm (an uncommon event) may be brought about by pregnancy-induced hypertension. Also called congenital aneurysm (a misnomer, for only the defect is present at birth, not the aneurysm).

dissecting a. Aneurysm resulting from a tear of the inner layer of the arterial wall, which allows blood to flow into, between, and along the layers of the wall; it commonly occurs in the aorta. See also dissecting aneurysm of aorta.

dissecting a. of aorta Dissecting aneurysm usually occurring in the ascending aorta, in the descending thoracic aorta just below the ligamentum arteriosum, and in the abdominal aorta below the renal arteries; the most common predisposing conditions are Marfan's syndrome, coarctation of the aorta, and congenital heart valve anomalies; it occurs only rarely in pregnancy, usually during the third trimester. Also called aortic dissection.

splenic artery a. Aneurysm of the splenic artery; if present during pregnancy, it may rupture spontaneously, especially during the last trimester.

syphilitic a. A spindle-shaped aneurysm occurring in the last stage of syphilis (tertiary stage), usually in the thoracic aorta.

angio-, angi- Combining forms meaning vessel, especially a blood vessel.

angioblast (an'je-o-blast) An embryonic cell that gives rise to a blood vessel.

angiogenesis (an-je-o-jen'ĕ-sis) Development of blood vessels.

angiography (an-je-og'ră-fe) The process of recording images of blood vessels on x-ray film or tape after intravenous injection of a radiopaque solution.

selective a. Introduction of the radiopaque solution through a catheter directly into vessels of the area to be studied.

angioid (an'je-oid) Resembling a blood vessel.

angiokeratoma (an-je-o-ker-ă-to'mă) A small, dark lesion on the skin composed of scales over an excess of capillaries. Also called telangiectatic wart.

angioma (an-je-o'mă) A lesion of the skin or subcutaneous tissues resulting from proliferation of blood or lymph vessels. See also hemangioma; lymphangioma.

spider a. See spider telangiectasia, under telangiectasia.

angioplasty (an'je-o-plas-te) Surgical restructuring of a blood vessel.

balloon a. See percutaneous transluminal angioplasty.

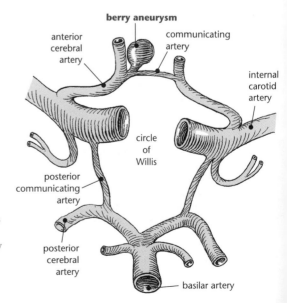

berry aneurysm

anterior cerebral artery

communicating artery

internal carotid artery

circle of Willis

posterior communicating artery

posterior cerebral artery

basilar artery

percutaneous transluminal a. (PCTA) Enlargement of the lumen of a partially occluded artery. A balloon-tipped catheter is introduced into the vessel to the site of occlusion; then the balloon is inflated to flatten the plaque or the hyperplastic area against the vessel wall and enlarge the lumen. Also called balloon angioplasty.

angiosarcoma (an-je-o-sar-ko'mă) An uncommon, malignant, rapidly growing fleshy mass that may occur anywhere in the body, usually the skin, breast, liver, and spleen. Also called hemangiosarcoma.

angiotensin (an-je-o-ten'sin) One of a family of peptides involved in regulating blood pressure. *Angiotensin I*, an inactive form, is split off from the precursor, angiotensinogen, by the enzyme renin and is converted to the active form, angiotensin II, by a converting enzyme. *Angiotensin II* causes narrowing of the blood vessels and stimulates production and release of the hormone aldosterone from the adrenal cortex. *Angiotensin III* is a derivative of angiotensin II and performs similar but weaker actions.

angiotome (an'je-o-tōm) A segment of the vascular system of the embryo.

angle (ang'gl) The figure formed by two lines or planes diverging from, or meeting at, a common point; the space enclosed by them.

   acromial a. The angle formed where the spine of the shoulder blade (scapula) ends and the acromion begins, forming the bony prominence at the upper back of the shoulder joint.

   carrying a. A characterization of the position of the arms in relation to the torso.

   lumbosacral a. Angle between the long axes of the lumbar and sacral portions of the vertebral column.

   popliteal a. In neonatology, a measurement of the popliteal angle (behind the knee) for neuromuscular maturity rating of the newborn. The thigh is held in the knee-chest position by the examiner's index finger, with the thumb supporting the knee; the leg is then extended by gentle pressure from the examiner's other index finger behind the ankle; the angle so formed is then measured. Used to determine postnatal gestational age.

anicteric (an-ik-ter'ik) Not associated with jaundice.

aniridia (an-ĭ-rid'e-ă) Developmental defect of the eye in which the iris is absent, either partly or completely.

aniso- Combining form meaning unequal.

ankylo- Combining form meaning bent; fused; adhered.

ankyrin (ang'kĭ-rin) A protein present on the cell membrane of erythrocytes, anchoring the contractile protein spectrin to the plasma membrane.

anlage (an'laj), pl. anlagen The earliest indication of a developing organ or structure of the body, when embryonic cells begin to group in a definite pattern; generally denoting a theoretical stage earlier than primordium.

anogenital (ă-no-jen'ĭ-tal) Relating to the anus and genitals.

anomaly (ă-nom'ă-le) Deviation from what is accepted as normal of form, shape, or position of a tissue, organ, or structure.

   chromosomal a. See chromosomal aberration, under aberration.

   developmental a. Anomaly occurring or originating during intrauterine life.

   Ebstein's a. Malformation of the tricuspid (right atrioventricular) valve of the heart; the valve is distorted and displaced downward into the right ventricle; if severe, the condition may lead to obstruction of blood flow out of the right ventricle. It is frequently associated with an atrial septal defect (ASD). Also called Ebstein's malformation.

   Hegglin's a. An autosomal dominant inheritance characterized by faulty maturation of platelets, thrombocytopenia, and the presence of basophilic structures (Döhle bodies) in neutrophils and eosinophils. Also called May-Hegglin anomaly.

   May-Hegglin a. See Hegglin's anomaly.

anorchia (an-or'ke-ă) See anorchism.

anorchism (an-or'kizm) Congenital absence of one or both testes. Also called anorchia.

anorectic (an-o-rek'tik) **1.** A substance that tends to depress the appetite. **2.** Relating to anorexia nervosa.

anorexia (an-o-rek'se-ă) Loss of appetite.

   a. nervosa An eating disorder seen predominantly in teenage girls; characterized by excessive loss of appetite and body weight, accompanied by metabolic derangement and serious neurotic symptoms centered around an abnormal fear of becoming fat, undiminished even after the patient becomes emaciated.

anovular, anovulatory (an-ov'u-lar, an-ov'u-lă-to-re) Denoting a menstrual period that is not accompanied by release of an ovum from the ovary (ovulation).

anovulation (an-ov-u-la'shun) Absence of ovulation.

anoxemia (an-ok-se'me-ă) Marked deficiency of

oxygen in arterial blood.

anoxia (ă-nok'se-ă) Without oxygen.

ansa (an'să), pl. ansae Any anatomic structure shaped like a loop or hook.

    a. cervicalis A loop of nerves located in the neck, formed by fibers from three cervical nerves (Cl, C2, C3) and the hypoglossal nerve. Formerly called ansa hypoglossi.

    a. hypoglossi See ansa cervicalis.

antacid (ant-as'id) **1.** Neutralizing acidity. **2.** Any agent that has such properties (e.g., aluminum hydroxide, magnesium hydroxide, calcium carbonate).

antagonism (an-tag'o-nizm) A state of mutual resistance, opposition, or competition.

    chemical a. Direct chemical interaction between an agonist and an antagonist, producing an inactive product.

    competitive a. Lessening of the action of an agonist because of competition with a nonactivating antagonist for a receptor site on a cell membrane.

    functional a. The offsetting of the effect of one agonist by the opposite effect of another agonist acting on different receptor sites (e.g., acetylcholine, which constricts the pupil, and epinephrine, which dilates it). Also called physiologic antagonism.

    physiologic a. See functional antagonism.

antagonist (an-tag'o-nist) **1.** Any structure or substance that opposes or counteracts the action of another structure or substance. **2.** In pharmacology, a chemical that occupies a receptor site on the cell membrane but does not initiate the biologic reaction associated with occupation of the site by an agonist; in effect, an antagonist interferes with the formation of an agonist–receptor complex, the mechanism by which most pharmacologic effects are produced.

    competitive a. (1) A drug that interacts reversibly with the same receptors as the active drug (agonist) to form a complex; the complex, however, does not elicit a biologic response and can be displaced from these receptor sites by increasing concentrations of the active drug. (2) See antimetabolite.

    folic acid a. A substance that interferes with the action of folic acid. Some folic acid antagonists are associated with severe malformations, spontaneous abortions, stillbirths, and small-for-gestational age infants.

    purine a. A substance (e.g., mercaptoprine, azathioprine) that is a false metabolite structurally similar to the natural purines hypoxanthine or guanine, and which interferes with DNA and RNA synthesis; used in cancer chemotherapy.

    pyrimidine a. An antimetabolite of a pyrimidine (the fundamental substance of several organic bases, some of which are components of nucleic acids). See also antimetabolite.

ante- Prefix meaning before.

anteflexion (an-te-flek'shun) Displacement of an organ or structure characterized by an abnormal forward bending (e.g., the forward flexion of the uterus at the isthmus).

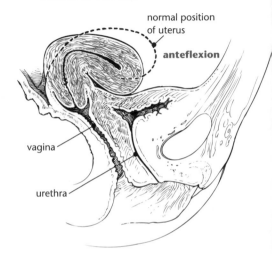

normal position of uterus

anteflexion

vagina

urethra

antegrade (an'te-grād) See anterograde.

antenatal (an-te-na'tal) See prenatal.

antepartum (an-te-par'tum) Before the onset of labor.

anterior (an-te're-or) **1.** Located or related to the front surface of the body or limbs. **2.** Located on or near the front of an organ.

antero- Combining form meaning before; forward; anterior.

anterograde (an'ter-o-grād) Moving or extending forward. Also called antegrade.

anteroinferior (an-ter-o-in-fēr'e-or) In front and below.

anterolateral (an-ter-o-lat'er-al) In front and to one side of the midline.

anteromedial (an-ter-o-me'de-al) In front and toward the midline.

anteroposterior (an-ter-o-pos-tēr'e-or) In a direction from front to back.

anterosuperior (an-ter-o-su-pēr'e-or) In front and above.

anteversion (an-te-ver'zhun) The tilting forward of an organ.

anteverted (an-te-vert'ed) Tilted forward.

anti- Prefix meaning opposing; against; counteracting.

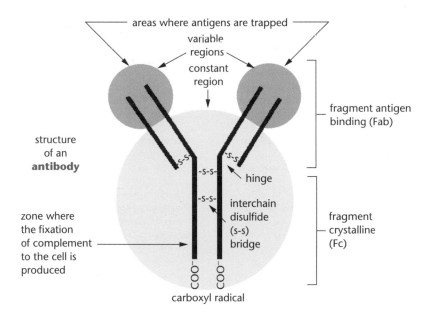

areas where antigens are trapped

variable regions

constant region

structure of an **antibody**

fragment antigen binding (Fab)

-s-s-

-s-s-

hinge

-s-s-

interchain disulfide (s-s) bridge

zone where the fixation of complement to the cell is produced

fragment crystalline (Fc)

COO⁻ COO⁻

carboxyl radical

antiadrenergic (an-tĭ-ă-dren-er'jik) **1.** Blocking the adrenergic action of the sympathetic nervous system. **2.** Any drug having such properties.

antiandrogen (an-tĭ-an'dro-jen) A substance that can diminish the effects of masculinizing (androgenic) hormone.

antibiotic (an-tĭ-bi-ot'ik) Any of a group of drugs, derived from fungi or bacteria, or produced synthetically, that kill or inhibit the growth of a variety of microorganisms. Antibiotics vary widely in structure and mode of action.

broad-spectrum a. An antibiotic that has a wide range of activity; effective against both Gram-positive and Gram-negative bacteria.

antibody (an'tĭ-bod-e) (Ab) A protein, found in the blood and other body fluids; its formation can be incited by the presence of antigen (microorganisms, nonself proteins, and tissue cells), and it has a destructive influence on the specific antigen that stimulated its formation. See also immunoglobin.

anticardiolipin a. An antibody that reacts with phospholipid antigens and may be elevated in acquired immune deficiency syndrome (AIDS) and systemic lupus erythematosus (SLE).

anti-D a. An antibody used as prophylaxis during, or shortly after, pregnancy to prevent sensitization to Rh factor D. See also Rh₀ immune globulin, under globulin.

antinuclear a. (ANA) An antibody that acts on components of the cell nucleus; it occurs in systemic lupus erythematosus and other connective-tissue disorders.

anti-P a. An antibody against a minor blood group called P; it has an important role in reproductive failure.

antiplatelet a. An antibody that is specific for blood platelets and may be implicated in infertility.

antisperm a.'s (ASAs) Antibodies (predominantly IgA type) that immobilize spermatozoa or interfere with spermatozoan activity. They are found in the serum of both males and females and act locally (in the testicles and the vagina); level of their activity fluctuates.

blocking a. An antibody that, by combining with antigen, stops further activity of that antigen.

complement-fixing a. (CF antibody) An antibody that, when combined with antigen, activates complement (material in normal serum that helps to destroy pathogens).

cytophilic a.'s See cytotropic antibodies.

cytotropic a.'s Antibodies that have an affinity for certain other cells in addition to, and independent of, the specific antigens that triggered their production.

fluorescent a. Antibody to which a fluorescent dye has been attached.

monoclonal a.'s Artificially produced antibodies that are chemically and immunologically homogeneous; produced in the laboratory to react with a specific antigen; used experimentally in the treatment of some forms of cancer.

treponema-immobilizing a. An antibody present in the serum of patients with syphilis (active or inactive); it has a specific affinity for *Treponema pallidum* (the causative agent of syphilis) and, in the presence of complement, immobilizes the microorganism.

anticholinergic (an-tĭ-ko-lin-er'jik) Blocking the passage of impulses through nerves of the parasympathetic system by inhibiting the action of the neurotransmitter acetylcholine.

anticoagulant (an-tĭ-ko-ag'u-lant) Any substance that prevents blood clotting.

circulating a. An inhibitor of factor VIII (usually an IgG antibody) that interferes with coagulation reactions. Circulating anticoagulants can cause various degrees of bleeding, from mild to severe hemorrhage.

lupus a. (LA, LAC) A circulating anticoagulant, one of a family of antiphospholipid antibodies, characterized by a prolonged partial thromboplastin time; it is present in a variety of clinical conditions; has been found in 10 to 15% of patients with systemic lupus erythematosus and is often associated with adverse pregnancy outcomes (e.g., abortions, fetal growth retardation, and fetal death).

anticonvulsant (an-tĭ-kon-vul'sant) Any substance that prevents or arrests seizures.

antidepressant (an-tĭ-de-pres'sant) An agent that alleviates depression.

tricyclic a.'s A class of antidepressants (e.g., imipramine and amitriptyline) that are closely related to the phenothiazines in structure and pharmaceutical effects; used in the outpatient treatment of depression; patients respond with mood elevation, improved sleep patterns, and a reduction in preoccupation with self-destruction; may cause fetal malformations, withdrawal symptoms, and urine retention when taken during pregnancy.

antidiuresis (an-tĭ-di-u-re'sis) Reducing urine formation.

antidiuretic (an-tĭ-di-u-ret'ik) Any agent that causes reduction of urine formation.

antidromic (an-tĭ-drom'ik) Conducting nerve impulses in a reverse direction to the normal.

antiemetic (an-te-ĕ-met'ik) An agent that prevents or relieves nausea and vomiting.

antiepileptic (an-te-ĕp-ĭ-lep'tik) 1. Tending to prevent or control epileptic convulsions. 2. Denoting a drug that has such a property.

antiestrogen (an-te-es'tro-jen) Any agent that is capable of blocking the action of estrogens in the body.

antifebrile (an-tĭ-feb'ril) See antipyretic.

antifibrinolysin (an-tĭ-fi-brĭ-nol'ĭ sin) A substance that inhibits the disintegration of fibrin, thereby retarding the dissolution of a blood clot.

antifol (an'tĭ-fol) A folic acid antagonist.

Baker's a. A chemotherapeutic agent used in the treatment of squamous cell carcinoma of the cervix; it has a response rate greater or equal to 10%.

antifolate (an-tĭ-fo'lāt) 1. Interfering with the action of folic acid. 2. An agent producing such action.

antifungal (an-tĭ-fung'al) Any agent that is destructive to fungi.

antigalactagogue (an-tĭ-ga-lak'tă-gog) An agent that suppresses the production of milk.

antigen (an'tĭ-jen) (Ag) Any material capable of triggering in an individual the production of specific antibody or the formation of a specific population of lymphocytes (a type of white blood cell), which react with that material. Antigens may be proteins, toxins, microorganisms, or tissue cells. Whether any material is an antigen in a person depends on whether the material is foreign to the person, the genetic make-up of the person, and the dose of the material. See also CA 15-3; CA 19-9; CA 125.

Australia a., Au a. See hepatitis B surface antigen.

carcinoembryonic a. (CEA) A glycoprotein constituent of normal gastrointestinal tissues of the fetus; present in the adult only in certain types of cancer, such as cancer of the colon. Also called oncofetal antigen.

CD4 a. A glycoprotein on the membrane of T-expressor cells.

CD8 a. A glycoprotein on the membrane of T-helper cells.

common acute lymphoblastic leukemia a. (CALLA) A tumor-associated antigen occurring in a high percentage (80%) of patients with acute lymphoblastic leukemia (ALL).

Forssman a. An antigen that is present in red blood cells of sheep and in organ tissues (but not blood) of many other species. The antibodies formed in patients with infectious mononucleosis react specifically with Forssman antigens.

hepatitis B core a. (HB$_c$Ag) Antigen associated with the core of the hepatitis B virus; present in complete virons (Dane particles) and in the nuclei of infected liver cells. HB$_c$Ag and its antibodies are detectable by various laboratory techniques.

hepatitis B e a. (HB$_e$Ag) A core antigen of hepatitis B virus (Dane particle) present in the blood of infected persons, associated with transmission of the infection. HB$_e$Ag and its antibodies are detectable by various laboratory techniques.

hepatitis B surface a. (HB$_S$Ag) Antigen of the outer coat of the complete hepatitis virus (Dane particle) and in smaller spherical and filamentous particles. HB$_S$Ag and its antibodies are detectable by various laboratory techniques. The presence of antibodies to HB$_S$AG connotes immunity; persistence of HB$_S$Ag in the blood denotes an infectious carrier state. Also called Australia antigen; Au antigen.

heterogenetic a. See heterophil antigen.

heterophil a. Any antigen that occurs in more than one species (e.g., Forssman antigen). Also called heterogenetic antigen.

histocompatibility a. Any of the genetically determined antigens, present on nucleated cells of most tissues, that induce an immune response (rejection) when transplanted from the donor into a genetically different recipient. Also called transplantation antigen.

HLA a.'s A group of histocompatibility antigens controlled by a region of chromosome 6 and its genetic sites (loci); they are polypeptides or glycoproteins responsible for rejection of tissue transplants in humans and are associated with certain diseases.

human leukocyte a.'s Antigens encoded by genes of the HLA complex (the major histocompatibility genetic region in humans); they are categorized into classes I, II, and III. Classes I and II are cell surface glycoproteins and have an important role in determining tissue transplant rejection. Class III are soluble molecules; they have no role in tissue transplantation.

H-Y a. A cell-surface protein encoded by a structured gene on the short arm of the Y chromosome, near the centromere; it is thought to induce the embryonic gonad to develop into a testis.

H-Y histocompatibility a. A protein formerly suggested as Y-encoded, gene-expressed, testis-determining factor (i.e., responsible for the differentiation of the human embryo into a male). The hypothesis has been abandoned due to inconsistencies of the antigen's expression in various cell types and its absence in indisputable males with testes.

I a. See I blood group.

oncofetal a. (OFA) See carcinoembryonic antigen.

squamous cell carcinoma a. A purified subfraction of the tumor antigen-4 (TA-4), a glycoprotein of approximately 48 kilodaltons isolated from cervical tissue.

transplantation a. Histocompatibility antigen.

tumor-associated a. (TAA) An antigen that is found on cells undergoing neoplastic transformation.

tumor-specific a. (TSA) Any antigen that can be detected only on the surface of tumor cells and not on the normal host cells.

antigenic (an-tĭ-jen'ik) Having the properties of an antigen (i.e., capable of inciting the formation of antibody).

antigenicity (an-tĭ-je-nisĭ-te) The state of being antigenic. Also called immunogenicity.

antihypertensive (an-tĭ-hi-per-ten'siv) Tending to reduce high blood pressure.

antimetabolite (an-tĭ-mĕ-tab'o-līt) Any structural analog of a metabolite (a naturally occurring substance essential for normal physiologic functioning); each antimetabolite competes with, replaces, or interferes with the activity of a particular metabolite.

antimicrobial (an-tĭ-mi-kro'be-al) A drug that destroys microorganisms.

beta-lactam a. A class of broad-spectrum antibiotics that are related, structurally and pharmaceutically, to the penicillins and cephalosporins.

antimutagen (an-tĭ-mu'tă-jen) Any factor that reduces the rate of mutation (e.g., by interfering with the action of a mutagen, or by rendering genetic elements less susceptible to change).

antineoplastic (an-tĭ-ne-o-plas'tik) Any agent that interferes with the growth of a tumor.

antiprogestin (an-tĭ-pro-jes'tin) A substance that inhibits the formation or action of progesterone.

antiprostaglandin (an-tĭ-pros-tă-glan'din) See prostaglandin inhibitor, under inhibitor.

antiprothrombin (an-tĭ-pro-throm'bin) A substance that inhibits the conversion of prothrombin (plasma protein) into thrombin (enzyme), thus preventing blood clot formation.

antipruritic (an-tĭ-proo-rit'ik) An agent that alleviates itching.

antipsychotic (an-tĭ-si-kot'ik) **1.** Relieving symptoms of mental disorders. **2.** Any agent having such an effect.

antipyretic (an-tĭ-pi-ret'ik) Any agent that reduces fever. Also called antifebrile; antithermic.

antiserum (an-tĭ-se'rum) Human or animal serum containing antibodies that are specific for one or more antigens.

antithrombin (an-tĭ-throm'bin) Any substance (occurring naturally or administered

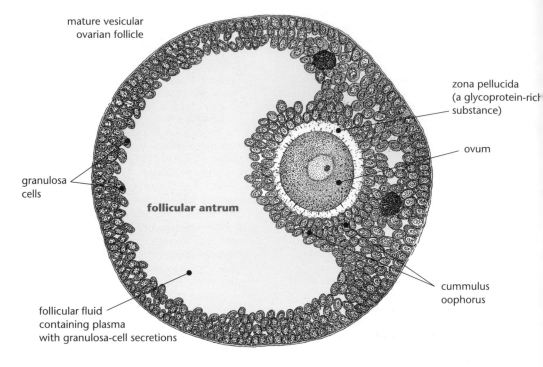

mature vesicular
ovarian follicle

zona pellucida
(a glycoprotein-rich
substance)

ovum

granulosa
cells

follicular antrum

cummulus
oophorus

follicular fluid
containing plasma
with granulosa-cell secretions

therapeutically) that prevents blood clotting by inhibiting the action of thrombin.

antithyroid (an-tǐ-thi'roid) An agent that counteracts the functioning of the thyroid gland, especially in producing thyroid hormone.

antitreponemal (an-tǐ-trep-o-ne'mal) See treponemicidal.

antro- Combining form meaning cavity.

antrum (an'trum), pl. antra **1.** A cavity within a bone. **2.** The normal, enlarged portion of a hollow organ.

> **follicular a.** The fluid-filled cavity within an ovarian follicle.

anuresis (an-u-re'sis) Total retention of urine in the bladder; inability to urinate.

anuretic (an-u-ret'ik) Relating to anuresis.

anuria (an-u're-ǎ) Inability to produce urine; in clinical use, denoting a 24-h urine volume of less than 100 cm³ for an adult of average size.

anuric (an-u'rik) Relating to anuria.

anus (a'nus) The terminal opening of the digestive tract. Also called the anal orifice.

> **imperforate a.** Congenital absence of the anus; sometimes associated with abnormal openings of the anal canal into the urethra or vagina. Also called anal atresia; proctatresia.

anxiety (ang-zi'ě-te) An effect characterized chiefly by a state of uneasiness, apprehension, and dread of impending internal or external danger, heightened vigilance, exhausting muscular tension, and autonomic hyperactivity accompanied by physical symptoms (e.g., dizziness, profuse sweating, trembling, or rapid heart beat).

aorta (a-or'tǎ), pl. aortas, aortae The largest and main trunk of the arterial system of the body; it begins at the upper part of the left ventricle of the heart, from which it receives blood for delivery to all tissues except the lungs. See also

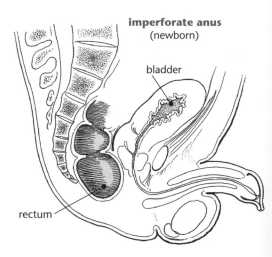

imperforate anus
(newborn)

bladder

rectum

arch of aorta, under arch.

abdominal a. The portion of the descending aorta from the diaphragm to the pelvis, where it divides into two branches (common iliac arteries).

ascending a. The part of the aorta beginning at the top of the left ventricle and directed toward the head before it curves to form the arch of the aorta.

descending a. The part of the aorta directed downward, from the arch of the aorta to its division into the two common iliac arteries, including the abdominal aorta.

overriding a. A developmental anomaly in which the aorta straddles the ventricular septum, thereby receiving ejected blood from both right and left ventricles of the heart.

thoracic a. The portion of the descending aorta from the arch of the aorta to the diaphragm.

aortic (a-or'tik) Relating to the aorta.

aortitis (a-or-ti'tis) Inflammation of the aorta; may result in weakening of vessel walls and aneurysm formation.

syphilitic a. An uncommon condition resulting from untreated syphilis and occurring in the tertiary stage of the disease, often several decades after the primary infection.

aperistalsis (a-per-ĭ-stal'sis) Absence of normal contractions of the digestive tract.

esophageal a. See achalasia.

aperture (ap'er-chūr) An opening.

inferior a. of minor pelvis See pelvic plane of outlet, under plane.

lateral a. of fourth ventricle One of two lateral openings on the roof of the fourth ventricle of the brain; it leads to the subarachnoid cavity. Also called the foramen of Luschka.

median a. of fourth ventricle An opening in the midline of the roof of the fourth ventricle of the brain; it leads to the subarachnoid space. Also called the foramen of Magendie.

superior a. of minor pelvis See pelvic plane of inlet, under plane.

aphagia (ă-fa'je-ă) Inability or refusal to eat.

apico- Combining form meaning a summit or tip.

aplasia cutis (ă-pla'se-ă ku'tis) A fetal scalp defect characterized by absence, or defective development, of a circumscribed area of the scalp; may occur subsequent to the use of the thyroid inhibitor methimazole during pregnancy for the treatment of hyperthyroidism.

apnea (ap-ne'ă) Temporary cessation of respiration.

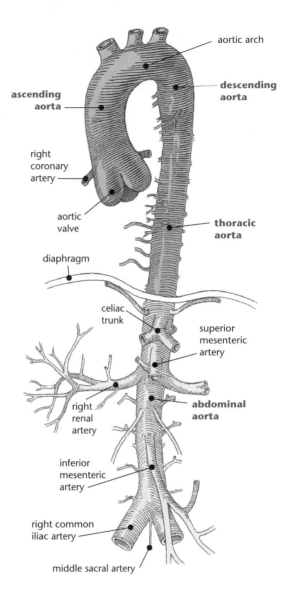

sleep a. Episodes of apnea occurring during sleep and lasting 10 s or longer; may be central, associated with depression of respiratory drive, or obstructive, caused by blockage of airflow at the nose or mouth.

apneic (ap'ne-ik) Relating to apnea.

apo- Prefix meaning separation; derived from.

apodia (a-po'de-ă) Congenital absence of feet.

apolipoprotein (ap-o-lip-o-pro'tēn) (apo) Any of the protein components of lipoproteins normally circulating in human blood plasma.

aponeurosis (ap-o-nu-ro'sis), pl. aponeuroses A

broad, often thin tendinous sheet of fibrous tissue; it connects a muscle to its attachment.

apoplexy (ap'o-plek-se) **1.** Rupture of a vessel into an organ. **2.** Obsolete term for stroke.

    uteroplacental a. See Couvelaire uterus, under uterus.

apoprotein (ap-o-pro'tēn) Protein on the surface of a lipoprotein molecule; it is the site that binds to the lipoprotein receptor on a cell surface.

apoptosis (ap-op-to'sis) Programmed cell death (i.e., it occurs naturally from internal perturbations).

apparatus (ap-ă-ră'tus), pl. apparatuses **1.** A group of instruments used together or in succession to perform a particular task. **2.** A group of organs or structures that collectively perform a common function.

    urogenital a. The combination of the organs concerned in the production and passage of urine, together with the organs of reproduction. Also called urogenital tract; genitourinary tract.

appendage (ă-pen'dij) Any part in close but subordinate relation to a principal structure.

    testicular a. See appendix of testis, under appendix.

    vesicular a. See vesicular appendix, under appendix.

appendix (ă-pen'diks), pl. appendices **1.** An appendage or accessory part attached to a main structure. **2.** The vermiform appendix.

    a. of epididymis A small, stalked, oval body situated on the head of the epididymis; a vestige of the mesonephros.

    a. of testis A minute oval body situated at the upper end of the testis; a normal remnant of the embryonic paramesonephric (mullerian) duct. Also called testicular appendage.

    Morgagni's a. See vesicular appendix.

    vermiform a. A slender, finger-shaped, tubular structure branching off the blind end of the cecum (beginning part of the large intestine), about 2 cm below the junction of the cecum and the ileum (terminal part of the small intestine). It has a thick wall with an ample supply of lymphoid tissue, which provides local protection against infection. Also called appendix.

    vesicular a. A minute fluid-filled structure attached to the fimbriated open end of the fallopian (uterine) tube; a normal remnant of the embryonic mesonephric duct. Also called vesicular appendage; Morgagni's appendix.

approximator (ă-prok'si-ma-tor) Instrument used in surgical procedures for bringing tissue edges into close apposition for suturing.

    microsurgical a. A noncrushing instrument designed to hold both ends of severed structures (e.g., blood vessels, nerves) for repair under magnification of a surgical microscope.

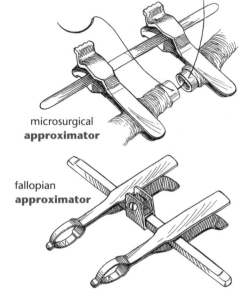

microsurgical **approximator**

fallopian **approximator**

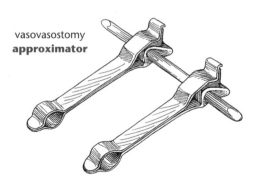

vasovasostomy **approximator**

apron (a'prun) **1.** A garment or device worn to protect clothing or the body. **2.** An anatomic structure resembling an apron in appearance or function, such as the omentum.

    leaded a. A shield of lead rubber that protects patients or health care workers from needless radiation exposure during radiography. Also called lead-rubber apron; protective apron.

    lead-rubber a. See leaded apron.

    protective a. See leaded apron.

aqueduct (ak'we-dukt) A passage or canal.

   a. of cerebrum See cerebral aqueduct.

   a. of Sylvius, sylvian a. See cerebral aqueduct.

   cerebral a. A small passage between the third and fourth ventricles of the brain, through which passes cerebrospinal fluid. Also called aqueduct of Sylvius; sylvian aqueduct; aqueduct of cerebrum; canal of midbrain.

   vestibular a. A canal in the internal ear extending from the medial wall of the vestibule to the posterior surface of the petrous portion of the temporal bone; it houses the endolymphatic duct.

arabinosylcytosine (ă-ră-bin-o-sil-si'to-sēn) See cytarabine.

ara-C See cytarabine.

arachidonic acid (ă-ră-kĭ-don'ik as'id) A polyunsaturated fatty acid that is essential for human nutrition; it is present abundantly in the amnion and amniotic fluid.

arborization (ar-bor-ĭ-za'shun) **1.** The branching termination of a nerve or blood vessel. **2.** The fern pattern sometimes formed by mucus from the uterine cervix when allowed to dry on a glass slide for inspection under the microscope. Seen in the proliferative phase of the menstrual cycle and in the presence of leaking amniotic fluid.

arch (arch) Any curved structure of the body.

   aortic a.'s The six arterial channels surrounding the pharynx of the embryo; some are functional only in the very young embryo, others develop into adult arteries. They never exist all at the same time.

   a. of aorta, aortic a. The curved part of the aorta, between the ascending and descending portions.

   neural a. See vertebral arch.

   pharyngeal a. One of a series of five mesodermal arches (bars) in the neck region of the embryo from which several structures of the head and neck develop.

   pubic a. The arch of the pelvis formed by the inferior pubic rami of both sides.

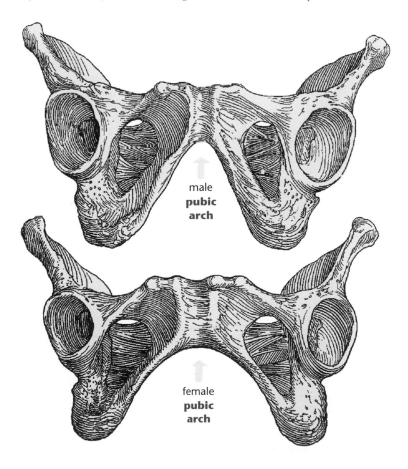

male
pubic arch

female
pubic arch

tendinous a. of levator ani muscle A linear thickening of the obturator fascia that extends in a curved fashion from the posterior surface of the pubic bone to the ischial spine; it provides origin to part of the levator ani muscle. Also called arcus tendineus musculi levatoris ani.

tendinous a. of pelvic fascia A linear thickening of the superior fascia of the pelvic diaphragm; it extends from the posterior surface of the pubic bone to the spine of the ischium, along the bladder and vagina, and provides attachment to ligaments of the pelvic organs. Also called arcus tendineus fasciae pelvis.

vertebral a. The arch of the dorsal or posterior side of the vertebra that forms the vertebral foramen for passage of the spinal cord. Also called neural arch.

archenteron (ar-ken′ter-on) The primitive digestive tract of the embryo. Also called primary gut.

arctation (ark-ta′shun) A narrowing in a hollow tubular structure.

arcus (ar′kus) Latin for arch.

a. tendineus fasciae pelvis See tendinous arch of pelvic fascia, under arch.

a. tendineus musculi levatoris ani See tendinous arch of levator ani muscle, under arch.

areflexia (ă-re-flek′se-ă) Absence of reflexes.

areola (ă-re′o-lă), pl. areolae **1.** A small space within a tissue. **2.** A circular pigmented area surrounding a central point, such as the nipple of the breast.

areolar (ă-re′o-lar) Relating to an areola.

arm (arm) The portion of the upper limb from the shoulder to the elbow; commonly used to mean the entire upper limb.

nuchal a. A fetal arm that is positioned around the back of the neck; sometimes seen in breech deliveries.

aromatase (ă-ro′mă-tās) Enzyme involved in synthesizing estrogens by promoting the conversion of androstenedione to estrone and the conversion of testosterone to estradiol.

arrest (ă-rest′) **1.** A state of inactivity; a cessation. **2.** To stop.

cardiac a. (CA) Sudden stoppage of effective heart action; may be due to absence of ventricular contractions (asystole) or to ineffective, uncoordinated contractions (fibrillation).

circulatory a. Cessation of blood circulation usually caused by cardiac arrest.

deep transverse a. Cessation of labor while the fetal head is in the transverse position, down deep in the pelvis with the occiput below the level of the maternal ischial spines.

a. disorders of labor See under disorder.

midpelvic a. Arrest of the fetal head's advance through the maternal midpelvis resulting from various factors, including (a) fetal malposition, occurring either in the occiput anterior (OA) position, or in the occiput posterior (OP) position; (b) failure of uterine forces of contraction; or (c) borderline cephalopelvic disproportion.

sinus a. A temporary cessation of cardiac activity due to a brief failure of the sinoatrial (S-A) node of the heart to send impulses to the atria.

sperm maturation a. Failure of the germinal cells in the testes to attain full maturity; may occur at any stage in the process of spermatozoon development (e.g., the stage when the primary spermatocyte [with a diploid chromosome content] divides to form two secondary spermatocytes [each with a haploid complement of chromosomes]).

arrhenoblastoma (ă-re-no-blas-to′mă) An uncommon benign tumor of the ovary occurring in young women. It secretes male hormones (androgens), causing development of male

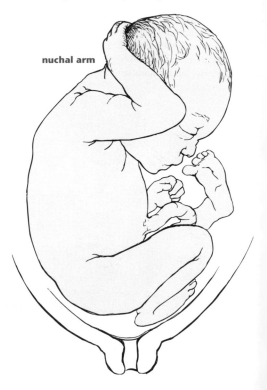

nuchal arm

characteristics (masculinization). Also called ovarian tubular adenoma.

arrhythmia (ă-rith'me-ă) Any variation from the regular rhythm of the heartbeat; may appear in the presence or absence of heart disease. Causes range widely, but basically arrhythmias are due to a disturbance either to the site of origin of the impulse or to the conduction system of the impulse through the heart wall.

arrhythmic (ă-rith'mik) Related to arrhythmia.

arterio-, arteri- Combining forms meaning artery.

arteriogram (ar-te're-o-gram) An x-ray image of an artery, obtained after injecting a radiopaque solution into it.

arteriography (ar-te-re-og'ră-fe) X-ray visualization of an artery after introducing a radiopaque solution into it.

    coronary a. Arteriography of the arteries supplying blood to the heart muscle.

arteriovenous (ar-te-re-o-ve'nus) Relating to both arteries and veins.

arteritis (ar-tĕ-ri'tis) Inflammation of an artery.

    cranial a. See temporal arteritis.

    giant cell a. See temporal arteritis.

    Takayasu's a. Uncommon disease of medium- and large-sized arteries, characterized by inflammation of the vessels and narrowing of their lumen; it affects all arteries but has a strong predilection for the aortic arch and its branches; most commonly involves the subclavian arteries, followed by the aortic arch, ascending aorta, carotid arteries, and femoral arteries. Symptoms include fever, night sweats, joint pain, appetite and weight loss, and general malaise; pulses are usually absent in the involved arteries. The condition is most prevalent in adolescent girls and young women. Also called aortic arch syndrome; pulseless disease.

    temporal a. Inflammation of the medium- and large-sized arteries, typically involving one or more branches of the carotid arteries, especially the temporal arteries and those of the scalp; it may also affect arteries in multiple areas, including the femoral arteries. Headache is the chief complaint; other symptoms include fever, appetite and weight loss, and joint pain. In advanced stages, the retinal arteries may become occluded, causing blindness. The condition primarily affects people over 50 years of age. Also called cranial arteritis; giant cell arteritis.

artery (ar'ter-e) A vessel conveying blood from the heart to all body parts. All arteries transport oxygenated blood except those from the heart to the lungs (pulmonary arteries).

    appendicular a. *Origin:* ileocolic artery. *Branches:* none. *Distribution:* vermiform appendix.

    arcuate a.'s of uterus *Origin:* uterine artery. *Branches:* radial arteries. *Distribution:* myometrium, endometrium.

    axillary a. *Origin:* continuation of subclavian artery in axilla. *Branches:* highest thoracic, thoracoacromial, lateral thoracic, subscapular, posterior humeral circumflex, anterior humeral circumflex; continues as brachial artery. *Distribution:* pectoralis major and minor muscles, deltoid, serratus anterior,

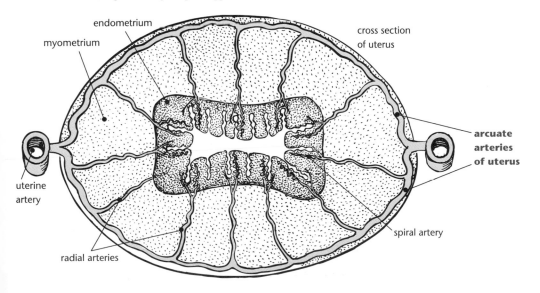

endometrium

myometrium

cross section of uterus

arcuate arteries of uterus

uterine artery

spiral artery

radial arteries

subscapularis, long head of biceps muscles, teres major and minor muscles, acromion, sternoclavicular joint, mammary gland, shoulder joint, head of humerus.

azygos a.'s of vagina, anterior and posterior *Origin:* uterine artery. *Branches:* anastomotic. *Distribution:* anterior and posterior walls of vagina.

basal a.'s of uterus *Origin:* radial arteries. *Branches:* none. *Distribution:* deep (basal) portion of endometrium.

a. of bulb of vestibule *Origin:* internal pudendal artery. *Branches:* none. *Distribution:* bulb of vestibule, greater vestibular glands.

a. of clitoris *Origin:* internal pudendal artery. *Branches:* deep artery of clitoris. *Distribution:* erectile tissues.

a. of clitoris, deep *Origin:* internal pudendal artery (via artery of clitoris). *Branches:* none. *Distribution:* corpus cavernosum of clitoris.

a. of clitoris, dorsal *Origin:* internal pudendal artery (via artery of clitoris). *Branches:* none. *Distribution:* dorsum, glans, and prepuce of clitoris.

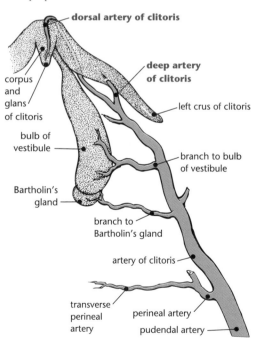

colic a., left *Origin:* inferior mesenteric artery. *Branches:* ascending, descending. *Distribution:* descending colon, left half of transverse colon.

colic a., right *Origin:* superior mesenteric

artery or ileocolic artery. *Branches:* none. *Distribution:* ascending colon.

epigastric a., inferior *Origin:* external iliac immediately above inguinal ligament. *Branches:* pubic, artery of round ligament of uterus. *Distribution:* rectus abdominis, skin.

epigastric a., superficial *Origin:* femoral artery about 1 cm below inguinal ligament. *Branches:* none. *Distribution:* lower part of abdominal wall, superficial inguinal lymph nodes, overlying skin.

epigastric a., superior *Origin:* internal thoracic artery. *Branches:* none. *Distribution:* rectus abdominis and diaphragm muscles, skin of the abdomen.

femoral a. *Origin:* continuation of external iliac artery immediately below the level of the inguinal ligament. *Branches:* superficial epigastric, superficial circumflex iliac, external pudendal, deep femoral, descending genicular. *Distribution:* lower abdominal wall, external genitalia, muscles of thigh, superficial inguinal lymph nodes.

gluteal a., inferior *Origin:* internal iliac artery (anterior division). *Branches:* muscular, coccygeal, sciatic, vesical, articular, anastomotic. *Distribution:* muscles of buttock and back of thigh.

gluteal a., superior *Origin:* internal iliac artery (posterior division). *Branches:* superficial, deep. *Distribution:* muscles of buttock, ilium.

hypogastric a. See internal iliac artery.

iliac a., common *Origin:* abdominal aorta about the level of the fourth lumbar vertebra. *Branches:* internal iliac, external iliac. *Distribution:* pelvis, gluteal region, perineum, lower limb, lower abdominal wall.

iliac a., external *Origin:* common iliac artery. *Branches:* inferior epigastric, deep circumflex iliac. *Distribution:* abdominal wall, external genitalia, cremasteric muscle, lower limb.

iliac a., internal *Origin:* bifurcation of common iliac artery. *Branches:* (anterior trunk) inferior vesical, middle rectal, uterine, obturator, internal pudendal, inferior gluteal, vaginal, umbilical; (posterior trunk) iliolumbar, lateral sacral, superior gluteal. *Distribution:* wall and viscera of pelvis, external genitalia, buttock, medial side of thigh.

iliolumbar a. *Origin:* internal iliac artery (posterior division). *Branches:* iliac, lumbar. *Distribution:* greater psoas and quadratus lumborum muscles, gluteal and abdominal walls, ilium, cauda equina.

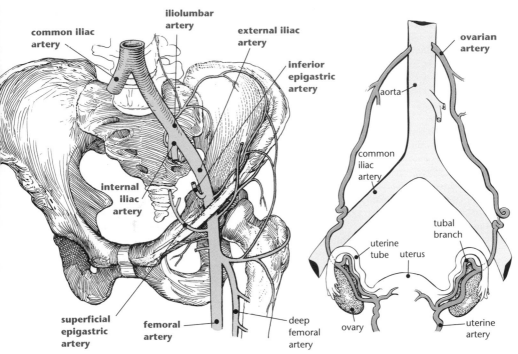

intercostal a.'s, anterior *Origin:* internal thoracic artery, musculophrenic artery. *Branches:* muscular, cutaneous. *Distribution:* upper six intercostal spaces, pectoralis major and minor muscles, skin of breast.

intercostal a.'s I and II, posterior *Origin:* highest intercostal artery. *Branches:* dorsal. *Distribution:* upper thoracic wall.

intercostal a.'s III-XI, posterior *Origin:* thoracic aorta. *Branches:* dorsal, collateral, lateral cutaneous. *Distribution:* nine lower intercostal spaces, anterior serratus muscle, pectoralis major and minor muscles, mammary gland.

intercostal a., highest *Origin:* costocervical trunk. *Branches:* first and second posterior intercostal. *Distribution:* first and second intercostal spaces.

lumbar a.'s *Origin:* abdominal aorta. *Branches:* dorsal, spinal. *Distribution:* lumbar vertebrae, back muscles, spinal cord.

lumbar a., lowest *Origin:* middle sacral artery. *Branches:* none. *Distribution:* sacrum.

mesenteric a., inferior *Origin:* abdominal aorta at level of third and fourth lumbar vertebrae. *Branches:* left colic, sigmoid, superior rectal. *Distribution:* transverse, descending, and sigmoid colon, rectum.

obturator a. *Origin:* internal iliac artery (anterior division). *Branches:* pubic, acetabular,

iliac, vesical, anterior, posterior. *Distribution:* pelvic muscles, hip joint, bladder, iliac fossa.

ovarian a. *Origin:* abdominal aorta at level of second lumbar vertebra. *Branches:* ureteric, capsular, tubal (lateral, middle, medial). *Distribution:* ovary, ureter.

perineal a. *Origin:* internal pudendal artery. *Branches:* transverse perineal artery. *Distribution:* posterior labial, superficial structures of perineum.

pudendal a., external *Origin:* femoral artery. *Branches:* anterior labial, inguinal. *Distribution:* skin of lower abdomen, skin of labium majus.

pudendal a., internal *Origin:* internal iliac artery (anterior division). *Branches:* inferior rectal, perineal, artery of the vestibule, posterior labial, urethral, bulb of vestibule, deep artery of clitoris, dorsal artery of clitoris. *Distribution:* external genitalia, muscles of perineum, anus.

pulmonary a., left *Origin:* pulmonary trunk. *Branches:* branches are named according to the segment that they supply (e.g., apical, anterior descending, posterior, anterior ascending). *Distribution:* left lung.

pulmonary a., right *Origin:* pulmonary trunk. *Branches:* branches are named according to the segment that they supply (e.g., apical, posterior descending, posterior ascending). *Distribution:* right lung.

radial a.'s of uterus *Origin:* arcuate arteries. *Branches:* basal, spiral. *Distribution:* myometrium, endometrium.

rectal a., inferior *Origin:* internal pudendal artery. *Branches:* none. *Distribution:* rectum, muscles and skin of anal region.

rectal a., middle *Origin:* internal iliac artery. *Branches:* vaginal. *Distribution:* rectal musculature.

rectal a., superior *Origin:* continuation of inferior mesenteric artery. *Branches:* none. *Distribution:* rectal musculature.

renal a. *Origin:* abdominal aorta at about level of first lumbar vertebra. *Branches:* inferior suprarenal, anterior branch, posterior branch, ureteral. *Distribution:* kidney, adrenal gland, ureter.

sacral a.'s, lateral *Origin:* internal iliac artery (posterior division). *Branches:* spinal. *Distribution:* sacrum, sacral canal.

sacral a., middle *Origin:* abdominal aorta at bifurcation. *Branches:* lower lumbar artery. *Distribution:* sacrum, rectum.

sigmoid a.'s *Origin:* inferior mesenteric artery. *Branches:* none. *Distribution:* sigmoid colon, lower part of descending colon.

spinal a., anterior *Origin:* vertebral artery near termination. *Branches:* central. *Distribution:* spinal cord.

spinal a., posterior *Origin:* posterior inferior cerebellar artery or vertebral artery. *Branches:* dorsal, ventral. *Distribution:* spinal cord.

spiral a.'s *Origin:* radial arteries. *Branches:* none. *Distribution:* superficial two-thirds of endometrium.

splenic a. *Origin:* celiac trunk. *Branches:* pancreatic, splenic, short gastric, left gastroepiploic (omental). *Distribution:* spleen, pancreas, stomach, greater omentum.

suprascapular a. *Origin:* thyrocervical trunk. *Branches:* suprasternal, articular, acromial, nutrient, supraspinous, infraspinous. *Distribution:* clavicle, scapula, skin of chest, muscles of scapula region, acromioclavicular and shoulder joints.

thoracic a., internal *Origin:* subclavian artery. *Branches:* pericardiacophrenic, mediastinal, sternal, perforating, anterior intercostal, musculophrenic, superior epigastric, thymus. *Distribution:* anterior thoracic wall, structures in mediastinum such as lymph nodes, diaphragm.

thoracic a., lateral *Origin:* axillary artery. *Branches:* lateral mammary. *Distribution:* pectoralis major and minor muscles, serratus anterior and subscapularis muscles, mammary

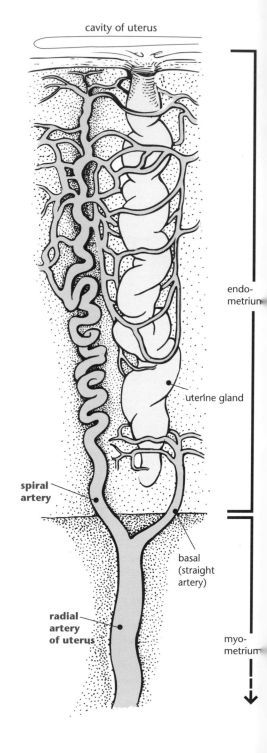

cavity of uterus

endo-
metrium

uterine gland

spiral
artery

basal
(straight
artery)

radial
artery
of uterus

myo-
metrium

gland, axillary lymph nodes.

thoracic a., highest *Origin:* axillary artery. *Branches:* none. *Distribution:* pectoralis major, pectoralis minor, anterior serratus, and intercostal muscles.

thoracoacromial a. *Origin:* axillary artery. *Branches:* pectoral, acromial, deltoid, clavicular. *Distribution:* pectoralis major and minor muscles, subclavius and deltoid muscles, sternoclavicular joint, acromion.

umbilical a. *Origin:* internal iliac artery. *Branches:* superior vesical, middle vesical. *Distribution:* base of bladder.

urethral a. *Origin:* internal pudendal artery. *Branches:* none. *Distribution:* urethra.

uterine a. *Origin:* internal iliac artery (anterior division). *Branches:* arcuate, vaginal, cervical, round ligament, tubal, ovarian. *Distribution:* upper part of vagina, cervix, uterus, round ligament of uterus, medial part of uterine tube. Provides maternal blood circulation to placenta during pregnancy.

vaginal a. *Origin:* internal iliac artery (anterior division) or uterine artery. *Branches:* none. *Distribution:* vagina, bulb of vestibule, base of bladder, rectum.

those of opposite side. *Distribution:* ureter, upper part of bladder.

arthritis (ar-thri'tis), pl. arthritides Inflammation of a joint or joints. The condition has no effect on pregnancy, unless antiprostaglandin medication is administered, which may prolong the duration of the pregnancy.

gonococcal a. A form associated with gonorrhea, involving one or several joints, especially of the knees, ankles, and wrists; *Neisseria gonorrhoeae* can be isolated from the joint fluid.

juvenile a., juvenile rheumatoid a. (JRA) Rheumatoid arthritis of childhood affecting one or a few large joints, with enlargement of the liver, spleen, and lymph nodes; may also involve the cervical spine or cause inflammation of the iris. Complete remission may occur at puberty.

rheumatoid a. (RA) A chronic disease of unknown cause characterized by progressive inflammation of small joints, especially those of the fingers; marked by swelling, slow thickening of connective tissues, erosion of articular cartilage, and potential deformity and disability.

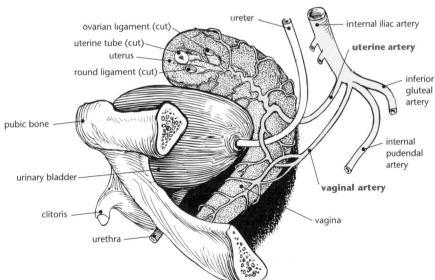

vesical a., inferior *Origin:* internal iliac artery. *Branches:* anastomosing with those of opposite side. *Distribution:* base of bladder, lower ureter.

vesical a., middle *Origin:* umbilical artery. *Branches:* none. *Distribution:* bladder.

vesical a.'s, superior *Origin:* umbilical artery. *Branches:* ureteric, anastomosing with

syphilitic a. (1) Mild chronic effusion into the knee joints (Clutton's joints) occurring during puberty in congenital syphilis. (2) Painful, stiff, tender joints with transient swelling ocurring with secondary syphilis; inflammation of adjacent periosteum usually occurs.

arthro-, arthr- Combining forms meaning joint;

articulation.

-ase Suffix meaning enzyme; added to the name of the substance upon which it acts (e.g., proteinase).

aspermatogenesis (a-sper-mă-to-jen'ĕ-sis) Absence of spermatozoa formation.

aspermatogenic (a-sper-mă-to-jen'ik) Failing to produce spermatozoa.

aspermia (ă-sper'me-ă) Failure to produce or ejaculate sperm.

asphygmia (as-fig'me-ă) Temporary absence of the pulse.

asphyxia (as-fik'se-ă) Suffocation due to interference with the oxygen supply of the blood; may be caused by obstruction of the airway by a foreign body, a lack of oxygen in the air (e.g., within a plastic bag), or inhalation of a gas (e.g., carbon monoxide) that prevents the uptake of oxygen into the bloodstream.

    a. neonatorum Breathing failure of the newborn infant.

    perinatal a. Imprecise term implying metabolic acidemia; the severity and associated factors necessary to cause fetal damage are not precisely determined. Metabolic acidosis, neonatal depression (including low Apgar scores), and neonatal neurologic and systemic symptoms may have causes other than asphyxia.

asphyxiant (as-fik'se-ant) Anything that suffocates.

asphyxiate (as-fik'se-āt) **1.** To induce suffocation. **2.** To undergo suffocation.

asphyxiation (as-fik-se-a'shun) The process of bringing about suffocation.

aspirate (as'pĭ-rāt) **1.** To withdraw (usually fluid) from a body cavity by suction. **2.** The withdrawn material.

aspiration (as-pĭ-ra'shun) **1.** Removal of material by suction. **2.** Intake of foreign material into the lungs while breathing.

    egg a. In *in vitro* fertilization, aspiration of preovulatory follicles from the ovary, performed approximately 34 hours after an injection of the hormone human chorionic gonadotropin (hCG), or 24 hours before the beginning of the natural burst of luteinizing hormone secretion (LH surge); may be performed under direct visualization with a laparoscope (laparoscopic aspiration) or under the guidance of an ultrasound scanner (ultrasound aspiration).

    endocervical a. Removal of mucus from the canal of the cervix for microscopic examination of cast-off cells (exfoliative cytology) for diagnostic purposes.

    meconium a. Inhalation of meconium-contaminated amniotic fluid by an infant taking its first breath at birth; the material may pass from the upper to the lower respiratory tract, causing meconium blockage of the airways and lung damage.

    menstrual a. Aspiration of the endometrium with a flexible 5- or 6-mm Karman cannula and syringe, performed 1 to 3 weeks after failure to menstruate. Also called atraumatic abortion; menstrual extraction; menstrual induction; miniabortion; instant period.

aspirator (as-pĭ-ra'tor) Any apparatus used in removing material from body cavities by means of suction.

    Vabra a. A suction curette, 3 to 4 mm in diameter, attached to a vacuum pump; used to obtain samples of the endometrium for histologic examination.

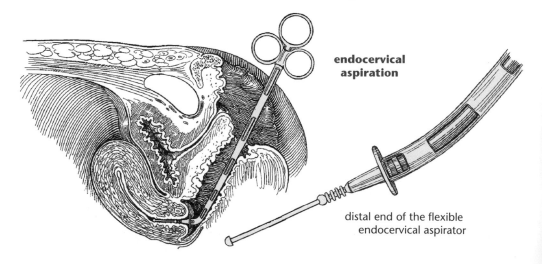

endocervical aspiration

distal end of the flexible endocervical aspirator

vacuum a. Aspirator used to remove the product of conception from the uterine cavity.

assault (ă-salt') An intentional act to make the victim apprehensive of immediate harmful or offensive bodily contact, even though contact may not actually occur.

aggravated sexual a. See rape.

sexual a. See rape.

assay (as'a) Analysis to determine the presence of a substance, its quantity, or its effects on an organism; a test; a trial.

biological a. See bioassay.

clonogenic a. See stem cell assay.

competitive protein-binding a. Assay in which labeled and unlabeled ligand compete for sites in a binder that has the same affinity for both. Also called saturation analysis.

enzyme-linked immunosorbent a. (ELISA) A laboratory blood test employed in the diagnosis of infectious diseases (e.g., AIDS and hepatitis A and B). The antigen of interest is fixed to a solid-state immunosorbent and incubated in a medium containing a test antibody raised against the antigen; then a second incubation is conducted with an enzyme-tagged detector antibody raised against the test antibody; finally, a substrate is added, which is digested by the enzyme, producing a color that can be measured by spectrophotometry.

hamster egg a. See sperm penetration assay.

human zona binding a. A male fertility test to determine the ability of sperm to pass through, or bind to, the zona pellucida of the ovum; two sperm samples, one from a donor and one from the patient, are exposed to different portions of surgically removed zona pellucida from ovarian tissue.

immunoradiometric a. (IRMA) A form of radioimmunoassay in which radioactively labeled antibody is added directly to the antigen being measured.

radioreceptor a. A competitive binding assay using a radioactively labeled hormone to measure the specific cellular receptor sites for the hormone; used as a pregnancy test.

sperm penetration a. A laboratory test of sperm function in which human spermatozoa, after special treatment, are allowed to incubate with denuded ova usually from the golden hamster. Presence of a swollen sperm head in the cytoplasm of the ovum is evidence of successful penetration. The implication is made that there is good sperm fertilizing ability. However, there is a controversy over the prognostic value of this test. Also called hamster egg assay, hamster egg test.

stem cell a. A laboratory test to measure the sensitivity of tumor cells to various chemotherapeutic agents. It measures the number of colonies of tumor cells formed in cell cultures treated with various dilutions of drugs, much like antibiotic sensitivities are determined for bacteria. It has not proven of great practical use and serves primarily as a general guide to therapy in individual patients. It has provided insights into tumor cell heterogeneity in drug resistance. Also called clonogenic assay.

Weisenthal DiSC a. Assay in which the specimen to be tested contains the total cell population (i.e., both dividing and nondividing cells); the specimen is examined after 4 days of exposure to the test drugs for damage to the total cell population.

assessment (ă-ses'ment) Evaluation.

child abuse a. (1) Determination of the validity of a reported case of suspected child abuse or neglect through investigatory interviews with persons involved. (2) Determination of the treatment potential and treatment plan for confirmed cases of child abuse.

assignment (ă-sīn'ment) The act of designating or characterizing.

sex a. The act of designating as male or female a newborn infant born with ambiguity of the genitalia.

asthenospermia (as-the-no-sper'me-ă) Reduced motility of spermatozoa; one of the causes of infertility.

asthma (az'mă) A reversible respiratory condition marked by recurrent airflow obstruction, causing intermittent cough with phlegm production. Severe asthma is associated with increased rates of perinatal morbidity and mortality due to alkalosis, hypoxemia, reduced blood flow to the uterus, and birth defects caused by drugs used for treatment. When the term is used alone, it usually denotes allergic asthma.

allergic a. Recurrent acute narrowing of the large and small air passages within the lungs (bronchi and bronchioles), resulting in difficult breathing, intermittent wheezing, and coughing; due to spasm of bronchial smooth muscle, swelling of mucous membranes, and overproduction of thick sticky mucus. Often simply called asthma.

bronchial a. See allergic asthma.

asymptomatic (a-simp-to-mat'ik) Without symptoms (i.e., without indications of disease that are usually noticed by the patient).

asynclitism (ă-sin'klĭ-tizm) A situation during childbirth in which the sagittal suture of the fetal head is tilted either anteriorly or posteriorly, instead of being aligned with the pelvic planes of the mother.

> **anterior a.** Deflection of the fetal head posteriorly; the sagittal suture approaches the maternal sacral promontory and the anterior parietal bone presents itself to the examining fingers. Also called anterior parietal presentation. Formerly called Nägele's obliquity.

> **posterior a.** Deflection of the fetal head anteriorly; the sagittal suture lies close to the maternal symphysis and the posterior parietal bone presents itself to the examining fingers. Also called posterior parietal presentation. Formerly called Litzmann's obliquity.

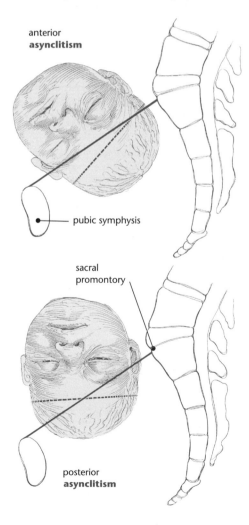

anterior
asynclitism

pubic symphysis

sacral
promontory

posterior
asynclitism

asystole (a-sis'to-le) Absence of the heartbeat; cardiac arrest.

atelectasis (at-e-lek'ta-sis) A shrunken and airless state of a lung, or of a portion of it; may be caused by obstruction of the air passages or by escape of air from the lung through a puncture of its covering membrane (the pleura).

> **primary a.** Failure of the lungs to expand and establish respiration immediately after birth; may be due to fetal oxygen deficiency, prematurity, excessive intrapulmonary secretions, or pneumonia. Lack of surfactant, especially in premature infants, is a prime cause.

> **secondary a.** Collapse of the lungs occurring at any age but seen most commonly in newborn infants suffering from respiratory distress syndrome; may also occur in patients recovering from abdominal surgery.

ateliosis (ă-te-le-o'sis) Incomplete development.

ateliotic (ă-te-le-ot'ik) Incompletely developed.

atenolol (ă-ten'o-lŏl) A beta-adrenergic blocking compound commonly used to treat high blood pressure and chest pain due to impaired blood supply to the heart muscle (angina pectoris). Intrauterine exposure causes neonatal low blood pressure and an abnormally slow heartbeat (bradycardia).

athymia (ă-thim'e-ă) Absence of the thymus gland.

atlantoaxial (at-lan-to-ak'se-al) Relating to the first and second cervical vertebrae (atlas and axis).

atlanto-occipital (at-lan'to ok-sip'ĭ-tal) Relating to the first cervical vertebra (atlas) and the occipital bone (of the skull).

atlanto-odontoid (at-lan'to o-don'toid) Relating to the first cervical vertebra (atlas) and the central articulating process (dens) of the second cervical vertebra (axis).

atlas (at'las) The first cervical vertebra; located next to the skull; articulates with the occipital bone above and the second cervical vertebra (axis) below.

atocia (ă-to'se-ă) Sterility in the female.

atonia (ă -to'ne-ă) See atony.

atonic (ă-ton'ik) Devoid of normal strength; applied to a muscle.

atony (at'o-ne) Lack of tone or tension; flaccidity. Also called atonia.

atopic (ă-top'ik) Relating to atopy.

atresia (ă-tre'ze-ă) Absence of a body opening or canal resulting from failure of development during fetal life. Most require, and are usually corrected by, early surgical intervention.

> **anal a.** See imperforate anus, under anus.

biliary a. Absence of one or more bile ducts; the most common cause of jaundice of newborn infants; believed to be caused by an intrauterine infection.

cervical a. Absence of the cervical canal (i.e., the channel communicating the interiors of the uterus and vagina).

duodenal a. Atresia of the duodenum, usually involving the distal portion; may be diagnosed prenatally by demonstration of the double-bubble sign, which indicates distention of the stomach and the proximal portion of the duodenum. See also double-bubble sign, under sign.

esophageal a. Lack of continuity of the esophagus, usually associated with an abnormal opening into the trachea.

gastrointestinal a. A rare anomaly in which the lumen in one or more portions of the alimentary canal is closed.

pulmonary a. Congenital narrowing of the opening between the pulmonary trunk and the right ventricle of the heart; marked by reduced blood flow to the lungs, heart enlargement, and atrophy of the right ventricle; usually accompanied by cardiovascular anomalies, especially tetralogy of Fallot and transposition of the great vessels.

tricuspid a. A developmental defect characterized by the absence, or fusion, of the tricuspid valve leaflets; associated with patency of the oval foramen, ventricular septal defect, underdevelopment of the right ventricle, and enlargement of the left ventricle.

atretic (ă-tret'ik) Relating to atresia.

atria (a'tre-ă) Plural of atrium.

atrial (a'tre-al) Relating to an atrium or atria.

atrioseptopexy (ă-tre-o-sep-to-pek'se) Surgical closure of an abnormal opening between the two atria of the heart.

atriotomy (a-tre-ot'o-me) A surgical cut into an atrium of the heart.

atrioventricular (a-tre-o-ven-trik'u-lar) (A-V) Relating to the atria and ventricles of the heart.

atrium (a'tre-um) **1.** Any anatomic chamber that opens into another space or structure. **2.** Either one of two (right and left) upper chambers of the heart that receive blood from the body tissues; the right atrium receives deoxygenated blood through the vena cavae, the left atrium receives oxygenated blood through the pulmonary veins; blood passes to each corresponding ventricle through atrioventricular heart valves, the tricuspid on the right side and the mitral on the left side of the heart.

atrophia (ă-tro'fe-ă) See atrophy.

atrophic (ă-trof'ik) Relating to atrophy.

atrophied (at'ro-fed) Wasted; shrunk.

atrophy (at'ro-fe) A decrease in the size of any tissue or part of the body resulting from a reduction either in the size of individual cells or in the number of cells composing the tissue or part. Also called atrophia.

acute yellow a. See acute fatty liver of pregnancy, under liver.

infantile muscular a. See Werdnig-Hoffmann disease, under disease.

infantile progressive spinal muscular a. See Werdnig-Hoffmann disease, under disease.

atropine (at'ro-pēn) An alkaloid derived from *Atropa belladonna* or produced synthetically; used systemically to produce relaxation of smooth muscles, and locally in the eye to dilate the pupil.

attack (ă-tak') The sudden onset of a process.

heart a. Popular term for describing an episode affecting the heart, especially a myocardial infarction. See under infarction.

panic a. A sudden episode of an overwhelming sense of impending doom, occurring unexpectedly and for no apparent reason, and accompanied by a variety of physical symptoms (e.g., rapid heartbeat, fast breathing, gasping for air); it often includes sweating, weakness, and feelings of unreality.

attitude (at'ĭ-tōod) **1.** Posture; the relative position of the body as a whole. **2.** A tendency to react in a particular way toward other people, institutions, or issues.

fetal a. The characteristic posture of the fetus within the uterus in the later months of pregnancy, generally with the head flexed and chin almost touching the chest, thighs flexed toward the abdomen, and legs bent at the knees. Also called fetal posture; fetal habitus. See also lie; position; presentation.

military a. See bregma presentation, under presentation.

atypia (a-tip'e-ă) The condition of not being typical; different.

atypical (a-tip'ĭ-kal) Differing from the usual.

auri- Combining form meaning the ear.

auscultate (aws'kul-tāt) To examine the chest or abdomen by listening to sounds made by the underlying organs.

auscultation (aws-kul-ta'shun) The act of listening to sounds made by a patient's organs as an aid to diagnosis.

auscultatory (aws-kul'tă-to-re) Relating to auscultation.

autakoid (aw'tă-koid) Any substance that produces some type of local effect on the body's biochemical and physiologic activities (e.g., prostaglandins, endothelins, serotonin).

auto-, aut- Prefixes meaning self.

autoantibody (aw-to-an'tĭ-bod-e) An antibody that is formed in response to, and reacts with, a tissue component (antigen) of the same person or animal.

autoantigen (aw-to-an'tĭ-jen) A tisssue component that triggers the formation of autoantibodies within the same individual.

autochthonous (aw-tok'tho-nus) Found at the site of origin.

autoerotism (aw-to-er'o-tizm) Self-arousal and self-gratification of sexual desire.

autoimmunity (aw-to-ĭ-mu'nĭ-te) Condition in which a person's immune system subjects that person's own tissues to injurious action; the basis of autoimmune disease.

autonomic (aw-to-nom'ik) Relating to the autonomic nervous system.

autosomal (aw-to-so'mal) Located on, or transmitted by, an autosome.

autosome (aw'to-sōm) Any chromosome that is not a sex chromosome. Autosomes normally occur in pairs in all cell nuclei except in the nuclei of the two sex cells or gametes (ovum and sperm), where they occur singly.

autotransfusion (aw-to-trans-fu'zhun) Transfusion of the patient's own blood or blood products.

avascular (ă-vas'ku-lar) Without blood supply.

axilla (ak-sil'ă) The pyramidal area at the junction of the arm and the chest; it contains the axillary blood and lymph vessels, a large number of lymph nodes, brachial plexus, and muscles. Commonly called armpit.

axillary (ak'sĭ-lar-e) Relating to the axilla.

axis (ak'sis), pl. axes **1.** A line, real or imaginary, used as a point of reference and about which a body or body part may rotate. **2.** The second cervical vertebra. **3.** Any centrally located anatomic structure.

> **long a.** A line passing lengthwise through the center of a structure.

> **pelvic a.** A hypothetical curved line passing through the center point of each of the four planes of the pelvis.

azathioprine (ă-za-thi'o-prēn) A compound used primarily to suppress the action of the immune system in order to prevent rejection of a transplant or to treat an autoimmune disorder, such as rheumatoid arthritis, in which the immune system attacks the body's own tissues; also used to treat inflammatory bowel disease. The drug has been found to interfere with the effectiveness of intrauterine contraceptive devices. Complications during pregnancy include increased incidence of urinary tract infections.

azithromycin (az-ith-ro-mi'sin) An antibiotic, erythromycin analog, effective against genital and ocular *Chlamydia trachomatis* infection.

azoospermia (a-zo-o-sper'me-ă) Absence of spermatozoa in the semen; a cause of male sterility.

azygos (az'ĭ-gos) An unpaired body structure (e.g., the azygos vein).

azygous (az'ĭ-gus) Unpaired.

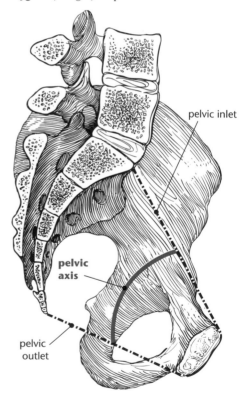

pelvic inlet

pelvic axis

pelvic outlet

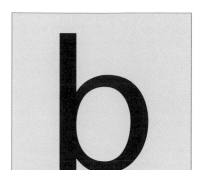

baby (ba´be) An infant.

   blue b. An infant born with a bluish
(cyanotic) tint of the skin due to inadequate
supply of oxygen in the blood; caused by a
developmental defect, either an abnormal
opening within the heart or transposition of
the main arteries leaving the heart. The defect
allows mixing of arterial and venous blood;
some of the deoxygenated blood returning to
the right side of the heart is pumped directly
back into the general circulation instead of
first passing through the lungs to receive
oxygen.

   blueberry muffin b. The occurrence of
yellowish and purple patches on the skin of a
newborn; it may be the result of an
intrauterine viral infection transmitted from
the mother through the placenta.

   collodion b. A newborn infant with a thick,
shiny, membranous skin that cracks and peels.
The condition may disappear completely or
may evolve into congenital ichthyosis,
especially lamellar ichthyosis, or it may cause
death of the infant.

   test-tube b. Popular term for an infant
born from an egg fertilized *in vitro* (in a Petri
dish) and then implanted in the mother's
uterus.

baby blues See postpartum depression, under
depresssion.

babygram (ba´be-gram) An x-ray film that
includes the chest and abdomen of a newborn
baby.

Bacillus (bă-sil´us) A genus of rod-shaped,
aerobic, Gram-positive bacteria (family
Bacillaceae); found usually in soil; some species
cause disease.

bacillus (bă-sil´us), pl. bacilli **1.** General term for
any microorganism of the genus *Bacillus*. **2.** Term
used to denote any rod-shaped bacterium.

   Calmette-Guérin b. An attenuated strain of
the bacterium *Mycobacterium bovis,* used in the
preparation of the Bacille Calmette-Guerin
(BCG) vaccine.

   Döderlein's b. A bacterium occurring in
normal vaginal secretions; believed to be
identical to *Lactobacillus acidophilus.*

   Ducrey's b. See *Haemophilus ducreyi,* under
Haemophilus.

   gas b. See *Clostridium perfringens,* under
Clostridium.

   Welch's b. See *Clostridium perfringens,* under
Clostridium.

backache (bak´āk) Pain in the back, especially the
lower (lumbosacral) portion.

backbone (bak´bōn) **1.** See vertebral column,
under column. **2.** Atoms in a polymer that are
common to all its molecules. **3.** The main chain
of a polypeptide.

backscatter (bak´skat-er) In radiology, radiation
deflected more than 90° from the main beam of
radiation.

bacteremia (bak-ter-e´me-ă) The presence of
viable bacteria in the bloodstream.

   MAC b. See *Mycobacterium avium* complex
bacteremia.

   ***Mycobacterium avium* complex b.**
Disseminated infection of the blood with a
complex of bacteria that includes several
strains of *Mycobacterium avium* and the closely
related *Mycobacterium intracellulare;* it occurs as
a common complication of advanced HIV
infection, frequently as a patient's first AIDS-
defining opportunistic disease, and causing a
significantly increased incidence of fatigue,
weight loss, fever, diarrhea, anemia, and a
shortened life span. Also called MAC
bacteremia.

bacteria (bak-te´re-ă) Plural of bacterium.

bacterial (bak-te´re-al) Relating to bacteria.

bactericidal (bak-tēr-ĭ-si´dal) Capable of
destroying bacteria.

bactericide (bak-tēr´ĭ-sīd) An agent that kills
bacteria.

bacteriology (bak-te-re-ol´o-je) The branch of
microbiology concerned with the study of
bacteria, especially in relation to medicine and
agriculture.

bacterium (bak-te´re-um), pl. bacteria Any of
several unicellular organisms of the plant
kingdom, existing as free-living organisms or as
parasites, multiplying by cell division, and having
a wide range of biochemical (including
pathogenic) properties. They may be rod-shaped
(bacilli), spherical (cocci), spiral-shaped
(spirilla), or comma-shaped (vibrios).

bacteriuria (bak-te-re-u´re-ă) The presence of

bacteria in the urine.

asymptomatic b. The presence of persistent, actively multiplying bacteria within the urinary tract without producing symptoms. Also called covert bacteriuria.

covert b. See asymptomatic bacteriuria.

Bacteroides (bak-ter-oi´dēz) A genus of bacteria (family Bacteroidaceae) composed of Gram-negative, mostly nonmotile, anaerobic organisms which may normally inhabit the oral cavity and intestinal tract of humans and animals. Some species are pathogenic, constituting an important source of infection in patients with damaged tissues and weakened immune systems.

B. fragilis A species causing urinary tract infections; also found in puerperal infections, such as pelvic abscesses, cesarean section wound infections, and septic pelvic thrombophlebitis.

bag (bag) A sac or pouch.

b. of waters Popular name for the amniochorion.

balance (bal´ans) **1.** A state of body stability achieved by the harmonious functional performance of its parts. **2.** The measured relationship between the body's input and output of a substance.

acid–base b. The normal ratio of acid and base elements in blood plasma, expressed in the hydrogen ion concentration or pH. Also called acid–base equilibrium.

fluid b. State of the body in relation to the intake and loss of water and electrolytes. Also called water balance.

thromboxane/prostacyclin b. Balance between the production of thromboxane A_2 (inducer of platelet aggregation and constrictor of blood vessels) and prostacyclin (inhibitor of platelet aggregation). After delivery of a baby, the maternal balance may possibly shift toward a thromboxane A_2 dominance.

water b. See fluid balance.

balloon (bă-lōon´) **1.** An inflatable, nonporous device that can be inserted in a body cavity or tube to provide support, to maintain a catheter in place, or to increase the lumen of the tubular structure. **2.** To expand a cavity with air to facilitate its examination. **3.** To distend an organ or vessel with gas or fluid.

balloonseptostomy (bă-lōon-sep-tos´to-me) The surgical creation of an opening in the wall between the two atria of the heart by catheterization and passing of an inflated balloon through the foramen ovale; used in the surgical treatment of transposition of the great vessels

and in atresia of the tricuspid (right atrioventricular) valve.

ballottement (bă-lot´ment) A method of physical examination to determine the size and mobility of an organ or mass in the body, especially one surrounded by fluid; the mass is pushed so as to rebound against the wall of the fluid-filled space. In obstetrics, the maneuver is used to palpate the fetus in the amniotic sac.

band (band) **1.** Any ribbon-shaped anatomic structure. **2.** Any device used to encircle a body structure or connect one structure with another.

amniotic b.'s Abnormal strands of tissue that sometimes develop between the fetus and the sac (amniochorion) containing the fetus, believed by some to cause fetal deformities.

chromosome b. A portion of a chromosome distinguishable from adjacent segments by a difference in staining intensity.

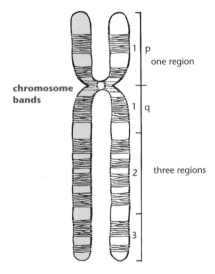

chromosome bands

one region

three regions

omphalomesenteric b. An abnormal persistent band from the intestine to the navel, representing a remnant of the embryonic omphalomesenteric (vitelline) duct that failed to obliterate; it occasionally results in small bowel obstruction when intestines loop around it.

silastic b. See Falope ring, under ring.

banding (band´ing) The staining of chromosomes to make visible their characteristic cross bands, thus allowing identification of each chromosome in a cell. The bands are consistent for all like chromosomes of an individual.

C b., centromeric b. Banding by heating preparations in saline solution to temperatures just below boiling and staining with Giemsa stain; useful for staining material near centromeres.

chromosome b. See banding.

G b., Giemsa b. Banding by incubating preparations in saline solution and staining with Giemsa stain; it is the most commonly used technique.

NOR (nucleolar organization region) b. Banding with a silver stain, useful for staining satellites and stalks of acrocentric chromosomes.

Q b., quinacrine b. Banding with quinacrine fluorescent stain.

R b., reverse b. Banding by incubating preparations in buffer solution at high temperatures and staining with Giemsa stain.

bank (bank) A place for collecting and storing certain donated organs, tissues, or cells in a viable condition, and for future use.

blood b. A place where blood is collected and typed for use in transfusions.

sperm b. A place where sperm is preserved in a frozen state and stored for future use in artificial insemination. Liquid nitrogen at 196°C is used to arrest molecular movement and preserve the cell vitality.

barbiturate (bar-bit´u-rāt) Any derivative of barbituric acid (e.g., phenobarbital, amobarbital, pentobarbital, secobarbital, and thiopental) that acts as an anesthetic and depressant of the central nervous system; used primarily for sedation or the treatment of convulsive disorders. Some have a potential for abuse.

barium (bar´e-um) A silvery-white metallic element; symbol Ba, atomic number 56, atomic weight 137.34.

baro- Combining form meaning pressure; weight.

baroceptor (bar-o-sep´tor) See baroreceptor.

baroreceptor (bar-o-re-sep´tor) A sensory-nerve terminal that is stimulated by increased blood pressure within an artery. Also called baroceptor; pressoreceptor.

barrel (bar´el) A cylinder or hollow shaft.

vaginal b. The vaginal cavity extending from the uterus to the vulva.

barren (bar´en) Popular term for sterile; unable to produce offspring.

barrier (bar´e-er) An obstruction or obstacle.

blood–air b. The thin layer of tissues in the lung that separates capillary blood from alveolar air, and through which exchange of gases occurs; composed of endothelium (lining the capillaries), basal membrane, and alveolar epithelium.

blood–brain b. (BBB) The tight junction between endothelial cells of capillary walls that normally permits only a limited exchange between blood in the capillaries on the one hand and cerebrospinal fluid and extracellular fluid in the brain on the other.

blood–testis b. The tight junction between Sertoli cells of the seminiferous tubules that prevents substances in the circulating blood from entering the lumen of the tubules, where the spermatozoa are developing.

incest b. In psychoanalysis, the learning of parental and social prohibitions against incest.

placental b. The semipermeable epithelial layer of the placenta separating maternal and fetal blood.

bartholinitis (bar-tho-lin-i´tis) Inflammation of the Bartholin's (greater vestibular) glands.

base (bās) **1.** A supporting part of a structure. **2.** The principal ingredient of a mixture. **3.** A hydrogen ion acceptor; a substance that turns litmus indicators blue and combines with an acid to form a salt. **4.** The area opposite the apex (e.g., the base of the heart). **5.** In molecular genetics, the chemical units: adenine, guanine, thymine, uracil, and cytosine, or their derivatives, as they occur bound to sugars in DNA and RNA molecules.

delta b. A calculated number that serves as a measure of the change in buffering capacity of bicarbonate in the blood.

basial (ba´se-al) Relating to the basion.

basicranial (ba-sĭ-kra´ne-al) Relating to the base of the skull.

basion (ba´se-on) A craniometric landmark; the middle point on the anterior margin of the foramen magnum, the large opening at the base of the skull.

baso-, basio-, basi- Combining forms meaning base.

basophil (ba´so-fil) A cell, especially a white blood cell, containing large granules that stain readily with basic dyes.

bath (bath) Any fluid in which the body, or any of its parts, is immersed for therapeutic or cleansing purposes.

douche b. The local application of a stream of water.

sitz b. Immersion of only the hips and buttocks in a tub of water.

battery (bat´er-e) The touching of one person by another without the consent of the person touched; intent to cause harm is not required. In medical malpractice, surgical operations are most commonly cited (e.g., removal of two ovaries when permission was obtained for removal of one only).

sexual b. See rape.

bearing down (bar´ing down) The expulsive effort made by a woman during the second stage of labor.

beat (bēt) 1. A pulsation (e.g., of the heart or an artery). 2. To pulsate.

becquerel (bek´rel) (Bq) The unit of radioactivity in the International System of Units (SI), equal to one disintegration per second. It replaces the curie.

belly (bel´e) 1. The abdomen. 2. The fleshy part of a muscle.

belly button (bel´e but´on) Umbilicus; navel.

benign (be-nīn´) Essentially harmless; regarding a tumor, one that neither invades adjacent tissues nor metastasizes to distant areas of the body.

benzthiazide (benz-thĭ´ă-zīd) A diuretic drug administered orally for the treatment of high blood pressure. It may have adverse effects on the pregnant woman and her child, including inhibition of labor and, if taken during the first trimester, increased risk of congenital defects.

bestiality (bes-te-al´ĭ-te) Sexual activities between a human and an animal.

beta-blocker (ba´tă blok´er) See beta-adrenergic blocking agent, under agent.

beta-fetoprotein (ba´tă fe-to-pro´tēn) A liver protein normally found in the fetus; it has been found in adults with liver disease. See also alphafetoprotein.

betamethasone (ba´tă-meth´ă-sōn) A potent anti-inflammatory glucocorticoid agent administered orally or as a topical application to the skin. Adverse effects of topical application include thinning of the skin; oral administration is associated with more serious adverse effects common to all steroids (e.g., enhanced susceptibility to infections, fluid retention, and high blood pressure).

bethanechol chloride (bě-than´ě-kol klor´īd) A parasympathomimetic drug used in the treatment of constipation, paralytic ileus, and urinary retention.

bi-, bin- Prefix meaning two; twice.

bicarbonate (bi-kar´bo-nāt) The ion HCO_3^- or any of its salts.

    standard b. The portion of bicarbonate in plasma that is derived from nonrespiratory sources; it is the bicarbonate concentration in the plasma of a whole blood sample that has been equilibrated at a 37°C temperature with a carbon dioxide pressure of 40 mm Hg. Metabolic alkalosis and acidosis are reflected in abnormally high or low levels, respectively.

bicornate, bicornuate (bi-kor´nāt, bi-kor´nu-āt) Having two horn-shaped parts.

bifid (bi´fid) Separated into two parts (e.g., a bifid uterus).

bigeminal (bi-jem´ĭ-nal) Paired; double.

bigeminy (bi-jem´ĭ-ne) Occurring in pairs, especially two heart beats occurring in rapid succession followed by a pause before the next two beats.

bigerminal (bi-jer´mĭ-nal) Relating to two ova.

bilateral (bi-lat´er-al) Having two sides.

bilirubin (bil-ĭ-roo´bin) An orange-red bile pigment formed from the normal breakdown of the red blood cell pigment (hemoglobin). Accumulation of bilirubin in the blood and tissues causes jaundice (e.g., in liver disease or in excessive destruction of red blood cells).

bilirubinuria (bil-ĭ-roo-bĭ-nu´re-ă) The presence of bilirubin in the urine.

bimanual (bi-man´u-al) Performed with both hands (e.g., bimanual palpation).

binder (bīnd´dr) A broad bandage.

    abdominal b. A binder placed around a lax and pendulous abdomen to support and maintain the enlarging pregnant uterus in an approximately normal position.

bio- Combining form meaning life.

bioassay (bi-o-as´a) The evaluation of a substance (e.g., a hormone or a vitamin) by comparing its effects on a living organism, or an *in vitro* organ preparation, with those of a standard preparation. Also called biological assay. See also biological monitoring, under monitoring.

bioengineering (bi-o-en-jin-er´ing) See biomedical engineering, under engineering.

biofeedback (bi-o-fēd´bak) A technique for training a person to exercise some control over a normally involuntary body function (e.g., blood pressure), or a voluntary muscular activity (e.g., to improve control over the anal sphincter mechanism in cases of anal incontinence). The patient is connected to a recording instrument, from which she receives information regarding fluctuations in the body function (feedback), and through which she endeavors to control the function.

biological, biologic (bi-o-loj´ě-kal, bi-o-loj´ik) Relating to biology.

biology (bi-ol´ŏ-je) The science concerned with living organisms.

bionosis (bi-o-no´sis) Any disease caused by a living organism.

biopsy (bi´op-se) (BX, Bx) 1. Diagnostic procedure in which cells or tissues from the living body are removed for gross and microscopic examination. 2. A popular name for the specimen itself.

    aspiration b. See needle biopsy.

    brush b. Removal of cells with a brush-

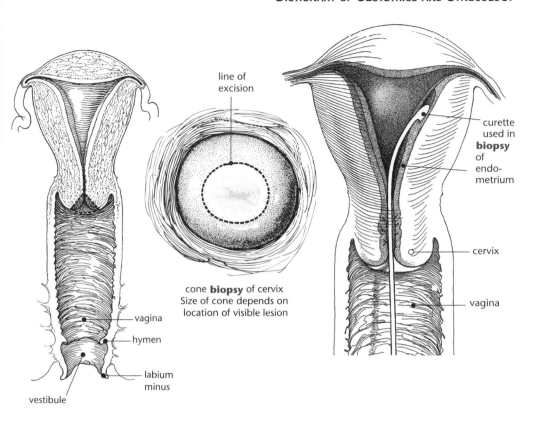

line of
excision

curette
used in
biopsy
of
endo-
metrium

cervix

vagina

cone **biopsy** of cervix
Size of cone depends on
location of visible lesion

vagina

hymen

labium
minus

vestibule

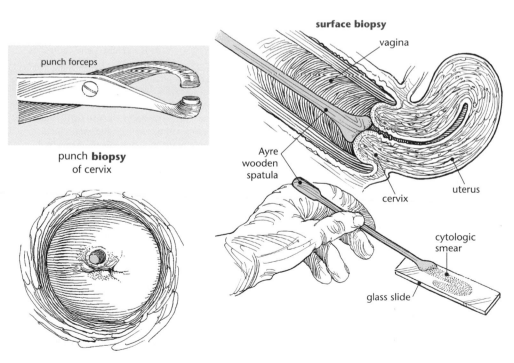

surface biopsy

vagina

punch forceps

punch **biopsy**
of cervix

Ayre
wooden
spatula

uterus

cervix

cytologic
smear

glass slide

tipped instrument; the cells of interest are entrapped in the bristles by manipulating the instrument against the suspected area of disease (e.g., within a ureter).

endoscopic b. Biopsy performed with a viewing instrument (endoscope) equipped with an attachment, either a forceps or a brush, for removing tissue or cells, respectively, from the lining of a hollow organ (e.g., the stomach, esophagus, or colon).

excisional b. The removal of an entire lesion (e.g., a lump) and a margin of surrounding normal tissue for gross and microscopic examination.

needle b. Biopsy performed with a needle attached to a syringe and inserted through the skin into the target tissue; the specimen is sucked out through the needle. Also called aspiration biopsy.

open b. Biopsy carried out during a surgical operation so that the organ may be visualized at the time of biopsy; performed when there is a need to avoid dangerously close structures, to ascertain proper sampling, or to avoid undue bleeding.

punch b. Removal of a plug of tissue by pressing down and twisting a special cutting instrument with a cylindrical sharp end. Also called trephine biopsy.

shave b. Biopsy in which a scalpel is used to cut through the base of an elevated lesion in one smooth motion.

surface b. The scraping of tissue from a surface as from the opening of the uterine cervix for the detection of cancer.

timed endometrial b. In artificial insemination, a biopsy of the endometrium performed approximately in mid-cycle (at the time of ovulation) to determine whether the endometrium is in its secretory phase, capable of participating in implantation of the fertilized egg. Also called timed uterine-wall biopsy.

timed uterine-wall b. See timed endometrial biopsy.

trephine b. See punch biopsy.

wedge b. Excision of a triangular specimen.

biorhythm (bi´o-rithm) A biologically determined cyclic occurrence in an organism (e.g., the sleep cycle).

biosensor (bi-o-sen´sor) Any of several probes for measuring the presence and concentration of molecules, cells, and microorganisms; they translate a biochemical interaction at the probe surface into a quantifiable physical signal (e.g., a change in temperature).

biostatistics (bi-o-stă-tis´tiks) The application of statistical methods to the analysis and interpretation of biological and medical phenomena.

biosynthesis (bi-o-sin´thĕ-sis) The formation of chemical compounds by and within living organisms.

biotechnology (bi-o-tek-nol´ŏ-je) The research and development concerned with the use of organisms, cells, or cell-derived constituents to develop products that are technically, scientifically, and clinically useful. The chief focus of biotechnology is the DNA molecule and the alteration of biologic function at the molecular level. Its laboratory methods include transfection and cloning techniques; sequence and structure analysis algorithms; computer databases; and function, analysis, and prediction of gene and protein structure. See also biomedical engineering and genetic engineering, under engineering; recombinant DNA, under DNA.

biotelemetry (bi-o-tel-em´ĕ-tre) The recording and measuring of vital processes of an individual located at a place remote from the measuring device; the data are transmitted without wires.

biotic (bi-ot´ik) Relating to life.

biotin (bi´o-tin) A growth factor present in minute quantities in every living cell; it is relatively abundant in such organs as the liver, kidney, and pancreas; also found in yeast and milk.

biparietal (bi-pă-ri´e-tal) Relating to both parietal bones of the skull.

biparous (bip´ă-rus) Having borne twins.

bipolar (bi-po´lar) Having two poles or extremes.

birth (birth) The act of being born.

live b. The complete expulsion or extraction of a fetus from the mother, regardless of the duration of pregnancy, which, after such separation, breathes or shows other evidence of life (e.g., pulsation of the umbilical cord, beating of the heart, and definite movements of involuntary muscles) regardless of whether the umbilical cord has been cut or the placenta has detached.

premature b. The birth of an infant after 20 weeks of gestation but before full term is achieved.

birthmark (birth´mark) Popular name for any area of discolored skin or growth present at birth (e.g., a nevus).

bis- Prefix meaning twice; double.

bisexual (bi-sek´shoo-al) An individual who has sexual interests in both males and females. Also called ambisexual.

bis in die (bis in de´a) (b.i.d.) Latin for twice a day.

bitemporal (bi-tem´po-ral) Relating to both temples or temporal bones.

bivalent (bi-va´lent) **1.** Having the combining power of two hydrogen atoms. **2.** In cytogenetics, composed of two homologous chromosomes.

bladder (blad´der) A distendable musculomembranous sac serving as a receptacle for a fluid. When used alone, the term designates the urinary bladder.

    atonic b. A flaccid, distended bladder that is unable to contract, usually due to paralysis of the motor nerves innervating it.

    Christmas tree b. The characteristic appearance of a spastic bladder, caused by lesions of the upper motor nerve supply of the bladder (at the 12th thoracic or 1st lumbar level).

    ileal b. See ileal conduit, under conduit.

    nervous b. Popular term for a functional bladder condition in which a person has a constant desire to urinate but is unable to empty the bladder completely.

    neurogenic b. Any disturbance of bladder function originating from an impaired nerve supply to the bladder, caused either by lesions of the spinal cord or of the nerves themselves.

    urinary b. The reservoir for urine located in the anterior area of the pelvic cavity. It receives urine from the kidneys via the ureters and discharges it through the urethra. Usually called the bladder.

-blast Suffix meaning immature; applied to cells (e.g., erythroblast).

blastema (blas-te´mă) In embryology, a group of cells from which develops an organ or part.

    metanephric b. In embryology, a caplike cellular mass located over the ampullar end of the ureteric bud and from which develop the excretory units of the kidney.

blasto- Combining form meaning early stage.

blastocele (blas´to-sēl) The fluid-filled cavity of a blastocyst.

blastocyst (blas´to-sist) The embryo at the time of implantation into the inner wall of the uterus. It consists of a single layer of outer cells (trophoblast), a fluid-filled cavity (blastocele), and a mass of inner cells (embryoblast). Also called blastodermic vesicle.

blastoma (blas-to´mă) Malignant tumor composed of embryonic, undifferentiated cells.

blastomere (blas´to-mēr) One of the cells into which the fertilized egg divides.

blastopore (blas´to-pōr) A small opening into the archenteron (primitive digestive cavity) of the embryo at the gastrula stage.

blastula (blas´tu-lă) Early stage in the development of an embryo consisting of a spherical structure formed by a single layer of cells that encloses a fluid-filled cavity.

blastulation (blas-tu-la´shun) Formation of a blastula.

bleb (bleb) A blister.

bleeder (bled´er) **1.** Popular name for a person whose integrity has been breached with

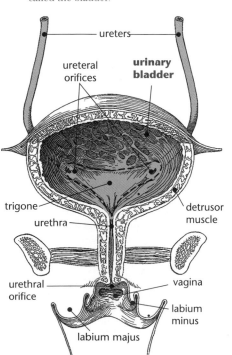

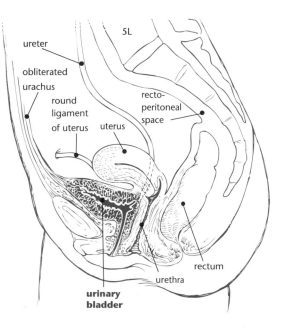

hemophilia or any other bleeding disorder. **2.** A blood vessel usually requiring surgical measures to achieve hemostasis.

bleeding (blēd´ing) The escape of blood.

abnormal uterine b. Any unusual bleeding from the uterus; may be caused by endocrine disturbances (dysfunctional bleeding), pregnancy, systemic disease, or cancer.

contact b. Bleeding occurring after sexual intercourse; may be caused by cervical cancer, eversion, polyps, or infection. Also called postcoital bleeding.

dysfunctional uterine b. (DUB) Bleeding from the uterus due to a disturbance of endocrine glands, when no pathologic uterine lesions are present.

implantation b. Slight uterine bleeding frequently occurring at the time of implantation of the fertilized ovum onto the uterine wall; caused by disruption of blood vessels at the implantation site.

intermenstrual b. See metrorrhagia.

occult b. Escape of blood in such minute amounts that it can only be detected by special tests.

postcoital b. See contact bleeding.

postmenopausal b. Uterine bleeding occurring after 12 months of absent menses; may be caused by disease (e.g., endometrial carcinoma).

withdrawal b. Bleeding from the uterus occurring when estrogen therapy is discontinued.

blennadenitis (blen-ad-ĕ-ni´tis) Inflammation of mucous glands.

blennorrhea (blen-no-re´ă) Any profuse discharge of secretions containing mucus, especially from the vagina or urethra.

inclusion b. See inclusion conjunctivitis, under conjunctivitis.

blennorrheal (blen-no-re´al) Relating to blennorrhea.

bleomycin (ble-o-mi´sin) An antibiotic produced by fermentation of a strain of *Streptomyces verticillus;* used as an antineoplastic in the form of bleomycin sulfate. May be contraindicated in the first trimester of pregnancy.

block (blok) **1.** An obstruction to passage. **2.** An interruption of nerve impulses.

atrioventricular b., A-V b. Impairment of the normal conduction of impulses between the atria and ventricles of the heart; classified in three degrees: *first degree,* conduction time is prolonged but all impulses from the atria reach the ventricles; *second degree,* some but not all atrial impulses fail to reach the ventricles,

therefore some ventricular beats are dropped; *third degree,* all atrial impulses are blocked.

caudal b. See caudal anesthesia, under anesthesia.

epidural b. See epidural anesthesia, under anesthesia.

heart b. See atrioventricular block.

lochia b. See lochiometra.

Mobitz type I b. A type of second-degree atrioventricular block in which a dropped beat occurs periodically after a series of increasingly prolonged P-R intervals.

Mobitz type II b. A type of second-degree atrioventricular block in which a dropped beat occurs periodically without previously prolonged P-R intervals.

paracervical b. See paracervical block anesthesia, under anesthesia.

pudendal nerve b. See pudendal anesthesia, under anesthesia.

spinal b. See spinal anesthesia, under anesthesia.

subarachnoid b. See spinal anesthesia (1), under anesthesia.

blocker (blok´er) See blocking agent, under agent.

calcium channel b. See calcium channel-blocking agent, under agent.

blood (blud) The fluid circulated through a closed circuit composed of the heart and blood vessels. It consists of a pale-yellow fluid (plasma) in which are suspended red blood cells (erythrocytes), white blood cells (leukocytes), and platelets.

arterial b. The relatively bright red blood that has been oxygenated in the lungs and is within the left chambers of the heart and the arteries.

cord b. Blood within the umbilical cord.

occult b. Blood present in amounts too small to be seen with the naked eye.

venous b. The dark red blood within the veins; it loses oxygen and gains carbon dioxide by passing through metabolically active tissues.

whole b. Donated blood that has not been separated into its components.

blood bank (blud bangk) See under bank.

blood count (blud kount) See under count.

blood group (blud grōōp) Any of various immunologically distinct and genetically determined classes of human blood, identified clinically by characteristic agglutination reactions. Blood groups are used in genetic, medicolegal, and anthropologic investigations. For individual blood groups, see specific names.

blood grouping (blud grōōp´ing) Classification of blood samples according to their agglutinating properties. Also called blood typing.

blood type (blud tīp) The specific reaction pattern of red blood cells of a person to the antisera of a blood group. See also blood group.

blood typing (blud ti´ping) See blood grouping.

bloody show (blud´e shō) Popular term for the vaginal discharge of blood-tinged mucus, indicating the onset of active labor; it represents expulsion of the mucus plug that has filled the cervical canal during pregnancy; the slight shedding of blood results from dilatation of the cervix with tearing of small blood vessels. A bloody show may also be caused by prior vaginal or rectal examination.

blotting (blot´ing) The process of transferring electrophoretically separated particles (such as proteins and DNA fragments) onto special filters, papers, or membranes for analysis. See also Northern, Southern, and Western blot analysis, under analysis.

   dot b., slot b. Blotting by placing a drop of the cell extract directly on filter paper, without using electrophoresis.

body (bod´e) **1.** The entire material structure of man and animal. **2.** The principal part of anything. **3.** Any small mass of material.

   acetone b.'s See ketone bodies.

   adipose b. of the cheek See sucking pad, under pad.

   Barr chromatin b., Barr b. See sex chromatin, under chromatin.

   Call-Exner b.'s Extracellular multilaminated bodies containing an accumulation of densely staining material; they are located among the granulosa cells in maturing ovarian follicles.

   Donovan b. See *Calymmatobacterium granulomatis*, under *Calymmatobacterium*.

   ketone b.'s Collective name for the end products of improper and excessive breakdown of stored fat in the liver. These substances are acetoacetic acid, acetone, and beta-hydroxybutyrate; they accumulate in the blood and spill over in the urine in such conditions as uncontrolled or undiagnosed diabetes and in severe starvation. Also called ketones.

   perineal b. A pyramidal mass of muscular and fibrous tissue located in the median plane of the perineum and, in the female, between the anal canal and the lower quarter of the vagina; in the male, between the anal canal and the membranous urethra and bulb of the penis. The perineal body provides attachment to the following muscles: bulbospongiosus, transverse perineal, levator ani, and external anal sphincter. Also called central tendon of perineum.

   polar b.'s The two normally nonfunctional cells formed in the ovum during its maturation. The *first polar b.* results from unequal division of the primary oocyte. The *second polar b.*, formed from unequal division of the secondary oocyte, occurs after the ovum is discharged from the ovary and fertilized.

   psammoma b.'s Spherical deposits of calcified material generally found in papillary cancer. Also called sand bodies.

   sex chromatin b. See sex chromatin, under chromatin.

   b. of uterus The upper two thirds of the uterus, above the constricted lower portion (isthmus).

   b. of vertebra The cylindrical anterior (ventral) portion of a vertebra, which is separated from the bodies of adjacent vertebrae by fibrocartilaginous pads (intervertebral discs).

   wolffian b. See mesonephros.

   X-chromatin b. See sex chromatin, under chromatin.

bomb (bom) An apparatus containing a radioactive material for therapeutic application to a circumscribed area of the body.

bombard (bom-bard´) To expose to a beam of ionizing radiation.

bonding (bond´ing) An emotional attachment to a person or a pet; especially the result of the process of attachment between two people, such as mother and child, whose identities are significantly affected by their mutual interaction; or the development of mutual attachment between mother and newborn during the sensitive period after birth, aided by visual and physical contact between the two.

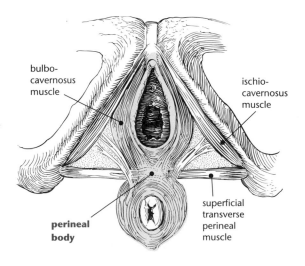

bulbo-cavernosus muscle

ischio-cavernosus muscle

superficial transverse perineal muscle

perineal body

bone (bōn) **1.** The special mineralized connective tissue forming the skeleton of vertebrates. **2.** Any of the units forming the skeleton.

    brittle b.'s See osteogenesis imperfecta, under osteogenesis.

    cancellous b. See spongy bone.

    collar b. See clavicle.

    compact b. A dense, ivory-like type forming the outer (cortical) layer of bones; it contains minute spaces and channels. Also called dense bone; cortical substance of bone; compact substance of bone.

    cranial b.'s The 21 bones forming the skull; the paired inferior nasal concha, lacrimal, maxilla, nasal, palatine, parietal, temporal, and zygomatic; and the unpaired ethmoid, frontal, occipital, sphetnoid, and vomer.

    dense b. See compact bone.

    flank b. See ilium.

    hip b. See hipbone.

    innominate b. See hipbone.

    pubic b. The anterior portion of the hipbone; it is surrounded by cartilage in early life and eventually ossifies, fusing with the ilium and ischium to form the hipbone; along with the ilium and ischium, it contributes to the formation of the acetabulum (the cup-shaped cavity into which the head of the femur fits to form the hip joint). Anteriorly, it articulates with the pubic bone of the opposite side by means of the pubic symphysis. Also called pubis. See also ilium; ischium; pelvis.

    spongy b. The inner portion of a bone, consisting of a meshwork of bony intercommunications separated by numerous spaces filled with vascular tissue, fat, and bone marrow. Spongy bone is surrounded by an outer layer of compact bone. Also called cancellous bone; spongy substance of bone.

bone marrow purging (bōn mar´o purj´ing) Elimination of subpopulations of cells (usually residual tumor cells) from bone marrow after it has been removed for transplantation; used in both autologous and allogeneic bone marrow transplantation.

borreliosis (bo-rel-e-o´sis) Any disease caused by bacteria of the genus *Borrelia*.

    Lyme b. See Lyme disease, under disease.

botryoid (bot´re-oid) Resembling a bunch of grapes.

bout (bout) An episode.

    periodic drinking b.'s A form of alcoholism in which the person overindulges in alcoholic drinks continuously for days or weeks, then recovers and abstains for several weeks or months before the next bout. Also called paroxysmal alcoholism.

bowel (bow´el) Common name for the intestine.

    large b. See large intestine, under intestine.

    small b. See small intestine, under intestine.

brachia (bra´ke-ă) Plural of brachium.

brachial (bra´ke-al) Relating to the arm.

brachialgia (bra-ke-al´je-ă) Pain in one or both arms. See also thoracic outlet syndrome, under syndrome.

brachio-, brachi- Combining forms meaning arm.

brachium (bra´ke-um), pl. brachia **1.** The arm. **2.** Any armlike structure.

brachy- Combining form meaning short.

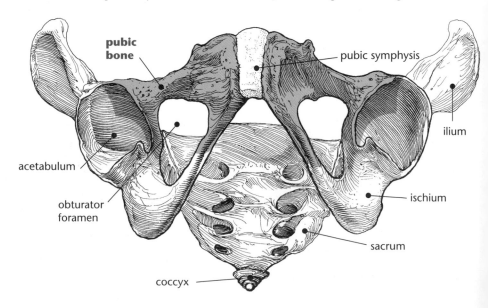

brachycephalic (brak-e-sĕ-fal´ik) Characterized by brachycephaly.

brachycephaly (brak-e-sef´ă-le) A disproportionate shortness and broadness of the head (i.e., an abnormally flattened anteroposterior plane of the skull); usually caused by a premature union of the coronal suture in infancy.

brachydactyly (brak-e-dak´tĭ-le) Abnormal shortness of the fingers and toes.

brachygnathia (brak-ig-na´the-ă) Abnormal shortness of the lower jaw (mandible).

brachymelia (brak-e-me´le-ă) Disproportionate shortness of the arms and legs.

brachysyndactyly (brak-e-sin-dak´tĭ-le) A combined shortness and webbing of fingers or toes.

brachytherapy (brak-e-ther´ă-pe) Treatment by local application of radiation in which a small sealed (or partly sealed) radiation source is placed directly on or near the tissues under treatment; may be a surface application, a body cavity application (intracavitary), or placement into the tissue (interstitial). Brachytherapy permits the use of high radiation doses to restricted tissue volumes (e.g., a small tumor with well-defined margins). Also called internal radiation therapy.

brady- Combining form meaning slow.

bradyarrhythmia (brad-e-ă-rith´me-ă) A slow and irregular heartbeat.

bradycardia (brad-e-kar´de-ă) Excessive slowness in the action of the heart (i.e., a heart rate below 60 beats per minute).

    fetal b. A baseline fetal heart rate under 120 beats per minute, lasting 15 minutes or longer. A rate of 80 to 100 beats per minute is considered moderate; a rate less than 80 beats per minute, lasting 3 minutes or longer, is considered severe.

bradycrotic (brad-e-krot´ik) Relating to a slow pulse.

bradypnea (brad-ip-ne´ă, brad-ip´ne-ă) Abnormally slow rate of breathing.

brain (brān) The portion of the central nervous system that is responsible for the coordination and control of all vital body activities; it is located within the skull, surrounded by cerebrospinal fluid, and composed of the forebrain (cerebrum and diencephalon), the midbrain (mesencephalon), and the hindbrain (cerebellum, pons, and medulla oblongata); it is continuous below with the spinal cord. The brain of the average adult weighs approximately 1.36 kg. Also called encephalon.

breach of duty In medical liability claims, a physician's violation of responsibilities owed to a patient to provide medical care within accepted standards of medical practice.

breast (brest) **1.** One of the two structures attached to the fascia covering the chest muscles. In the male, breasts are rudimentary; in the female, they are the organs of lactation. The adult female breast consists of fifteen to twenty glandular lobes and their ducts (the mammary gland proper, which secretes milk), fibrous tissue binding the glandular lobes, and fatty tissue in the spaces between the lobes; also present are blood vessels, nerves, and lymph vessels. Multiple fibrous bands pass forward to the skin and nipple, forming the Cooper's (suspensory) ligament for supporting the breast in its upright position. When distorted by a tumor, these bands cause dimpling of the skin surface. Also called mamma. See also mammary gland, under gland. **2.** The chest.

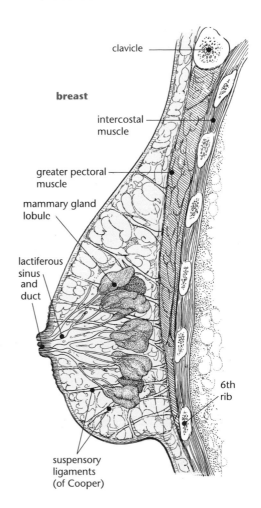

clavicle

breast

intercostal muscle

greater pectoral muscle

mammary gland lobule

lactiferous sinus and duct

6th rib

suspensory ligaments (of Cooper)

accessory b. See polymastia.

caked b.'s See breast engorgement, under engorgement.

secondary b. See polymastia.

supernumerary b. See polymastia.

breastbone (brest´bōn) See sternum.

breast-feeding (brest fēd´ing) The nursing of a baby at the mother's breast.

breathing (brēth´ing) The process of taking in and expelling air from the lungs to allow blood to take up oxygen and release carbon dioxide.

continuous positive pressure b. (CPPB) See continuous positive pressure ventilation, under ventilation.

intermittent positive pressure b. (IPPB) See intermittent positive pressure ventilation, under ventilation.

breech (brēch) The buttocks (nates). See also breech presentation, under presentation.

bregma (breg´mă) A craniometric landmark on the upper surface of the skull at the point where the sagittal and coronal sutures meet.

bregmatic (breg-mat´ik) Relating to the bregma.

bretylium (bre-til´e-um) An antiarrhythmic drug used in the treatment of ventricular fibrillation. When used during pregnancy, it may cause maternal hypotension with potential fetal risk from reduced blood flow.

brim (brim) The upper border of a hollow structure.

pelvic b. The circumference of the oblique plane dividing the major and minor pelves.

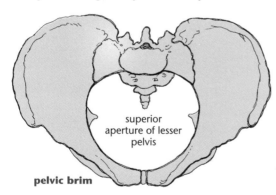

superior aperture of lesser pelvis

pelvic brim

broad-spectrum (brod spek´trum) Referring to antimicrobial drugs, effective against a wide variety of microorganisms.

bromide (bro´mīd) Any of a class of compounds containing bromine and another element or organic radical. Intrauterine exposure has a possible association with developmental malformations and diminished reflexes of the newborn.

bromocriptine (bro-mo-krip´tēn) An ergot derivative that suppresses secretion of the hormone prolactin from the adenohypophysis (anterior portion of the pituitary). Used in the treatment of conditions caused by excessive prolactin production, such as abnormal milk production (galactorrhea), formerly used for the suppression of puerperal lactation.

bronchi (brong´ki) Plural of bronchus.

bronchial (brong´ke-al) Relating to the bronchi.

bronchiectasis (brong-ke-ek´tă-sis) Persistent and irreversible dilatation and distortion of medium-sized bronchi.

bronchiole (brong´ke-ōl) One of the numerous small airways branching off the bronchi within the lungs. Also called bronchiolus.

terminal b. The last portion of a bronchiole, without the final outpouchings (alveoli).

bruxism (bruk´sizm) Forceful clenching and grinding of the teeth, especially during sleep; may be a manifestation of severe stress.

bubo (bu´bo) A swollen, inflamed lymph node, especially of the groin.

tropical b. See lymphogranuloma venereum.

venereal b. Bubo associated with a venereal disease.

bubonic (bu-bon´ik) Relating to swollen lymph nodes, especially of the groin (buboes).

bud (bud) In embryology, a small mass that has the potential for growth and differentiation.

bronchial b. One of several outgrowths from the embryonic lateral and stem bronchi that become the air passages within the lungs.

limb b. A swelling on the trunk of an embryo that gives rise to an arm or leg.

metanephric b. An outgrowth from the wolffian (mesonephric) duct that gives rise to the calyces and pelvis of the kidney, the straight collecting tubules, and the ureter. Also called ureteric bud.

ureteric b. See metanephric bud.

buffer (buf´er) **1.** Any substance that maintains the relative concentrations of hydrogen and hydroxyl ions in a solution by neutralizing added acid or alkali. **2.** To add a buffer to a solution.

buffering (buf´er-ing) The process by which hydrogen ion concentration is maintained constant.

bulb (bulb) An expanded or spherical structure or prosthesis.

Krause's end b. A sense organ situated at the end of some sensory nerve fibers; it responds to cold stimuli. Also called Krause's corpuscle.

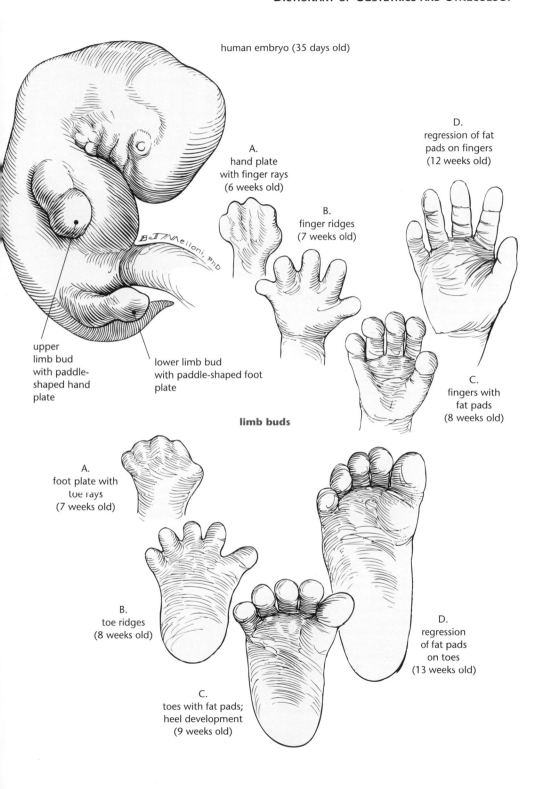

human embryo (35 days old)

upper
limb bud
with paddle-
shaped hand
plate

lower limb bud
with paddle-shaped foot
plate

limb buds

A.
hand plate
with finger rays
(6 weeks old)

B.
finger ridges
(7 weeks old)

C.
fingers with
fat pads
(8 weeks old)

D.
regression of fat
pads on fingers
(12 weeks old)

A.
foot plate with
toe rays
(7 weeks old)

B.
toe ridges
(8 weeks old)

C.
toes with fat pads;
heel development
(9 weeks old)

D.
regression
of fat pads
on toes
(13 weeks old)

sinovaginal b.'s In embryology, the paired sacculations of the female urogenital sinus that eventually develop into the lower part of the vagina.

b. of vestibule of vagina A structure composed of erectile tissue; it consists of two elongated masses, located on each side of the vaginal opening and connected by a band that enlarges at the midline to form the glans of the clitoris.

bulimia (bu-lim′e-ă) Eating disorder occurring chiefly in young women; characterized by binge–purge cycles, i.e., episodes of overeating (binges), generally beyond voluntary control, followed by efforts to avoid weight gain by induced vomiting, laxative or diuretic abuse (purge), excessive exercise, and fasting. Bulimics usually have normal body weight. Long-term effects may include tooth decay and constant sore throat. Eventual pathologic effects are the consequences of vomiting (tears and bleeding in the esophagus and associated inflammation of the lungs) and of laxative abuse (usually resulting in alkalosis and hypokalemia, the latter sometimes severe enough to precipitate heart problems). Commonly called binge-and-purge syndrome.

bulimic (bu-lim′ik) Relating to bulimia.

buphthalmos (bŭf-thal′mos) An uncommon congenital glaucoma occurring in both eyes of an infant; increased fluid and pressure within the eyeball produce a larger than normal eye with a milky, protruding cornea. Also called hydrophthalmos.

bursa (ber′să), pl. bursae A closed, flattened sac of synovial membrane containing a viscid fluid; usually present over bony prominences, between and beneath tendons, and between certain movable structures; it serves to facilitate movement by diminishing friction and by creating discontinuity between tissues, thus allowing complete freedom of movement.

omental b. See lesser sac of peritoneum, under sac.

ovarian b. A peritoneal recess between the medial surface of the ovary and the overlapping mesosalpinx.

busulfan (bu-sul′fan) An antitumor alkylating drug used in the treatment of ovarian cancer. Its use during pregnancy is associated with fetal malformations and low birth weight.

butterfly (but′er-fli) **1.** Any material or device in the shape of a butterfly (e.g., a piece of tape for approximating the edges of a wound, or a wad of absorbent material used in gynecologic surgery). **2.** A butterfly-shaped rash on the cheeks and across the nose, characteristic of lupus erythematosus.

buttocks (but′oks) The protuberances formed by the gluteus muscles.

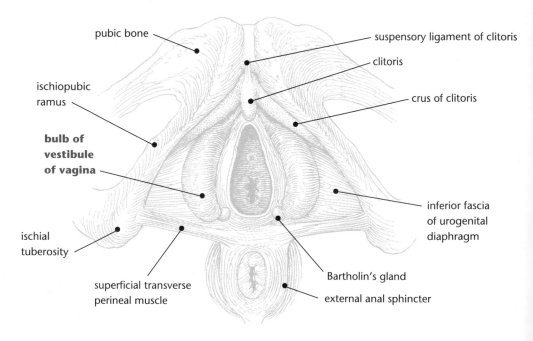

pubic bone

suspensory ligament of clitoris

clitoris

ischiopubic ramus

crus of clitoris

bulb of vestibule of vagina

inferior fascia of urogenital diaphragm

ischial tuberosity

superficial transverse perineal muscle

Bartholin's gland

external anal sphincter

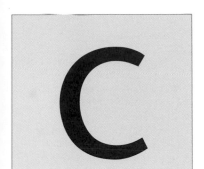

CA 15-3 An antigen often found in elevated levels in the serum of a high percentage of patients with metastatic cancer.

CA 19-9 An antigen often found in elevated levels in the serum of patients with ovarian mucinous cystadenocarcinomas, endometrial, tubal, and endocervical cancers, and in patients with metastatic pancreatic cancer. It is part of the Lewis blood group system.

CA 125 An antigen often found in elevated levels in the serum of patients with epithelial ovarian cancer, but can also be found in a variety of benign conditions such as endometriosis.

caffeine (kă-fēn') A bitter alkaloid compound present in various plants, e.g., tea *(Thea sinensis)*, coffee *(Coffea arabica)*, kola *(Cola nitida)*, cacao *(Theofroma cacao)*, and mate *(Ilex paragayensis)*; it stimulates the central nervous system, promotes an increased discharge of urine (diuresis), and stimulates dilatation of blood vessels (vasodilatation). Caffeine has been used in combination with other drugs to treat migraine.

caffeinism (kaf'ēn-izm) Condition resulting from ingesting excessive amounts of caffeine; marked by increased rate of the heartbeat (tachycardia), insomnia, and irritability.

calcification (kal-sĭ-fĭ-ka'shun) The process by which calcium salts are deposited in organic tissue; may be normal (e.g., in bone and tooth substance) or a pathologic process.

　　intracranial c. Minute areas of calcification in the brain and its covering membranes (meninges), caused by intrauterine infection either with cytomegalovirus (the herpesvirus causing cytomegalic inclusion disease) or with *Toxoplasma gondii* (the parasite causing toxoplasmosis).

calcitonin (kal-se-to'nin) A potent hormone produced in the thyroid gland that lowers calcium levels in the blood.

calcium (kal'se-um) Metallic element; symbol Ca, atomic number 20, atomic weight 40.08; component of bones and teeth; essential in regulating blood coagulation, muscle contraction, conduction of nerve impulses from nerve endings to muscle fibers, function of cell membranes, activity of enzymes, and in maintaining rhythmicity of the heartbeat.

　　c. gluconate A calcium salt of gluconic acid used as a calcium supplement and in the treatment of low-calcium tetany; also useful in the treatment of abnormally high magnesium content of the blood (hypermagnesemia) associated with the treatment of preeclampsia and eclampsia.

calcium channel blocker. See calcium channel-blocking agent, under agent.

calciuria (kal-se-u're-ă) The presence of calcium in the urine.

calculation (kal-ku-la'shun) An estimate based on probabilities.

　　Johnson's c. of fetal weight Fetal weight in vertex presentation: fw = fh – 12 (or 11) × 155; i.e., fetal weight (in grams) equals: fundal height (in centimeters measured from the pubic symphysis) minus 12 (if vertex is above ischial spines) or 11 (if vertex is below ischial spines), multiplied by 155. If the pregnant woman weighs more than 90 kg, 1 cm is subtracted from the fundal height.

calculi (kal'ku-li) Plural of calculus.

calculous (kal'ku-lus) Relating to calculus.

calculus (kal'ku-lus), pl. calculi An abnormal stony concretion usually composed of mineral salts, formed most frequently in the lumen of ducts and hollow organs. See also stone.

　　mulberry c. Calculus resembling a mulberry, composed mainly of calcium oxalate and formed in the bladder.

　　renal c. See kidney stone, under stone.

　　staghorn c. A large kidney stone with many branches lodged in and filling the pelvis and calices of the kidney.

　　urinary c. See urinary stone, under stone.

　　vesical c. See vesical stone, under stone.

calipers (kal'ĭ-perz) An instrument composed of two hinged parts used for measuring diameters,

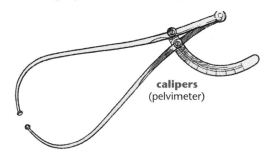

calipers
(pelvimeter)

such as the pelvic diameters.

calmodulin (kal-mod'u-lin) An intracellular calcium-binding regulatory protein that serves as a mediator of cellular responses to calcium. It is involved in contraction of smooth muscle cells of the uterus during labor.

calpain (kal'pān) A calcium-dependent enzyme (cysteine protease) that breaks down the amino acid cysteine and is activated during fertilization, allowing meiosis to resume.

Calymmatobacterium (kă-lim-ă-to-bac-tĕr'e-um) A genus of Gram-negative, pathogenic bacteria.

>   **C. granulomatis** A species causing granuloma inguinale. Also called Donovan body.

calvaria (kal-var'e-ă), pl. calvariae The upper, domelike part of the skull. Popularly called skullcap; roof of skull.

Campylobacter (kam-pǐ-lo-bak'ter) A genus of curved or spiral, Gram-negative bacteria; some species are pathogenic.

>   **C. fetus** A species that causes abortion in animals but not humans.

>   **C. jejuni** Species that is the major cause of enterocolitis ranging from self-limited mild intestinal disturbances to severe recurrent diarrhea with inflammatory changes resembling those of ulcerative colitis or Crohn's disease.

>   **C. pylori** See *Helicobacter pylori*, under *Helicobacter*.

canal (kă-nal') A tubular structure; a channel; a relatively narrow passage or conduit.

>   **Alcock's c.** See pudendal canal.

>   **alimentary c.** Canal consisting of the esophagus, stomach, and small and large intestines.

>   **anal c.** Canal beginning at the lower end of the rectum and passing downward and backward to the end of the anus; sphincter muscles normally keep the canal closed.

>   **atrioventricular c.** The canal in the embryonic heart leading from the common atrium to the primitive ventricle.

>   **birth c.** Canal through which the fetus passes at birth; consists of the uterine cervix, vagina, and vulva. Also called parturient canal; obstetric canal.

>   **caudal c.** See sacral canal.

>   **central c.** Canal extending through the lower half of the medulla oblongata (where it opens into the fourth ventricle of the brain) and throughout the entire length of the spinal cord. After the age of approximately 40 years, the lower portion of the canal tends to obliterate.

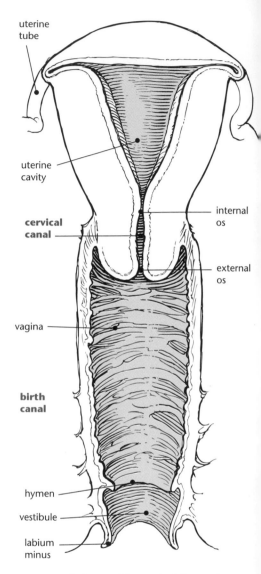

>   **cervical c., c. of the cervix** A flattened, normally closed, canal within the uterine cervix that connects the vagina to the cavity within the body of the uterus.

>   **femoral c.** The medial and smallest of the three compartments of the femoral sheath underlying the inguinal ligament at the groin; it is bounded posteriorly by the pectineus muscle, medially by the lacunar ligament, and laterally by the femoral vein; it is cone-shaped and contains extraperitoneal fatty and lymphoid tissue, which cushions any expansion of the femoral vein or artery as it traverses the intermediate and lateral compartments of the femoral sheath.

inguinal c. An obliquely directed passage through the layers of the lower abdominal wall on either side, through which pass the spermatic cord in the male and the round ligament of the uterus in the female.

c. of midbrain See cerebral aqueduct, under aqueduct.

c. of Nuck See persistent processus vaginalis peritonei, under processus.

obstetric c. See birth canal.

parturient c. See birth canal.

pudendal c. A fibrous tunnel formed by the splitting of the obturator fascia that lines the lateral wall of the ischiorectal fossa; it transmits the internal pudendal vessels and nerves. Also called Alcock's canal.

sacral c. The part of the spinal canal extending from the first sacral vertebra to the inferior end of the sacrum (sacral hiatus); it contains a collection of spinal roots (cauda equina), the terminal filament (filum terminale) that connects the end of the spinal cord to the coccyx, and the spinal membranes (meninges). Also called caudal canal.

spinal c. The canal formed by the foramina of successive vertebrae; it is large and triangular in the cervical and lumbar regions, small and circular in the thoracic region, and small and triangular in the sacral region; it encloses the spinal cord and its membranes (meninges). Also called vertebral canal.

vertebral c. See spinal canal.

cancer (kan'ser) (CA) General term for any of a group of diseases in which symptoms are due to unrestrained proliferation of abnormal, malignant cells in the body's organs or tissues. Unlike noncancerous (benign) tumors, this new growth (neoplasm) is invasive (i.e., it infiltrates and destroys adjacent tissues) or metastatic (i.e., it spreads via blood vessels and lymphatic channels to other sites of the body, creating new satellite tumors that grow independently); it has a tendency to recur after treatment, and, unless adequately treated, it causes death. The term includes carcinoma and sarcoma. Generally, it is used interchangeably with carcinoma. See also CA 15-3; CA 19-9; CA 125; carcinoma.

epidermoid c. See squamous cell carcinoma, under carcinoma.

glandular c. See adenocarcinoma.

occult c. An asymptomatic small cancer that has not been clinically detected but has invaded adjacent tissues or spread to other sites (metastasized).

cancericidal (kan-ser-ĭ-si'dal) See carcinolytic.

Cancer Information Service (CIS) A nationwide

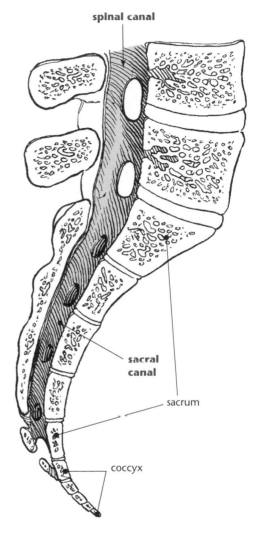

spinal canal

sacral canal

sacrum

coccyx

telephone service supported by the National Cancer Institute (NCI) that responds to inquiries from cancer patients and their families, health care professionals, and the general public.

CANCERLIT Cancer Literature. An online database on the MEDLARS system of the National Library of Medicine; sponsored by the National Cancer Institute of the National Institutes of Health (NIH). The database contains more than 600,000 references dealing with various aspects of cancer. It may be accessed by universities, medical schools, hospitals, government agencies, commercial and nonprofit organizations, and private individuals.

cancerous (kan'ser-us) Relating to malignant growths.

Candida (kan'dĭ-dă) A genus of yeastlike fungi.

C. albicans A species that normally inhabits the intestinal tract of humans but may cause disease under certain conditions (e.g., pregnancy, diabetes mellitus, obesity, and weakened immunity). Also called thrush fungus.

candidal (kan'dĭ-dal) Relating to or caused by *Candida.* Also called (incorrectly) monilial.

candidemia (kan-dĭ-de'me-ă) The presence of *Candida* fungus in the blood, usually due to systemic candidiasis.

candidiasis (kan-dĭ-di'ă-sis) Infection with fungi of the genus *Candida.* Also called candidosis. See also candidal vaginitis, under vaginitis.

cutaneous c. Candidiasis occurring as reddish, sometimes itchy, patches on the skin or the nails; predisposing factors include chronic maceration, as occurs in diaper rash and in friction of the scrotal area of the thighs of obese individuals.

oral c. An oropharyngeal manifestation of a candidal infection marked by plaques of white friable pseudomembranous material on a reddish base distributed over the tongue, palate, buccal mucosa, and gingivae. Immunocompromised patients appear particularly vulnerable to this infection.

vulvovaginal c. Candidiasis of the vulva and vagina; it produces itching and irritation and a scant to moderate discharge with white curd-like clumps; seen most commonly in pregnant women, especially during the third trimester, and in women infected with the human immunodeficiency virus (HIV).

candidosis (kan-dĭ-do'sis) See candidiasis.

cap (kap) Any structure or device that resembles or serves as a cover.

acrosomal c. See acrosome.

cervical c. A thimble-shaped contraceptive device, smaller than a diaphragm, that fits over the uterine cervix. See also contraceptive cap.

contraceptive c. Any of three latex devices (cervical, vault, and vimule caps) used to prevent pregnancy; designed to fit snugly over the uterine cervix, where it is held in place by suction; often used by women who cannot use a diaphragm due to anatomic changes (e.g., prolapse of the uterus, cystocele).

cradle c. The crusted seborrheic dermatitis of the scalp occurring in infants usually during the first 3 months of life.

vault c. A bowl-shaped contraceptive device smaller than a diaphragm. See also contraceptive cap.

vimule c. Contraceptive cap, smaller than a diaphragm, that includes features of both cervical and vault caps. See also contraceptive cap.

capacitation (kă-pas-ĭ-ta'shun) The morphologic, physiologic, and biochemical changes occurring in a spermatozoon secondary to enzymatic activation which prepare it to fertilize an ovum.

capacity (kă-pas'ĭ-te) **1.** The ability to hold or retain. **2.** A measure of such ability. **3.** A legal qualification, competence, or fitness. **4.** The ability to do something.

forced vital c. (FVC) The volume of air that is forcefully and rapidly expired from full inspiration. In testing, the patient inhales maximally to full lung capacity, then exhales into an apparatus (spirometer) as forcefully, as rapidly, and as completely as possible.

functional residual c. (FRC) The volume of air remaining in the lungs at the end of exhaling during normal breathing.

inspiratory c. (IC) The maximum volume of air that can be inhaled into the lungs after a normal expiration.

iron-binding c. (IBC) The maximum ability of plasma proteins to combine with iron.

maximum breathing c. (MBC) See maximum voluntary ventilation (MVV), under ventilation.

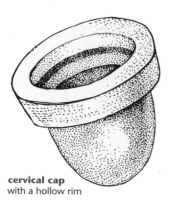

cervical cap
with a hollow rim

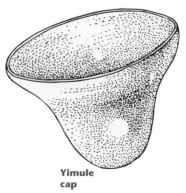

**Yimule
cap**

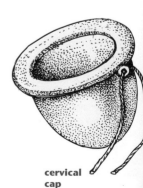

**cervical
cap**

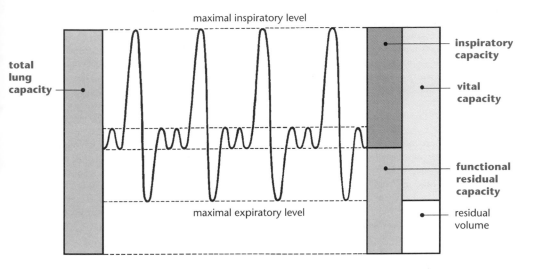

maximal inspiratory level

total lung capacity

inspiratory capacity

vital capacity

functional residual capacity

residual volume

maximal expiratory level

residual c. See residual volume (RV), under volume.

total iron-binding c. (TIBC) A quantitative measure of the content of transferrin, the iron-binding protein, in serum.

total lung c. (TLC) The volume of air contained in the lungs at full inflation (i.e., following maximum inspiration).

vital c. (VC) The maximum volume of air that can be exhaled from the lungs after a maximal inspiration.

capsule (kap'sul) **1.** A small, soluble, gelatinous container enclosing a dose of a drug. **2.** A saclike structure enveloping an organ, a part, or a tumor. **3.** In radiation therapy, a small, sealed metallic tube containing a radioactive material (e.g., radium), applied to a body surface or placed within a cavity. **4.** A mucopolysaccharide substance surrounding certain bacteria; it is secreted by the organisms and remains in intimate contact with them.

Bowman's c. See glomerular capsule.

glomerular c. A double-walled, spherical, pouchlike structure enveloping a tuft of capillaries (glomerulus) in the kidney; it comprises the beginning of a renal tubule. Also called Bowman's capsule.

captopril (kap'to-pril) A member of a group of drugs known as ACE inhibitors (angiotensin-converting enzyme inhibitors); it acts to prevent the formation of angiotensin II and to lower blood pressure. Captopril has been associated with fetal malformation and uterine growth retardation when taken during pregnancy.

caput (kap'ut), pl. **capita 1.** Latin for head. **2.** Any rounded prominence of an organ or structure.

c. succedaneum A subcutaneous soft swelling on the presenting area of the head of a newborn infant, due to collection of fluid just beneath the scalp between the membrane covering the skull (periosteum) and the scalp; it typically disappears a few days after birth. The swelling results from mild trauma caused by the pressures to which the head is subjected as it passes through the birth canal, most commonly when the head encounters resistance in a rigid vaginal outlet; occurs also in prolonged labor when the cervix is incompletely dilated, or the maternal pelvis is contracted. Removal of fluid predisposes to infection and is not necessary. Compare with cephalhematoma.

caput succedaneum

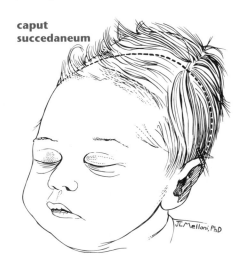

carbamazepine (kar-bă-maz'ĕ-pēn) An anticonvulsant drug used in the treatment of epilepsy. Prenatal exposure may cause craniofacial defects, underdevelopment of fingernails, and developmental delays; a 1% risk of spina bifida has been reported.

carboplatin (kar'bo-plat-in) An analog of cisplatin used in the treatment of epithelial ovarian cancer.

carcinoembryonic (kar-sin-o-em-bre-on'ik) Relating to substances that are associated with cancer in adults but are present normally in the embryo (e.g., carcinoembryonic antigen [CEA] and alpha-fetoprotein [AFP]).

carcinogen (kar-sin'ŏ-jen) Any cancer-causing agent.

    direct-contact c. See proximate carcinogen.

    proximate c. An industrial, agricultural, or household chemical that acts locally at the site of contact without having to undergo metabolic changes in the body. Also called direct-contact carcinogen.

    ultimate c. Chemicals that are metabolically converted in the body into active cancer-causing agents.

carcinogenesis (kar-sĭ-no-jen'ĕ-sis) Production of cancer.

    transplacental c. The passage of cancer-producing substances from the pregnant woman to her unborn child through the placental circulation (e.g., the intrauterine exposure to diethylstilbestrol [DES], which causes cancer of the cervix and vagina in the adult offspring).

carcinogenic (kar-sĭ-no-jen'ik) Causing cancer.

carcinogenicity (kar-sĭ-no-ge-nis'ĕ-te) The ability to produce or incite cancer.

carcinolytic (kar-sĭ-no-lit'ik) Destructive to cancerous cells.

carcinoma (kar-sĭ-no'mă), pl. carcinomas, carcinomata (CA) Any of various malignant tumors derived from epithelial cells (which form the surface layers and lining membranes of organs); characteristically carcinomas invade adjacent tissues, spread to distant sites of the body via the bloodstream (metastasize), and, unless adequately treated, tend to cause death.

    adenoid cystic c. A slow-growing carcinoma most commonly seen in salivary glands; marked by the presence of large epithelial masses containing spaces frequently filled with mucus; may occur, rarely, in a Bartholin gland with frequent local recurrences and metastasis after therapy.

    adenosquamous c. See adenoacanthoma.

    clear cell c. of kidney See renal adenocarcinoma, under adenocarcinoma.

    ductal c. in situ (DCIS) Preinvasive cancer developed within one or more milk-transporting ducts of the breast; it does not invade other breast tissues as long as it remains within the duct.

    embryonal c. A highly malignant type of carcinoma arising from primordial germ cells; composed of undifferentiated cells or occurring as part of mixed germ cell tumors; seen in young children and adolescents.

    embryonal c. of ovary Uncommon but most malignant of the cancers developing in the ovary; seen in young girls, especially those with hormonal abnormalities (e.g., precocious puberty, amenorrhea, and hirsutism); presenting symptom is usually a painful abdominal or pelvic mass.

    embryonal c. of vagina See embryonal rhabdomyosarcoma of vagina, under rhabdomyosarcoma.

    epidermoid c. See squamous cell carcinoma.

    hepatocellular c. (HCC) See hepatoma.

    infantile embryonal c. See yolk-sac tumor, under tumor.

    infiltrating breast c. Cancer of the breast that begins as a small and movable painless mass; it enlarges, sometimes rapidly, and in later stages becomes fixed to the chest wall and skin and ulcerates through the skin.

    c. in situ (CIS) Carcinoma that is confined to transformation of cells to abnormal patterns (typical of invasive cancer) within its original location and has not spread into surrounding tissues. Also called intraepithelial carcinoma, preinvasive carcinoma.

    intraductal c. Carcinoma derived from the lining membrane of a duct, especially a milk duct in the breast, forming masses that obliterate the duct's lumen.

    intraepithelial c. See carcinoma in situ.

    papillary c. A finger-shaped carcinoma.

    preinvasive c. See carcinoma in situ.

    primary c. Carcinoma at the site of origin.

    renal cell c. See renal adenocarcinoma, under adenocarcinoma.

    scirrhous c. A hard nodule containing a large amount of fibrous tissue; it usually develops in the breast. Also called fibrocarcinoma.

    squamous cell c. (SCC) Carcinoma derived from the superficial flattened cells of epithelium, appearing as thickened plaques that progress to nodules, ulcer formation, and eventual invasion of surrounding tissues and/or spread to distant sites (metastasis); may develop from normal tissue that has been made susceptible by long-term exposure to certain agents; commonly found in the lungs, oral cavity, sinuses, skin (including skin of the vulva), uterine cervix, and vagina (most commonly of postmenopausal women). Also called epidermoid carcinoma; epidermoid cancer.

 transitional cell c. Carcinoma derived from transitional cells of the urinary tract; most frequently occurring in the bladder and especially associated with cigarette smoking.

 verrucous c. of vulva A variant of squamous cell carcinoma; it is locally invasive but does not spread to the lymph nodes; it has a tendency to recur after excision.

carcinomata (k'ar-sĭ-no'mă-tă) Plural of carcinoma.

carcinomatoid (kar-sĭ-nom'ă-toid) Resembling carcinoma.

carcinomatosis (kar-sĭ-no-mă-to'sis) The presence of widely disseminated cancer in the body.

cardiolipin (kar-de-o-lip'in) A phospholipid that is the chief antigenic part of Wassermann-type antigens used in nontreponemal serologic tests for syphilis.

cardio-, cardi- Combining forms meaning the heart; the orifice between the esophagus and the stomach; the area of the stomach adjacent to the esophagus.

cardiomyopathy (kar-de-o-mi-op'ă-the) Primary disease of the muscular wall of the heart, characterized by enlargement of the ventricles in the absence of congenital, hypertensive, valvular, or ischemic heart disease. Also called myocardiopathy.

 hypertrophic c. (HCM) Inherited disease that is the most common cause of sudden death in the young (especially young athletes participating in strenuous sports); characterized by enlargement of the heart due to hypertrophy of the ventricles, involving the left ventricle more than the right one, resulting in poor diastolic relaxation, inadequate filling, and rapid emptying of the ventricle. The disease is an autosomal dominant inheritance, linked to a mutation of the beta-myosin heavy-chain gene located on chromosome 14; mutations involving the amino acid arginine are predictors of sudden death. Also called familial hypertrophic cardiomyopathy (FHCM). See also sudden cardiac death, under death.

cardiospasm (kar'de-o-spazm) See achalasia.

care (kār) General term used in medicine and public health to denote the application of knowledge to the benefit of an individual person or a community.

 critical c. The constant monitoring and immediate treatment of seriously ill patients by specially trained personnel using advanced technology at a hospital. Also called intensive care.

 intensive c. See critical care.

 medical c. The application of medical knowledge to the identification, treatment, and prevention of illness.

 ordinary c. In medical practice, the degree of care that a reasonable practitioner exercises to prevent risk of unreasonable harm to the patient; failure to exercise such care when under duty to do so constitutes negligence. Also called reasonable care.

 postoperative c. Care of a patient immediately following a surgical operation; it includes surveillance of: vital signs (blood pressure, pulse, respiration), body temperature, fluid balance, bleeding from surgical wounds, persisting anesthetic effects on the lungs and cardiovascular circulation (if general anesthesia was used), position of patient in bed, drainage tubes, renal and bladder function, medications, mobility, diet, and (if applicable) performance of special laboratory examinations.

 preconception c. A comprehensive program of health care that aims to identify and reduce a woman's reproductive risks before conception takes place (e.g., genetic counseling and testing, financial and family planning, medical assessment, and nutritional guidance); may include the male partner in providing counseling and educational information in preparation for fatherhood. Distinguished from prenatal care. Also called preconception counseling.

 prenatal c. Comprehensive care provided to the pregnant woman and her fetus throughout pregnancy to enhance their health and well-being, to prevent complications at delivery, and to decrease the incidence of disease and mortality of both; may include tests of both woman and fetus to detect disease, defects, or potential hazards, and guidance regarding diet and exercise.

 preoperative c. Care of a patient prior to a major surgical operation; it involves a diagnostic workup to determine the cause and extent of the illness, preoperative evaluation to assess the patient's overall health and preoperative preparation, consisting of procedures dictated by the findings of the diagnostic workup and preoperative evaluation and by the planned operative procedure.

primary medical c. Care given by the first member of the health professions approached by the patient. In general use, the term refers to care provided by a family physician, internal medicine specialist, or pediatrician, who may refer out for special-care needs.

reasonable c. See ordinary care.

secondary medical c. Care given by a medical specialist at the request of the professional who administered primary care.

tertiary medical c. Consultative care given by a specialist at a medical center (e.g., in specialized surgical procedures, critical care support).

carrier (kar'e-er) **1.** An individual who shows no signs of a disease but harbors infective microorganisms that cause disease in those to whom they are transmitted. **2.** In genetics, an individual who carries an abnormal gene in a recessive state (i.e., the person does not show signs of carrying the abnormality but can transmit it to an offspring who, when inheriting the same gene from the other parent, may develop the disease or abnormality of the gene). The abnormal gene may be detected by appropriate laboratory tests. **3.** A substance in a cell that is capable of accepting an atom or a subatomic particle, thus facilitating transport of organic solutes. **4.** In immunology, a molecule, or part of a molecule, capable of inducing an immune response that is recognized by T cells in an antibody response.

chronic c. A person who harbors disease-producing organisms for some time after recovery.

passive c. One who harbors infectious organisms without having had the disease.

cartilage (kar'tĭ-lij) A firm, slightly elastic connective tissue that constitutes the major portion of the fetal skeleton and is present in specialized areas of the adult body (e.g., in articular surfaces of bones, in the ear, auditory tube, nose, larynx, trachea, bronchi); it consists of specialized cells (chondrocytes) embedded in a ground substance (matrix), which is permeated by collagenous fibers; cartilage has no nerve or blood supply of its own.

cartilaginous (kar-tĭ-laj'ĭ-nus) Relating to cartilage.

caruncle (kar'ung-kl) A small soft nodule.

amniotic c.'s See amnion nodosum.

urethral c. A small protrusion just within the opening of the female urethra; it usually represents a varicosity of a vein within the lining tissue (mucosa).

cast (kast) **1.** A rigid dressing usually made by impregnating a gauze bandage with wet plaster of Paris, used to immobilize a body part. **2.** A cylindrical hardened material formed from discharges within tubular structures of the body as a product of certain disease processes; it is molded in the shape of the structure in which discharges accumulated.

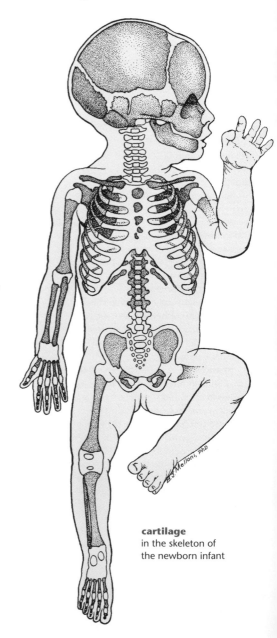

cartilage
in the skeleton of
the newborn infant

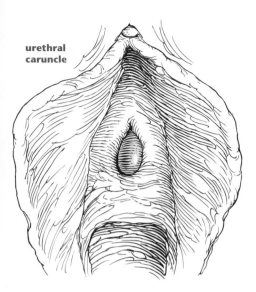
urethral caruncle

blood c. Cast composed of a thick material containing blood elements, usually formed in kidney tubules or in the smallest air passages in the lungs (bronchioles) as a result of bleeding into these structures; it is a characteristic finding of glomerulonephritis. Also called red blood cast.

decidual c. The degenerated decidua (pregnancy-modified endometrium) shed intact from the uterus upon the death of a fetus in a tubal pregnancy.

epithelial c. Cast containing cells from the inner lining (epithelium) of the tubular structure in which it was formed.

fatty c. Urinary cast containing fat globules with cholesterol esters.

granular c. Urinary cast containing particles of cellular debris from the kidney tubules.

hyaline c. A clear urinary cast composed chiefly of protein.

red blood cell c. See blood cast.

renal c. See urinary cast.

urinary c. Any cast formed in the kidney and discharged in the urine; usually they are indicative of kidney disease but occasionally some occur in healthy people. Also called renal cast.

waxy c. A light yellow urinary cast associated with reduced or lack of urinary output.

white blood cell c. A urinary cast composed of white blood cells; it occurs in interstitial nephritis.

castrate (kas'trāt) To remove the ovaries or testes by surgical means.

castration (kas-tra'shun) The removal of the testes (orchiectomy) or ovaries (oophorectomy), usually performed when these organs are diseased or in the treatment of cancer of the prostate or breast.

functional c. Rendering gonadal function clinically ineffective by medical means (e.g., hormones or chemotherapeutic agents) or physical means (e.g., radiation).

catagen (kat'ă-jen) The brief period in the cycle of (anagen) and the resting phase (telegen).

catamenia (kat-ă-me'ne-ă) The menses.

catamenial (kat-ă-me'ne-al) Relating to, or occurring during, menstruation; menstrual.

catamenogenic (kat-ă-me-no-jen'ik) Causing menstruation.

cataract (kat'ă-rakt) A cloudy or opaque condition of the normally transparent lens of the eye or its capsule; it obstructs passage of light rays and diminishes vision, partially or totally.

congenital c. Cataract present at birth due to faulty development of the fetus; may be caused by a maternal infection (especially rubella) during early pregnancy, or it may be associated with chromosomal abnormalities (e.g., Down's syndrome).

juvenile c., early onset c. Cataract occurring in a child or young adult; may result from a variety of conditions (e.g., from congenital syphilis, congenital rubella).

catecholamine (kat-ĕ-kol'ă-mēn) Any of a group of amine compounds, some of which (e.g., epinephrine, norepinephrine, dopamine) are important in transmission of nerve impulses and have an important influence on many metabolic processes.

catechol-O-methyltransferase (kat'e-kol o meth-il-trans'fer-ās) (COMT) A widely distributed enzyme, with highest concentration levels in the liver and kidneys; it is not present in nerve endings.

catgut (kat'gut) A sterilized suture material obtained from connective tissue of healthy animals; it is frequently impregnated with chromium trioxide to increase its strength. Also called catgut suture; surgical gut.

catheter (kath'ĕ-ter) A slender, usually flexible tube that is inserted into a body channel or cavity (e.g., blood vessel, bladder) to introduce diagnostic or therapeutic substances, to drain fluids, or to perform special procedures.

acorn-tipped c. A flexible catheter with a cone-shaped tip used to occlude the distal opening of the ureter during x-ray examination of the ureter and kidney pelvis.

Also called cone-tipped catheter.

balloon-tip c. A catheter with a balloon at its tip that can be inflated and deflated after insertion, usually into a blood vessel; used in diagnostic procedures and to dilate the lumen of a blood vessel (angioplasty).

cone-tipped c. See acorn-tipped catheter.

c. coudé See elbowed catheter.

double-channel c. A catheter with two lumens, which permit irrigation and drainage. Also called two-way catheter.

elbowed c. A catheter with a curved tip, which allows great mobility of the tip by simply twisting the catheter. Also called catheter coudé.

Foley c. A catheter held in place by an inflated balloon.

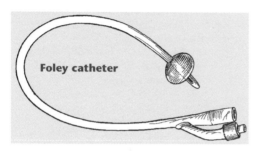

Foley catheter

indwelling c. A catheter designed to be left within a body cavity or passage for an extended period of time.

Swan-Ganz c. A multilumen, flow-directed catheter, used with or without a balloon at its tip for diagnosis and for hemodynamic and therapeutic monitoring (e.g., cardiopulmonary procedures) to measure pulmonary arterial pressure.

two-way c. See double-channel catheter.

Word c. A disposable device that has a small inflatable balloon at its distal end, the purpose of which is to allow drainage of accumulated secretions of a Bartholin cyst or abscess by creating an opening into the cyst or abscess cavity.

catheterization (kath-ĕ-ter-ĭ-za'shun) Introduction of a catheter into a body cavity to obtain data for diagnosis or for therapeutic purposes (e.g., to maintain patency).

in-and-out c. See straight catheterization.

straight c. Withdrawal of urine from a patient by inserting a catheter into the bladder through the urethra, holding it in place while the urine drains, then withdrawing it when the flow stops. Popularly called straight cath; occasionally called in-and-out catheterization.

urinary c. Insertion of a catheter into the bladder to drain urine.

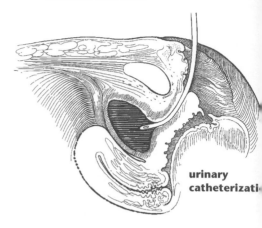

urinary catheterization

catheterize (kath'ĕ-ter-īz) To introduce a catheter into a body cavity.

cauda (kaw'dă), pl. caudae The tapered end of a structure.

c. equina A group of nerves from the lumbar, sacral, and coccygeal segments of the spinal cord; it extends beyond the end of the spinal cord and occupies the lower third of the vertebral canal.

caudad (kaw'dad) Directed toward the part of the body opposite the head.

caudal (kaw'dal) Relating to the part of the body opposite the head.

caudate (kaw'dāt) Having a tail or tail-like appearance.

caul (kawl) The portion of fetal membranes (amniochorion) that sometimes surrounds the head of a newborn at the time of birth; seen when the membranes remain intact until completion of delivery. Popularly called veil.

cauterization (kaw-ter-ĭ-za'shun) Destruction or searing of body tissues with heat, electricity, or caustic chemical to stop bleeding or to promote healing.

cauterize (kaw'ter-īz) To apply a cautery.

cautery (kaw'ter-e) **1.** A chemical agent or hot instrument used to destroy body tissues by scarring or burning. **2.** The application of such an agent or instrument.

cavitary (kav'ĭ-tar-e) Relating to a cavity.

cavitation (kav-ĭ-ta'shun) Formation of a cavity or cavities.

cavity (kav'ĭ-te) A hollow space within the body, often designating a potential space between layers of tissue or membranes.

abdominal c. The body cavity between the diaphragm above and the pelvis below.

abdominopelvic c. The abdominal and pelvic cavities considered as a unit.

amniotic c., amnionic c. The fluid-filled space inside the membranes (amniochorion) containing the embryo/fetus.

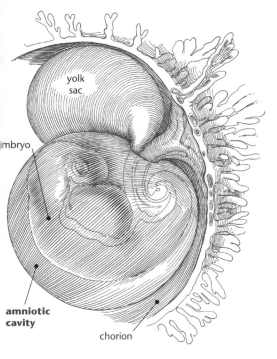

axillary c. The armpit.

cranial c. The space within the skull.

greater peritoneal c. See greater sac of peritoneum, under sac.

pelvic c. The short, wide, curved space within the bony framework of the minor pelvis, between the pelvic brim and the pelvic floor (pelvic diaphragm); it contains the pelvic colon, rectum, bladder, and some of the organs of reproduction.

pericardial c. The potential space between the two layers of membrane (pericardium) enclosing the heart.

pleural c. The potential space between the two layers of membrane (pleura) enclosing each lung.

thoracic c. The space between the neck and the respiratory diaphragm.

visceral c. Any of the body cavities that contain major organs: cranial, thoracic, abdominal, and pelvic.

cecum (se'kum) The saclike portion of intestine to which the vermiform appendix is attached; it is the widest and most proximal of the three parts of the large intestine (the other two being the colon and rectum) and is situated between the ileum proximally and the colon distally.

cell (sel) **1.** The smallest unit of living organisms capable of independent functioning, composed of a nucleus and organelle-containing cytoplasm enclosed within a semipermeable plasma membrane. **2.** In anatomy, any small hollow cavity or compartment.

alpha c.'s of hypophysis The acidophilic cells of the anterior pituitary (adenohypophysis); they secrete growth hormones, prolactin, and adrenocorticotropic hormone (ACTH).

amniogenic c.'s Cells lining the inner surface of trophoblasts during the early phase of blastocyst implantation; they are the precursors of the amniotic epithelium.

anaplastic c. An undifferentiated cell characteristic of carcinoma.

antigen-presenting c. (APC) A cell that helps to initiate an immune response by capturing antigen and carrying it on its cell membrane in a form that is recognized by T lymphocytes (T cells), thereby stimulating the lymphocytes' immune activity.

antigen-sensitive c. See immunocyte.

B c. See B lymphocyte, under lymphocyte.

balloon c. A large, degenerated squamous cell with abundant vacuolated cytoplasm and a perinucleal 'halo'; often seen in human papilloma virus infection.

beta c.'s of hypophysis The basophilic cells of the anterior pituitary (adenohypophysis); they secrete thyroid-stimulating hormone (TSH), follicle-stimulating hormone (FSH), and luteinizing hormone (LH).

clue c.'s Epithelial cells of a vaginal specimen by which bacterial infection with *Gardnerella vaginalis* can be detected; the bacteria attach themselves to the cells, covering the cytoplasmic membrane.

daughter c. Any cell resulting from the division of another (parent) cell.

effector c. In immunology, a T lymphocyte (T cell) capable of carrying out the end function of the immunologic process (e.g., cytotoxicity, suppression).

endothelial c. One of the thin, flat (squamous) cells lining the blood and lymph vessels as well as the chambers of the heart.

ependymal c.'s The cells constituting the lining membrane of the ventricles of the brain and of the central canal of the spinal cord (ependyma).

epithelial c. One of a variety of cells forming the surface epithelium of the skin, and alimentary, respiratory, and genitourinary passages, and their associated glands; it covers all free surfaces of the body except the synovial membranes and the bursae of joints.

follicular c.'s See granulosa cells.

follicular lutein c.'s See granulosa lutein cells.

germ c. An ovum or spermatozoon, or one of their precursors (immature stages). Also called reproductive cell; germinal cell.

germinal c.'s (1) See germ cell. (2) Cells from which other cells are derived, especially the dividing cells in the embryonic neural tube from which the nerve cells are derived by proliferation and migration.

granulosa c.'s Special epithelial cells surrounding the ovum within developing ovarian follicles. Also called follicular cells.

granulosa lutein c.'s Giant glandular cells forming the major part of the wall of a ruptured vesicular follicle (corpus luteum) in the ovary; formed by hypertrophy of the granulosa (follicular) cells of the old vesicular follicle; they produce the sex steroid progesterone. Also called follicular lutein cells.

HeLa c.'s The first documented, continuously cultured, human malignant cells, derived from a squamous cell carcinoma of the uterine cervix; often used in the culture of viruses.

helper c. Any of a subtype of T lymphocytes (T cells) that facilitate an immune response by stimulating conversion of B lymphocytes into antibody-producing cells. Also called helper T-lymphocyte.

Hofbauer c. One of many large, nearly round cells found in connective tissue of the chorionic villi of the placenta; thought to be a fetal macrophage.

I c. See immunocyte.

immunocompetent c. See immunocyte.

interstitial c.'s of testis See Leydig cells.

islet c.'s Any of the cells in the pancreatic islets (of Langerhans).

killer c.'s, K c.'s Small cells believed to be derived from T lymphocytes (T cells), which are able to attack target cells (e.g., tumor cells) after IgG antibodies have reacted with an antigen on the target cell; complement is not needed to kill the cell.

Langerhan's c. A specialized macrophage-type cell of the epidermis; an antigen-presenting cell in skin that migrates to neighboring lymph nodes to become dendritic cells active in stimulating T lymphocytes (T cells).

Langhans' c.'s Round cells with clear cytoplasm and light-staining nuclei forming the cytotrophoblast (the innermost layer of the trophoblast).

Leydig c.'s The endocrine interstitial cells of the testis that secrete androgens (mainly

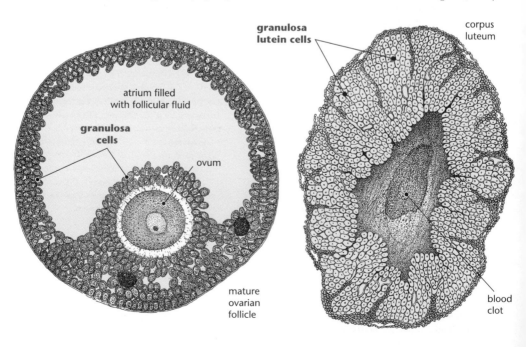

granulosa lutein cells

corpus luteum

atrium filled with follicular fluid

granulosa cells

ovum

mature ovarian follicle

blood clot

testosterone); situated between the seminiferous tubules. Also called interstitial cells of testis.

lymph c., lymphoid c. See lymphocyte.

memory B c. B cell that has already encountered antigen, undergone class switching, and returned to a resting state to be reactivated by a second challenge from the antigen it recognizes; during the second challenge, the cell mounts a more sustained response. Also called immunologic memory cell.

mesothelial c. A cell of mesodermal origin; one of the flat cells of the squamous epithelium (mesothelium) lining the pleural, pericardial, peritoneal, and scrotal cavities.

Mikulicz c.'s Large macrophages with rod-shaped cytoplasmic inclusion bodies present in lesions of granuloma inguinale.

mother c. See parent cell.

myoepithelial c. One of the smooth muscle cells of ectodermal origin, with processes that spiral around some of the epithelial cells of sweat, mammary, lacrimal, and salivary glands; their contraction forces the secretion of the glands toward the ducts.

natural killer c.'s See NK cells.

NK c.'s Lymphocytes that originate in bone marrow and do not have surface markers of either B or T lymphocytes (B or T cells); they comprise a small percentage of lymphocytes of normal blood and are cytotoxic against target cells without being specifically sensitized against them. NK cells can destroy a wide variety of tumor cells and probably provide natural resistance to tumor formation and against invasion by some microorganisms.

navicular c. A small ovoid cell containing a vesicular, elongated nucleus; found in small clusters throughout the vaginal epithelium during pregnancy.

permanent c. A fetal cell that is unable to divide mitotically in postnatal life.

parent c. A cell that undergoes division and gives rise to a new generation of (daughter) cells. Also called mother cell.

plasma c. A cell with RNA-rich cytoplasm and an eccentrically placed nucleus; the cytoplasm contains an extensive system of endoplasmic reticulum studded with ribosomes. The cell arises from the antigen-induced, terminal transformation of a B lymphocyte (B cell). It produces specific antibody against the antigen that induced its formation.

red blood c. (RBC) See erythrocyte.

reproductive c. See germ cell.

Sertoli c.'s The nonspermatogenic supporting cells in the seminiferous tubules of the testes, extending from the basal lamina to the lumen; they house the developing spermatogenic cells in deep recesses and produce sex hormone-binding globulin and androgens.

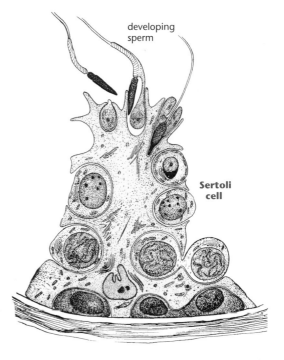

developing sperm

Sertoli cell

sickle c. An abnormal crescent-shaped red blood cell; the characteristic shape is caused by the presence of varying proportions of hemoglobin S; seen in sickle cell anemia.

signet-ring c. A cell engorged with mucin that pushes the cell's nucleus to one side; found in Krukenberg tumors (cancerous stomach tumors that frequently metastasize to the ovary).

sperm c. See spermatozoon.

squamous c. A flat, scalelike cell that is usually arranged in layers to form a lining (e.g., epithelium, endothelium, and mesothelium) of certain structures.

suppressor T c.'s In immunology, a subset of T lymphocytes (T cells) that inhibit antibody production by B lymphocytes (B cells) or inhibit other cellular immune reactions by effector cells.

T c. See T lymphocyte, under lymphocyte.

target c. (1) An abnormal red blood cell

that, when stained, shows a dark center surrounded by a light band encircled by a darker ring, resembling a bull's eye target; found in a variety of anemias, including thalassemia, and other blood disorders. Also called Mexican hat cell. (2) A cell displaying a foreign (nonself) antigen recognized by an effector T lymphocyte. (3) A cell containing specific receptors for circulating messengers such as hormones.

theca lutein c.'s Lutein cells located within the folds of the glandular corpus luteum of the ovary and derived from the theca interna; they produce estrogens.

white blood c.'s (WBC) Formed elements in the blood that include granular leukocytes (neutrophils, eosinophils, and basophils), lymphocytes (small and large), and monocytes.

cellular (sel'u-lar) 1. Relating to cells. 2. Having numerous compartments.

cellulitis (sel-u-li'tis) A rapidly spreading acute inflammation of subcutaneous tissue occurring as a complication of wound infection; the infective organism is usually *Streptococcus pyogenes*.

pelvic c. See parametritis.

celom (se'lom) The body cavity of the embryo, formed between the two layers of mesoderm after one unites with the ectoderm and the other with the endoderm.

celomic (se-lom'ik) Relating to the celom.

center (sen'ter) 1. The middle of an organ or structure. 2. A point or region at which a process begins. 3. A collection of nerve cells governing a particular function. 4. A place, agency, or group designated to serve the community.

birth c., birthing c. A facility that provides prenatal, childbirth, and postnatal care, and usually includes family-oriented maternity care concepts and practice.

germinal c. The area of antibody formation within a lymph nodule containing a large number of antibody-producing white blood cells (lymphocytes).

centesis (sen-te'sis) Perforating or puncturing a cavity.

centriole (sen'tri-ol) Either of two short, hollow, cylindrical bodies in the cytoplasm of animal cells and lower plant cells; its wall is composed of nine sets of microtubules. Centrioles are responsible for organizing the spindle apparatus during cell division.

centromere (sen'tro-mer) The constricted part of the chromosome to which spindle fibers attach during cell division (mitosis). Chromosome movement occurs about the centromere.

centrosome (sen'tro-som) A specialized area of cytoplasm, near the cell nucleus, which plays an important role in cell division (mitosis). Also called cytocentrum.

centrosphere (sen'tro-sfer) A clear specialized area of a cell containing the centrosome.

centrum (sen'trum), pl. centra The center of any anatomic structure.

cephalad (sef'a-lad) Directed toward the head.

cephalalgia (sef-a-lal'je) See headache.

cephalhematoma (sef-al-he-ma-to'ma) Blood cyst with palpable edges overriding a single cranial bone of a newborn infant; blood accumulates between the bone and its covering membrane (periosteum); it does not cross suture lines; may occur after an uneventful delivery with no apparent trauma, or may be caused by a periosteal injury during labor and delivery (e.g., from a vacuum extractor). Within 3 months, it is gradually absorbed, becoming firmer and smaller, and finally disappears. On rare occasions it calcifies, forming a bony protuberance that takes over 1 year to absorb. Compare with caput succedaneum, under caput.

cephalic (se-fal'ik) Relating to the head.

cephalization (sef-al-i-za'shun) Embryologic growth of structures and function of the head.

cephalo-, cephal- Combining forms meaning head.

cephalohematoma See cephalhematoma.

cephalomegaly (sef-a-lo-meg'a-le) Abnormal enlargement of the head.

cephalometry (sef-a-lom'e-tre) Measurement of the head.

ultrasonic c. Measurement of the fetal head by means of ultrasonography.

cephalosporins (sef-a-los-po'rins) A class of antibiotics that inhibit bacterial wall synthesis in a manner similar to penicillin. They are classified by the general features of their antimicrobial activity.

first generation c. Cephalosporins with good activity against Gram-positive bacteria and modest activity against Gram-negative bacteria, but no activity against enterococci or *Listeria* (e.g., cefazolin, cephalothin, and cephalexin).

second generation c. Cephalosporins that are less active against Gram-positive organisms; a few are active against *Bacteroides fragilis* (e.g., cefoxitin, cefotetan, and cefmetazole).

third generation c. Cephalosporins with more activity against Enterobacteriaceae; a few are active against *Pseudomonas aeruginosa* (e.g., ceftazidime and cefoperazone).

fourth generation c. Cephalosporins comparable to third generation cephalosporins but more resistant to some beta-lactamases (a group of bacterial enzymes).

-ceptor Suffix meaning receiver (e.g., proprioceptor).

cerclage (ser-klahzh') Encircling with a ring or loop (e.g., in the treatment of bone fractures, a detached retina, or an incompetent cervix).

> **Lash c.** A transabdominal surgical procedure used for the treatment of an incompetent cervix in which a suture, usually of permanent material, is placed around the lower portion of the uterus at the level of the internal os in an effort to prevent midtrimester pregnancy loss.

> **McDonald's c.** A transvaginal surgical procedure used for the treatment of an incompetent cervix in which a suture is placed in purse-string fashion around the cervix at the level of the internal os in an effort to prevent midtrimester pregnancy loss. Also called McDonald's operation.

> **Shirodkar's c.** A transvaginal surgical procedure used for the treatment of an incompetent cervix in which a suture is placed submucosally around the cervix at the level of the internal os. Also called Shirodkar's operation.

cerebro-, cerebr-, cerebri- Combining forms meaning cerebrum or brain.

cerebrospinal (ser-ĕ-bro-spi'nal) Relating to brain and spinal cord.

cerebrovascular (ser-e-bro-vas'ku-lar) Relating to the blood vessels or circulation of the brain.

cervical (ser'vĭ-kal) **1.** Relating to the neck. **2.** Relating to the uterine cervix.

cervical ripening Changes that occur in the smooth muscle, collagen, and extracellular matrix of the cervix in preparation for the first stage of parturition.

cervicectomy (ser-vĭ-sek'tŏ-me) Amputation of the uterine cervix. Also called trachelectomy.

cervicitis (ser-vĭ-si'tis) Inflammation of the uterine cervix, often caused by a sexually transmitted disease (e.g., gonorrhea, herpes, chlamydial infection) or by trauma (e.g., during childbirth). Also called trachelitis.

cervico- Combining form meaning neck; cervix.

cervico-occipital (ser'vĭ-ko ok-sip'ĭ-tal) Relating to the neck and the lower back of the head.

cervicovesical (ser-vĭ-ko-ves'ĭ-kal) Relating to the uterine cervix and the bladder.

cervix (ser'viks), pl. cervices Any constricted, necklike part of an organ or structure. The term is frequently used alone to denote the uterine cervix.

> **double c.** Two distinct cervices present in one individual; a developmental anomaly resulting from separate maturation of the mullerian ducts. Compare with septate cervix.

> **incompetent c.** In pregnancy, a cervix prone

McDonald's cerclage

purse-string suture placed at the junction of vaginal mucosa and cervix

vaginal mucosa

cross section of cervix with suture in place

Shirodkar's cerclage

suture placed within vaginal mucosa

anterior lip of cervix

longitudinal view of suture in place at level of internal os to dilate prematurely, usually resulting in midterm spontaneous abortion.

ripe c. Popular term for the softened condition of the cervix, which occurs in preparation for the onset of labor; it results from hormonal action upon collagen fibers that provide normal rigidity to the cervix.

septate c. Developmental anomaly in which the cervix is divided by a partition (septum), which is usually a downward continuation of a septum in the uterine cavity, or it may be an upward extension of a longitudinal vaginal septum; occasionally, it is a separate partition confined to the cervix. The cervical wall is formed by a single muscular ring. Compare with double cervix.

uterine c. The neck of the uterus; the cylindrical, lower portion of the uterus extending from the isthmus into the vagina; it contains a spindle-shaped canal or passage that is continuous with the interior of the uterus above and the vagina below. Frequently called cervix; popularly called neck of the womb.

cesarean (sĕ-za′re-an) See cesarean section, under section.

chancre (shang′ker) An ulcer formed at the site of initial invasion by the sexually transmitted *Treponema pallidum*, marking the beginning of the first stage of syphilis (primary syphilis). It begins as a dull red spot 14 to 30 days after infection, then it develops into a painless ulcer with an indurated base; usual sites are the penis (head or shaft) and the vulva; other sites include the cervix, scrotum, anus, rectum, and the lips or throat. Also called hard chancre; hard sore.

hard c. See chancre.

soft c. See chancroid.

chancroid (shang′kroid) A sexually transmitted disease caused by *Haemophilus ducreyi*, a Gram-negative bacillus; characterized by one or more painful ulcers on the genitals, with acute inflammation of lymph nodes of the groin. Also called soft chancre; soft sore; soft ulcer; venereal ulcer.

change (chānj) A modification.

fatty c. Accumulation of fats (lipids) within cells; it occurs in all organs, most frequently in the liver in cases of cirrhosis.

fibrocystic c. of breast Benign condition of the female breast characterized by formation of cysts, overgrowth of connective tissue and intraductal epithelium, and sclerosing of gland tissue. Formerly called fibrocystic disease of breast; cystic hyperplasia of breast; chronic cystic mastitis; mammary dysplasia.

c. of life Popular term for menopause.

channel (chan′el) A passageway, a canal.

character (kar′ak-ter) In genetics, the expression

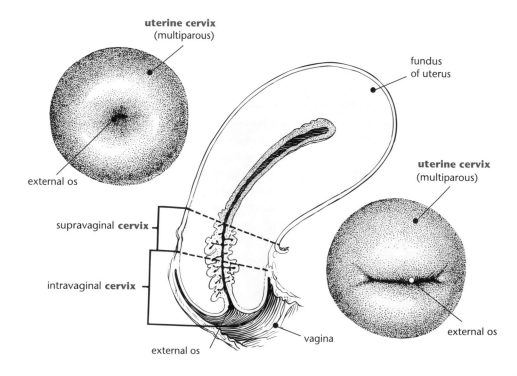

uterine cervix (multiparous)

fundus of uterus

uterine cervix (multiparous)

external os

supravaginal **cervix**

intravaginal **cervix**

external os

external os

vagina

of a gene or a group of genes.

characteristic (kar-ak-ter-is'tik) A distinctive feature, trait, or attribute.

    secondary sex c. The distinctive attributes normally developed at puberty (e.g., beard, breasts, pubic hair).

chart (chart) 1. The graphic or tabular presentation of data. 2. A record of the course of a patient's illness, including temperature, pulse, blood pressure, respiratory rate, urinary and fecal output, and comments from physicians and nurses. 3. To enter data into a patient's health record or to present data in graphic form.

    bleeding c. A written record of uterine bleeding, frequently used to characterize menstrual function.

charting (chart'ing) The process of recording data in a tabular or graphic form.

    basal temperature c. (BTC) A method of detecting the time of ovulation in the menstrual cycle by recording body temperature daily.

chem-, chemo- Combining forms meaning chemistry.

chemo (ke'mo) Popular shortened version of chemotherapy.

chemocautery (ke-mo-kaw'ter-e) Destruction of tissues with a caustic agent.

chemoprevention (ke-mo-pre-ven'shun) A program using natural and synthetic cancer inhibitors to suppress the development of cancer.

chemoprophylaxis (ke-mo-pro-fĭ-lak'sis) Prevention of a specific disease by administration of a chemical agent.

chemotherapeutic (ke-mo-ther-ă-pu'tik) Relating to chemotherapy.

chemotherapy (ke-mo-ther'a-pe) Treatment of disease with any drug (e.g., antimicrobial, antibiotic, and antitumor drugs). The term is usually applied to the treatment of cancer. Commonly called chemo.

    adjuvant c. Chemotherapy used after a malignant tumor has been removed by other methods (e.g., surgery).

    combination c. The simultaneous administration of two or more drugs for the treatment of cancer, especially for advanced stages of the disease. Also called multiple agent chemotherapy; polychemotherapy.

    intracavitary c. Delivery of chemotherapeutic drugs into a body cavity, such as the peritoneal cavity and pleural space, for the treatment of malignant tumors located within such areas. Since cavity walls do not have the abundant blood supply, typical of other body parts, to carry the drugs, the method supposedly delivers a higher drug concentration to the tumor than by systemic administration of the drugs.

    intraperitoneal c. Intracavitary chemotherapy applied to the peritoneal cavity.

    multiple agent c. See combination chemotherapy.

    salvage c. Any treatment regimen used when other methods have failed (e.g., second-line chemotherapy).

    second-line c. Treatment used when the initial chemotherapeutic regimen has failed; it consists of a drug, or combination of drugs, that were not used in the first treatment.

    single agent c. Treatment of cancer with one drug, usually an alkylating agent (e.g., hexamethylmelamine).

chest (chest) The thorax.

chickenpox (chik'en-poks) A contagious disease, mostly of childhood, caused by the varicella-zoster virus; characterized by skin eruption, fever, and mild constitutional symptoms. Complications may include corneal lesions causing visual impairment, pneumonia, and encephalitis. Also called varicella.

chignon (shen-yon) A large swelling (artificial caput) in the back of the head of a newborn infant resulting from the firm suction of a metal cup vacuum extractor applied to the head to create adequate traction during delivery.

childbearing (child'bār-ing) Pregnancy and parturition.

childbirth (child'birth) The process of giving birth to a child.

    natural c. Management of childbirth based on the concept that labor is easier for women who are relaxed and free of fear; this state is achieved by antepartum education that emphasizes elimination of anxiety and apprehension by knowledge of the natural physiologic processes taking place during pregnancy and parturition, exercises to promote relaxation, muscle and breathing control, and constant attendance of an obstetrical professional during labor and delivery who is skilled in providing reassurance and confidence. Also called physiological childbirth.

    physiological c. See natural childbirth.

chimera (ki-me'ra) 1. A person who has received genetically and immunologically different cell types, as in a graft or a bone marrow transplant. 2. In experimental genetics, an organism developed from cells or tissues from two different species.

chimerism (ki-mēr'izm) The state of being a chimera.

blood c. The presence of two blood types in one individual, occurring when the blood of one dizygotic twin fetus is transferred to the other twin through a common blood vessel. Blood chimerism occurs in the second twin.

Chlamydia (klă-mid'e-ă) A genus of bacteria (family Chlamydiaceae) consisting of Gram-negative, intracellular parasites; formerly considered viruses.

    C. pneumoniae A species causing pneumonia, most frequently in young adults. Formerly called TWAR organism.

    C. trachomatis A species causing infectious diseases in humans. Some strains cause eye infections (e.g., trachoma, conjunctivitis); other strains cause sexually transmitted diseases and infections of the genitourinary tract (e.g., lymphogranuloma venereum, nongonococcal urethritis, epididymitis, cervicitis, salpingitis, proctitis). The infection can be transmitted to the newborn during the birth process.

chlamydia (klă-mid'e-ă), pl. chlamydiae Any bacterium of the genus *Chlamydia*.

chloasma (klo-az'mă) See melasma.

    c. of pregnancy See melasma gravidarum, under melasma.

chlorambucil (klor-am'bu-sil) An anticancer drug prescribed to treat certain types of cancer (e.g., chronic lymphocytic leukemia and Hodgkin's disease). Cardiovascular anomalies and absence of a kidney and ureter have been reported as a result of intrauterine exposure to chlorambucil.

chloramphenicol (klor-am-fen'ĭ-kol) An antibiotic drug used selectively because it carries the risk of causing irreversible bone marrow suppression; a lactating woman can readily transmit the drug to her breast-feeding infant. It can be associated with 'gray syndrome' (pallid cyanosis, abdominal distention, vascular collapse, and death) when given to preterm infants after birth.

chlordiazepoxide (klor-di-az-ĕ-pok'sīd) A tranquilizer used mainly to treat anxiety; may cause dependence. When taken by a pregnant woman at term, the newborn may experience withdrawal symptoms and exhibit lack of muscle tone for up to 1 week.

2-chloroprocaine (klor-o-pro'kān) Local anesthetic formerly used extensively in obstetric and gynecologic patients; its toxic effects include inflammation of the arachnoid and associated neuropathies.

chlorothiazide (klor-o-thi'ă-zīd) A diuretic drug widely used to reduce fluid retention (commonly due to liver disease and congestive heart failure) and as an adjunct in the management of high blood pressure. Use during pregnancy is discouraged because it adversely affects placental perfusion. It may cause increased risk of congenital defects if taken during the first trimester.

chlorotrianisene (klor-o-tri-an'ĭ-sēn) A synthetic estrogen used for estrogen replacement therapy; formerly used for the suppression of puerperal lactation.

chlorpromazine (klor-pro'mă-zēn) One of the first antipsychotic drugs developed; used as a tranquilizer and to treat nausea and vomiting caused by pregnancy, chemotherapy, radiation therapy, and anesthesia. When administered in the last trimester of pregnancy, it may cause tremors and increased muscle tone in the newborn. Its use during pregnancy is contraindicated.

chlorpropamide (klor-pro'pă-mīd) An oral hypoglycemic agent used to reduce high blood sugar levels (hyperglycemia) in persons with non-insulin-dependent diabetes. Intrauterine exposure causes hyperinsulinism in the newborn, with resulting low blood sugar levels (hypoglycemia). Its use during pregnancy is contraindicated.

chlorthalidone (klor-thal'ĭ-dōn) A diuretic administered orally for the treatment of hypertension and tissue fluid retention; transmitted in milk to a breast-fed infant.

cholagogue (ko'lă-gog) An agent that stimulates the flow of bile into the intestine.

chole-, chol-, cholo- Combining forms meaning bile.

cholestasis (ko-le-sta'sis) Suppression of bile flow; may occur at any level, from the canaliculus in the liver to the duodenum; causes may include use of oral contraceptives, anabolic steroids, and oral antidiabetic drugs.

    intrahepatic c. Accumulation of bile acids in the liver and, later, in blood plasma, causing jaundice and itchiness (pruritis); in the absence of liver and gallbladder disease, it may be attributed to increased hormonal activity (i.e., of estrogen andt progesterone, as seen in oral contraceptive use and in pregnancy).

    intrahepatic c. of pregnancy Intrahepatic cholestasis limited to the pregnant state, with a tendency to recur in subsequent pregnancies; characterized clinically by generalized pruritis (without a skin rash) and, sometimes, mild jaundice; it occurs most commonly during the third trimester but may appear any time after the seventh week of gestation. The condition may be associated with a slight increase in preterm births, stillbirths, and maternal hemorrhage. Also called icterus gravidarum; recurrent jaundice of pregnancy.

cholestatic (ko-le-stat'ik) Tending to suppress bile flow.

cholinesterase (ko-lin-es'ter-ās) See acetylcholinesterase.

chondrosternal (kon-dro-ster'nal) Relating to a cartilage of the breastbone (sternum).

chorea (kor-e'a) Irregular, rapid, jerky, involuntary movements of the face and limbs; they disappear during sleep.

    c. gravidarum Any chorea that develops during pregnancy.

    Sydenham's c. Condition seen most commonly in children, characterized by an acute onset of emotional instability, involuntary movements, muscular weakness, incoordination, and slurred speech usually following (by many months) an episode of rheumatic fever. The individual attack of chorea is self-limited but may last up to 3 months. Formerly called St. Vitus dance.

choreic (ko-re'ik) Relating to chorea.

chorio- Combing form meaning membrane.

chorioadenocarcinoma (ko-re-o-ad'ĕ-no-kar-sĭ-no'mă) See invasive mole, under mole.

chorioadenoma destruens (ko-re-o-ad-ĕ-no'mă des-tru'ens) See invasive mole, under mole.

chorioamnionitis (ko-re-o-am-ne-on-i'tis) Inflammation of the fetal membranes, usually due to infection with microorganisms present in the vagina.

choriocarcinoma (ko-re-o-kar-sĭ-no'mă)
1. Gestational choriocarcinoma; an uncommon but highly malignant tumor of the placenta most often found in the uterus after any type of pregnancy (normal or ectopic), frequently as a complication of a hydatidiform mole; occasionally it occurs after an abortion, or it may develop months after the pregnancy; the tumor is derived from cells of the original placental tissues (trophoblast). Also called chorioepithelioma; chorionic epithelioma; trophoblastoma. **2.** A rare primary germ cell tumor of the ovary unrelated to gestational choriocarcinoma, associated with elevated levels of human chorionic gonadotropin (hCG).

chorioepithelioma (ko-re-o-ep-ĭ-the-le-o mă) See choriocarcinoma.

chorion (ko're-on) The cellular, outermost membrane enclosing the fetus.

    c. frondosum The fetal portion of the

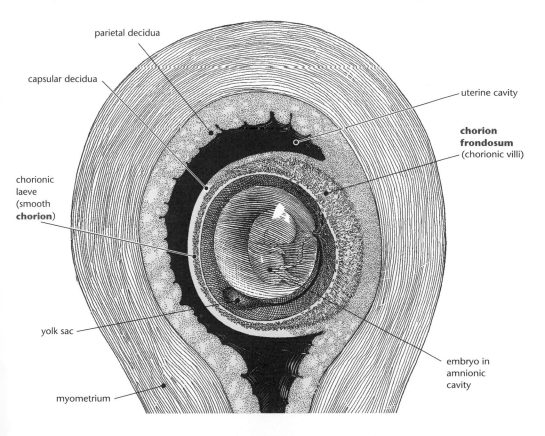

placenta containing numerous branching villi. Also called shaggy chorion; villous chorion.

c. laeve The avascular part of the chorion that is denuded of villi; it constitutes the greater portion of the chorion.

shaggy c. See chorion frondosum.

villous c. See chorion frondosum.

chorionic (ko-re-on'ik) Relating to the chorion.

chromatid (kro'mă-tid) One of two strands in the cell nucleus (joined by a single centromere) formed by longitudinal splitting of a chromosome during mitosis or meiosis. Eventually, each chromatid becomes a chromosome.

chromatin (kro'mă-tin) The irregular clumps of DNA proteins in a cell nucleus that are readily stainable by basic dyes and of which chromosomes are made.

sex c. The chromatin mass situated just inside the nuclear membrane in somatic (body) cells of the normal female. Its presence or absence in cells obtained from a smear of the inside of the cheek (buccal mucosa) has been used as an indicator of the sexual genotype of an individual. Also called Barr chromatin body; Barr body; sex chromatin body; X-chromatin body.

chromonema (kro-mo-ne'mă), pl. chromonemata In genetics, the coiled central filament extending throughout the length of the chromosome and containing the genes.

chromosome (kro'mo-sōm) In any cell, one of a group of threadlike structures that are located within the cell nucleus and contain DNA (deoxyribonucleic acid) encoding genetic information (hereditary material) from both parents. Normally, human cells contain 46 chromosomes.

fragile X c. An abnormal X chromosome that is associated with mental retardation. It has an area associated with chromosome breakage, discernible under special culture medium as a nonstaining band. Female carriers of the fragile X chromosome are usually not afflicted with mental retardation but they can transmit the condition through their daughters (some of whom may also be affected) to their grandchildren. See also fragile X syndrome, under syndrome.

ring c. A chromosome that has lost two fragments, one at each end, and has healed by fusing together the two ends, forming a ring.

sex c. A chromosome that has a major role in determining the sex of an individual; in humans and most animals, they are designated X or Y. Normally females have two X chromosomes (no Ys); males have one X and one Y chromosome.

X c. In humans, a large metacentric sex chromosome.

Y c. In humans, a small acrocentric sex chromosome.

yeast artificial c. (YAC) A DNA segment introduced into the yeast *Saccaromyces cerevisiae* for cloning DNA segments that are larger than those using bacteria as vectors.

chronic (kron'ik) Of slow development and long duration; applied to diseases; the opposite of acute.

ciliogenesis (sil-e-o-jen'ě-sis) The development of fine, short filaments (cilia) on the surface of certain cells.

cine-, cin- Combining forms meaning movement.

cineurography (sin-ě-u-rog'ră-fe) Motion pictures of the bladder in action.

circadian (sir-ka'de-an) Occurring approximately every 24 hours.

circhoral (sir-ko'ral) Occurring approximately once every hour.

circle (ser'kl) A ring-shaped anatomic structure.

arterial c. A ring of arteries formed by the connecting branches of the carotid and basilar arteries at the base of the brain; it is a common site of aneurysms. Also called circle of Willis.

c. of Willis See arterial circle.

circulation (sir-ku-la'shun) Movement through a circular course; unless otherwise specified, the term refers to blood circulation.

collateral c. Alternative circulation through small connecting blood vessels when the normally larger vessels are occluded.

coronary c. The blood flow through the vessels supplying the heart muscle.

enterohepatic c. Normal passage of substances through the liver, into the bile, through the intestines, and back to the liver.

extracorporeal c. Temporary diversion of blood through a special machine that performs the function of an organ (e.g., through a heart-lung machine for oxygen–carbon dioxide exchange, or through an artificial kidney for dialysis).

fetal c. The blood flow through the blood vessels of the fetus, carried to the placenta (by two arteries in the umbilical cord) and returned from the placenta to the fetus (by a vein in the umbilical cord).

lymphatic c. The flow of lymph from tissue spaces to the circulating blood; it begins in minute blind channels within spaces of many body tissues; contraction of surrounding muscles compresses the lymphatic channels, moving the lymph toward the lymph nodes; from the nodes, the lymph eventually reaches either the thoracic duct, which empties lymph into the left subclavian vein, or the right lymphatic duct, which empties lymph into the right subclavian vein.

placental c. The flow of blood through the intervillous space of the placenta, which

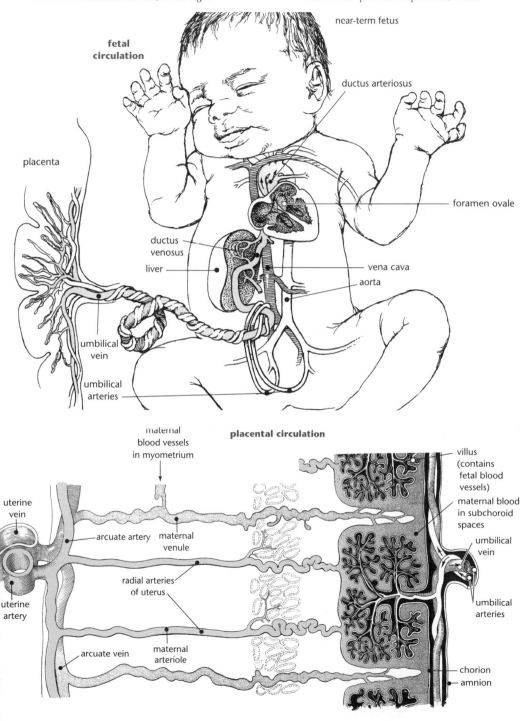

fetal circulation

near-term fetus

ductus arteriosus

placenta

foramen ovale

ductus venosus

liver

vena cava

aorta

umbilical vein

umbilical arteries

maternal blood vessels in myometrium

placental circulation

villus (contains fetal blood vessels)

maternal blood in subchoroid spaces

uterine vein

arcuate artery   maternal venule

umbilical vein

radial arteries of uterus

uterine artery

umbilical arteries

arcuate vein   maternal arteriole

chorion

amnion

transfers oxygen and nutritive materials from mother to fetus and carbon dioxide and waste products from fetus to mother.

portal c. (1) The blood flow through the spleen, pancreas, stomach, and intestines, carried to the liver via the portal vein. (2) In general, any blood circulation between the capillary beds of two organs before the blood returns to the heart (e.g., between the hypothalamus and pituitary in the brain).

pulmonary c. The flow of blood from the heart, through the pulmonary artery and lungs, and back to the heart through the pulmonary veins.

systemic c. Blood circulation through the whole body.

third c. See twin–twin transfusion syndrome, under syndrome.

circum- Prefix meaning around, surrounding, about.

circumanal (sir-kum-a'nal) See perianal.

circumcision (sir-kum-sizh'un) The cutting away of the foreskin of the penis or clitoris.

pharaonic c. See infibulation.

circumvolute (sir-kum-vo'lūt) Twisted around a central axis.

cirrhosis (sĭ-ro'sis) General term for any liver disease characterized by loss of the lobular architecture of the liver with formation of fibrous scars, nodules, and abnormal interconnections between arteries and veins; these abnormalities interfere with liver function and circulation. Symptoms may include appetite and weight loss, weakness, fatigue, diarrhea, and vomiting.

cis- 1. Prefix meaning on this side. 2. In genetics, prefix denoting the location of two genes on the same chromosome of a homologous pair.

cisplatin (sis'plat-in) A compound used in the treatment of cancer, especially of the testis and ovary; it may cause kidney damage. It is potentially hazardous to the fetus when taken during pregnancy.

cissa, citta (sis'ă, sit'ă) See pica.

Citrobacter (sit-ro-bak'ter) A genus of Gram-negative bacteria (family Enterobacteriaceae); a variety of species cause infections of the alimentary and urinary tracts, neonatal meningitis, and opportunistic infections in debilitated persons.

clamp (klamp) An instrument for compressing a part or tissue.

bulldog c. A small cross-action clamp for occluding cut blood vessels; the jaws are frequently covered with rubber tubing to prevent injury to the vascular wall. Also called bulldog forceps.

classification (klas-ĭ-fĭ-ka'shun) A systematic grouping according to established criteria.

Bethesda system of c. A system of classification used in cytopathology reports for describing results of the cytologic examination of a cervical/vaginal specimen (Pap smear). It is basically composed of three categories: *specimen adequacy* (e.g., satisfactory, satisfactory but limited, unsatisfactory); *general categorization* (e.g., within normal limits, benign cellular changes, epithelial cell abnormality); and *descriptive diagnosis* (e.g., low grade squamous intraepithelial lesion [mild dysplasia], high grade squamous intraepithelial lesion [severe dysplasia], cancer [adenocarcinoma, squamous cell carcinoma, etc.]. Sometimes simply called Bethesda system.

Breslow c. Classification of melanoma of the skin, including skin of the vulva, based on the depth of invasion. It includes six levels of depth, measured in millimeters from the epidermis through the subcutaneous fat tissue: 1.0 mm, 1.5 mm, 2 mm, 3 mm, 4 mm, and 5 mm.

Buttram and Gibbons c. of uterine anomalies A classification of uterine anomalies useful in assessing pregnancy performance.

Caldwell-Moloy c. Classification of the female pelvis as gynecoid, android, anthropoid, and platypelloid, based on anteroposterior and transverse dimensions of the pelvic inlet.

Clark's c. Classification of melanoma of the skin of the vulva, using five histologic depth levels of involvement. *Level I, in situ* melanoma in which all demonstrable malignant cells are in the epidermis, superficial to the basement membrane. *Level II*, tumor crosses the basement membrane and invades the papillary dermis. *Level III*, tumor fills the papillary dermis up to (but does not invade) the reticular dermis. *Level IV*, tumor invades the reticular dermis. *Level V*, tumor invades subcutaneous fat tissue.

Rutledge c. Classification of extended hysterectomy for the treatment of cervical cancer, based on the extent of tissue involvement. *Class I*, extrafascial hysterectomy with lateral deflection of the ureters through an incision in the pubocervical ligament, indicated for intraepithelial neoplasm and for early stromal invasion. *Class II*, moderately extended radical hysterectomy with removal of the medial half of the cardinal and uterosacral ligaments, and upper third of the vagina;

indicated for microinvasion beyond early stromal involvement and local postirradiation recurrence. *Class III*, wide incision, including entire cardinal and uterosacral ligaments and upper third of the vagina; indicated for stage Ib and IIa involvement. *Class IV*, extended radical hysterectomy with removal of all periureteral tissue, superior vesical artery, and

three fourths of the vagina; indicated for anterior central recurrences where preservation of the bladder is possible. *Class V*, removal of bladder and adjacent (distal) portions of the ureters; indicated for central recurrence of disease involving those structures.

Tanner c. Classification of female adolescent

THE BETHESDA SYSTEM OF CLASSIFICATION (Revised 1991)

I   Adequacy of Specimen
   A. Satisfactory for evaluation
   B. Satisfactory for evaluation but limited by ... (specify reason)
   C. Unsatisfactory for evaluation ... (specify reason)

II   General Categorization (optional)
   A. Within normal limits
   B. Benign cellular changes. See descriptive diagnosis
   C. Epithelial cell abnormality. See descriptive diagnosis

III Descriptive Diagnosis
   A. Benign Cellular Changes

      1. Infection
         a. *Trichomonas vaginalis*
         b. Fungal organisms morphologically consistent with *Candida* species
         c. Predominance of coccobacilli consistent with shift in vaginal flora
         d. Bacteria morphologically consistent with *Actinmyces* species
         e. Cellular changes associated with herpes simplex virus
         f. Other

      2. Reactive changes
         Reactive cellular changes associated with:
         a. Inflammation (includes typical repair)
         b. Atrophy with inflammation ("atrophic vaginitis")
         c. Radiation
         d. Intrauterine contraceptive device (IUD)
         e. Other

   B. Epithelial Cell Abnormalities

      1. Squamous cell
         a. Atypical squamous cells of undetermined significance: Qualify
         b. Low grade squamous intraepithelial lesion encompassing: HPV mild dysplasia/CIN 1
         c. High grade squamous intraepithelial lesion encompassing: moderate and severe dysplasia, CIS/CIN 2, and CIN 3
         d. Squamous cell carcinoma

      2. Glandular cell
         a. Endometrial cells, cytologically benign, in a postmenopausal woman
         b. Atypical glandular cells of undetermined significance: Qualify
         c. Endocervical adenocarcinoma
         d. Endometrial adenocarcinoma
         e. Extrauterine adenocarcinoma
         f. Adenocarcinoma, not otherwise specified

      3. Other malignant neoplasms: Specify

      4. Hormonal Evaluation (applies to vaginal smears only)
         a. Hormonal pattern compatible with age and history
         b. Hormonal pattern incompatible with age and history: Specify
         c. Hormonal evaluation not possible due to ... Specify

development into five stages based on development of secondary sexual characteristics (i.e., breasts and pubic hair).

White's c. of diabetes mellitus A scheme used in prenatal care for determining the fetal risk associated with the degenerative systemic effects of diabetes mellitus.

clathrin (klath'rin) A lattice of specific protein on cell membranes that facilitates receptor-mediated internalization of low density lipoprotein (LDL) and the uptake of such substances as insulin, epidermal growth factor (EGF), nerve growth factor (NGF), and a variety of viruses.

claustrum (klaws'trum) An anatomic structure resembling a barrier.

c. virginale See hymen.

clavicle (klav'ĭ-kl) The long, curved bone forming the anterior portion of the pectoral girdle; composed of: the sternal end, which articulates with the manubrium of the breastbone (sternum) and provides attachment for the sternohyoid, sternocleidomastiod, pectoralis major, and subclavius muscles; the acromial end, which articulates with the acromion at the shoulder joint and provides attachment for the deltoid and trapezius muscles; the body, the elongated portion of the bone.

clearance (klēr'ans) **1.** Removal of a substance from the body by an excretory organ (e.g., the kidney). **2.** The space between apposed structures (e.g., teeth). **3.** In toxicology, the rate at which a toxic agent is excreted, divided by the average concentration of the agent in the plasma. It is a measure of the volume of fluid that is freed of a toxic agent per unit time, rather than the amount of toxic substance removed.

creatinine c. Rate at which the kidney removes endogenous or exogenous creatinine from blood plasma; an approximate measure of glomerular filtration rate. Normal values are 100–125 ml/min for males and 85–125 ml/min for females of average size.

cleavage (klēv'ij) **1.** The series of cell divisions immediately after fertilization of the egg and formation of the zygote; one of these divisions. **2.** The splitting of a molecule into simpler ones.

cleft (kleft) A groove or slit.

branchial c.'s In mammalian embryology, a term loosely applied to bilateral ectodermal grooves (the equivalent of gills in aquatic animals); on rare occasions, they persist in the adult form as fistulas, sinus tracts, or cysts in the neck area.

vulvar c. The cleft between the major lips (labia majora) of the vulva. Also called rima pudendi; pudendal fissure; urogenital fissure.

cleidal (kli'dal) Relating to the collarbone (clavicle).

clido-, clid- Combining forms meaning collarbone (clavicle).

clidotomy (kli-dot'ome) Surgical division of the clavicles of a dead fetus to facilitate its delivery.

climacteric (kli-mak'ter-ik) The phase of the aging process during which a woman passes from the reproductive to the nonreproductive stage; symptoms correlate with the diminution of hormone production and ovarian function and may include hot flushes, headache, vulvar discomfort, painful sexual intercourse, and mental depression. Commonly called the change of life. The term is popularly used interchangeably with menopause.

climacterium (kli-mak-te're-um) See climacteric.

climax (kli'maks) **1.** The stage of greatest severity in the course of a disease. **2.** Orgasm.

clinic (klin'ik) **1.** A facility where treatment is given to patients not requiring hospitalization. **2.** Medical instruction given to students in which patients are examined and treated in their presence. **3.** An establishment run by medical specialists working cooperatively.

clinical (klin'ĭ-kal) **1.** Relating to the bedside observation of the course and symptoms of a disease. **2.** Relating to a clinic.

clip (klip) **1.** A device used in surgical procedures to approximate cut skin edges or to stop or prevent bleeding. **2.** A clasp.

aneurysmal c. Any of several noncrushing clips used in the surgical treatment of cerebral aneurysms; they usually have a spring mechanism that allows their removal, repositioning, and reapplication.

Filshie c. A rubber-lined, hinged clip used in female tubal sterilization. The clip is placed around the fallopian (uterine) tube to compress and destroy 4 mm of the tube.

Hulka-Clemens spring c. Clip designed to occlude and destroy 4 mm of a fallopian (uterine) tube for female sterilization; it consists of two hinged plastic jaws with teeth on opposing surfaces; a stainless steel spring sleeve keeps the clip closed once it is placed around the tube.

towel c. A forceps for clipping towels to the skin at the edge of the operative field. Also called towel forceps.

clitoral (klit'ŏ-ral) Relating to the clitoris.

clitoridectomy (klit-ŏ-rĭ-dek'to-me) Surgical removal of the clitoris.

clitorimegaly (klit-ŏ-rĭ-meg'ă-le) A clitoris measuring more than 10 mm in width.

clitoris (klit'ŏ-ris, kli'tor-is, klĭ-tor'is) The

homologue of the penis; a structure partially enclosed between the anterior ends of the labia minora and normally measuring 2 to 3 cm in length and 2 to 4 mm in width; it has a body, consisting of two corpora cavernosa that contain dense fibers enveloping erectile tissue, and a free extremity (glans clitoridis), a small rounded tubercle composed of erectile tissue.

clitorism (klit'ŏ-rizm) **1.** Prolonged, usually painful, erection of the clitoris. **2.** Abnormal large size of the clitoris.

clitoromegaly (klit-ŏ-ro-meg'ă-le) See clitorimegaly.

cloaca (klo-a'kă) In mammalian embryology, the common ending of the intestinal and genitourinary tracts of an early embryo.

clomiphene citrate (klo'mĭ-fēn ci'trāt) A weakly estrogenic nonsteroidal substance with a chemical structure similar to that of estrogen; it can be used to induce ovulation. Although it can increase sperm production, it does not increase fertility.

clonazepam (klo-naz'ĕ-pam) Anticonvulsant drug administered orally; may cause apnea; it is transmitted in breast milk to nursing infants, potentially causing the same effect.

cloning (klōn'ing) **1.** The asexual development of a colony of genetically identical cells from a single cell (common ancestor) by repeated cell divisions. **2.** Transplantation of the nucleus of a somatic (body) cell to an ovum for the purpose of developing an embryo through sexual reproduction.

    gene c. The process of making copies of a gene by first isolating it and then inserting it into cells and allowing it to multiply.

Clostridium (klos-trid'e-um) A genus of bacteria (family Bacillaceae) composed of Gram-positive, anaerobic or aerotolerant, rod-shaped organisms commonly found in soil. Some species cause putrefaction of proteins.

    C. difficile A species found in 25% of normal adults. Subsequent to antibiotic therapy, a pseudomembranous colitis may develop from the toxin of this bacterium.

    C. perfringens A species found in soil and milk; the causative agent of gas gangrene and postpartum infections (e.g., postpartum endometritis, puerperal fever) within the first 24 hours after childbirth or after an abortion; may also cause intestinal conditions (e.g., enteritis, appendicitis). Also called gas bacillus; Welch bacillus.

    C. sordelli A species that has been associated with toxic shock syndrome.

clot (klot) **1.** A thrombus or semisolid mass formed from a liquid. **2.** To form such a mass.

    blood c. An elastic mass containing fibrin, platelets, red blood cells, and white blood cells; the product of whole blood coagulation.

clotrimazole (klo-trim'ă-zol) A broad spectrum fungicidal agent used for the treatment of candidal and other fungal infections.

clubfoot (klub'foot) See *talipes equinovarus*.

coagulation (ko-ag-u-la'shun) **1.** The process of clot formation, especially of blood. **2.** A clot.

    disseminated intravascular c. (DIC) The presence of numerous widespread blood clots in minute blood vessels throughout the body, occurring as a complication of a variety of disorders, e.g., obstetric conditions (abruptio placentae, retained dead fetus in the uterus, septic abortion, amniotic fluid embolism), cancers, infectious diseases, massive trauma, extensive surgery and burns. Symptoms vary depending on the underlying disorder; may be acute (as in amniotic fluid embolism and major trauma) or chronic (as in retention of dead fetus and cancer). Outcome also varies.

coagulative (ko-ag'u-lă-tiv) Capable of causing clotting.

coagulopathy (ko-ag-u-lop'ă-the) Any disease that affects the blood-clotting mechanism.

    consumption c. A marked reduction of platelets and certain blood clotting factors in the blood, resulting from utilization of platelets in excessive blood clotting throughout the body.

coagulum (ko-ag'u-lum), pl. coagula A blood clot.

coarctation (ko-ark-ta'shun) A constriction, as of a blood vessel.

    c. of aorta Congenital defect characterized by a localized narrowing of the aorta (large artery leaving the left atrium of the heart), just beyond the point where the left subclavian artery branches off the vessel.

cobalt (ko'bawlt) Metallic element; symbol Co, atomic number 27, atomic weight 58.94.

cobalt 60 A radioactive isotope of cobalt used as a source of gamma rays in place of radium for the treatment of cancer and in radiography.

cocaine (ko'kān) A narcotic alkaloid extracted from coca leaves or synthesized from ergomine or its derivatives; when used habitually or in excess, it causes functional changes of the cardiovascular system, the central nervous system, the autonomic nervous system, and the gastrointestinal system, as well as psychosocial changes.

    crack c. The purified, potent form of cocaine; it is usually smoked (free-based), injected intravenously, or taken orally.

Popularly called crack.

cocarcinogen (ko-kar-sin'ŏ-jen) An agent that increases the activity of a cancer-producing substance.

coccyx (kok'siks), pl. coccyges The small triangular bone at the inferior end of the vertebral column; composed of three to five fused rudimentary vertebrae; it articulates with the sacrum and provides attachment to the lavator ani and coccygeus muscles on its pelvic surface and to the gluteus maximus and external sphincter ani muscles on its dorsal surface.

cocktail (kok'tāl) A liquid mixture of several ingredients.

Brompton c. A drink containing cocaine hydrochloride and morphine hydrochloride, given orally as a pain reliever to patients who are dying of cancer. Also called Brompton mixture.

code (kōd) **1.** A system of symbols or characters designed to transmit information. **2.** A set of rules establishing a standard. **3.** To assign a standard designation (e.g., a number) to a disease or a medical procedure. The use of numbers for standard nomenclature facilitates epidemiologic surveys; the numerical coding for procedures is the basis of billing third parties for services performed.

genetic c. The pattern of three adjacent nucleotides in a DNA molecule that controls protein synthesis.

codon (ko'don) The set of three adjacent nucleotides in DNA or RNA that codes the insertion of one specific amino acid in the synthesis of a protein chain; the term is also used for corresponding (and complementary) sequences of three nucleotides in messenger RNA into which the original DNA sequence is transcribed.

initiation c.'s Codons (AUG and sometimes GUG) that act as 'start' signals, coding for synthesis of polypeptide chains.

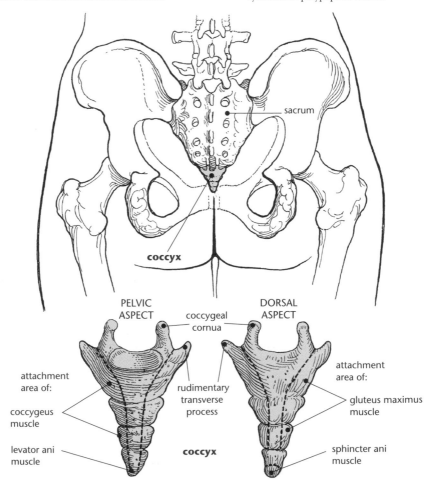

sacrum

coccyx

PELVIC ASPECT

DORSAL ASPECT

coccygeal cornua

attachment area of:

coccygeus muscle

levator ani muscle

rudimentary transverse process

coccyx

attachment area of:

gluteus maximus muscle

sphincter ani muscle

stop c.'s See termination codons.

termination c.'s Codons (UAA, UGA, UAG) that specify a stop of translation of RNA into protein. Also called stop codons.

coital (ko′ĭ-tal) Relating to vaginal sexual intercourse.

coitus (ko′ĭ-tus) Vaginal sexual intercourse between man and woman.

c. interruptus Withdrawal of the penis from the vagina just prior to ejaculation; used as a method of contraception. Also called onanism.

c. reservatus Coitus in which ejaculation is intentionally delayed or suppressed.

colectomy (ko-lek′to-me) Excision of the colon or parts thereof.

colitis (ko-li′tis) Inflammation of the colon.

granulomatous c. Colitis producing lesions in the wall of the colon similar to those seen in the small intestine in cases of regional enteritis.

infectious c. General term for acute inflammation of the colon caused by any of a variety of infectious microorganisms.

pseudomembranous c. An acute form of colitis characterized by formation of a membrane-like substance covering eroded areas of intestinal lining; the substance is composed of gray-yellow inflammatory debris, fibrin, and mucosal elements. Caused usually by toxin of the bacterium *Clostridium difficile*, especially in patients undergoing long-term antibiotic therapy; may also be caused by other infections.

ulcerative c. A recurrent, chronic disease of uncertain cause, affecting primarily the rectum and adjacent sigmoid colon; characterized by ulceration of the mucosa and submucosa; it causes lower abdominal pain and diarrhea with passage of blood and mucus in the stool.

colon (ko′lon) The longest and middle portion of the large intestine (the others being the cecum and the rectum); it is continuous proximally with the cecum and distally with the rectum.

ascending c. The part of the colon on the right side of the abdomen; it extends upward from the cecum toward the liver, where it curves sharply to the left, forming the right flexure of the colon. Also called right colon.

descending c. The part of the colon on the left side of the of the abdomen; it extends downward, from the left flexure to the pelvic brim. Also called left colon.

left c. See descending colon.

right c. See ascending colon.

pelvic c. See sigmoid colon.

sigmoid c. The S-shaped, terminal portion of the colon, situated in the pelvis between the descending colon and the rectum. Also called pelvic colon.

transverse c. The relatively horizontal portion of the colon; it crosses the upper part of the abdomen from the right flexure to the left side of the abdomen, where it curves sharply downward, forming the left flexure of the colon.

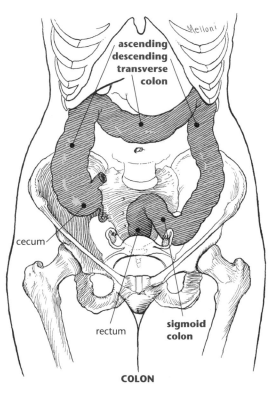

COLON

colotomy (ko-lot′o-me) Opening into the colon.

colostomy (ko-los′to-me) The surgical establishment of an opening (stoma) into the colon through the abdominal wall to allow evacuation of intestinal contents.

colostrorrhea (kŏ-los-tro-re′ă) An abundant discharge of colostrum.

colostrum (kŏ-los′trum) A sticky yellowish fluid produced by the breasts during late pregnancy and the first few days after delivery; it contains less fat and sugar, and more minerals and proteins than milk; it is rich in a certain type of white blood cells (lymphocytes) and antibodies (immunoglobulins), which help protect the newborn from infection. Popularly called foremilk.

colpalgia (kol-pal′jĕ) See vaginodynia.

colpatresia (kol-pă-tre'zě) Occlusion of the vagina.

colpectomy (kol-pek'tŏ-me) Surgical removal of the vagina.

colpitis (kol-pi'tis) Vaginitis.

    c. emphysematosa See emphysematous vaginitis, under vaginitis.

    c. macularis Condition of the vagina characterized by generalized redness with multiple small purplish 'strawberry' spots (petechiae); caused by infection with the flagellated protozoan *Trichonomas vaginalis*.

colpo-, colp- Combining forms meaning vagina.

colpocleisis (kol-po-kli'sis) Suturing of the vaginal canal to obliterate its lumen.

colpocystocele (kol-po-sis'to-sēl) See cystocele.

colpodynia (kol-po-din'e-ă) See vaginodynia.

colpohysterectomy (kol-po-his-ter-ek'to-me) See vaginal hysterectomy, under hysterectomy.

colpomicroscope (kol-po-mi'kro-skōp) A high-powered microscope, especially designed for insertion into the vagina, for direct examination of cells and tissues of the cervix *in situ*.

colpoplasty (kol'po-plas-te) See vaginoplasty.

colpopoiesis (kol-po-poi-e'sis) Surgical construction of a vagina, when none exists, by dissection and insertion of a split thickness graft.

colpoptosis (kol-po-to'sis) Prolapse of the vagina.

colporrhaphy (kol-por'ă-fe) 1. The suturing of a vaginal tear. 2. Restructuring of the vaginal wall.

    anterior c. (1) Surgical repair of a large cystocele by reconstructing and reinforcing the vesicovaginal tissues (anterior vaginal wall); often performed in combination with posterior colpoperineorrhaphy and vaginal hysterectomy to correct a coexisting rectocele and pelvic floor relaxation. (2) A transvaginal approach to the reconstruction of the endopelvic fascia supporting the bladder neck (the urethrovesical junction) for the treatment of stress urinary incontinence (SUI). Also called Kelly plication; Kennedy plication.

colporrhexis (kol-po-rek'sis) Laceration or tearing of the vagina.

colposcope (kol'po-skōp) A low-powered microscope with a built-in light source for

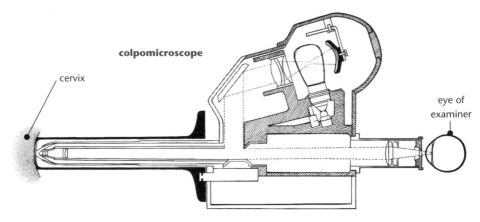

colpomicroscope

cervix

eye of examiner

colpomicroscopy (kol-po-mi-kros'ko-pe) Examination of cells of the cervix by means of a colpomicroscope.

colpoperineorrhaphy (kol-po-per-ĭ-ne-or'ă-fe) Surgical repair and reinforcement of a lacerated vagina and musculature of the pelvic floor. Also called vaginoperineorrhaphy.

    posterior c. Colpoperineorrhaphy performed for the correction of a large rectocele and a generalized relaxation of the pelvic floor; involves the reconstruction of the rectovaginal connective tissues and levator muscles; often performed in combination with an anterior colporraphy and vaginal hysterectomy.

colpopexy (kol'po-pek-se) See vaginopexy.

examination of the vagina and cervix under magnification.

colposcopy (kol-pos'kŏ-pe) Visualization of the cervical and vaginal tissues under magnification by means of a colposcope; performed after obtaining a positive Pap test or to evaluate suspicious lesions.

colpospasm (kol'po-spazm) See vaginismus.

colpostat (kol'po-stat) An intracavitary applicator containing radioactive material used in local irradiation of a gynecologic cancer.

colpostenosis (kol-po-stě-no'sis) Abnormal narrowing of the vaginal lumen.

colpotomy (kol-pot'ŏ-me) Incision through the vaginal wall (e.g., to drain a pelvic abscess). Also called vaginotomy.

colpourethropexy (kol-po-u-re-thro-peks'e) See urethrocystopexy.

colpoxerosis (kol-po-ze-ro'sis) Abnormal dryness of the vaginal lining.

column (kol'um) A cylindrical, pillar-shaped structure.

    spinal c. See vertebral column.

    vertebral c. The assemblage of vertebrae, from just below the skull through the coccyx, that encloses and provides flexible support to the spinal cord. Also called backbone; spinal column; spine.

coma (ko'mă) A condition of unresponsiveness from which the person cannot be aroused. See also stupor.

    diabetic c. Coma occurring almost exclusively in type I (insulin dependent) diabetes as a result of severe diabetic ketoacidosis. See also hypoglycemic coma.

    hypoglycemic c. Coma occurring in persons with type I (insulin-dependent) diabetes mellitus when the blood sugar (glucose) level becomes excessively low; it may occur when food consumed is less than the usual amount or due to overdosage of insulin.

comedocarcinoma (ko-me-do-kar-sĭ-no'mă) Carcinoma of the breast, filling and plugging the milk (lactiferous) ducts with a necrotic substance that can be expressed with slight pressure.

commissure (kom'ĭ-shur) **1.** The small area where corresponding parts meet (e.g., upper and lower eyelids, adjacent cusps of a heart valve). **2.** A bundle of fibers crossing the midline of the brain or spinal cord.

    anterior c. of labia The junction of the labia majora anteriorly, at the mons pubis.

commissurotomy (kom-ĭ-shūr-ot'ŏ-me) Surgical division of a commissure.

    mitral c. Surgical separation of the abnormally fused leaflet of a mitral (left atrioventricular) valve of the heart for the treatment of mitral stenosis.

communication (ko-mu-nĭ-ka'shun) **1.** The transmission of ideas, attitudes, or beliefs between individuals or groups by any means. **2.** The information transmitted. **3.** In anatomy, an access or connecting passage between two structures.

    autocrine c. The act whereby a single cell produces a regulatory substance that activates receptors on or within the same cell.

    intracrine c. The binding of an unsecreted substance to receptors located within the cell producing the substance.

    paracrine c. Diffusion of a regulatory substance from the cell that produces the

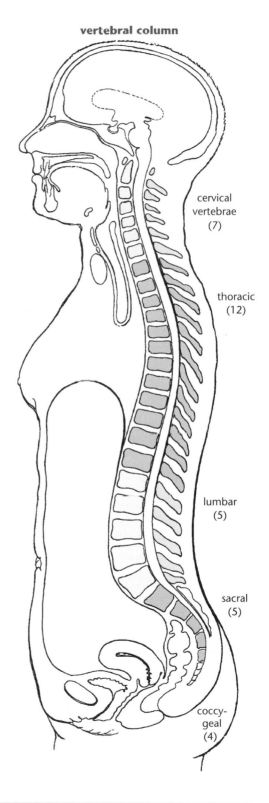

vertebral column

cervical vertebrae (7)

thoracic (12)

lumbar (5)

sacral (5)

coccygeal (4)

substance to other, adjacent, cells.

complement (kom'plĕ-ment) (C) In immunology, a group of proteins in normal serum that become involved in the control of inflammation, the activation of phagocytes (cells that engulf nonself particles, bacteria, and other cells), and the destructive attack on cell membranes. The reaction of the complement system can be activated by the body's immune system.

   c. component Any of the nine proteins participating in the sequential activities of complement (complement cascade). Each complement component takes its turn in the precise chain-reaction steps set in motion (like a domino effect) when the first protein in the complement series is activated. Complement components are named on the basis of functional activity by the symbols C1 through C9.

complex (kom'pleks) **1.** A collection of interrelated parts or factors. **2.** In electrocardiography, a group of deflections corresponding to a part of the heart cycle.

   AIDS-related c. A group of symptoms and signs representing a stage in the course of AIDS (i.e., manifestation of AIDS before the body is attacked by the pathogens of such opportunistic diseases as *Pneumocystis carinii* pneumonia, Kaposi's sarcoma, and others). See also AIDS.

   immune c. A complex composed of antigen and antibody molecules linked together in a lattice-like network; it may also contain proteins of the complement system.

   major histocompatibility c. (MHC) A cluster of closely linked gene loci on chromosome 6 coding for cell proteins that determine tissue type and transplant compatibility.

   Mycobacterium avium c. (MAC) A bacterial complex that includes several strains of *Mycobacterium avium* and the immunologically related *Mycobacterium intracellulare*; most frequently found in respiratory secretions from persons with a tuberculous-like lung disease; it is the cause of a disseminated blood infection (MAC bacteremia) in AIDS patients. Distinguished from *Mycobacterium avium*, which causes disease primarily in birds. See also *Mycobacterium avium* complex bacteremia, under bacteremia.

   oocyte-cumulus-corona c. (OCCC) In *in vitro* fertilization, the entirety of the egg and its accompanying cellular coverings harvested from the ovary.

compliance (kom-pli'ans) **1.** The quality of yielding to pressure. **2.** A measure of the ease

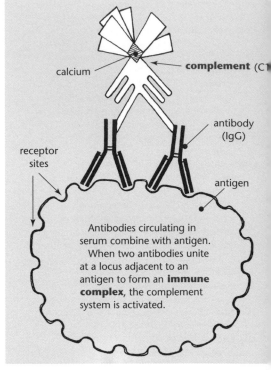

Antibodies circulating in serum combine with antigen. When two antibodies unite at a locus adjacent to an antigen to form an **immune complex**, the complement system is activated.

with which an air- or fluid-filled organ (e.g., lungs and bladder) may be distended. **3.** A patient's disposition to follow a specific regimen prescribed by a health professional.

compression (kom-presh'un) Pressing together.

   aortocaval c. Compression of the abdominal aorta and inferior vena cava by the weight of the uterus when the pregnant woman at term, or near term, lies on her back; compression is relieved when she lies on her side.

   digital c. Pressure applied with the fingers over a cut blood vessel to stop bleeding.

   uterine c. Bimanual procedure for controlling uterine hemorrhage immediately following delivery of the placenta. The uterus is compressed and massaged for 20 minutes or longer with one hand placed on the patient's abdomen and the other hand introduced into the vagina.

con- Prefix meaning with, together, in association.

concentration (kon-sen-tra'shun) **1.** The quantity of a specified substance in a unit (of volume or weight) of another substance. **2.** A pharmaceutical preparation that has had its strength increased by evaporation (e.g., by evaporating the solvent of a solution).

   mean cell hemoglobin c., mean corpuscle

hemoglobin c. (MCHC) The average hemoglobin concentration in a given volume of packed red blood cells, calculated by dividing the blood hemoglobin concentration by the hematocrit.

spermatozoa c. The number of spermatozoa in 1.0 ml of semen. Normal values range from 20 to 200 million sperms per 1 ml of semen. In most *in vitro* fertilization (IVF) programs, a semen specimen containing up to 40 million spermatozoa may be considered inadequate (hypofertile).

conception (kon-sep'shun) The fertilization of an ovum by a spermatozoon.

wrongful c. In medical negligence: (1) An unwanted pregnancy resulting from the physician's failure to inform the parents that a sterilization procedure might be unsuccessful, or a promise that the procedure would be successful. (2) Development of a genetically defective fetus resulting from the physician's failure to inform the parents of the genetic risk.

conceptus (kon-sep'tus) All the tissue products of conception from the time the ovum and sperm unite and form a zygote until birth; it includes the placenta, fetal membranes, and the embryo/fetus.

condom (kon'dum) A sheath, usually made of thin latex rubber or plastic; placed over the penis before intercourse to provide a barrier against conception and to provide both partners with protection against sexual transmission of disease. Also called contraceptive sheath; prophylactic.

bikini c. Device resembling a G-string panty with a rolled up condom within the panty crotch; the condom itself is composed of 0.12 mm latex with a water-based lubricant; the condom unrolls upon penile penetration.

female c. Any protective sheath worn by a woman during sexual intercourse as a contraceptive sheath and as protection against minute abrasions and transmission of disease. Also called vaginal pouch.

Reality c. A polyurethane sheath with two flexible rings, a closed one at one end to be fitted internally like a diaphragm and an open one at the other end to remain outside the vagina.

Women's Choice c. Sheath similar to a male condom (the same length but wider) with a thick latex dome and a 5 cm flexible ring at the open end; it is inserted with a tampon-like applicator.

conduct (kon'dukt) The manner in which a person acts.

criminal sexual c. See rape.

conduit (kon'doo-it) A channel.

ileal c. Intestinal conduit constructed from a segment of the ileum. Also called ileal bladder. See also intestinal conduit.

intestinal c. A surgically created channel made for discharging urine through the abdominal wall when the bladder has been removed. It consists of a detached segment of bowel into which the ureters are transplanted at one end; the other end of the segment opens to the exterior through a permanent opening (stoma). The segment may be of the small bowel (e.g., ileum) or large bowel (e.g., sigmoid colon, transverse colon).

conduplicato corpore (kon-doo-pli'-ka'to kor'po-re) The characteristic position of a very small fetus in transverse lie as it passes through the birth canal in spontaneous delivery. The fetus is doubled upon itself, its head and thorax passing through at the same time.

condyloma (kon-di'-lo'mă), pl. condylomata A wartlike growth.

c. acuminatum, pl. condylomata acuminata A soft, pointed, warty growth, or collection of growths, usually occurring around the anus and on the external genitalia of males or females, and in the uterine cervix; when numerous, they become confluent, resembling a cauliflower; caused by infection with human papillomavirus (HPV), usually types 6 and 11; chiefly transmitted through sexual contact; although almost always benign, a squamous carcinoma association, especially in the cervix, has been reported. Also called anorectal wart; genital wart; venereal wart; moist wart; pointed wart; fig wart; verruca acuminata; papilloma venereum; pointed condyloma.

c. latum The highly infectious lesion of the secondary stage of syphilis; it appears as a multiple, slightly elevated, disk-shaped or oval growth with a moist surface and occurs on the genitalia, around the anus, and on the inner thighs and buttocks. Also called moist papule.

pointed c. See condyloma acuminatum.

condylomatous (kon-di'-lo'ma-tus) Relating to a condyloma.

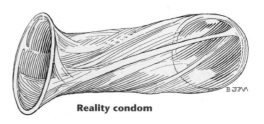

Reality condom

confinement (kon-fīn'ment) The period of childbirth.

congenital (kon-jen'ĭ-tal) Present at birth; denoting a condition manifested, or occurring, at the time of birth; may or may not be genetic. Compare with genetic.

congestion (kon-jest'chun) Abnormal accumulation of blood in a body part resulting from impaired outflow of venous blood with distention of veins, venules, and capillaries; the affected part appears reddish blue and, often, swollen; it may be localized, caused by obstruction of a vein, or generalized (systemic) as seen in heart failure. Sometimes called passive hyperemia.

    hypostatic c. See venous stasis, under stasis.

conization (kon-ĭ-za'shun) Surgical removal of a conical portion of tissue.

    cervical c. Conization of the uterine cervix up to the lower portion of the cervical canal with a scalpel, cautery, laser, or loop electrocautery procedure; usually performed to obtain tissue for diagnosis or to treat small lacerations.

conjugata vera (kon-jōō-ga'tă ver'ă) See true conjugate, under conjugate.

conjugate (kon-jōō-gāt) Coupled, paired.

    diagonal c. The distance between the sacral promontory and the lower border of the pubic symphysis.

    obstetric c. The distance between the sacral promontory and the inner surface of the pubic symphysis (a few millimeters below the upper border of the symphysis), representing the shortest anteroposterior diameter through which the fetal head must pass in its descent through the pelvic inlet. It is determined by subtracting 1.5 to 2 cm from the diagonal conjugate.

    true c. The anteroposterior diameter of the pelvic inlet from the sacral promontory to the upper border of the pubic symphysis. Also called conjugata vera; anteroposterior diameter of pelvic inlet.

conjunctivitis (kon-junk-tĭ-vi'tis) Inflammation of the conjunctiva.

    adult inclusion c. See inclusion conjunctivitis.

fundus of uterus

uterine cavity

cervical conization

cervix

line of excision

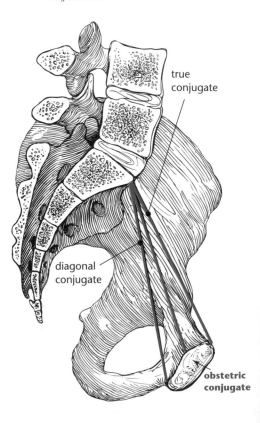

true conjugate

diagonal conjugate

obstetric conjugate

gonococcal c. Acute conjunctivitis characterized by a profuse purulent discharge and edematous eyelids; caused by *Neisseria gonorrhea*, the bacterium causing gonorrhea. Also called gonorrheal conjunctivitis.

gonorrheal c. See gonococcal conjunctivitis.

inclusion c. Acute chlamydial conjunctivitis caused by *Chlamydia oculogenitalis*, occurring most frequently in sexually active people exposed to infected genital secretions; indirect transmission in inadequately chlorinated swimming pools has occasionally been reported; newborn infants usually acquire the infection by direct contact with secretions from an infected birth canal. Also called inclusion blennorrhea; swimming pool conjunctivitis; adult inclusion conjunctivitis.

neonatal c. See ophthalmia neonatorum.

swimming pool c. See inclusion conjunctivitis.

connexin (kŏ-nek'sin) The specific gap-junction protein forming connexons.

connexon (kŏ-nek'son) An assemblage of protein joining its counterpart on the membrane of an adjoining cell, forming a tubelike channel across the intercellular gap; it provides the means of transport of small molecules and ions between cells.

consanguineous (kon-san-gwin'e-us) Genetically related, of the same blood.

consanguinity (kon-san-gwin'ĭ-te) Genetic relationship between individuals that is attributable to a common ancestor; blood relationship.

consciousness (kon'shus-nes) A state of awareness of, and responsiveness to, one's environment.

consent (kon-sent) Voluntary agreement to medical care or treatment by one with the capacity to do so.

informed c. Voluntary permission given by a patient or patient's legal representative for medical, surgical, or experimental treatment, based on full discussion between physician and patient (or patient's representative) of the purpose and potential benefits of the treatment, the risks involved, the possible complications and adverse effects, the consequences of withholding permission, and alternative methods of treatment; the physician is legally obligated to disclose fully to the patient (or patient's representative) all information necessary for a reasoned decision except in a medical emergency; the informed consent obtained from the patient is usually documented in the medical record.

conservative (kon-ser'vă-tiv) Denoting therapeutic practice that is based on cautious methods.

consultand (kon-sul'tand) The person seeking, or referred for, genetic counseling; one whose genetic constitution is in question. Compare with proband.

consultant (kon-sul'tant) A person called upon for expert or professional advice.

medical c. A physician who is called upon to give advice regarding diagnosis or treatment of a patient's illness.

consultation (kon-sul-ta'shun) In medical practice, a meeting of two or more physicians to determine or evaluate the diagnosis or therapy of a patient's condition.

contact (kon'takt) 1. The point or area at which two adjacent structures touch. 2. A person who has been exposed to the causative agent of an infectious disease.

contact tracing Identification of persons or animals who have had an association with an infected person, animal, or contaminated environment and who, through such an association, have had the opportunity to acquire the infection; contact tracing is an accepted method of controlling sexually transmitted diseases.

contagion (kon-ta'jun) The direct or indirect transmission of an infectious disease.

contagious (kon-ta'jus) Transmissible by direct or indirect means. Popularly called catching.

contagium (kon-ta'je-um) The causative agent of a disease.

continence (kon'tĭ-nens) Self-control (e.g., ability to delay urination or defecation).

contraception (kon-tră-sep'shun) The use of drugs, chemicals, devices, methods, or procedures that diminish the likelihood of, or prevent, conception.

contraceptive (kon-tră-sep'tiv) 1. Preventing conception. 2. Anything that prevents conception.

barrier c. See barrier method, under method.

chemical c. An agent (e.g., cream, foam, gel, jelly, suppository) containing a spermicidal substance (e.g., nonoxynol-9) and introduced into the vagina before sexual intercourse.

intrauterine c. See intrauterine device (IUD), under device.

oral c. Any synthetic steroid that is similar to the female hormones, estrogen and progesterone, and is taken orally by regular doses to prevent conception. Oral contraceptives alter the woman's hormonal balance, thereby inhibiting ovulation and preventing pregnancy. Also called birth-control pill. Popularly called the pill.

postcoital c. Oral contraceptive taken within 72 hours after sexual intercourse (coitus); usually a combination of hormones (a progestin and an estrogen). Also called morning-after pill; postcoital pill.

contract (kon-tract') **1.** To compress or shorten (e.g., a muscle). **2.** To acquire (e.g., a disease).

contraction (kon-trak'shun) (C) **1.** A shortening or increase of tension (e.g., of a functioning muscle). **2.** A shrinkage or reduced size. **3.** A heart beat.

Braxton Hicks c.'s Short, relatively painless contractions of the pregnant uterus, usually beginning at irregular intervals during early pregnancy and becoming more frequent and rhythmic as pregnancy advances, especially during the last 2 weeks of gestation, when they may be mistaken for labor pains; they occasionally occur without pregnancy (e.g., in the presence of soft tumors of the uterine wall). See also disordered labor, under labor.

c. of midpelvis Contraction of the midpelvis indicated when the sum of the interspinous and posterior sagittal diameters is 13.5 cm or less.

hourglass c. Narrowing of a hollow organ (e.g., uterus) around its middle area.

c. of pelvic inlet A pelvic inlet with a diagonal conjugate of less than 11.5 cm. Also called inlet disproportion.

c. of pelvic outlet A reduction of the transverse diameter of the pelvic outlet to 8 cm or less. Also called outlet disproportion.

premature c. A premature heart beat.

contraindication (kon-tra-in-dĭ-ka'shun) Any factor in a patient's condition that renders a particular course of treatment undesirable, unwise, or improper.

control (kon-trōl') **1.** An individual or a group used in an experiment or study as a standard against which observations are evaluated. **2.** To verify or evaluate results of an experiment or study against a standard. **3.** Limitation of certain events.

birth c. Deliberate use of contraceptive measures to limit the number of children conceived.

coracoacromial (kor-ă-ko-ă-kro'me-al) Relating to the coracoid and acromial processes of the shoulder blade (scapula). Also called acromiocoracoid.

coracobrachial (kor-ă-ko-bra'ke-al) Relating to the coracoid process of the shoulder blade

(scapula) and the arm.

coracoclavicular (kor-ă-ko-klă-vik'u-lar) Relating to the coracoid process of the shoulder blade (scapula) and the collarbone (clavicle).

cord (kord) Any stringlike structure.

nephrogenic c. A longitudinal mass, derived from the embryonic urogenital ridge, which gives rise to the mesonephric and metanephric tubules of the embryo.

nuchal c. A coil of umbilical cord encircling the fetal neck.

prolapsed c. See funic presentation, under presentation.

spermatic c. The cord extending from the deep inguinal ring to the testis within the scrotum; it contains the deferent duct and associated arteries, veins, nerves, and lymphatic vessels held together within a sheath of connective tissue.

spinal c. The elongated portion of the central nervous system enclosed by the vertebral column.

testicular c.'s An interconnected network of cords of the embryonic testis.

umbilical c. The dull white, slender structure connecting the fetus to the fetal side of the placenta; it consists of a sheet of amnion encasing the umbilical vessels (one vein, carrying oxygenated blood to the fetus, and two arteries carrying deoxygenated blood from the fetus to the placenta) and Wharton's jelly (a connective tissue in which the vessels are embedded); at birth, the cord's dimensions range from 30 to 100 cm in length and 0.8 to 2.0 cm in diameter.

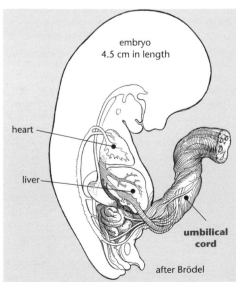

embryo
4.5 cm in length

heart

liver

umbilical cord

after Brödel

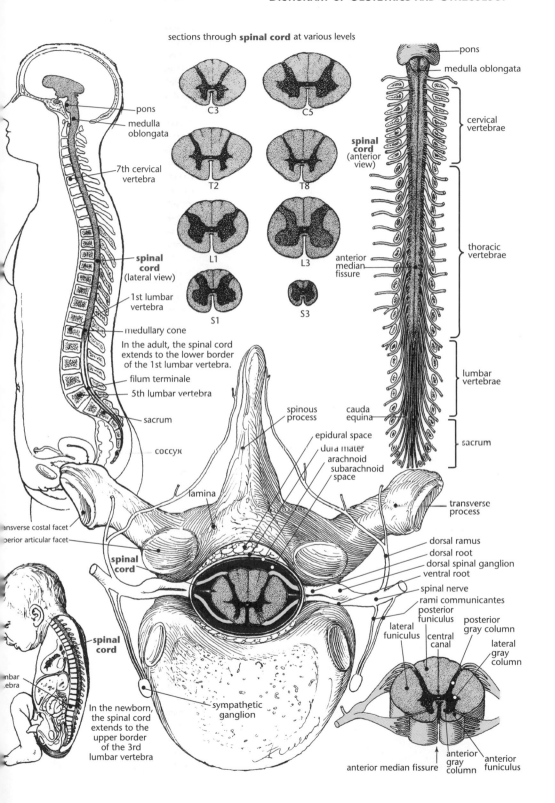

sections through **spinal cord** at various levels

pons

medulla oblongata

spinal cord (anterior view)

cervical vertebrae

thoracic vertebrae

lumbar vertebrae

sacrum

C3

C5

T2

T8

L1

L3

S1

S3

anterior median fissure

pons

medulla oblongata

7th cervical vertebra

spinal cord (lateral view)

1st lumbar vertebra

medullary cone

In the adult, the spinal cord extends to the lower border of the 1st lumbar vertebra.

filum terminale

5th lumbar vertebra

sacrum

coccyx

spinous process

epidural space

dura mater
arachnoid
subarachnoid space

cauda equina

sacrum

lamina

transverse process

transverse costal facet

superior articular facet

spinal cord

spinal cord

lumbar vertebra

In the newborn, the spinal cord extends to the upper border of the 3rd lumbar vertebra

sympathetic ganglion

dorsal ramus
dorsal root
dorsal spinal ganglion
ventral root

spinal nerve
rami communicantes
posterior funiculus

lateral funiculus

central canal

posterior gray column

lateral gray column

anterior median fissure

anterior gray column

anterior funiculus

cord pH The acid–base status of fetal blood as determined by umbilical blood sampling.

cordocentesis (kor-do-sen-te'sis) See percutaneous umbilical cord sampling, under sampling.

corniculate (kor-nik'u-lāt) **1.** Having the shape of a small horn. **2.** Having a horn or hornlike processes.

cornification (kor-nĭ-fĭ-ka'shun) **1.** Changing into keratin, a hornlike substance. **2.** Conversion of epithelium into a keratinized layer of cells.

cornu (kor'noo), pl. cornua **1.** Any horn-shaped anatomic structure. Also called horn. **2.** Any structure composed of hornlike material or tissue.

> **coccygeal cornua** Bilateral extensions from the posterior upper part of the first coccygeal vertebra; they articulate with the cornua of the sacrum. Also called coccygeal horns.

> **sacral cornua** Bilateral processes extending downward from the arch of the fifth or last sacral vertebra; they articulate with the cornua of the coccyx. Also called sacral horns.

> **uterine cornua** See lateral horns of uterus, under horn.

corona (ko-ro'nă), pl. coronas or coronae Any anatomic structure surrounding another, resembling a crown or a wreath.

> **c. radiata** The thin layer of cells from the cumulus oophorus left attached to, and surrounding, the ovum after it is released from the ovary.

coronal (kŏ-ron'al) **1.** Relating to the crown of the head. **2.** Relating to the side-to-side plane of the head or any vertical plane parallel to it.

coronion (kŏ-ro'ne-on) A craniometric point at the tip of the coronoid process of the lower jaw

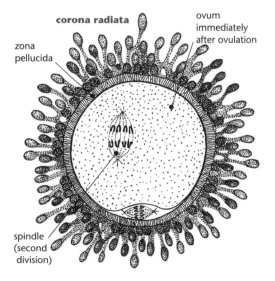

corona radiata
ovum immediately after ovulation
zona pellucida
spindle (second division)

(mandible).

corpus (kor'pus), pl. corpora **1.** The body. **2.** The principal portion of a structure, especially if it can be delimited from its surroundings.

> **c. albicans** The yellowish white, fibrous tissue that replaces the corpus luteum when conception does not occur.

> **c. atreticum** A follicle of the ovary that was unable to mature.

> **c. cavernosum** One of two columns of erectile tissue forming the greater part of the body of the penis (and clitoris); posteriorly, it is continuous with the crus; anteriorly, it inserts into an acorn-shaped cap formed by the glans.

> **c. hemorrhagicum** A blood clot formed in the cavity left by a ruptured ovarian follicle after ovulation (i.e., after the normal rupture of a mature ovarian follicle and release of the ovum).

> **c. luteum** A secretory structure in the ovary formed at the site of a ruptured vesicular ovarian follicle after it has discharged its ovum; it consists of a large mass of lipid-rich cells containing a yellow pigment (lutein); it secretes estrogens and progesterone, the hormones that cause thickening of the uterine lining in preparation for the implantation of the fertilized ovum; if pregnancy occurs, it continues to grow for 13 weeks before slowly regressing; if pregnancy fails to occur, the corpus luteum regresses to a mass of scar tissue (corpus albicans).

> **c. spongiosum** The median cylindrical mass of erectile tissue of the penis, situated between and inferior to the corpora cavernosa and surrounding the urethra; it is continuous with the bulb of the penis posteriorly and the glans penis anteriorly.

corpuscle (kor'pusl) **1.** A small, discrete anatomic structure, such as a microscopic encapsulated nerve ending. **2.** A cell in the body, either one capable of moving freely or restricted to a particular structure. **3.** A primary particle such as a photon or electron.

> **colostral c.** A large, round cellular body containing cytoplasmic fat globules, present in breast secretion occurring in the later stages of pregnancy and for a few days after childbirth; thought to be a phagocytic cell of the mammary gland. Also called galactoblast.

> **Dogiel's c.** See genital corpuscles.

> **genital c.'s** Specialized encapsulated sensory nerve endings, found in the mucous membrane of the external genitalia, in the skin around the nipple and, along with

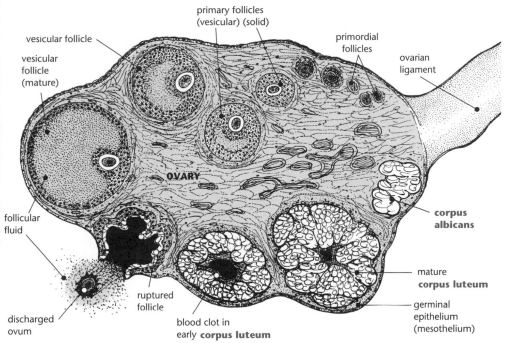

primary follicles
(vesicular) (solid)

vesicular follicle

vesicular
follicle
(mature)

primordial
follicles

ovarian
ligament

OVARY

follicular
fluid

corpus
albicans

discharged
ovum

ruptured
follicle

blood clot in
early **corpus luteum**

mature
corpus luteum

germinal
epithelium
(mesothelium)

Krause's end-bulbs, in the endocervix;
sometimes found in the broad ligament and
around the uterine arteries as they enter the
uterus. Also called Dogiel's corpuscle.

Krause's c. See Krause's end-bulb, under
bulb.

lamellated c.'s Encapsulated nerve endings
(receptor terminals) that possess
circumferential, concentric layers of
connective tissue around the terminal part of
the nerve. Examples include the pacinian
corpuscle, Krause's corpuscle, and genital
corpuscle.

Meissner's c. A small, oval encapsulated
nerve ending with a central core, seen in the
papillae of the skin of the hand and foot, in
the lips, palpebral conjunctiva and the mucous
membrane of the most anterior part of the
tongue; functions as a low-threshold receptor
for the sensation of discriminative touch. Also
called oval corpuscle; tactile corpuscle of
Meissner; corpuscle of touch.

oval c. See corpuscle of Meissner.

pacinian c. A relatively large (up to 2 mm in
length) receptor nerve ending composed of a
capsule with approximately 25 to 35
concentrically arranged lamellae of flattened
cells and a core consisting of approximately 50
to 60 closely packed lamellae positioned on
both sides of a central unmyelinated nerve
terminal; it responds to pressure stimuli from

touch or vibrations and is present in
subcutaneous tissue, fascial planes around
joints and tendons, and in the mesentery
about the pancreas; especially numerous in the
palm of the hand, sole of the foot, and genital
organs; may also be present in the broad
ligament; occasionally seen in the outer coat of
the aorta. Also called Vater-Pacini corpuscle.

Ruffini's c. Encapsulated nerve ending
concerned with the perception of pressure and
of warmth; found in the dermis of hairy skin
and in the superficial layers of the articular
capsules of joints. Also called Ruffini's nerve
ending.

tactile c. of Meissner See Meissner's
corpuscle.

c. of touch See Meissner's corpuscle.

Vater-Pacini c. See pacinian corpuscle.

cortex (kor'teks), pl. cortices The outer layer of an
organ (e.g., of the brain, kidney, or adrenal
gland); distinguished from the inner medullary
substance.

cortical (kor'tĭ-kal) Relating to the cortex.

corticoid (kor'tĭ-koid) See corticosteroid.

corticosteroid (kor-tĭ-ko-ster'oid) Any of the
hormones produced by the cortex of the adrenal
(suprarenal) gland, or a synthetic substitute. Also
called corticoid.

corticosterone (kor-tĭ-kos'ter-ōn) A hormone
that induces deposition of the simple sugar
glycogen in the liver, some retention of sodium,

and excretion of potassium; it is produced in the adrenal cortex.

corticotropin (kor-tĭ-ko-tro'pin) See adrenocorticotropic hormone (ACTH), under hormone.

cortisone (kor'tĭ-sōn) A hormone produced in minute amounts by the adrenal cortex in response to the action of a pituitary hormone (adrenocorticotropic hormone); also produced synthetically.

Corynebacterium parvum (ko-rĭ-ne-bak-te're-um par'vum) **1.** Former name for *Propionibacterium acnes* (an anaerobic bacterium). **2.** A preparation of heat-killed and formaldehyde-treated *Corynebacterium parvum (Propionibacterium acnes)*; used as an immunotherapy agent to stimulate macrophages and depress T cell function.

costal (kos'tal) Relating to a rib.

cotinine (ko'tĭ-nēn) A major byproduct of nicotine; it is rapidly eliminated by the kidneys and excreted in the urine; thought to be an indicator of the amount of tobacco smoke a person has inhaled; has been found excreted in cervical mucus, where it adversely affects immunologic response to infection, and also in the urine of nonsmokers exposed to tobacco smoke.

cotyledon (kot-ĭ-le'don) One of the 15 to 20 subdivisions of the placenta, on the maternal side (i.e., the side that is attached to the uterine wall).

coumarin (koo'mă-rin) An anticoagulant that acts by inhibiting vitamin K-dependent coagulation factors. Coumarin has a significant risk of causing fetal defects; may also cause maternal hemorrhage.

counseling (kown'sel-ing) A type of professional service that includes guidance in psychosocial situations and gives a person an understanding of his or her problems and potentialities.

    genetic c. A professional service that provides individuals and families having a genetic disorder, or at risk of such a disorder, with information about their condition; it also provides information that would allow couples at risk to make informed decisions about having children. See also preconception care, under care.

    preconception c. See preconception care, under care.

count (kount) **1.** The total number of items in a sample (e.g., of blood cells or pollutant particles). **2.** The process of obtaining such a number.

    blood c. The determination of the number of red or white blood cells (RBC or WBC) in a cubic millimeter of blood.

    complete blood c. (CBC) A combination of laboratory tests including red blood cell count, white blood cell count, differential white cell count, hemoglobin concentration, hematocrit, and stained red cell examination; may also include platelet count.

    cornification c. The percentage of precornified and cornified cells in a vaginal cytologic smear; used to assess estrogenic activity.

    differential white cell c. Determination of the percentage of various types of white blood cells that make up the total white blood cell count.

    'kick' c. See fetal movement counting, under counting.

    mitotic c. A histologic criterion for diagnosing leiomyosarcoma of the uterus based on the mitotic activity observed in

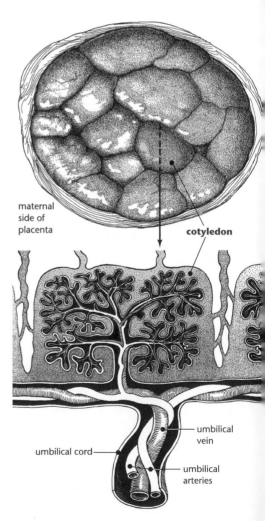

maternal side of placenta

cotyledon

umbilical cord

umbilical vein

umbilical arteries

sample tissue. Malignancy is generally diagnosed if 5 to 9 or more mitoses per 10 HPF (high power field) are present in the histologic sample.

platelet p. Determination of the total number of platelets per cubic millimeter.

reticulocyte c. The number of reticulocytes present in a whole blood sample, expressed as a percentage of the total red cell count; it is normally elevated in pregnancy after 20 weeks of gestation.

sperm c. The total number of sperms (spermatozoa) in the ejaculate. The human ejaculate generally measures 3 to 5 milliliters, with about 50 to 150 million sperms per milliliter. If the ejaculate has fewer than 20 million sperms per milliliter, the male is likely to be infertile.

counting (kount'ing) The act of enumerating.

fetal movement c. (FMC) The daily counting of fetal movements during a 15-minute time frame between 8 a.m. and 8 p.m. (usually after eating a meal or drinking a cold drink to stimulate movement), recording the sum, and noting the time in which 10 movements occur.

coupling (kup'ling) A regular succession of paired heartbeats, a normal beat followed by a premature beat.

cramps, menstrual cramps (kramps, mens'tru-al kramps) Popular terms for dysmenorrhea.

cranio-, crani- Combining forms meaning the cranium.

craniocele (kra'ne-o-sēl) See encephalocele.

craniometric (kra-ne-o-met'rik) Relating to craniometry.

craniometry (kra-ne-om'ĕ-tre) Measurement of the distances between standard points on the skull, and the study of their proportions.

craniopagus (kra-ne-op'ă-gus) Conjoined twins with fused skulls.

craniopuncture (kra'ne-o-punk-chur) Puncture of the skull.

craniorachischisis (kra-ne-o-ră-kis'kĭ-sis) The presence of a fissure or open slit in the skull and vertebral column; a congenital defect.

cranioschisis (kra-ne-os'kĭ-sis) The presence of a congenital fissure or open slit in the skull; a congenital defect.

craniotomy (kra-ne-ot'ŏ-me) **1.** Surgical opening into the skull. **2.** Procedure in which the head of a fetus is punctured with a craniotome and its contents evacuated to allow a vaginal delivery; performed either to deliver a dead fetus or in partial-birth abortion (PBA).

cranium (kra'ne-um), pl. crania The skull; in general, the bones of the head; in particular, the

bones enclosing the brain, excluding the bones of the face.

crease (krēs) A slight linear depression.

plantar c.'s Creases on the soles of a newborn infant, ranging from zero to several creases covering the entire sole; their number and character indicate the degree of the infant's physical maturity.

simian c. A major flexion crease across the entire palm of the hand, formed by fusion of the proximal and distal palmar creases; most frequently seen in persons afflicted with Down's syndrome but it occasionally occurs in normal individuals. Also called simian line.

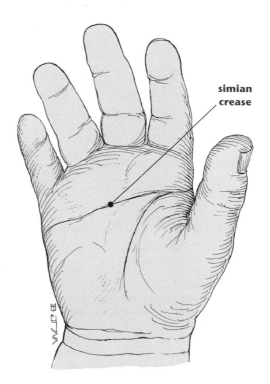

simian crease

creatinine (kre-at'ĭ-nin) (Cr) A product of creatine metabolism and a normal metabolic waste; it is removed from the blood by glomerular filtration in the kidneys and excreted in the urine. Since creatinine is usually produced at a constant rate, the clearance rate and the serum level are used as an index of kidney function.

creatinuria (kre-at-ĭ-nu're-ă) An increased amount of creatine in the urine.

crest (krest) **1.** A bony ridge. **2.** A linear elevation of soft tissue.

ganglionic c. See neural crests.

iliac c. The long, curved upper and outer border of the ilium.

neural c.'s The two bands of ectodermal cells flanking the neural plate of the early embryo; eventually they give rise to the nerve cells of sensory and autonomic ganglia. Also called ganglionic crests.

pubic c. The rough, upper anterior border of the pubic bone.

coma and, occasionally, heart failure. The crisis occurs in patients afflicted with thyrotoxicosis, precipitated by events that cause marked release of thyroid hormone such as thyroid surgery, radioactive thyroid therapy, childbirth, or during a severe illness. Also called thyroid storm; thyroid crisis.

criterion (kri-tēr'e-on), pl. criteria A standard for judging.

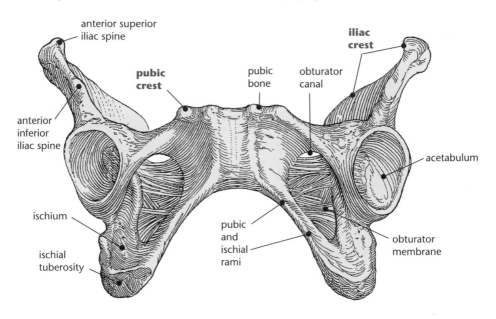

anterior superior iliac spine

iliac crest

pubic crest

pubic bone

obturator canal

anterior inferior iliac spine

acetabulum

ischium

ischial tuberosity

pubic and ischial rami

obturator membrane

urethral c. In the female, a longitudinal fold of mucous membrane on the posterior wall of the urethral canal; the site where many small mucous urethral glands open. In the male, a narrow median longitudinal elevation on the posterior wall of the urethral canal passing vertically through the prostate; the site where the two ejaculatory ducts open.

crisis (kri'sis), pl. crises **1.** A sudden change, for better or worse, in the course of a disease. **2.** A sudden paroxysmal attack of pain or distress.

aplastic c. Transient disappearance of erythroblasts (immature red blood cells) from bone marrow, developing suddenly in patients with such conditions as infections and chronic hemolytic disease.

thyroid c. See thyrotoxic crisis.

thyrotoxic c. A life-threatening flare of thyrotoxicosis, characterized by high fever, rapid pulse, a rise in basic metabolic rate, nausea, vomiting, diarrhea, agitation, delirium,

Spielberg's criteria Criteria used for diagnosis of ovarian pregnancy: *(a)* The uterine tube on the affected side must be intact; *(b)* the amniotic sac must occupy the position of the ovary; *(c)* the amniotic sac must be connected to the uterus by the ovarian ligament; *(d)* ovarian tissue must be present in the wall of the amniotic sac.

critical (krit'ĭ-kl) **1.** Relating to a crisis. **2.** Denoting the state of a patient's illness in which death is possible or imminent.

crown (krown) The top of a structure, as of the head or a tooth.

crowning (krown'ing) In obstetrics, the end of the second stage of labor when the head of the baby is visible, its largest diameter encircled by the stretched vulva.

crura (kroo'rǎ) Plural of crus.

crural (kroor'al) Relating to the leg or thigh.

crus (krus), pl. crura **1.** In anatomic nomenclature, the leg; the region between the

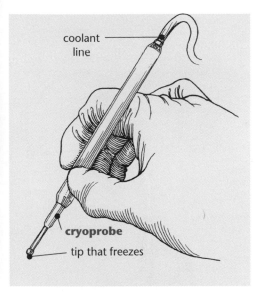

coolant line

cryoprobe

tip that freezes

knee joint and ankle joint. **2.** Any elongated process or leglike structure.

crura of clitoris Two extensions of the corpora cavernosa of the clitoris, attached to the pubic and ischial rami; they converge anteriorly to form the greater part of the body of the clitoris.

c. of inguinal ring Either of two bands forming the margins of the superficial inguinal ring: *Lateral (inferior)*, a curved band forming the lateral (inferior) margin of the superficial inguinal ring; composed of fibers of the inguinal ligament. *Medial (superior)*, a thin, flat band forming the medial (superior) margin of the superficial inguinal ring; composed of the aponeurosis of the external abdominal oblique muscle.

cryo-, cry- Combining forms meaning cold.

cryocautery (kri-o-kaw'ter-e) Destruction of tissue by application of extreme cold.

cryoconization (kri-o-kon-ĭ-za'shun) Removal of a cone of tissue with a freezing instrument (cryoprobe) for diagnostic or therapeutic purposes.

cryopreservation (kri-o-prez-er-va'shun) The preservation of viable cells by freezing.

c. of embryos The freezing of *in vitro* fertilized embryos in liquid nitrogen to allow their implantation at a later date.

cryoprobe (kri'o-prōb) A blunt surgical instrument with a tip that can be maintained at below freezing temperatures; used in cryosurgery (i.e., for destroying tissue or to cause tissue to adhere to the instrument for removal).

cryosurgery (kri-o-sur'jer-e) Surgery performed by the application of freezing temperatures with a cryoprobe.

crypt (kript) A pitlike depression on a surface.

anal c. See anal sinus, under sinus.

crypto-, crypt- Combining forms meaning obscured, without apparent cause, concealed.

cryptogenic (krip-to-jen'ik) Of obscure origin.

cryptolith (krip'to-lith) A concretion present in a crypt or follicle.

cryptomenorrhea (krip-to-men-o-re'ă) The monthly occurrence of menstrual symptoms without a flow of blood, as seen in imperforate hymen and large cervical obstructions.

cuff (kuf) A bandlike structure encircling a part of the body.

vaginal c. The upper end of the vagina surrounding the vaginal portion of the uterine cervix. See also vaginal cuff operation, under operation.

cul-de-sac (kul-de-sak') A pouch or saclike space.

Douglas' c. See rectouterine pouch, under pouch.

culdocentesis (kul-do-sen-te'sis) A needle aspiration of fluid from the retrouterine pouch through the posterior vaginal wall, just posterior to the cervix.

culdoscope (kul do-skōp) Endoscopic instrument for viewing the pelvic cavity and its contents.

culdoscopy (kul-dos'ko-pe) Visual examination of the uterus, ovaries, and fallopian (uterine) tubes with a culdoscope, introduced into the pelvic cavity through the posterior vaginal fornix in the region of the cul-de-sac (rectouterine pouch).

culture (kul'chur) A colony of microorganisms or cells, or of tissues grown in a suitable nutrient medium in the laboratory.

culdoscope

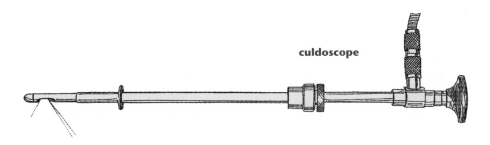

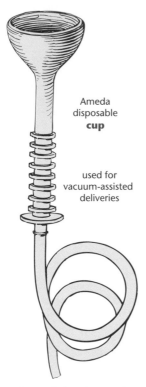

Ameda
disposable
cup

used for
vacuum-assisted
deliveries

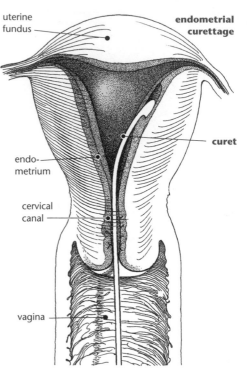

endometrial curettage

uterine fundus

endo-metrium

cervical canal

vagina

curet

cumulus oophorus (ku'mu-lus ooph'orus) The mass of cells surrounding the egg in the vesicular ovarian follicle; when the follicle ruptures and releases the egg during ovulation, the cells of the cumulus, now termed corona radiata, still surround the egg. The cumulus oophorus remains attached when the egg is harvested for *in vitro* fertilization (IVF); its presence and appearance is an important criterion in the evaluation of harvested eggs for IVF. Also called cumulus ovaricus.

cunnilingus (kun-ĭ-ling'us) Oral stimulation of the female genitals.

cunnus (kun'us) Latin for vulva.

cup (kup) **1.** Any anatomic or pathologic hollow space. **2.** A cuplike device.

curet (ku-ret') Tubular instrument with a spoon-shaped tip for scraping the inner wall or lining of a body cavity. The spoon-shaped end may have sharp or blunt edges. Also spelled curette.

curettage (ku-rĕ-tazh') The removal of tissue from the inner wall of a cavity (e.g., uterus) with a spoon-shaped instrument (curet); may be used to remove abnormal tissue, to obtain a specimen for histologic examination and diagnosis, or in abortion procedures.

    endocervical c. Curettage of the cervical

canal, up to the level of the internal os, with a small, slightly curved curet (e.g., a Gusberg curet).

    endometrial c. Scraping of the interior lining of the uterus with a sharp-edge curet.

    fractional c. Separate curettage of the cervical canal and the uterine lining.

    suction c. See vacuum aspiration curettage.

    vacuum aspiration c. Removal of uterine contents or samples with a suction curet.

curette (ku-ret') See curet.

curie (ku're) (Ci) A unit of radioactivity equal to 3.7 × 10^10 disintegrations per second. See also becquerel.

curve (kurv) **1.** A deviation from a straight line. **2.** Representation of plotted data on a graph.

    c. of Carus The curve of the birth canal, which corresponds to the axis of the pelvic cavity. See also pelvic axis, under axis.

    dose-response c., dose-effect c. A curve showing the relationship between a dose of a chemical or ionizing radiation and its influence on a biological process.

    isodose c.'s In radiation therapy, a pattern of curves on the body delineating the quantities of radiation delivered to the tissues.

    oxyhemoglobin dissociation c. Curve representing the percentage of hemoglobin that is saturated with oxygen as a function of the partial pressures of oxygen and carbon dioxide. Major factors influencing the position of the curve are hydrogen ion concentration, body temperature, and 2,3-diphosphoglycerate in red blood cells.

receiver-operating-characteristic (ROC) c. 1. A curve indicating true positive versus false positive results from data usually obtained in a trial of a diagnostic test. **2.** A curve for assessing the capability of a screening test to distinguish between healthy persons and those who are afflicted with a disease.

Starling c. See ventricular function curve.

ventricular function c. A graphic representation of cardiac output against atrial pressure; used to assess myocardial performance. Also called Starling curve.

cutdown (kut'doun) A small incision made over a vein to gain access into the vessel for introduction of intravenous fluids.

cyano-, cyan- Combining forms meaning blue.

cyanosis (si-ă-no'sis) A bluish discoloration of the skin, mucous membranes, and nail beds occurring when there is insufficient oxygen in the blood; caused by the presence of 5 g reduced (deoxygenated) hemoglobin or more per 100 ml blood; seen in certain malformations of the heart (e.g., tetralogy of Fallot) and in respiratory disease.

cyanotic (si-ă-not'ik) Relating to cyanosis.

cycle (si'kl) A recurrent series of phenomena usually occurring at regular intervals.

anovulatory c. A sexual cycle in which no ovum is produced.

cardiac c. The complete round of events occurring in the period between the beginning of one heartbeat and the beginning of the next.

endometrial c. See menstrual cycle.

menstrual c. The sequence of normal changes taking place (about every 28 days) in the endometrium, culminating with shedding of uterine mucosa and bleeding (menstruation); the changes correspond to changes in the ovary (ovarian cycle) and occur in response to hormonal activity. In popular usage, the term encompasses all ovarian and uterine changes. Also called endometrial cycle.

ovarian c. The recurrent sequence of events taking place in the ovary, including production and release of the ovum, in response to hormone activity.

sexual s. The physiologic changes recurring in the female genital organs when pregnancy does not take place.

cyclo-, cycl- Combining forms meaning round; recurring.

menstrual cycle

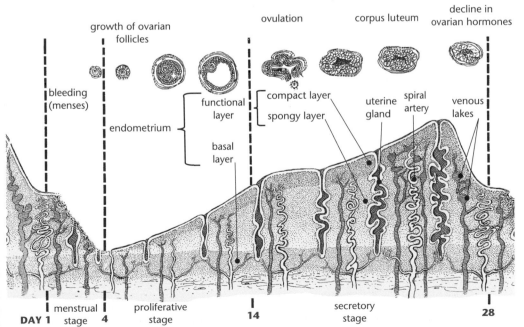

cyclophosphamide (si-klo-fos'fă-mĭd) A compound with antitumor properties, used to treat autoimmune diseases. First trimester intrauterine exposure may cause fetal malformations and low birth weight; paternal intake prior to conception may also cause fetal malformations.

cyst (sĭst) **1.** An abnormal saclike, epithelium-lined cavity within the body containing fluid or gas. **2.** A bladder.

    allantoic c. See urachal cyst.

    amnionic c.'s Cysts in the inner layer of the fetal membranes (amnion), resulting from fusion of amnionic folds and subsequent retention of fluid.

    apocrine gland c.'s See Fox-Fordyce disease, under disease.

    Bartholin's c. A common cyst of the vulva, containing secretions from a Bartholin's (greater vestibular) gland; caused by obstruction of a major duct of the gland.

    chocolate c. Ovarian cyst containing a thick, dark brown fluid typically occurring in endometriosis. Also called endometrioma.

    choroid plexus c. A cyst formed in the tufts of minute blood vessels located within the ventricles of the brain. It is usually a transient condition of the fetus; occasionally, it may be associated with trisomy 18 syndrome.

    corpus luteum c. Ovarian cyst containing a serous accumulation developed when the corpus luteum fails to regress normally during the ovarian cycle. Also called granulosa lutein cyst.

    dermoid c. A common ovarian cyst, often bilateral, lined with skin and containing displaced skin elements (e.g., hair and sebaceous glands, well-formed teeth, and mandibular bone). Also called mature benign teratoma; benign cystic teratoma; dermoid.

    distention c. See retention cyst.

    follicle c. A common type of ovarian cyst resulting from failure of resorption of the fluid in a maturing graafian follicle; may be associated with a short menstrual cycle or a prolonged intermenstrual interval; if large, it may cause pelvic pain, painful sexual intercourse, and abnormal uterine bleeding.

    functional ovarian c. Any of three types of benign masses of the ovary: follicle cyst, corpus luteum cyst, and theca lutein cyst.

    Gartner's c.'s Cystic or tubular structures sometimes observed along the sides of the uterus and vagina; they are embryonic vestiges of the mesonephric duct.

    granulosa lutein c. See corpus luteum cyst.

    lacteal c. See milk-retention cyst.

    lutein c. A cyst of the ovary arising from a corpus luteum (e.g., corpus luteum cyst and theca lutein cyst).

    milk-retention c., milk c. A cystic dilatation of one or more milk ducts in the breast, caused by occlusion of these ducts during lactation. Also called lacteal cyst; galactocele; lactocele.

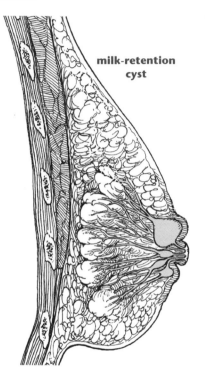

milk-retention cyst

    mucous c. Retention cyst resulting from an obstructed duct of a mucous gland.

    nabothian c.'s Cysts on the uterine cervix due to compression of the ducts of nabothian glands, frequently occurring in chronic cervicitis. Sometimes called nabothian follicles.

    ovarian c. Any cyst of the ovary, usually implying a noncancerous condition.

    paramesonephric c. An uncommon cyst accompanying a unicornuate uterus; it extends along the lateral side of the vaginal wall, on the opposite side of the anomalous uterus. Endometrium lines the upper portion of the cyst and bleeds at menarche; blood accumulates in the lower portion of the cyst, forming a mass that protrudes into the vagina.

    paratubal c. A symptomless, clear fluid-filled cyst, about 1 cm in diameter, commonly found at the fimbriated end of the fallopian (uterine) tube.

parovarian c. A large serous cyst of low malignancy potential; found most frequently in the broad ligament.

piliferous c. A dermoid cyst containing hair.

pilonidal c. A superficial cyst connected to the skin surface by a narrow sinus tract; it contains hair follicles and is usually located in the sacrococcygeal area.

retention c. Cyst caused by obstruction or compression of a duct draining a gland. Also called distention cyst; secretory cyst.

sebaceous c. Cyst of the skin or scalp containing sebum and keratin, caused by obstruction of the duct of a sebaceous gland; sebaceous cysts are frequently found in the labia majora.

secretory c. See retention cyst.

serous c. Cyst containing a clear or translucent fluid.

squamous c. A flat, scalelike cell that is usually arranged in layers to form a lining (e.g., epithelium, endothelium, and mesothelium) of certain structures.

theca-lutein c.'s Small, usually bilateral, cysts containing a clear yellowish fluid; may be associated with hydatidiform mole, polycystic disease of the ovary, or clomiphene therapy.

urachal c. An abdominal cyst, which may communicate with the bladder or with the umbilicus, resulting from persistent patency of a segment of the urachus (i.e., it failed to obliterate completely during intrauterine life). Also called allantoic cyst.

vaginal inclusion c. One of several cysts sometimes formed in the vaginal wall of

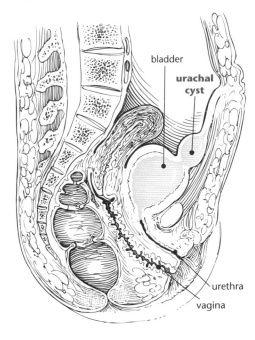

parous women; they arise from mucosal fragments that become embedded in the vaginal connective tissue during repair of vaginal lacerations after delivery.

cystadenocarcinoma (sis-tad-ĕ-no-kar-sĭ-no'mă) A malignant tumor derived from glandular epithelium and composed of cystic cavities filled with fluid secretions and solid masses; found most frequently in the ovary.

cystadenoma (sis-tad-ĕ-no'mă) Benign tumor containing large cystic masses lined with epithelium and filled with retained secretions; typically found in the ovary and pancreas.

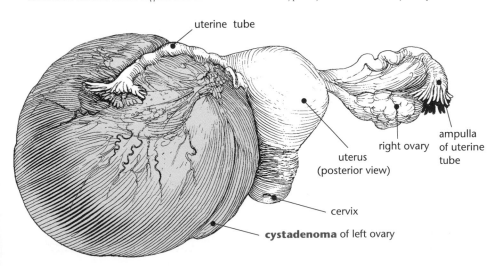

cystadenoma of left ovary

cystectomy (sis-tec'tŏ-me) Removal of a portion of the bladder.

cystic (sis'tik) **1.** Relating to cysts. **2.** Relating to the urinary bladder or the gallbladder.

cystitis (sis-ti'tis) Inflammation of the urinary bladder.

> **acute c.** Cystitis caused by a microbe, usually a bacterium; onset in women frequently follows sexual intercourse.

> **chronic c.** Cystitis that may be unresolved or persistent, or that occurs in separate but frequent bouts (e.g., three episodes in 1 year).

> **eosinophilic c.** Cystitis characterized by the presence of a large number of eosinophils (a type of white blood cell) in the urine.

> **hemorrhagic c.** Cystitis and bleeding from the urinary bladder; caused by radiation treatment (e.g., for cancers of the bladder and cervix), by treatment with antitumor drugs excreted via the urine (e.g., cyclophosphamide) or occasionally by bacterial infection.

> **interstitial c.** A chronic, intensely symptomatic cystitis of unknown cause involving the lining and musculature of the lower urinary bladder; symptoms include suprapubic pain brought on by bladder distention and relieved upon urination.

> **radiation c.** Cystitis occurring as a complication of radiation treatment (e.g., for cancer of the cervix). Symptoms may develop months after termination of treatment.

cysto-, cyst- Combining forms meaning bladder; cyst.

cystocele (sis'to-sēl) Prolapse of the urinary bladder wall into the vagina due to weakening of the supporting pelvic musculature. Also called colpocystocele; vesicocele.

cystoid (sis'toid) Having the shape and consistency of a cyst but lacking an enclosed wall.

cystolith (sis'to-lith) A bladder stone.

cystolithectomy (sis-to-lĭ-thek'tŏ-me) See cystolithotomy.

cystolithiasis (sis-to-lĭ-thi'ă-sis) The presence of one or more stones in the bladder. Also called vesicolithiasis.

cystolithotomy (sis-to-lĭ-thot'ŏ-me) Surgical removal of bladder stones. Also called cystolithectomy; vesicolithotomy.

cystoma (sis-to'mă) A tumor containing cysts.

cystometer (sis-tom'ĕ-ter) Device used to measure the tone of the bladder musculature in relation to the volume of fluid in the bladder.

cystometrogram (sis-to-met'ro-gram) A graphic recording made by a cystometer.

cystometry (sis-tom'ĕ-tre) A method of evaluating

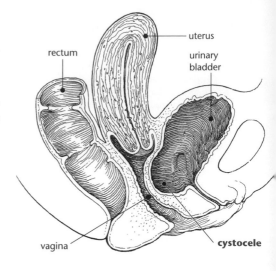

rectum · uterus · urinary bladder · vagina · **cystocele**

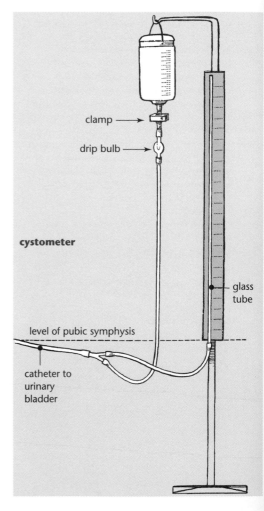

clamp · drip bulb · **cystometer** · glass tube · level of pubic symphysis · catheter to urinary bladder

bladder function by means of a cystometer; it includes measurements of total bladder capacity, of the pressure changes within the bladder during filling and voiding, and of the amount of residual urine after voiding.

cystoplasty (sis'to-plas-te) Any reconstructive operation of the bladder.

cystoplegia (sis-to-ple'jĕ) Paralysis of the bladder.

cystoptosis (sis-top-to'sis) Prolapse of the inner lining of the bladder into the urethra.

cystorrhagia (sis-to-ra'jĕ) Bleeding from the bladder.

cystorrhea (sis-to-re'ă) Mucous discharge from the bladder.

cystoscope (sis'to-skōp) A tubular instrument, equipped with a light, for visual examination of the interior of the bladder.

cystoscopy (sis-tos'kŏ-pe) Visual examination of the interior of the bladder with the aid of a cystoscope.

cystospasm (sis'to-spazm) Spasmodic contraction of the bladder muscles.

cystostomy (sis-tos'tŏ-me) Creation of an opening into the bladder through the abdominal wall for the purpose of draining the bladder when drainage with a catheter via the urethra is not possible or advisable. Also called vesicostomy.

cystotomy (sis-tot'ŏ-me) Surgical cutting or opening into the bladder. Also called vesicotomy.

cystoureteritis (sis-to-u-re-ter-i'tis) Inflammation of the bladder and one or both tubes (ureters) leading from the kidneys to the bladder.

cystourethritis (sis-to-u-re-thri'tis) Inflammation of the bladder and the urethra.

cystourethrocele (sis-to-u-re'thro-sēl) Prolapse of the neck of the bladder and urethra toward the vagina.

cystourethropexy (sis-to-u-re-thro-peks'e) See urethrocystopexy.

cytarabine (si-tar'ă-bēn) A chemotherapeutic agent generally used as part of a combination regimen in the treatment of ovarian carcinoma and certain leukemias. Also called a-C; ara-C; arabinosylcytosine.

cyto-, cyt- Combining forms meaning cell.

cytocentrum (si-to-sen'trum) See centrosome.

cytogenetics (si-to-je-net'iks) The field of science derived from both genetics and cytology concerned with the study of physical components of heredity; it concentrates on the chromosome, especially its structure, replication, and recombination.

   clinical c. The study of the relationship between aberrations of chromosome structure and abnormal or pathologic conditions.

cytology (si-tol'ŏ-je) The science concerned with the study and identification of cells. Also called cell biology; cytobiology.

   vaginal c. Microscopic examination of desquamated cells from the vaginal epithelium for diagnostic purposes.

cytomegalovirus (si-to-meg'ă-lo-vi'rus) (CMV) Any of a group of herpesviruses infecting humans, rodents, and other mammals, producing enlargement of cells and development of characteristic inclusions in the cytoplasm or nucleus of the cell; they cause a variety of disorders in humans, including cytomegalovirus mononucleosis (a mononucleosis-like disease), hepatitis, pneumonia, and cytomegalic inclusion disease (in the newborn); the species causing human diseases is also called human herpesvirus 5 (HHV-5). See also herpesvirus.

cytometry (si-tom'ĕ-tre) The counting of blood cells.

   flow c. A technique to measure the responses of specially prepared cells in a cell suspension to an excitation (laser or mercury arc lamp) beam.

cytosmear (si'to-smēr) See cytologic smear, under smear.

cytostatic (si-to stat'ik) Capable of stopping cell growth.

cytotoxic (si-to-tok'sik) Capable of killing cells.

cytotoxin (si-to-tok'sin) A substance that destroys cells.

cytotrophoblast (si-to-trof'o-blast) The layer of round cells (Langhan's cells) forming the innermost portion of the wall of the trophoblast; the syntrophoblast (a multinucleated mass of cytoplasm) forms the outer portion of the wall.

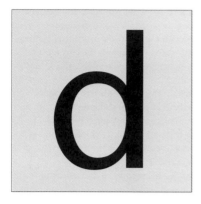

dactinomycin (dak-tĭ-no-mi'sin) An antineoplastic agent used for the treatment of malignant tumors, including choriocarcinoma; adverse effects include ulceration of the oral mucosa and bone marrow depression; normal infants have been delivered after intrauterine exposure to the drug but stillbirths and low-birthweight infants have also been reported.

danazol (dan'ă-zol) An anterior pituitary suppressant, chiefly used in the treatment of endometriosis; intrauterine exposure before the eighth week of gestation does not appear to have a deleterious effect on the fetus; cases of enlarged clitoris and partial labial fusion have been reported when exposure occurs after the eighth week of gestation.

dance (dans) In medical parlance, abnormal movements, especially of the limbs, associated with brain lesions.

    hilar d. Strong pulsations of the pulmonary arteries observed on fluoroscopic examination in patients with congenital left-to-right shunt.

    St. Vitus' d. See Sydenham's chorea, under chorea.

daunorubicin (daw-no-roo'bĭ-sin) An antitumor antibiotic with birth defect potential when taken by either parent.

D and C See dilatation and curettage.

D and E See dilatation and evacuation.

death (deth) Death as described by The Uniform Determination of Death Act passed by the US Congress (1981), which states that an individual is dead if there is (1) irreversible cessation of circulatory and respiratory functions or (2) irreversible cessation of all functions of the entire brain, including the brainstem.

    brain d. An irreversible state persisting after a specified length of time (usually 6–24 hours) in which there is total cessation of brain function (i.e., complete unresponsiveness to all stimuli, including painful stimuli such as hard pinching), absence of brainstem reflexes

(e.g., pupils are dilated and unresponsive to light), and disappearance of the electroencephalogram pattern (electrocerebral silence; i.e., a 'flat' electroencephalogram); heartbeat and breathing may continue only with the assistance of a respirator. Two conditions are excluded: hypothermia and depression of the central nervous system by drugs (e.g., barbiturates or alcohol). Although the use of confirmatory tests makes it possible to shorten the observation period in adults, in the case of infants and young children a full 24-hour observation period is recommended. Also called cerebral death.

    cell d. The termination of a cell's ability to carry out vital functions (i.e., metabolism, growth, reproduction, and adaptability).

    cerebral d. See brain death.

    clinically unexplained d. (1) Death of a patient whose prolonged, complex illness was extensively studied but a satisfactory diagnosis was not established. (2) Death of a patient whose illness was of such brief duration that there was little or no opportunity for medical observation or studies to provide a reasonable explanation.

    fetal d. Intrauterine death of a fetus; in early pregnancy, the first sign is absence of uterine enlargement; in later pregnancy, the first sign is absence of fetal movement.

    infant d. Death of a baby under the age of 1 year.

    maternal d. Death of a woman occurring during pregnancy, labor, or the puerperium (i.e., within 42 days of termination of pregnancy). *Direct maternal d;* death that results from obstetric complications of pregnancy, labor, or the puerperium; or from any intervention, incorrect treatment, or omission; or from any sequence of events derived from any of the above. *Indirect maternal d;* death caused by a previously existing medical condition, or one developed during pregnancy, that was aggravated by the natural physiologic burdens of pregnancy and the additional demands of labor and delivery.

    neonatal d. Death of an infant during the first 28 days of life; usually designated *early* when it occurs during the first 7 days and *late* thereafter.

    nonmaternal d. Death of a pregnant woman unrelated to the pregnant state (e.g., from an automobile accident).

    perinatal d. Death occurring during the perinatal period (i.e., from completion of 20 weeks of gestation through the first 28 days after delivery).

sudden cardiac d. (SCD) Unexpected cessation of cardiac contraction occurring within 1 hour of the onset of symptoms; most commonly caused by obstruction of one or more coronary arteries; other causes include constriction of the aortic valve, abnormalities of the conduction system in the heart muscle, and prolapse of the mitral (left atrioventricular) valve. In young people (especially young athletes participating in strenuous sports), it may be caused by hypertrophic cardiomyopathy (HCM) resulting from a genetic defect (a mutation in the myosin gene). See also hypertrophic cardiomyopathy, under cardiomyopathy.

debulking (de-bulk'ing) Operative removal of portions of a large malignant tumor to reduce its size; oxygenate the tumor tissues (oxygen is often toxic to malignant cells); and provide space to encourage proliferation of malignant cells, thus rendering the tumor more susceptible to destruction by chemotherapy (quiescent cells are not as susceptible).

deca- Prefix used in the International System of Units (SI) meaning 10.

decarboxylase (de-kar-bok'sĭ-lās) Any enzyme that accelerates removal of carbon dioxide from a compound.

deceleration (de-sel-er-a'shun) **1.** Decrease in velocity. **2.** A transient fall in the fetal heart rate below the baseline rate (120–160 beats per minute), determined by internal electronic fetal monitoring. Nomenclature depends chiefly on either of two criteria: timing of the deceleration in relation to a uterine contraction, or the pathophysiologic events considered most likely to cause the decelerations.

early d. Deceleration of the fetal heart rate in the second stage of labor, at the beginning of a uterine contraction and returning to baseline levels at the end of the contraction; believed to be triggered by compression of the fetal head.

late d. Decrease in fetal heart rate beginning at, or after, the peak of a uterine contraction and returning to baseline levels well after the contraction has ended; believed to be caused by any factor compromising uteroplacental gas exchange.

variable d. Deceleration of the fetal heart rate occurring irregularly at different times during a uterine contraction and varying in intensity and duration; most common cause is compression of the umbilical cord.

deci- Prefix used in the International System of Units (SI) meaning one-tenth (10^{-1}).

decidua (de-sid'u-ă) The inner lining of the pregnant uterus, which has become thick and vascular, forming a receptive environment for implantation of the blastocyst and development of the embryo/fetus and its membranes. It is shed at childbirth except the deepest layer. Also called decidual membrane; decidua of pregnancy.

basal d. The area of the decidua directly beneath the site of blastocyst implantation; it develops into the maternal part of the

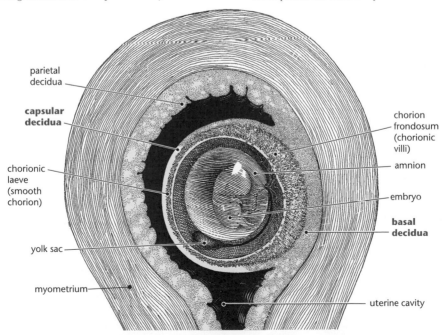

parietal decidua

capsular decidua

chorionic laeve (smooth chorion)

yolk sac

myometrium

chorion frondosum (chorionic villi)

amnion

embryo

basal decidua

uterine cavity

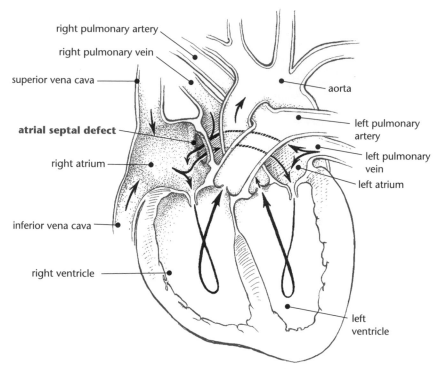

right pulmonary artery

right pulmonary vein

superior vena cava

atrial septal defect

right atrium

inferior vena cava

right ventricle

aorta

left pulmonary artery

left pulmonary vein

left atrium

left ventricle

placenta.

capsular d. The part of the endometrium that seals the implanted conceptus from the uterine cavity; it stretches as the blastocyst grows, then (from about the fourth month of pregnancy) it undergoes rapid regression, thereby allowing the nonvillous part of the chorion to make direct contact with the parietal decidua. Also called reflex decidua.

menstrual d. The engorged (hyperemic) endothelial mucosa of the nonpregnant uterus that is shed during the menstrual period.

parietal d. The entire endometrium lining the cavity of the pregnant uterus except at the site of attachment of the conceptus. Also called decidua vera; true decidua.

d. polyposa Hyperplasia of the uterine decidua with projections on its surface resembling polyps.

d. of pregnancy See decidua.

reflex d. See capsular decidua.

true d. See parietal decidua.

d. vera See parietal decidua.

decidual (dĕ-sid'u-al) Relating to decidua.

decidualization (de-sid-u-ă-lĭ'za'shun) Term used to describe the changes occurring in tissues in which the fertilized ovum implants; these changes (which occur normally within the uterine lining under the influence of hormones)

culminate in the formation of the highly specialized endometrium (decidua) in preparation for the blastocyst implantation; may occur also in tissues in which ectopic pregnancies take place (e.g., the mucosal lining of uterine tubes, the peritoneum, and the ovaries).

deciduation (dĕ-sid-u-a'shun) The casting off of endometrial tissue after childbirth.

deciduoma (dĕ-sid-u-o'mă) A mass of decidual tissue in the uterus.

deciduous (dĕ-sid'u-us) Temporary; not permanent.

defect (de'fekt) Malformation; mutation.

atrial septal d. (ASD) An abnormal hole in the septum dividing the two atria of the heart.

body wall d. Malformation of the fetal body wall; caused by chronic deficiency of amniotic fluid, resulting in a reduced size of the uterine cavity, which restricts proper positioning of the enlarging fetus.

neural tube d. Any developmental anomaly resulting from failure of the neural tube to close normally by day 26 to 28 of embryonic life (e.g., spina bifida, anencephaly, meningocele).

single-gene d. A single mutant gene present either on one chromosome of a pair (one copy), or on both chromosomes of the pair at a single locus (two copies).

ventricular septal d. (VSD) An abnormal hole in the septum between the two ventricles of the heart.

defeminization (de-fem-ĭ-nĭ-za'shun) The loss or decrease of female characteristics.

deferentectomy (def-er-en-tek'to-me) See vasectomy.

deficiency (de-fish'en-se) An insufficient state; a lack.

> **attenuated 21-hydroxylase d.** See late-onset 21-hydroxylase deficiency.

> **glucose-6-phosphate dehydrogenase (G6PD) d.** A sex-linked inherited deficiency characterized by low levels of the enzyme G6PD in red blood cells, which renders the cells susceptible to destruction when exposed to certain drugs and toxic substances (e.g., sulfa drugs, antimalarials, nitrofurantoin, naphthalene). In pregnancy, treatment of urinary tract infections with sulfa drugs may precipitate fetal hemolysis and death of a G6PD-deficient fetus.

> **21-hydroxylase (P450c21) d.** An autosomal recessive inheritance causing scant production of P450c21 (the steroid enzyme that triggers the production of cortisol); the result is a compensatory hypersecretion of corticotropin (ACTH) by the adrenal cortex, with subsequent adrenal hyperplasia and excessive androgen production; congenital deficiency of P450c21 is one of the enzyme deficiencies responsible for ambiguous genitalia of the female; it is a frequent cause of neonatal death when left untreated.

> **immune d.** See immunodeficiency.

> **late-onset 21-hydroxylase (P450c21) d.** A nonclassic form of P450c21 deficiency that manifests itself later in life, causing various symptoms of excessive androgen production, ranging from female hirsutism to sterility. Also called attenuated 21-hydroxylase deficiency.

> **luteal phase d.** A condition associated with infertility, manifesting itself as pregnancy loss (miscarriage). It is descriptive of an ovarian problem. The ovary is the site of the underlying pathophysiology; the endometrium is quite normal.

> **ornithine transcarbamoylase (OTC) d.** A dominantly inherited deficiency of OTC (an enzyme important in urea synthesis in the liver); it affects mostly males, most of whom die in infancy; those who survive (usually females) may be physically and mentally retarded, may display a gradual developmental regression, or may have only mild symptoms; defects are related to the degree of deficiency.

placental aromatase d. Reduced activity of the enzyme aromatase in the placenta, with subsequent accumulation of the fetal androgen precursors that produce placental estrogens; associated with virilization and low estrogen levels of the pregnant woman and masculinization of the newborn (if the infant is a female).

> **placental sulfatase d.** An X-linked disorder (all affected fetuses are males) that causes very low estrogen levels in otherwise normal pregnancies by precluding the hydrolysis of C_{19}-steroid sulfate precursors of estrogen, the first enzymatic step in the placental use of circulating prehormones for estrogen biosynthesis. It is associated with dry scaliness of the skin (ichthyosis), which may be present at birth or appear later in life.

deficit (def'ĭ-sit) A deficiency, usually temporary.

> **base d.** A decrease of bicarbonate (HCO_3) concentration below normal levels in a newborn infant.

degeneration (dejen-er-a'shun) **1.** Any deterioration or process of worsening. **2.** The process of deterioration of tissues with corresponding functional impairment as a result of injury or disease; the process may advance to an irreversible stage and eventually cause death of the tissues (necrosis).

> **adipose d.** See fatty degeneration.

> **atrophic d. of leiomyoma** A reduction in size of a uterine leiomyoma (commonly called fibroid) after menopause or pregnancy; associated with reduced estrogenic activity.

> **calcareous d.** Deposition of insoluble calcium salts in tissues that have deteriorated by other processes; especially seen in subserous uterine leiomyomas affected by reduced circulation. Also called calcific degeneration.

> **calcific d.** See calcareous degeneration.

> **carneous d.** Degeneration of a uterine leiomyoma, usually occurring during pregnancy associated with potential preterm labor; characterized by formation of soft, dark red areas of hemorrhage and necrosis; symptoms include pain, tenderness on palpation, and low-grade fever. Also called red degeneration.

> **cystic d.** Degeneration with formation of cysts.

> **fatty d.** Any abnormal accumulation of fat within cells forming the substance of an organ. Also called adipose degeneration.

> **hyaline d.** A regressive cellular change in which the cytoplasm becomes glossy and homogeneous; may be due to viral inclusions

or to injury that causes coagulation of proteins; may occur in an old leiomyoma, causing no symptoms.

mucoid medial d. See cystic medial necrosis, under necrosis.

red d. See carneous degeneration.

dehiscence (de-his'ens) **1.** A splitting along a line or slit. **2.** Separation of any of the suture layers of an operative wound at any stage of healing. Compare with evisceration (3).

uterine d. An uncommon postoperative complication of cesarean section, associated with adhesions between the abdominal wall and the uterus; symptoms include spiking temperatures, pain, and intestinal obstruction.

deliver (de-liv'er) **1.** To assist a woman in childbirth. **2.** To remove or extract (e.g., a tumor or a cataract).

delivery (de-liv'er-e) The mode of actual expulsion of the infant and placenta from the uterus.

abdominal d. See cesarean section, under section.

breech d. Vaginal delivery of a baby whose pelvis or lower limb is the presenting part.

failed forceps d. An unsuccessful attempt at forceps delivery, with opting for a cesarean section instead.

forceps d. The use of forceps for delivery of a fetus in vertex presentation (i.e., when the top-back of the skull is foremost within the birth canal).

high forceps d. Application of forceps to the fetal head before its engagement (i.e., before its biparietal plane has descended to a level below that of the pelvic inlet). Also called high forceps.

low forceps d. Application of forceps to the fetal head when the leading point of the head is at a station +2 cm or more and not on the pelvic floor; includes two subdivisions: (1) rotation is 45 degrees or less (left or right occipitoanterior to occiput anterior, or left occipitoposterior to occiput posterior); (2) rotation is greater than 45 degrees. Also called low forceps.

midforceps d. Application of forceps to the fetal head when the leading point of the head is above station +2 cm but the head is engaged (i.e., the parietal plane of the head has descended to a level below that of the pelvic inlet). Also called midforceps.

operative d. Any obstetric delivery effected by means of active measures, including forceps procedures and cesarean section.

outlet forceps d. Application of forceps to the fetal head when (a) the scalp is visible at the introitus without separating the labia, (b) the fetal skull has reached the pelvic floor, (c) the sagittal suture is in the anteroposterior diameter (or in the right or left occiput anterior or posterior position), and (d) the fetal head is at or on the perineum. Also called outlet forceps.

postmortem d. Delivery of a fetus after the death of its mother.

premature d. The birth of a fetus before 34 weeks of gestation.

prophylactic d. The performance of an episiotomy along with an outlet forceps delivery when the only obstacle for delivery is a marked resistance of the perineum and vaginal opening. Also called prophylactic forceps.

trial forceps d. An attempt at a low or midforceps delivery with the full intention of switching to a cesarean section if undue resistance is encountered, which may be incompatible with the safety of the fetus. Also called trial forceps.

vaginal d. Delivery of an infant through the birth canal and vaginal orifice.

demineralization (de-min-er-al-ĭ-za'shun) A reduction of the mineral constituent of tissues; applied especially to calcium depletion of bones.

denidation (den-ĭ-da'shun) Disintegration and expulsion of the superficial layer of the uterine lining.

density (den'sĭ-te) **1.** The state of compactness; the quantity of matter per unit volume, expressed in grams per cubic centimeter. **2.** A measure of the degree of resistance to the speed of transmission of light.

bone d. In clinical practice, the amount of mineral per square centimeter of bone; usually measured by photon absorptiometry or by x-ray computed tomography. Actual bone density is expressed in grams per milliliter.

deoxycorticosterone, desoxycorticosterone (de-ok'se-kor-tĭ-kos'ter-ōn, des-ok'se-kor-tĭ-kos'terōn) (DOC) A steroid hormone with mineralocorticoid activity formed in the cortex of the adrenal (suprarenal) gland; maternal plasma levels of DOC increase markedly during pregnancy.

depo-bromocriptine (de'po bro-mo-krip'tēn) The long-acting form of bromocriptine, administered intramuscularly. See also bromocriptine.

dependence (dĕ-pen'dens) The state of being subordinated to, or controlled by, someone or something greatly desired.

alcohol d. See alcoholism.

drug d. General term for a condition in which the user of a drug has a compelling desire to continue taking the drug either to experience its effects or to avoid the discomfort that occurs when it is not taken. The dependence may be: *psychologic,* characterized by an emotional drive to continue taking a drug, which the user believes is necessary to maintain a sense of optimal well-being; or *physical,* characterized by an adaptive physiologic state resulting from the repeated use of a drug (i.e., the body has adapted to the presence of the drug). Formerly called drug addiction; drug habituation.

deportation (dĕ-por-ta'shun) The act of carrying away.

    trophoblastic d. See trophoblastic embolization, under embolization.

depot (de'po) An organ or tissue in which drugs or biologic substances are deposited and stored by the body.

depressant (de-pres'ant) 1. Reducing functional activity. 2. An agent that has such a property.

depressed (de-prest') 1. Pressed down or sunk below the level of a surrounding surface. 2. Below normal functional level. 3. Dejected; afflicted by depression.

depression (de-presh'un) 1. Emotional dejection and reduction of functioning; a morbid sadness accompanied by lack of interest in surroundings and reduced energy; may range from mild to major. 2. A pressed down area, lower than the surrounding level. 3. A reduction or lessening of functional activity (e.g., of bone marrow).

    endogenous d. Depressive disorder occurring without predominant psychosocial causative factors and thus presumed to be somatic in origin; symptoms include disturbances of sleep, appetite, sexual interest, and motor regulation as well as depressed mood.

    major d. A syndrome that, every day for at least 2 weeks, includes at least four of the following symptoms: *(a)* decreased or increased appetite with corresponding change in weight; *(b)* insomnia (especially very early awakening) or sleeping for excessively long periods; *(c)* motor retardation, or agitation; *(d)* loss of interest and pleasure in surroundings and decreased sexual drive; *(e)* feelings of excessive guilt, self reproach, or worthlessness; *(f)* decreased ability to make decisions; *(g)* fatigue; and *(h)* recurrent suicidal thinking or attempts.

    postpartum d. A temporary mood disturbance experienced by some women, usually 3 to 10 days after delivery; characterized by crying, irritability, anxiety, forgetfulness, and mood swings from sadness to elation. Commonly called baby blues; postnatal blues; three-day blues.

-derm Combining form meaning layer (e.g., ectoderm).

dermatitis (der-ma-ti'tis), pl. dermatitides Inflammation of the skin.

    contact d. Dermatitis resulting from contact with any of a variety of natural or manufactured substances and occurring as a delayed allergic reaction to the substance.

    papular d. An uncommon dermatitis occurring in late pregnancy, characterized by a generalized intensely pruritic eruption of soft reddish papules; some become excoriated, healing with a hemorrhagic crust.

dermato-, dermo-, derm- Combining forms meaning skin.

dermatomycosis (der-mă-to-mi-ko'sis) Any fungal infection of the skin.

dermatomyositis (der-mă-to-mi-o-si'tis) A disorder of skin and muscle characterized by a blue-violet rash on the face (especially around the eyes) and on the back of the hands and fingers, with muscle weakness especially in the shoulder and pelvic areas; two varieties are known, affecting children or adults; the adult form is sometimes associated with an occult internal cancer.

dermatophytosis (der-mă-to-fi-to'sis) Any superficial fungal infection of the skin, such as athlete's foot (tinea pedis), ringworm (tinea corporis), and tinea versicolor, which occasionally affects the vulvar skin.

dermatosis (der-mă-to'sis), pl. dermatoses General term for any disease of the skin.

    dermatoses of pregnancy Skin eruptions that are unique to the pregnant state; they include pruritis gravidarum, pruritis urticarial papules and plaques of pregnancy (PUPPP), herpes gestationis, and papular eruptions.

dermoid (der'moid) 1. Resembling skin. 2. See dermoid cyst, under cyst.

descensus (de-sen'sus) Latin for descent.

    d. uteri See prolapse of uterus, under prolapse.

descent (de-sent') The process of moving downward; in obstetrics, the passage of the fetal presenting part through the birth canal.

    precipitate d. See precipitate labor disorder, under disorder.

    protracted d. See protraction disorder, under disorder.

desmo-, desm- Combining forms meaning ligament.

desmoid (dez'moid) A locally aggressive nodule formed by proliferation of fibrous tissue of muscle sheaths; most common site is the abdominal rectus muscle, especially in women after pregnancy; it does not spread to other sites but tends to recur after surgical removal unless a wide margin of healthy tissue is included in the resection. Also called aggressive fibromatosis; desmoid tumor.

desmopressin acetate (des-mo-pres'in as'ĕ-tāt) A synthetic analog of the natural pituitary hormone vasopressin, an antidiuretic hormone (ADH) affecting renal water conservation; used in the treatment of diabetes insipidus; also used to treat von Willebrand's disease type I and hemophilia A.

detachment (de-tach'ment) **1.** Separation of a structure from its support. **2.** In psychiatry, the condition of being free from emotional involvement.

    retinal d. Separation of the neural layer of the retina from its pigment epithelium, causing altered vision.

determinant (de-ter'mĭ-nant) Some factor that establishes the characteristics or occurrence of an event.

    antigenic d. The exact site on the surface of an antigen molecule or a hapten (smaller molecule) to which attaches a specific antibody produced by the host's immune system; a single antigen molecule may have several determinants recognized separately and specifically by the host's immune system. Also called epitope.

determination (de-ter-mĭ-na'shun) **1.** The process of measuring a quantity of scientific, laboratory, or forensic investigations. **2.** A conclusion reached after deliberation as to the nature of a disease or the cause of death.

detrusor (de-troo'sor) Denoting a muscle that effects an expulsion or pushing out of something (e.g., the detrusor muscle of the bladder). See also detrusor instability, under instability; detrusor loop, under loop.

deutoplasm (doo'to-plazm) The inactive, nonliving material in cytoplasm, especially the yolk granules in the ovum.

deviation (de-ve-a'shun) **1.** A turning aside. **2.** Departure from a norm, rule, or accepted course of behavior.

    standard d. (SD) A statistic that describes the degree of variation among the individual observations in a sample.

device (de-vīs') Something constructed for a

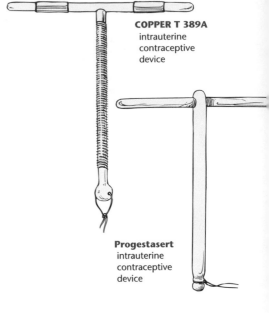

COPPER T 389A intrauterine contraceptive device

Progestasert intrauterine contraceptive device

particular purpose.

    contraceptive d. Any device for preventing conception. See also barrier method, under method.

    COPPER T 380A d. A T-shaped intrauterine contraceptive device composed of polyethylene and barium sulfate with 314 mm^2 of fine copper wire wound around the stem and 33 mm^2 around each arm.

    intrauterine d. (IUD) A device made of plastic or metal inserted into the uterus to prevent conception. Also called intrauterine contraceptive device.

    intrauterine contraceptive d. (IUCD) See intrauterine device.

    Progestasert d. A T-shaped intrauterine contraceptive device 36 mm long and 32 mm wide, made of ethylene vinyl acetate co-polymer; the vertical stem contains 38 mg of progesterone and barium sulfate.

dexter (deks'ter) (D) Latin for right.

dextrad (deks'trad) Toward the right.

dextroamphetamine sulfate (deks-tro-am-fet'ă-mēn sul'fāt) A stimulant of the central nervous system and an appetite depressant; intrauterine exposure may cause congenital defects and withdrawal syndrome in the newborn infant; may also be transmitted in the milk to breast-feeding infants. Dextroamphetamine is one of the drugs of abuse popularly known as 'uppers'.

dextrocardia (deks-tro-kar'de-ă) **1.** Abnormal congenital position of the heart on the right side of the chest with or without mirror-image transposition of the right and left heart chambers. Also called dextroposition of heart. **2.** An acquired condition in which the major portion of the heart is displaced to the right side, as may occur in collapse of the right lung.

dextroposition (deks-tro-pŏ-zish'un) Abnormal right-sided location of an organ normally located on the left side.

    d. of heart See dextrocardia.

dextroversion (deks-tro-ver'shun) A displacement toward the right.

di- Prefix meaning two.

dia- Prefix meaning through.

diabetes (di-ă-be'tēz) General term for metabolic disorders characterized by excessive excretion of urine (polyuria); when used alone, the term refers to diabetes mellitus.

    d. 1 See type 1 diabetes mellitus.

    d. 2 See type 2 diabetes mellitus.

    adult-onset d. See type 2 diabetes mellitus.

    brittle d. See labile diabetes.

    gestational d. mellitus (GDM) Glucose intolerance detected by a glucose tolerance test during pregnancy in the absence of clinical evidence usually associated with overt carbohydrate intolerance; although limited to pregnancy, patients who develop gestational diabetes are at increased risk of developing diabetes mellitus subsequently in the nonpregnant state. Also called pregnancy-induced glucose intolerance.

    d. insipidus A comparatively rare form of diabetes characterized by excessive thirst and the passage of large amounts of dilute urine (of low specific gravity), due to an inadequate production of antidiuretic hormone (vasopressin) by the posterior lobe of the pituitary; normally, the antidiuretic hormone curtails the amount of water the kidney releases in the urine. Compare with nephrogenic diabetes insipidus.

    insulin-dependent d. mellitus (IDDM) See type 1 diabetes mellitus.

    juvenile d., juvenile-onset d. Former terms for type 1 diabetes mellitus.

    labile d. Diabetes mellitus that is difficult to control, with unpredictable and frequent episodes of hyper- and hypoglycemia. Formerly called brittle diabetes.

    latent d. mellitus See impaired glucose tolerance, under tolerance.

    maturity-onset d. mellitus See type 2 diabetes mellitus.

    maturity-onset d. of youth (MODY) A subtype of type 2 diabetes mellitus characterized by a gradual onset during late adolescence or early adulthood.

    d. mellitus (DM) A chronic systemic disease of disordered metabolism of carbohydrate, protein, and fat; its primary feature is inappropriately high levels of glucose in the blood (hyperglycemia), from which the term *mellitus* (Latin for honeyed) was derived. The condition has been classified into two major categories (type 1 diabetes mellitus and type 2 diabetes mellitus). Pregnancy in diabetic women whose condition is poorly controlled may have deleterious effects in both mother and child. Maternal effects can include: the likelihood of preeclampsia–eclampsia, increased risk of acquiring bacterial infections, birth canal injuries (due to abnormally large size of the fetus), cesarean delivery (with increased risk of complications), and large volume of amniotic fluid (with attending cardiorespiratory symptoms). Fetal and neonatal effects include: increased incidence of perinatal death, malformations, preterm delivery, and neonatal morbidity (e.g., birth injury due to large size, respiratory distress, metabolic disturbances).

    nephrogenic d. insipidus A rare familial form of diabetes insipidus due to severely diminished ability of the kidney tubules to reabsorb water; it does not respond to the administration of antidiuretic hormone. Also called vasopressin resistant diabetes.

    non-insulin-dependent d. mellitus (NIDDM) See type 2 diabetes mellitus.

    preclinical d. mellitus See impaired glucose tolerance, under tolerance.

    pregestational d. Diabetes mellitus known to be present in a woman before pregnancy occurs.

    subclinical d. mellitus See impaired glucose tolerance, under tolerance.

    type 1 d. mellitus An often severe type of diabetes mellitus characterized by a sudden onset of insulin deficiency, with a tendency to develop ketoacidosis; may occur at any age, but is most common in childhood and adolescence (peak age of onset is 11–15 years); the disorder is due to destruction of the beta cells of the islets of Langerhans in the pancreas, possibly by a viral infection and autoimmune reactions; symptoms and signs include elevated blood glucose levels (hyperglycemia), excessive urination (polyuria), chronic excessive thirst (polydipsia), excessive eating (polyphagia), weight loss, and irritability; affected persons must have injections of insulin to survive. Also called diabetes **1.** Formerly called juvenile diabetes; juvenile-onset diabetes; insulin-dependent diabetes mellitus (IDDM); diabetes mellitus type I.

type 2 d. mellitus A relatively mild form of diabetes mellitus characterized by a gradual onset that may occur at any age but is most common in adults over the age of 40 years, especially those with a tendency to obesity (peak age of onset is 50–60 years); may be due to a tissue insensitivity to insulin, or to a delayed insulin release from the pancreas in response to glucose intake; a genetic predisposition is noted when it occurs in young people. Also called diabetes **2.** Formerly called adult-onset diabetes mellitus; maturity-onset diabetes mellitus; non-insulin-dependent diabetes mellitus (NIDDM); diabetes mellitus type II.

vasopressin-resistant d. See nephrogenic diabetes insipidus.

diabetic (di-ă-bet'ik) Relating to diabetes.

diabetogenic (di-ă-bet-o-jen'ik) Causing diabetes.

diacetylmorphine (di-ă-se-til-mor'fēn) See heroin.

diameter (di-am'ĕ-ter) **1.** A straight line passing through the center of any circular anatomic structure or space; frequently used to specify certain dimensions of the female pelvis and fetal head. **2.** The distance along such a line. **3.** The thickness or width of any structure or opening.

anteroposterior d. of midpelvis The distance between the pubic symphysis and sacrum at the junction of the fourth and fifth vertebrae; it is on the midplane or plane of least pelvic dimensions.

anteroposterior d. of pelvic inlet See diagonal conjugate and true conjugate, under conjugate.

anteroposterior d. of pelvic outlet The distance between the lower rim of the pubic symphysis and the sacrococcygeal junction. Sometimes the tip of the coccyx is used for the posterior point.

biischial d. of pelvic outlet See transverse diameter of pelvic outlet.

biparietal d. The transverse distance between the two parietal eminences of the skull, representing the maximal cranial breadth.

bispinous d. See interspinous diameter.

bitemporal d. The distance between the two temporal sutures of the fetal skull at term, usually around 8.0 cm.

bituberous d. See transverse diameter of pelvic outlet.

fronto-occipital d. See occipitofrontal diameter.

interspinous d. The transverse diameter of the midpelvis between the two ischial spines; usually the smallest diameter of the pelvis. Also called bispinous diameter.

intertuberous d. See transverse diameter of pelvic outlet.

mento-occipital d. See occipitomental diameter.

oblique d.'s of pelvis (1) Of the inlet: two diameters, each measured from one sacroiliac joint to the opposite junction of the iliac and pubic rami (iliopubic eminence). (2) Of the outlet: the distance from the midpoint of the sacrotuberous ligament to the opposite junction of the iliac and pubic rami (ilio pubic eminence).

occipitofrontal d. The diameter of the skull from the frontal bone between the eyebrows (glabella) to the external occipital protuberance (furthest point at occiput); it represents the maximal cranial diameter. The greatest circumference of the head corresponds to the plane of the occipitofrontal diameter. Also called fronto-occipital diameter.

occipitomental d. The distance on the skull from the chin to the most prominent portion of the occipital bone (external occipital protuberance). Also called mento-occipital diameter.

posterior sagittal d. of inlet The posterior segment of the obstetric conjugate (i.e., the distance between the promontory of the sacrum to the midpoint on the transverse diameter of the pelvic inlet, about 4 cm in front of the promontory).

posterior sagittal d. of midpelvis The posterior segment of the anteroposterior diameter of the midpelvis (i.e., the distance between the midpoint on the interspinous diameter and a point on the sacrum on the same plane).

posterior sagittal d. of pelvic outlet The posterior segment of the anteroposterior diameter of the pelvic outlet (i.e., the distance between the midpoint on the transverse diameter of the pelvic outlet and the sacrococcygeal junction).

suboccipitobregmatic d. The diameter of a fetal skull at term from the middle of the anterior fontanel to the under surface of the occipital bone, just where it joins the neck. The smallest circumference of the fetal head corresponds to the plane of the suboccipitobregmatic diameter.

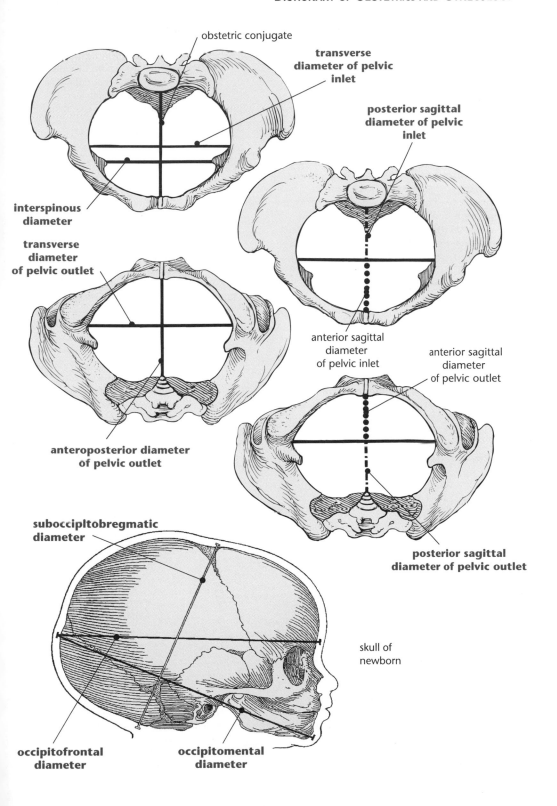

obstetric conjugate

transverse
diameter of pelvic
inlet

posterior sagittal
diameter of pelvic
inlet

interspinous
diameter

transverse
diameter
of pelvic outlet

anterior sagittal
diameter
of pelvic inlet

anterior sagittal
diameter
of pelvic outlet

anteroposterior diameter
of pelvic outlet

posterior sagittal
diameter of pelvic outlet

suboccipltobregmatic
diameter

skull of
newborn

occipitofrontal
diameter

occipitomental
diameter

transverse d. of midpelvis See interspinous diameter.

transverse d. of pelvic inlet The greatest distance between opposite sides of the pelvic brim (i.e., between the iliopectineal lines on either side).

transverse d. of pelvic outlet The distance between the two ischial tuberosities. Also called bituberous diameter; intertuberous diameter; biischial diameter.

diamine oxidase (di-ă-mēn ok'sĭ-dās) An enzyme that promotes the metabolism of the polyamine putrescine; its activity in decidual tissues is enhanced by progesterone action.

diaphragm (di'ă-fram) 1. A dome-shaped, musculofibrous structure separating the thoracic and abdominal cavities and functioning in such activities as respiration, defecation, and parturition; its periphery consists of muscular fibers attached to the circumference of the thoracic outlet, namely, to the back of the xiphoid process, to the internal surface of the lower six ribs and their cartilages, to the arcuate ligaments, and to the lumbar vertebrae; the fibers converge toward a central tendon, a thin but strong aponeurosis located immediately below the fibrous covering of the heart (pericardium), with which it is partly blended. Also called thoracoabdominal diaphragm. 2. Any anatomic partition. 3. Any device serving as a partition. 4. The adjustable grid of lead strips used for minimizing radiation exposure to patients when taking x-ray pictures.

contraceptive d. A dome-shaped, individually fitted, rubber disk coated with a spermicidal agent just prior to each use; it is inserted into the vagina prior to sexual intercourse in order to cover the uterine cervix and thus prevent pregnancy.

pelvic d. The part of the pelvic floor formed by the paired levator ani and coccygeus muscles and their fasciae.

thoracoabdominal d. See diaphragm (1).

urogenital d. A strong musculomembranous structure stretched across the anterior half of the pelvic outlet between the ischiopubic rami; it is composed of the sphincter muscle of the membranous urethra, and the right and left deep transverse muscle of the perineum and fascia. In the female, it is primarily pierced by the urethra and vagina; in the male, by the membranous urethra and the ducts of the Cowper's (bulbourethral) glands.

diaplacental (di-ă-plă-sen'tal) Through the placenta.

diarrhea (di-ă-re'ă) An increase in the looseness or fluidity and frequency of bowel movements beyond what is normal for the person.

traveler's d. Diarrhea occurring in a person who lives in an industrialized country and travels to a developing country, usually in tropical or semitropical areas; caused by a variety of bacterial and viral microorganisms; may occur suddenly while traveling, lasting 1 to 3 days and causing the passage of at least three unformed stools in a 24-hour period,

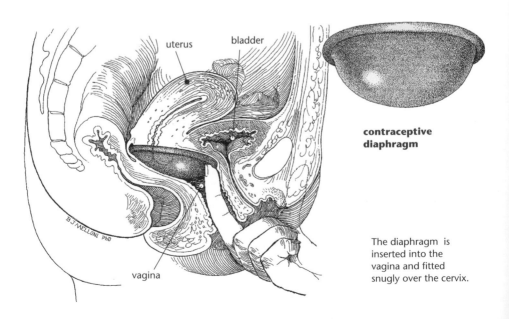

contraceptive diaphragm

The diaphragm is inserted into the vagina and fitted snugly over the cervix.

accompanied by nausea, vomiting, abdominal cramps, fecal urgency, or the passage of bloody or mucoid stools; or it may occur during the first 7 to 10 days after returning home, causing the passage of 3 to 10 unformed stools daily for 3 to 5 days, usually accompanied by abdominal cramps and, sometimes, fever, vomiting, and bloody stools. Colloquially called turista.

diastasis (di-as'tă-sis) Abnormal separation of two normally joined structures.

    d. recti Separation of the two abdominal rectus muscles along the midline, sometimes occurring in pregnancy or abdominal surgery.

diathesis (di-ath'ĕ-sis) An inherited predisposition to a disease or abnormality; a constitutional susceptibility.

    cystic d. A susceptibility to formation of cysts in an organ.

diazepam (di-az'ĕ-pam) A nondiuretic thiazide derivative with addiction potential, used primarily as an antianxiety agent and as an adjunct in the treatment of muscle spasms; also used in the management of alcohol withdrawal symptoms; intrauterine exposure may cause adverse effects on the neonate (e.g., lethargy, sucking difficulties, withdrawal syndrome, apnea, delayed motor development). Trade name: Valium.

diazoxide (di-az-ok'sīd) A nondiuretic thiazide derivative used intravenously to lower blood pressure in the management of a hypertensive crisis; intrauterine exposure may cause transient slowing of the fetal heart and increased blood sugar level.

dicephalous (di-sef'ă-lus) Having two heads; applied to certain conjoined twins.

diet (di'et) **1.** Bodily nourishment, daily sustenance. **2.** Regulated nourishment, including or excluding certain items of food, especially as prescribed for health reasons. **3.** To follow a specific dietary plan, especially for reduction of body weight by limitation of caloric intake. **4.** Anything taken regularly.

differentiation (dif-er-en-she-a'shun) **1.** In biology, the process of developing into specialized organs; applied to embryonic tissues. **2.** See differential diagnosis, under diagnosis.

    cell d. In embryology, the progressive restriction of developmental potential and the increasing specialization of function occurring during development of the embryo, leading to formation of tissues and organs.

dihydrotestosterone (di-hi-dro-tes-tos'ter-ōn) (DHT) A potent androgenic hormone, secreted by both the ovary and adrenal (suprarenal) glands but primarily formed in peripheral tissues (e.g., hair follicles) by the action of the enzyme 5α-reductase upon testosterone; believed to play a significant role in somatic virilization during embryonic development.

dilatation (dil-ă-ta'shun) The condition of being enlarged or stretched by normal or artificial processes or as a result of disease; applied to a tubular structure, a cavity, or an opening. Also called dilation.

    gastric d. An uncommon, life-threatening complication of surgery, characterized by massive distention of the stomach due to accumulation of fluid with secondary bleeding; may follow untreated gastric gas distention; predisposing factors may include asthma, absence of spleen, and conditions associated with low cardiac output.

dilatation and curettage (dil-ă-ta'shun and ku-rĕ-tazh') (D and C) Dilatation of the uterine cervix and scraping of the uterine lining with either a sharp or blunt curet, or with a vacuum aspirator; used for diagnosis and treatment, or after childbirth or an early spontaneous abortion to remove any residual placenta. See also vacuum aspiration curettage, under curettage.

dilatation and evacuation (dil-a-ta'shun and e-vak-u-a'shun) (D and E) Induced abortion performed after 16 weeks of gestation by wide dilatation of the uterine cervix (e.g., by serial application of *Laminaria* tents), followed by mechanical fetal destruction and removal of fetal parts; the placenta and remaining pregnancy products are then removed with a large bore vacuum curet.

dilatation and extraction (dil-a-ta'shun and eks-trak'-shun) (D and X) See dilatation and evacuation.

dilate (di-lāt') To enlarge; to stretch.

dilation (di-la'shun) See dilatation.

dilator (di-la'tor) Instrument for enlarging a passage, cavity, or opening.

    cervical d. Any device used to expand the cervical canal.

    Hank's d. A cylindrical implement with a sharply tapered end for gradual dilatation of the cervix.

    Hegar's d.'s A series of cylindrical, blunt, curved implements of graduated diameters, each with a number designation corresponding to its diameter in millimeters; used sequentially (from thinner to thicker) to gently and slowly dilate the cervical canal, especially in dilatation and curettage operations, and for digitally palpating the uterine cavity.

    hygroscopic d. An absorbent material,

organic or synthetic, that expands gradually upon exposure to moisture (e.g., *Laminaria* tents and synthetic sponges); used to soften, dilate, and efface the cervix prior to a vaginal delivery or an abortion.

pneumatic d. An inflatable tube used for stretching a muscular constriction (achalasia) of the esophagus.

diltiazem (dil-ti'ă-zem) A calcium channel blocking agent of the benzothiazepine class used in the treatment of angina pectoris and hypertension. Adverse effects include swelling of the ankles, headache, and constipation.

dimenhydrinate (di-men-hi'drĭ-nāt) An antihistamine drug used in the prevention and treatment of motion sickness. Trade name: Dramamine.

dioxin (di-oks'in) A toxic chlorinated hydrocarbon; a herbicide contaminant; also formed at incineration sites; causes birth defects and cancer in laboratory animals and possibly in humans.

dipalmitoylphosphatidylcholine (di-pal-mĭ-to'il-fos-fă-ti-dil-ko'lēn) (DPPC) A phospholipid which is the major component of surfactant.

diphenhydramine hydrochloride (di-fen-hi'dră-mēn hi-dro-klo'rīd) An antihistamine drug used in the treatment of allergies. Adverse effects include drowsiness and dry mouth. Trade name: Benadryl.

diplegia (di-ple'ge-ă) Paralysis of corresponding parts on both sides of the body. Also called bilateral paralysis.

diplo- Combining form meaning double.

diplotene (dip'lo-tēn) In meiosis, the stage in the prophase of the first meiotic division in which paired chromosomes separate longitudinally. See also leptotene; pachytene; zygotene.

diprosopus dipygus (di-pros'o-pus di-pi'gus) Conjoined twins attached either at the upper or lower half of the body with incomplete double development of parts.

dis- Prefix meaning opposite of, not, apart.

disease (dĭ-zēz') Any abnormal condition that affects either the whole body or any of its parts, is manifested by a characteristic set of symptoms and signs, and impairs normal functioning.

ABO hemolytic d. See hemolytic disease of the newborn.

Addison's d. Chronic deficiency of hormones that are concerned with mineral and glucose metabolism, due to destruction of the adrenal cortex; findings include a bronzelike pigmentation of skin and mucous membranes, anemia, low blood pressure, and low concentration of sodium in the blood. In pregnancy, the most reliable signs include

persistent nausea and vomiting and appetite and weight loss.

Bart d. See alpha thalassemia, under thalassemia.

brittle bone d. See osteogenesis imperfecta, under osteogenesis.

Bourneville's d. See tuberous sclerosis, under sclerosis.

Bowen's d. Noninvasive squamous cell carcinoma of the skin involving only the superficial layer (epidermis), appearing as pink-to-brown papules or plaques covered with gray-white encrustations; occurs in multiple sites, especially in sun-exposed areas of the body and in the genitals of both males and females over 35 years; associated with increased (25%) incidence of cancer of internal organs.

cerebrovascular d. Any brain dysfunction due to a disruption of the blood supply to the brain.

chronic obstructive lung d. (COLD) See chronic obstructive pulmonary disease.

chronic obstructive pulmonary d. (COPD) The combination of chronic bronchitis and emphysema with increased resistance to air flow in the lungs. Also called chronic obstructive lung disease (COLD).

coronary artery d. (CAD) Occlusion of the coronary arteries, which supply blood to the heart muscle, by formation of fatty-fibrous plaques in the arterial walls (atherosclerosis); may cause angina pectoris, myocardial infarction, and sudden death. Also called coronary heart disease (CHD).

coronary heart d. (CHD) See coronary artery disease.

Crohn's d. Chronic inflammation of the gastrointestinal tract; it most commonly affects the ileum but may involve the entire gut from mouth to anus; characterized by formation of sharply demarcated deep ulcers separated by normal (skip) areas, with thickening of the walls, narrowing of the lumen, and perforations with connections into adjacent structures (e.g., other bowel segments, bladder, vagina) or abdominal skin; symptoms may be precipitated by periods of emotional or physical stress and include diarrhea, fever, and pain in the lower right area of the abdomen. Also called regional enteritis; terminal ileitis; distal ileitis.

Cushing's d. Overactivity of the adrenal cortex and increased production of cortisone; caused by excessive secretion of adrenocorticotropic hormone (ACTH) from the pituitary. Also called hypercortisolism. See also Cushing's syndrome, under syndrome.

cyanotic heart d. Any of a group of disorders (e.g., tetralogy of Fallot and Ebstein's anomaly) characterized by the presence of congenital heart defects associated with right-to-left shunting of blood, resulting in discoloration of the skin and mucous membranes (cyanosis).

cystic d. of the breast See fibrocystic change of the breast, under change.

cytomegalic inclusion d. Disease caused by infection with cytomegalovirus (CMV), a herpesvirus that remains dormant indefinitely in the tissues of the infected person and may be reactivated. Symptoms depend on the organs affected, or the disease may be asymptomatic. It may be acquired through sexual contact, transfusion of infected blood, or transplantation of an infected organ. An infected pregnant woman can transmit the disease to her fetus through the placenta, or during childbirth as the infant passes through the birth canal, or via breast milk. The infected infant may develop enlargement of the liver and spleen, jaundice, superficial hemorrhages (purpura), central nervous system involvement, and mental retardation. People undergoing immunosuppressive therapy and those afflicted with acquired immune deficiency syndrome (AIDS) are susceptible to infection with the virus or its reactivation.

diverticular d. of colon Condition occurring most commonly in people over 60 years old; characterized by formation of outpouchings of the mucous lining of the colon, which protrude through defects in the muscular wall of the bowel at points of blood vessel entry; may be asymptomatic or may cause intermittent cramping pain and bleeding; occasionally may undergo inflammatory changes and infection. Also called diverticulosis. See also diverticulitis.

extramammary Paget's d. See Paget's disease of vulva.

fibrocystic d. (FCD) of breast See fibrocystic change of the breast, under change.

fifth d. See erythema infectiosum, under erythema.

Fox-Fordyce d. An uncommon disorder affecting mainly women, characterized by eruptions of dry, intensely itchy papules in the breasts, armpits, and pubic area.

genetic d. General term for any inherited disease caused by a defective gene.

gestational trophoblastic d. (GTD) Any of a group of pregnancy-related tumors or tumor-like conditions that have a progressive potential for becoming cancerous; characterized by proliferation of trophoblastic tissue; the lesions include invasive mole, hydatidiform mole, choriocarcinoma, and placental-site tumors. Also called gestational trophoblastic neoplasia (GTN).

graft-versus-host d. (GVHD) A type of incompatibility reaction in which the T lymphocytes of the graft react against the host tissues; it is the major cause of mortality in bone marrow transplantation.

hemolytic H d. See alpha thalassemia, under thalassemia.

hemolytic d. of the newborn A condition resulting from an incompatibility of fetal and maternal red blood cell groups in which fetal red blood cells (antigens) are destroyed by the transplacental passage of maternal antibodies of the IgG type. Although most often caused by Rh factor incompatibility, it occurs with other less common blood groups, such as Kell and Duffy. ABO blood group incompatibility may also cause a milder form of this disease, and is usually manifest in the neonatal period.

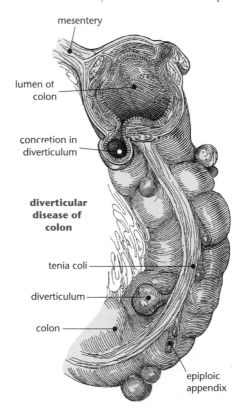

mesentery

lumen of colon

concretion in diverticulum

diverticular disease of colon

tenia coli

diverticulum

colon

epiploic appendix

Also called ABO hemolytic disease; erythroblastosis fetalis; fetal erythroblastosis; hemolytic anemia of the newborn.

hemorrhagic d. of newborn Deficiency of vitamin K-dependent clotting factors (II, VII, IX, X), causing bleeding in an infant in the first days of life; sites of bleeding usually include the gastrointestinal tract, umbilical stump, circumcision site, and nose.

hereditary d. Disease transmitted genetically from parent to offspring.

Hirschsprung's d. See congenital megacolon, under megacolon.

hookworm d. Infection with either of two hookworm species, *Ancylostoma duodenale* or *Necator americanus*; the parasites' larvae penetrate the host's skin and eventually migrate through the lungs to the small intestine, where they mature while remaining attached to the intestinal lining. Severe or prolonged infections may cause iron-deficiency anemia and, occasionally, a reduction of albumin in the blood.

hyaline membrane d. See respiratory distress syndrome of the newborn, under syndrome.

immune complex d. (ICD) Any of a group of conditions caused by circulating immune complexes (i.e., antibody and antigen molecules tightly bound together and sometimes including protein), which become trapped within the walls of small blood vessels, especially within the filtering units (glomeruli) of the kidney, thereby triggering a hypersensitivity reaction; they include systemic lupus erythematosus, rheumatoid arthritis, dermatomyositis, Sjögren's syndrome, Behçet's syndrome, and several vasculitis syndromes; high blood pressure is a common occurrence, which may be aggravated during pregnancy, necessitating an early delivery. Also called connective tissue disorder; collagen-vascular disorder.

inflammatory bowel d. (IBD) General term for a group of chronic conditions of the gastrointestinal tract. See also Crohn's disease; ulcerative colitis, under colitis.

ischemic heart d. (IHD) Any of a group of heart conditions having in common an imbalance of oxygen supply and demand; most commonly caused by reduced blood flow to the heart due to coronary artery occlusion; may also be caused by abnormally increased oxygen demand (e.g., in ventricular hypertrophy due to hypertension), or by a reduction in the oxygen-carrying capacity of

the blood (e.g., in severe anemia), or by a combination of the two.

kyphoscoliotic heart d. Impairment of heart and lung function due to severe deformation of the chest cavity by an abnormal backward and lateral curvature of the spine (kyphoscoliosis); may be aggravated during pregnancy due to the typically increased oxygen demands and cardiac workload of the pregnant state.

Lou Gehrig's d. See amyotrophic lateral sclerosis, under sclerosis.

Lyme d. A multisystem disease involving the skin, heart, nervous system, and joints, caused by a corkscrew-shaped microorganism *(Borrelia burgdorferi)*. Field mice and white-tailed deer are the most common reservoirs of the microorganisms, which are transmitted to humans by the bite of infected ixodid ticks (especially *Ixodes dammini*). In most cases, the disease progresses in three stages. Stage 1: *Localized infection,* manifested, 1 to 4 weeks after the bite of an infected tick, by the appearance of the characteristic skin lesion (erythema migrans), which sometimes expands into a reddened area several inches across and may be accompanied by flu-like symptoms. Stage 2: *Disemminated infection*; other symptoms occur days or weeks later; may include secondary annular skin lesions, muscle and joint pains, fever, headache, neuritis, meningitis, lethargy, irregular heartbeat, dizziness, and fainting. Stage 3: *Persistent infection*; arthritis of one or more large joints, especially of the knee, is a predominant feature, appearing months to years later; it may become chronic, lasting weeks or months with recurrences. Pregnancy complications may include preterm labor or fetal death; a rash-like illness has been reported in the newborn. Also called Lyme borreliosis.

mitral valve d. Any disease of the left atrioventricular (mitral) valve of the heart. See mitral prolapse, under prolapse; mitral regurgitation, under regurgitation; mitral stenosis, under stenosis.

notifiable d. A disease that, by statutory requirements, must be reported to public health officials of the proper jurisdiction (federal, state, or local) when diagnosis is made and is deemed important to human health. Also called reportable disease.

Osler-Weber-Rendu d. See hereditary hemorrhagic telangiectasia, under telangiectasia.

Paget's d. of breast Carcinoma of the

breast arising within the major excretory ducts of the nipple-areola complex and extending to the overlying skin; initial symptoms are minimal; they usually include itching and burning of the nipple with superficial eczematoid changes and, often, a nipple discharge.

Paget's d. of vulva A red, crusted, maplike area usually restricted to the epithelium of the vulva, predominantly on the labia majora; sometimes it extends to the perianal and inguinal areas, buttocks, and mons; initial symptoms are itching and tenderness; unlike Paget's disease of the breast, it is not usually associated with underlying cancer of vulvar glands. Also called extramammary Paget's disease.

pelvic inflammatory d. (PID) Acute or chronic inflammation of the female reproductive organs and associated structures; may not have obvious causes; often caused by sexually transmitted diseases (e.g., gonorrhea, *Chlamydia* and *Mycoplasma* infections; may also occur after induced abortion, miscarriage, or childbirth.

polycystic ovary d., PCO d. Disorder affecting young women characterized by bilaterally enlarged ovaries with multiple cysts, chronic failure to release ova, secondary absent or scanty menstruation (amenorrhea or oligomenorrhea), and infertility. Also called polycystic ovary syndrome.

polygenic d. Any disease resulting from the interaction of multiple genes that alone produce relatively minor effects.

preinvasive d. See cervical intraepithelial neoplasia, vaginal intraepithelial neoplasia, vulvar intraepithelial neoplasia, under neoplasia.

proliferative breast d. (PBD) Condition marked by benign but excessive multiplication of cells in mammary tissue; the cells do not lose their distinctive characteristics or invade other tissues as do cancerous cells. The condition occurs as an inherited trait in families that have a high prevalence of either premenopausal or postmenopausal breast cancer.

pulseless d. See Takayasu's arteritis, under arteritis.

Recklinghausen's d. See neurofibromatosis I.

reportable d. See notifiable disease.

runt d. Condition characterized by failure to thrive, enlargement of liver and spleen, lymph node atrophy, anemia, and diarrhea; a graft-versus-host disease occurring in an immunologically immature experimental animal after injection of mature immunologically competent cells from a donor of the same species.

severe combined immunodeficiency d. (SCID) A severe form of congenital immunodeficiency characterized by failure of T and B lymphocyte functions and deficiency of lymphoid tissue; development of the thymus gland is typically arrested in fetal life; caused by a defect of the lymphoid stem cells; inherited in a variable pattern, either as an autosomal recessive or an X-linked recessive inheritance. Death usually occurs from opportunistic infections within the first year of life.

sexually transmitted d.'s (STDs) Disorders spread by intimate contact (including sexual intercourse, kissing, cunnilingus, anilingus, fellatio, mouth–breast contact, and anal intercourse); many can be acquired transplacentally by the fetus or through contact with maternal secretions by the newborn; causative microorganisms include herpesvirus 1 and 2, cytomegalovirus, *Chlamydia*, group *B Streptococcus*, molluscum contagiosum virus, *Sarcoptes scabiei*, hepatitis viruses, and human immunodeficiency virus (HIV). Also called venereal diseases.

sickle cell d. See sickle cell anemia, under anemia.

sickle cell C d. Disease characterized by anemia, blood vessel occlusion, chronic leg ulcers, and bone deformities; caused by a genetically determined abnormality of red blood cells, which contain hemoglobin S and hemoglobin C.

Simmonds' d. See panhypopituitarism.

slapped cheek d. See erythema infectiosum, under erythema.

social d. Obsolete term for any sexually transmitted disease.

venereal d.'s See sexually transmitted diseases.

von Willebrand's d. Hemorrhagic disease transmitted as an autosomal inheritance, characterized by spontaneous bleeding from mucous membranes (especially the gums and gastrointestinal tract), excessive bleeding from wounds, and profuse or prolonged menstrual flow; the abnormal bleeding occurs in the presence of normal platelet count and normal clot retraction; caused by partial and variable deficiency of factor VIII, a blood clotting factor.

Werdnig-Hoffmann d. A rare disease of newborns inherited as an autosomal trait; it affects the motor nerve cells of the spinal cord, causing floppiness and paralysis of muscle (including those involved in breathing and feeding). Death usually occurs before the child is 3 years old. Cause is unknown. The infant's mother sometimes recalls being aware of reduced fetal movements during pregnancy. Also called infantile muscular atrophy; infantile progressive spinal muscular atrophy; (colloquially) floppy infant.

disengagement (dis-en-gāj'ment) In childbirth, the emergence of the presenting part of the fetus through the vulva.

disk (disk) Any platelike structure, usually circular in form. Also spelled disc.

    ectodermal d. In the embryo, an elongated mass of epithelial cells developed from the inner cell mass about 1 week after fertilization.

    herniated d. Posterior rupture of the inner portion of an intervertebral disk, causing pressure on the nerve roots with resulting pain; occurring most commonly in the lower back. Also called ruptured disk; prolapsed disk; slipped disk.

    interpubic d. A midline plate of

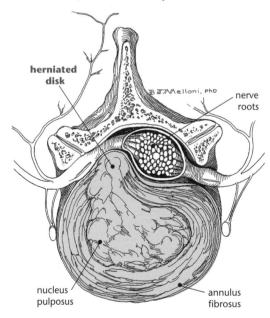

fibrocartilage between the pubic bones at the symphysis.

    intervertebral d.'s The fibrocartilaginous pads interposed between the bodies of adjacent vertebrae, from the axis (second cervical vertebra) to the sacrum, consisting of a jelly-like center (nucleus pulposus)

surrounded by a fibrous ring (annulus fibrosus). They act as elastic buffers to absorb the daily mechanical shocks sustained by the spinal column. The disks are lacking between the atlas (first cervical vertebra) and the axis, and between the atlas and the lower part of the skull (occiput).

    Merkel tactile d. See tactile disk.

    prolapsed d. See herniated disk.

    ruptured d. See herniated disk.

    slipped d. Popular name for herniated disk.

    tactile d. The saucer-shaped termination of specialized sensory nerve fibers in contact with a single, modified epithelial cell in the deep layer of the epidermis, in hair follicles, and in the hard palate; it functions as a touch receptor. Also called Merkel tactile disk.

dislocate (dis'lo-kāt) To shift from the usual or normal position, especially to displace a bone from its socket.

dislocation (dis-lo-ka'shun) Displacement of a body part from its normal location, especially of a bone from its socket or joint.

    closed d. Dislocation of a bone occurring without an external wound. Also called simple dislocation.

    compound d. See open dislocation.

    congenital d. of hip Dislocation present at birth, thought to be caused by chronic deficiency of amniotic fluid, resulting in an inadequately small uterine cavity that does not allow proper positioning of the enlarging fetus.

    open d. Dislocation of a bone occurring in conjunction with an open wound. Also called compound dislocation.

    simple d. See closed dislocation.

disomy (di'so-me) The normal presence of two members of a chromosome in each of the 23 pairs, each member of the pair acquired from each parent.

    uniparental d. The abnormal presence of two members of a chromosome pair acquired from one of the parents.

disorder (dis-or'der) An abnormality of function.

    anxiety d.'s A group of disorders characterized by persistent apprehension and worry as the predominant disturbance and by the onset of anxiety when the person attempts to confront his symptoms. See also anxiety.

    arrest d. of labor Any of four abnormal patterns of labor, often reflective of dystocia, and diagnosed on the basis of gravidity and labor progress: *prolonged deceleration phase* (lasts more than 3 hours in nulliparas or 1 hour in multiparas); *secondary arrest of dilatation* (no progression of cervical dilatation occurs in the active phase of labor for 2 or more hours); *arrest of descent* (fetal descent stops for 1 or more hours); *failure of descent* (no fetal descent occurs during deceleration phase of dilatation and second stage of labor). Causes include fetopelvic disproportion, fetal malposition, excessive sedation, and inappropriately administered anesthesia.

bleeding d. Popular name for any condition associated with spontaneous bleeding or with abnormally prolonged or excessive bleeding after injury (e.g., hemophilia and von Willebrand's disease).

collagen-vascular d. See immune complex disease, under disease.

connective tissue d. See immune complex disease, under disease.

eating d. Any of a group of disorders characterized by abnormalities of appetite, food intake, or both, including bulimia, anorexia nervosa, and pica.

genetic d. Any disorder due entirely or in part to a defective gene; distinguished from congenital, although a disorder may be both genetic and congenital.

immunoproliferative d. Proliferation of cells of the lymphoreticular system associated with autoallergic disturbances or gamma-globulin abnormalities.

mendelian d. See single-gene disorder.

obsessive-compulsive d. (OCD) Anxiety disorder characterized by obsessions (recurrent ideas, thoughts, or impulses) and compulsions (repetitive behaviors designed to produce or prevent some future situation) which are experienced as distressful and interfere with social functioning.

panic d. Anxiety disorder characterized by panic attacks. See also panic attack, under attack.

posttraumatic stress d. (PTSD) Anxiety disorder resulting from having experienced an overwhelming stress or trauma (e.g., rape or assault), characterized by recurrent nightmares, flashbacks, intrusive recollections, general detachment, excessive startle response, and abnormal response to stimuli that recall the traumatic event. Also called posttraumatic neurosis; posttraumatic stress syndrome.

precipitate labor d. Condition in which labor and delivery occur at an extremely rapid rate (i.e., when the presenting part descends about 5 cm or more per hour in a nullipara, or about 10 cm or more per hour in a multipara); may be caused by abnormally strong uterine contractions or abnormally low resistance of the birth canal.

protraction d. In obstetrics, any of two abnormally slow patterns of labor: *prolonged active-phase dilatation* (dilatation of the cervix occurring less than 1.2 cm/h in nulliparas or less than 1.5 cm/h in multiparas); *prolonged descent of the fetus* (fetal descent occurring less than 1 cm/h in nulliparas or less than 2 cm/h in multiparas).

PATTERNS OF DISORDERED LABOR

Labor Pattern	Nullipara	Multipara
Prolonged latent-phase disorder	> 20 hrs	> 14hrs
Protraction disorders		
Protracted active-phase dilatation	< 1.2 cm/hr	< 1.5 cm/hr
Protracted descent	< 1.0 cm/hr	< 2.0 cm/hr
Arrest disorders		
Prolonged deceleration phase	> 3 hrs	> 1 hr
Secondary arrest of dilatation	> 2 hrs	> 2 hrs
Arrest of descent	> 1 hr	> 1 hr
Failure of descent	no descent in deceleration phase or second stage	no descent in desceleration phase or second stage

---

psychosexual d.'s A group of disorders of sexual functioning caused primarily by psychological factors; includes gender identity disorders such as transsexualism, the paraphilias (e.g., fetishes, voyeurism, exhibitionism, sexual sadism, sexual masochism), and psychosexual dysfunctions.

single-gene d. Any disorder (e.g., cystic fibrosis, fragile X syndrome, hemophilia A) that is caused by the occurrence of a mutant gene present either on only one chromosome of a pair or on both chromosomes of the pair at a single locus (i.e., a single-gene defect). Sometimes called mendelian disorder.

dispermy (di'sper-me) The entrance of two spermatozoa into one ovum.

disproportion (dis-pro-por'shun) Absence of due relationship, as of size.

cephalopelvic d. Disproportion in size between the fetal head and the maternal pelvis, precluding vaginal delivery. Designated *absolute cephalopelvic d.* when it occurs regardless of whether the fetal head presents its largest diameters; *relative cephalopelvic d.* when the fetal head presents its largest diameters and consequently cannot pass through the maternal pelvis.

inlet d. See contraction of pelvic inlet, under contraction.

outlet d. See contraction of pelvic outlet, under contraction.

fetopelvic d. Disproportion in size between the presenting part of the fetus and the maternal pelvis, precluding vaginal delivery. The term is commonly used to characterize a situation in which the presenting part is the breech.

disruption (dis-rup'shun) Deformity of a body part resulting from breakdown of, or interference with, an originally normal developmental process.

wound d. See dehiscence.

dissection (dĭ-sek'shun) The act of dissecting.

aortic d. See dissecting aneurysm of aorta, under aneurysm.

disseminated (dĭ-sem'ĭ-nāt-ed) Widely distributed; widespread.

distention (dis-ten'shun) The state of being stretched as from internal pressure.

acute gastric d. Massive distention of the stomach caused by accumulation of air; commonly seen as a postoperative complication.

distress (dis-tres') Physical or mental anguish or pain.

fetal d. A complex of signs reflecting the response of the fetus to stress; may be acute or chronic.

diuresis (di-u-re'sis) Discharge of increased amounts of urine.

alcohol d. Diuresis induced by consumption of alcoholic beverages.

osmotic d. Diuresis caused by filtration into the kidney tubules of substances that limit water reabsorption.

water d. Diuresis caused by a reduced release of antidiuretic hormone from the pituitary in response to lower osmotic pressure in the blood after administration of water.

diuretic (di-u-ret'ik) An agent that increases the volume flow of urine.

diurnal (di-er'nal) **1.** Occurring during the day; opposite of nocturnal. **2.** Occurring once every 24 hours (e.g., a rhythm).

divarication (di-var-ĭ-ka'shun) Diversion, separation (e.g., of muscles or muscle fibers).

diverticula (di-ver-tik'u-lă) Plural of diverticulum.

diverticular (di-ver-tik'u-lar) Relating to a diverticulum.

diverticulectomy (di-ver-tik-u-lek'tŏ-me) Removal of one or more diverticula.

diverticulitis (di-ver-tik-u-li'tis) Inflammatory changes occurring in diverticular disease of the colon; the saccular outpouchings of the intestinal wall become impacted with feces; infection follows; bowel perforation, abscess formation, or peritonitis may also occur; most common symptoms include acute abdominal pain and tenderness, fever, and nausea. See also diverticular disease of colon, under disease.

diverticulosis (di-ver-tik-u-lo'sis) See diverticular disease of colon, under disease.

diverticulum (di-ver-tik'u-lum), pl. diverticula A saccular dilatation of variable size protruding from the wall of a tubular organ or structure; may be a normal structure or may be a herniation through the muscular coat of a tubular organ.

intestinal d. A herniation of the mucous membrane through a defect in the muscular layer of the intestinal wall.

Meckel's d. A congenital sacculation or appendage of the distal part of the small intestine (ileum); it is derived from the yolk stalk (omphalomesenteric duct) that failed to obliterate normally during intrauterine life.

Nuck's d. See persistent processus vaginalis peritonei, under processus.

division (dĭ-vizh'on) Separation.

first meiotic d. See meiosis.

reduction d. See meiosis.

second meiotic d. See meiosis.

dol (dōl) A unit of measure of pain intensity.

dolicho- Combining form meaning long.

dolichocephalic, dolichocephalous (dol-ĭ-ko-sě-fal'ik, dol ĭ ko-sef'ă-lus) Having an abnormally long head; denoting a skull with a cephalic index below 80.

dolichopelvic (dol-ĭ-ko-pel'vik) Having a long narrow pelvis.

dolorific (do-lor-if'ik) Producing pain.

domain (do-mān') One of the regions of a peptide molecule having a coherent structure of functional significance that distinguishes it from other regions of the same molecule.

dominance (dom'ĭ-nans) The state of being dominant.

> **fundal d.** The greater intensity of uterine contractions in the uterine fundus relative to those in the mid- or lower portions of the uterus; observed in the normal process of labor.

dominant (dom'ĭ-nant) **1.** Exerting control. **2.** In genetics, denoting a characteristic that is apparent even when the gene for it is inherited from only one parent.

donor (do'nor) **1.** One who gives blood for transfusion, organs for transplantation, or spermatozoa for artificial insemination. **2.** In chemistry, a substance that yields part of itself to another substance.

dorsal (dor'sal) Relating to the back of the body or to the posterior part of an anatomic structure.

dorsiflexion (dor-sĭ-flek'shun) Flexion or bending upward, as of the foot or toes.

dorsolumbar (dor-so-lum'bar) Relating to the back of the body between the upper lumbar and lower thoracic regions.

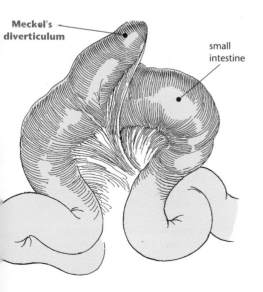

Meckel's diverticulum

small intestine

dosage (do'sij) The determination and formulation of doses (e.g., of medications or radioactivity).

dose (dōs) (D) **1.** A specified amount given at one time or at stated intervals. **2.** In genetics, the number of copies of a particular gene present in a chromosome.

> **absorbed d.** The amount of ionizing radiation absorbed by the tissues at one time. In radiation therapy, the former unit is the rad; the current (SI) unit is the gray (Gy).

> **booster d.** A supplementary dose of an immunizing agent given to maintain immunity.

> **curative d.** The amount of any therapeutic substance required to cure a disease or correct a deficiency.

> **daily d.** The total amount of a medication taken during a 24-hour period.

> **divided d.** A portion of the dose of a drug given repeatedly at short intervals to add up to the full dose within a specified period of time.

> **effective d.** (ED) (1) The quantity of a drug that produces the desired effects. (2) In radiation protection, the sum of the equivalent doses in all body tissues weighted for tissue effects of radiation. The effective dose (SI) unit is the sievert (Sv).

> **equivalent d.** In radiation protection, the absorbed dose averaged over a tissue and weighted for the quality of the radiation of interest. The equivalent dose (SI) unit is the sievert (Sv).

> **erythema d.** The minimal safe amount of radiation required to produce redness of the skin within 10 days to 2 weeks.

> **exposure d.** The radiation dose delivered at a point in free air; expressed in roentgens.

> **gonad d., gonadal d.** The exposure dose delivered to the ovaries or testes, usually from secondary (scattered) radiation in diagnostic or therapeutic irradiation, or from whole-body exposure.

> **initial d.** A relatively large dose administered at the beginning of a treatment. Also called loading dose.

> **loading d.** See initial dose.

> **maintenance d.** The amount of medication administered to keep the patient under the influence of the drug after larger amounts have been given previously.

> **maximal permissible d.** (MPD) The greatest amount of radiation to which a person may be exposed without causing harmful effects.

> **minimal infective d.** (MID) The smallest amount of infective material that produces disease.

skin d. (SD) The amount of radiation received on the skin surface.

dosimetry (do-sim'ĕ-tre) Determination of correct dosages.

dosimetrist (do-sim'ĕ-trist) A person who plans and calculates the proper radiation dose necessary for treatment in radiation therapy.

douche (dōōsh) A stream of liquid, vapor, or gas directed into a cavity of the body, especially the rinsing of the vagina with a liquid.

down-regulation (doun reg-u-la'shun) A decrease in the number of active receptors on the cell surface in response to an excess of a homologous hormone or neurotransmitter.

doxorubicin (dok-so-roo'bĭ-sin) An anticancer antibiotic drug administered intravenously, either in single-agent chemotherapy or in combination with other chemotherapeutic agents, for the treatment of a wide variety of cancers, including gynecologic cancers; adverse effects are those usually common to all, or most, antibiotic chemotherapeutic agents (anthracyclines); although normal infants have been delivered after intrauterine exposure, some fetal malformations have also been reported.

doxycycline (dok-se-si'klēn) An antibiotic agent of the tetracycline group used to treat a wide variety of microbial infections, especially sexually transmitted infections caused by such bacteria as *Chlamydia trachomatis* and *Neisseria gonorrhoeae;* adverse effects of intrauterine exposure include permanent discoloration of teeth, enamel dysplasia, and growth inhibition.

drainage (drān'ij) **1.** The continuous draining of fluid from a body cavity or wound. **2.** The fluid drained off.

    capillary d. Drainage effected by means of a wick of gauze or other material.

    closed d. Drainage of a cavity (e.g., of the chest) carried out with protection against entrance of outside air into the cavity.

    open d. Drainage of a cavity without sealing off the wound against entrance of outside air.

    tidal d. Drainage of a paralyzed bladder by means of an irrigation apparatus.

drug (drug) Any chemical agent capable of affecting living processes.

    d.'s of abuse A group of substances most frequently taken for the effects they produce on the brain and spinal cord; usually they belong to the psychoactive group of drugs and include alcohol, sedative-hypnotics, opiates and opioids, stimulants, and hallucinogenics.

    d. abuse See substance abuse, under abuse.

    d. addiction See drug dependence, under dependence.

    analgesic d. A medication that relieves pain without causing loss of consciousness.

    anesthetic d. A drug that produces a reversible loss of sensation.

    cell phase-specific d.'s, cell cycle-specific d.'s A group of anticancer drugs that produce their greatest cytotoxic effects on tumors when the tumor cells are actively dividing; they kill the largest number of cells when administered in multiple repeated fractions rather than a large single dose. Some of these drugs, such as fluorouracil, may cause fetal malformation and low birth weight.

    cell phase-nonspecific d.'s, cell cycle-nonspecific d.'s A group of anticancer drugs effective in the treatment of large tumors; they are most effective when administered in one single bolus dose.

    d. dependence See under dependence.

    designer d.'s A group of highly potent drugs of abuse produced in clandestine laboratories; they are either analogs of such narcotic analgesics and stimulants as meperidine, fentanyl, and amphetamines, or are variants of phencyclidine; they are manufactured in such a way that their chemical structures do not fall within the federal laws controlling manufacture and distribution of drugs listed under the Controlled Substances Act.

    d. habituation See drug dependence, under dependence.

    psychoactive d.'s A group of substances that exert a direct action on the central nervous system (CNS) and produce profound effects on mood, feeling, and behavior.

    recreational d., social d. A drug usually with euphoric effects taken for self-gratification rather than for medical reasons.

    d. resistance See drug resistance, under resistance.

    stimulant d. Any drug that increases the excitability of the central nervous system (CNS), either as its principal action or as a side or adverse effect.

    d. tolerance See drug tolerance, under tolerance.

drug-fast (drug' fast) See drug resistance, under resistance.

duct (dukt) A channel or tube, usually for conveying fluid, such as secretions from a gland to another part of the body.

    adipose d. See sebaceous duct.

    arterial d. See ductus arteriosus, under ductus.

    deferent d. The duct that conveys sperm

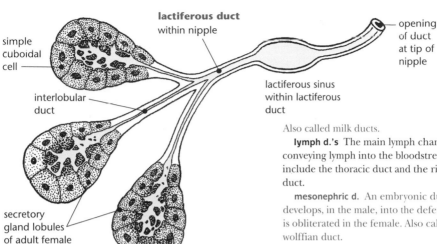

simple cuboidal cell

lactiferous duct within nipple

opening of duct at tip of nipple

interlobular duct

lactiferous sinus within lactiferous duct

secretory gland lobules of adult female breast

from the tail of the epididymis in the testis to the base of the prostate gland where it is joined by the seminal vesicle duct to form the ejaculatory duct. Also called vas deferens; ductus deferens; spermatic duct.

ejaculatory d. One of two tubes formed by the union of the terminal part of the deferent duct with the seminal vesicle duct; after passing through the prostate gland, it opens into the prostatic urethra.

lactiferous d.'s About 20 to 25 main ducts in the breast that drain milk from the lobes of the mammary gland and open on the nipple.

Also called milk ducts.

lymph d.'s The main lymph channels conveying lymph into the bloodstream; they include the thoracic duct and the right lymph duct.

mesonephric d. An embryonic duct that develops, in the male, into the deferent duct; is obliterated in the female. Also called wolffian duct.

milk d.'s See lactiferous ducts.

mullerian d. See paramesonephric duct.

paramesonephric d. In the female, either of the two embryonic tubes that develop into the uterine tubes, vagina, and uterus; it disappears in the male. Also called mullerian duct.

paraurethral d. In the female, one of two ducts formed from the union of minute excretory channels leaving the many small mucous urethral (Skene's) glands; each opens into the lateral margin of the external urethral orifice. Also called Skene's duct.

right lymph d. The smaller of two terminal lymphatic channels (about 1 cm long); it conveys lymph from the right side of the head

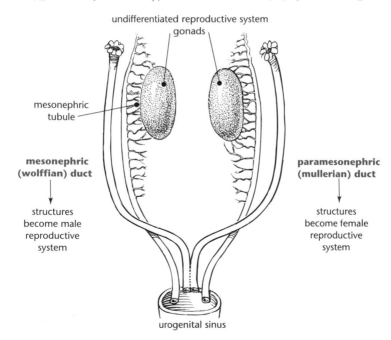

undifferentiated reproductive system

gonads

mesonephric tubule

mesonephric (wolffian) duct

↓

structures become male reproductive system

paramesonephric (mullerian) duct

↓

structures become female reproductive system

urogenital sinus

and neck, the right upper limb, and the right side of the chest, and ends by opening into the junction of the right subclavian and internal jugular veins.

sebaceous d. A duct that emerges from a sebaceous gland and opens most frequently into the distal part of the hair follicle, but occurs in most parts of the dermis, especially around the apertures of the anus, mouth, nose, and ear; it does not occur in the palms of the hand and soles of the feet; it conveys an oily secretion (sebum). Also called adipose duct.

seminal vesicle d. The short, narrow, straight tube at the lower end of the seminal vesicle that joins the deferent duct to form the ejaculatory duct.

Skene's d. See paraurethral duct.

spermatic d. See deferent duct.

urogenital d.'s The mesonephric (wolffian) and the paramesonephric (mullerian) ducts.

wolffian d. See mesonephric duct.

ductule (dukt'ūl) A small duct.

ductus (duk'tus), pl. ductus Latin for duct, a tubular structure.

d. arteriosus A communicating channel between the pulmonary artery and the beginning of the descending aorta in the fetus, directing the major output of the right ventricle into the aorta; it closes spontaneously in full-term infants by 4 days of age, remaining as a fibrous remnant (ligamentum arteriosum). Also called arterial duct.

d. deferens See deferent duct, under duct.

patent d. arteriosus (PDA) A ductus arteriosus that remains abnormally open (patent) beyond a few weeks after birth, with blood flowing from the aorta to the pulmonary artery, resulting in recirculation of oxygenated blood through the lungs; the signs of PDA include an active precordium, increased peripheral pulses, and a widened pulse pressure; the abnormal condition can be confirmed by echocardiography; seen in some children born to mothers who had German measles (rubella) during the first trimester of pregnancy and in a high percentage of premature infants weighing less then 1500 grams. Also called persistent ductus arteriosus.

persistent d. arteriosus See patent ductus arteriosus.

reversed d. arteriosus Patent ductus arteriosus accompanied by obstruction of the small vessels of the lungs, resulting in reversed blood flow from the pulmonary artery to the aorta.

d. venosus A major blood channel in the fetal liver created by the union of the left umbilical vein and the left branch of the portal vein in the liver; it is later joined by the left hepatic vein immediately before the ductus venosus terminates by opening into the inferior vena cava, below the right atrium of the heart. At birth, when the umbilical cord is severed, the ductus venosus obliterates and its fibrous remnant is termed the ligamentum venosum of the liver; the umbilical vein also obliterates and its fibrous remnant is termed the ligamentum teres of the liver.

Duffy blood group (duf'e blud groop) A blood group composed mainly of antigens Fy^a and Fy^b Named after the patient in whose blood it was first detected.

duodenum (du-od'e-num, du-o-de'num) The first of three portions of the small intestine (the others being the jejunum and the ileum); it extends from the lower (pyloric) end of the stomach to the jejunum and forms a constant C-shaped curve surrounding the head of the pancreas; it lies entirely above the level of the umbilicus.

duplication of chromosomes (doo-plĭ-ka'shun of kro'mo-sōms) A chromosome aberration characterized by the presence of an extra, distinct portion of chromosome, usually resulting from unequal exchange of fragments between homologous chromosomes (unequal crossing over) during the first meiotic division.

dwarf (dwarf) A very small person for whom there is no expectation of reaching a size in the range typical for people of like race and sex. Also called nanus; person of short stature.

dwarfism (dwarf'izm) In a broad sense, failure to achieve full growth potential; an abnormal condition of being very undersized, due to arrested growth; may be induced by ecological factors (e.g., dietary intake, systemic disease), by genetic factors, or by endocrine factors; diminished height is only one of the resulting features. Also called nanosomia.

achondroplastic d. Dwarfism caused by congenital abnormality in the ossification process of cartilage at the ends of long bones; affected individuals have a relatively elongated trunk, short limbs, and a large head.

acromelic d. Dwarfism characterized by extremely short distal segments of the limbs.

campomelic d. Dwarfism characterized by short limbs, affecting mainly the lower limbs, with anterior bowing of the femur and tibia, enlarged upper portion of the skull, small face with wideset eyes, depressed nasal bridge, lowset ears and, frequently, cleft palate. Females are mostly affected, some are chromosomal males (46,XY) with female or ambiguous genitalia. Death usually occurs during the neonatal period (i.e., the first 4 weeks after birth).

diastrophic d. An autosomal recessive inheritance affecting cartilage; characterized by short limbs, club feet, short broad hands deviated toward the ulnar side, fingers with limited flexion ability, ossification of ear cartilage, progressive joint contractures, and scoliosis.

Laron-type d. Dwarfism associated with ineffectiveness of growth hormone due to deficiency or absence of somatomedin, a peptide that mediates the action of growth hormone on cartilage; plasma contains high or normal levels of the growth hormone.

thanatophoric d. Dwarfism thought to be caused by a dominant mutation; characterized by markedly short limbs (covered with many skin folds), narrow thorax with short ribs, and vertebral bodies that are poorly developed and greatly reduced in height. Death usually occurs a few hours after birth.

dyad (di'ad) **1.** A pair. **2.** One pair of chromosomes formed after disjunction of a tetrad in the first meiotic division.

dynorphin (di-nor'fin) An endogenous opioid peptide present in the nervous system; it suppresses hypothalamic secretion of gonadotropin-releasing hormone (GnRH).

dys- Combining form meaning defective, bad, difficult.

dyscephaly (dis-sef'ă-le) Malformation of the head and face.

dyschondrogenesis (dis-kon-dro-jen'ĕ-sis) Defective formation of cartilage.

dysfibrinogenemia (dis-fi-brin-oje-ne'me-ă) An autosomal dominant inheritance usually affecting 50% of the offspring; characterized by a functional abnormality of fibrinogen, a plasma protein involved in blood clotting; an acquired form has been reported as a complication of certain pregnancy conditions, causing an increased risk of abortion. See also hypofibrinogenemia.

dysfunction (dis-funk'shun) An impaired or disordered functioning of an organ or body system.

erectile d. Term suggested as more precise than impotence for describing the inability to attain and/or maintain erection of the penis sufficient for satisfactory sexual intercourse, which is considered part of the overall

multifaceted process of male sexual function; causes may be organic (from the nervous or vascular systems) or psychological, but they most commonly appear to derive from problems in all three areas acting in concert; assessment and treatment of the dysfunction may require a multidisciplinary approach. Also called impotence.

hypertonic uterine d. A greatly elevated tone of the uterus typically occurring in the latent phase of labor, causing frequent, intense, yet ineffective contractions; may be due to contraction of the mid-segment of the uterus with a force that is greater than that of the uterine fundus, or to a complete lack of synchronism of nerve impulses, or to a combination of the two; may cause precipitate labor. Also called incoordinate uterine dysfunction.

hypotonic uterine d. Uterine dysfunction usually occurring during the active phase of labor, after the cervix has dilated to more than 4 cm; contractions are usually irregular and lack sufficient force to dilate the cervix at a satisfactory rate.

incoordinate uterine d. See hypertonic uterine dysfunction.

orgasmic d. In regard to women, inability to reach orgasm; designated *primary,* when orgasm has never been achieved, even after prolonged sexual stimulation and adequate lubrication; or *secondary,* when the dysfunction occurs after a period of normal functioning.

dysgenic (disjen'ik) Relating to dysgenesis.

dysgenesis (dis jen'ĕ-sis) Abnormal differentiation of the mass of embryonic cells (anlage) leading to the formation of structurally abnormal organs.

gonadal d. Defective or deficient development of the ovaries or testes. See also Turner's syndrome and Swyer syndrome, under syndrome.

mixed gonadal d. Condition in which individuals with a 45,X/46,XY karyotype have one streak gonad on one side and one dysgenetic testis on the other. They usually have ambiguous external genitalia and mullerian derivatives (e.g., uterus, uterine tubes, vagina).

mullerian d. Developmental anomalies of genitourinary organs (e.g., uterus, vagina, ureter, kidney) due to defective development of one or both mullerian ducts (embryologic structures from which those organs are derived).

dysgerminoma (dis-jer-mĭ-no'mă) An

uncommon malignant tumor of the ovary composed of undifferentiated germinal epithelium; it occurs usually in the young (20–30 years) age group, and occasionally in children.

dysmelia (dis-me'le-ă) Congenital absence of a portion of one or more extremities.

dysmenorrhea (dis-men-o-re'ă) Painful menstrual periods. Popularly called menstrual cramps, cramps.

> **functional d.** See primary dysmenorrhea.

> **membranous d.** A rare form of dysmenorrhea due to the passage of massive portions of endometrium through the undilated cervix.

> **primary d.** Dysmenorrhea occurring in the absence of organic disease. Also called functional dysmenorrhea.

> **secondary d.** Dysmenorrhea caused by inflammation, tumor, infection, or anatomic factors.

dysmorphism (dis-mor'fizm) Abnormalities of shape, as seen in syndromes of genetic and environmental origin.

dysmorphology (dis-mor-fol'ŏ-je) The area of clinical genetics dealing with the diagnosis and interpretation of abnormal development of body structures.

dysontogenesis (dis-on-to-jen'e-sis) Abnormal development.

dyspareunia (dis-pă-roo'ne-ă) Painful intercourse.

> **deep d.** Discomfort during sexual intercourse associated with penile thrusting; it may be associated with organic conditions such as uterine displacement, endometriosis, or postinflammatory adhesive disease of internal female pelvic organs.

> **superficial d.** Discomfort associated with penile intromission during sexual intercourse, usually secondary to insufficient vulvovaginal lubrication.

dysphagia (dis-fa'je-ă) Difficulty in swallowing.

> **sideropenic d.** See Plummer-Vinson syndrome, under syndrome.

dysplasia (dis-pla'se-ă) **1.** In pathology, abnormality of cell growth in which some cells in a tissue have some of the characteristics of malignancy but not enough for a diagnosis of an early cancer; unlike cancer (which is irreversible), dysplastic tissue may sometimes reverse spontaneously to normal. **2.** In embryology, abnormal or altered development of a body part.

> **cervical d.** Dysplasia involving the

superficial layer (epithelium) of the uterine cervix; it is considered a precancerous lesion. Depending on the thickness of the involved epithelium, it is designated mild (CIN I), moderate (CIN II), or severe (CIN III). The human papilloma virus (HPV) has been implicated as a causative agent, especially types 16, 18, and 31. Also called cervical intraepithelial neoplasia (CIN).

> **mammary d.** See fibrocystic change of breast, under change.

> **vulvar d.** Dysplasia of the vulva characterized by multicentric mucosal lesions; graded as mild (VIN I), moderate (VIN II), or severe (VIN III), depending on the degree of involvement; it is associated with the presence of human papilloma virus (HPV), especially types 16 and 18 (in 80–90% of cases). Also called vulvar intraepithelial neoplasia (VIN). See also Bowen's disease, under disease.

dysplastic (dis-plas'tik) Relating to dysplasia.

dyssynergia (dis-sin-er'je-ă) Disturbance of muscle coordination.

> **detrusor d.** See detrusor instability, under instability.

dystocia (dis-to'se-ă) Difficult labor.

> **fetal d.** Difficult labor due to excessive fetal size, malposition, malpresentation, or multiple fetuses.

> **maternal d.** Difficult labor caused by a variety of factors, including aberrations of pelvic architecture, soft tissue abnormalities of the birth canal, tumors, aberrant location of the placenta, and ineffective uterine activity.

> **shoulder d.** Inability to deliver the fetal shoulders, even after routine obstetric procedures have been performed; contributing factors include fetal macrosomia (i.e., excessive body size relative to the head size), postterm pregnancy, maternal obesity, and diabetes mellitus.

> **soft tissue d.** Dystocia caused by abnormalities of the uterus or birth canal such as scarring, adhesions, pelvic masses, malformations (e.g., bicornuate uterus, vaginal transverse septa), and low implantation of the placenta.

dystopia (dis-to'pe-ă) Malposition; faulty position.

dystrophy (dis'tro-fe) Disorder caused by faulty nutrition or by lesions of the pituitary and/or other parts of the brain.

dysuria (dis-ure-ă) Painful or difficult urination.

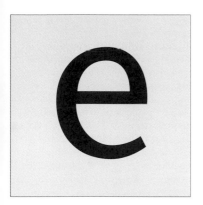

ecchymosis (ek-ĭ-mo'sis), pl. ecchymoses
Bleeding within the skin, causing an area of
bluish-black discoloration.

    periumbilical e. See Cullen's sign, under
sign.

eccyesis (ek-si-e'sis) See ectopic pregnancy, under
pregnancy.

echocardiogram (ek-o-kar'de-o-gram) The
graphic record produced by echocardiography.

echocardiography (ek-o-kar-de-og'rǎ-fe) The
placing of an ultrasonic device on the chest wall
to send sound impulses toward the walls of the
heart, which in turn bounce the sounds back; the
patterns produced are graphically displayed for
interpretation; used for determining the
movement patterns of the heart and its valves,
chamber size, wall thickness, and the presence of
pericardial fluid; also useful for differentiating
the typical physiologic murmurs of pregnancy
from the murmurs of heart disease (acquired or
congenital).

echogram (ek'o-gram) See ultrasonogram.
echograph (ek'o-graf) See ultrasonograph.
eclampsia (ě-klamp'se-ǎ) An acute disorder
occurring in pregnant and puerperal women,
representing a progression of preeclampsia;
characterized by one or more seizures occurring,
with no warning signs (aura), most commonly
before delivery, usually after the 20th week of
gestation; most postpartum episodes occur in the
first 48 hours after delivery, but may occur as late
as 6 weeks. Seizure-induced complications may
include pulmonary edema and retinal
detachment. Fever is an unfavorable prognostic
sign.

    puerperal e. Eclampsia occurring within six
weeks after childbirth.

eclamptic (ě-klamp'tik) Relating to eclampsia.
eclamptogenic (ě-klamp-tojen'ik) Causing
eclampsia.

ectasia, ectasis (ek-ta'ze-ǎ, ek'tǎ-sis) Dilatation

of a tubular structure.

    mammary duct e. Breast condition affecting
multiparous women 50 to 60 years of age;
characterized by thickening of secretions
within major excretory ducts, duct dilatation,
and periductal inflammation; the condition
may superficially resemble cancer of the
breast.

ectatic (ek-tat'ik) Relating to ectasia.
ecto- Prefix meaning on the outside.
ectoblast (ek'to-blast) See ectoderm.
ectocardia (ek-to-kar'de-ǎ) Abnormal position of
the heart.
ectocervix (ek-to-ser'viks) The lowest portion of
the uterine cervix that extends into the lumen of
the vagina.
ectocervical (ek-to-ser'vĭ-kal) Relating to the
vaginal portion of the uterine cervix.
ectoderm (ek'to-derm) The outermost of three
germ layers of the embryo; it gives rise mainly to
the nervous system and to the skin and its
derivatives (e.g., hair, lens of the eye). Sometimes
called ectoblast.

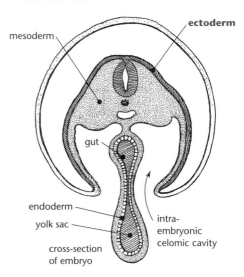

cross-section
of embryo

ectodermal, ectodermic (ek-to-der'mal, ek-to-
der'-mik) Relating to the ectoderm.
ectodermatosis (ek-to-der-mǎ-to'sis) See
ectodermosis.
ectodermosis (ek-to-der-mo'sis) Any disorder of
a tissue derived from the ectoderm (e.g., skin,
neural tissues). Also called ectodermatosis.
ectomere (ek'to-mēr) Any of the cells derived
from division of the fertilized ovum that
participates in the formation of the ectoderm.
-ectomy Combining form meaning removal (e.g.,
hysterectomy).

ectopia (ek-to'pe-ă) **1.** Congenital displacement of a body part. Also called ectopy. **2.** In cardiology, a state in which heart beats originate at some point in the heart other than the sinoatrial node (ectopic heart beats).

> **e. vesicae** See exstrophy of bladder, under exstrophy.

ectopic (ek-top'ik) **1.** The occurrence of a structurally normal tissue or organ in an abnormal location. Also called heterotopic. **2.** Arising from a site other than normal (e.g., a heart beat). **3.** Used in the vernacular as a noun (an 'ectopic') to characterize an ectopic pregnancy. See ectopic pregnancy, under pregnancy.

ectoplacental (ek-to-plă-sen'tal) Outside of, or adjacent to, the placenta.

ectopy (ek'to-pe) See ectopia.

ectro- Combining form meaning congenital absence.

ectrodactyly (ek-tro-daktĭ-le) Congenital absence of fingers and toes.

ectrogeny (ek-troj'ĕ-ne) Congenital absence of a body part.

ectromelia (ek-tro-me'le-ă) Congenital absence of one or more limbs.

ectropion (ek-tro'pe-on) A turning outward.

> **mucosal e.** A growth-like protrusion of the urethral mucous membrane, occurring in the distal portion of the urethra.

ectrosyndactyly (ek-tro-sin-dak'tĭ-le) Congenital absence of one or more digits and the fusion of the rest.

edema (ĕ-de'mă) Soft tissue swelling due to collection of fluid in the intercellular spaces.

> **cerebral e.** Edema of the brain; may be caused by tumors, infarction, abscesses, concussions, certain toxic conditions, or an obstruction in the cerebrospinal fluid circulation.

> **dependent e.** Subcutaneous edema localized in dependent areas, especially the feet, ankles, and lower legs (when the person is upright).

> **generalized e.** Edema of most or all regions of the body usually caused by advanced heart, kidney, or liver disease; may also be caused by drugs (e.g., steroids, estrogen, vasodilators), pregnancy, or starvation.

> **interstitial e.** Edema associated with hydrocephalus, characterized by the presence of increased fluid within brain tissues.

> **localized e.** Edema originating from, or occurring in, a restricted area of the body (seen in inflammation and venous or lymphatic obstruction).

> **menstrual e.** Water retention during or just prior to menstruation.

> **pulmonary e.** Escape of fluid into the air sacs (alveoli) and intercellular spaces of the lungs; causes include left ventricular failure (left-sided heart failure), narrowing of the mitral valve (mitral stenosis), and the presence of chemicals that are toxic to the lungs.

> **pulmonary interstitial e.** (PIE) Leakage of air into the perivascular tissues of the lungs (especially around the veins), resulting from overdistention and rupture of the lung's air sacs (alveoli), or of the smallest airways (bronchioles); occurs almost exclusively in premature and very-low-birthweight infants who have been placed on ventilatory support.

> **vulvar e.** Edema of the vulva; may be due to a variety of conditions, such as accidental trauma, circulatory changes in the lower genital tract before or during labor, or obstruction of blood or lymph circulation by a tumor or infection; it may be associated with systemic disorders (e.g., pre-eclampsia), or (when acute) it may be an allergic reaction.

edematous (ĕ-dem'ă-tus) Characterized by edema.

effacement (ĕ-fās'ment) Obliteration; a taking up.

> **cervical e.** The shortening or flattening of the cervical canal during the first stage of labor, occurring as the muscle fibers around the internal os are pulled up toward the lower uterine segment; as a result, the cervical canal is reduced from about 2 cm in length to a flat, almost paper-thin structure, while the external os remains temporarily the same.

effect (ĕ-fekt') The result of an action.

> **adverse e.** A deleterious secondary response to the normal dose of a drug.

> **Bohr e.** The observation that changes in the pH of blood influence the oxygen carrying capacity of hemoglobin.

> **cytopathic e.** A degenerative change in cells, such as that produced by a viral infection.

> **inotropic e.** The increased force of cardiac muscular contractions occurring during pregnancy to compensate for the need for an increased cardiac output, which is typical of the pregnant state.

> **photoelectric e.** The proportionately higher radiation levels absorbed by those tissues having constituent elements of higher atomic numbers (e.g., bone calcium).

> **Poseiro e.** Obstruction of the blood supply to the pregnant uterus by its contracted state when the woman lies on her back; occurs during the third trimester.

side e. A result or consequence other than that for which a drug or therapy is administered; the term applies to an additional or secondary effect and usually (although not always) refers to an undesirable or adverse result. It is not applied to the toxic consequences of a drug overdose.

toxic e. An effect of a drug on a living organism that is harmful to the well-being or life of the organism.

effort (ef'ert) Deliberate expenditure of physical and mental energy to achieve something.

expulsive e. The two or three final pushing efforts made by a woman in labor, which lead to expulsion of the fetus from the birth canal; they occur during the second stage of labor (i.e., between complete dilatation of the cervix and the birth of the child).

impaired expulsive e. Feeble, inadequate, and ineffective pushing by a woman during the second stage of labor; may be caused by conduction analgesia, excessive sedation, exhaustion, neurologic dysfunction (e.g., paraplegia or hemiplegia), or psychiatric disorders.

effusion (ĕ-fu'zhun) 1. Escape of fluid into a body space or cavity (e.g., pleural, pericardial, or joint cavities). 2. The fluid effused.

pleural e. Fluid appearing in the space surrounding the lung; if in large quantities, it may impede respiration; causes include congestive heart failure (beginning usually as a right-sided effusion), infection (e.g., pneumonia, tuberculosis) or tumor involving the pleural surface.

egg (eg) See ovum.

fertilized e. See zygote.

ejaculate (e-jak'u-lāt) 1. To discharge suddenly, especially semen. 2. The material so discharged. Also called ejaculum.

ejaculation (e-jak-u-la'shun) The propulsion of semen out of the urethra at orgasm.

inhibited e. A rare condition in which erection is normal (or prolonged) but ejaculation does not occur.

premature e. Discharge of the semen prior to or immediately upon engaging in sexual intercourse.

retrograde e. Condition in which semen is forced backwards into the bladder due to failure of the sphincter muscle of the bladder to close at orgasm; may result from neurological disease, a surgical operation upon the neck of the bladder and prostatic urethra, or certain antihypertensive medications.

ejaculatory (e-jak'u-lă-to-re) Relating to ejaculation.

ejaculum (e-jak'u-lum) See ejaculate.

elective (e-lek'tiv) Nonurgent; applied especially to surgical procedures that, although advisable, do not pose imminent problems to the health of the patient if not carried out.

electrocardiogram (e-lek-tro-kar'de-o-gram) (ECG, EKG) A graphic record (made with an electrocardiograph) of the variations in voltage produced by the heart muscle during the different phases of the cardiac cycle.

electrocardiograph (e-lek-tro-kar'de-o-graf) Instrument for making an electrocardiogram.

electrocardiography (e-lek-tro-kar-de-og'ră-fe) A method of recording the conduction, magnitude, and duration of the electric current generated by the activity of the heart muscle.

fetal e. Electrocardiography of a fetus while in the uterus.

electrocoagulation (e-lek-tro-ko-ag-u-la'shun) Coagulation of tissues with a bipolar electric current.

electrolyte (e-lek'tro-līt) A substance that, when in solution, splits into constituent ions, thereby becoming capable of transmitting electricity.

electrophoresis (e-lek-tro-fŏ-re'sis) A process in which particles with an electric charge in a solution migrate under the influence of an applied electric current; used as a means of separating substances in a diffusing medium. Also called phoresis.

hemoglobin e. Electrophoresis performed to determine the kind and amount of hemoglobin present in red blood cells. Especially useful in detecting abnormal hemoglobins and diagnosing hemoglobinopathies (e.g., hemoglobin A [thalassemias] or hemoglobin S [sickle cell disease]).

electrosurgery (e-lek-tro-sur'jer-e) The surgical use of high frequency current delivered by needles, wire loops, or blades.

embolism (em'bo-lizm) Blockage of a blood vessel by an abnormal solid or gaseous mass (embolus) that is transported by the bloodstream to that site from another location in the body.

amniotic fluid e. (AFE) A rare complication of childbirth in which amniotic fluid (usually containing particulate matter) enters the blood circulation of the woman in labor through ruptured uterine veins, causing hemorrhage, shock, pulmonary embolism and, frequently, maternal death; principal predisposing factors include tumultuous uterine contractions, premature detachment of the placenta, and a dead fetus; other precipitating factors may include trauma caused by abdominal injuries, operative delivery of the infant, and introduction of an intrauterine catheter for monitoring uterine contractions. Consideration has been given to an immunologic etiology of this entity and renaming it 'anaphylactoid syndrome of pregnancy'.

    pulmonary e. (PE) Clogging of one or more arteries supplying blood to the lungs by detached fragments of a blood clot (thrombus), most frequently located in a deep vein of a leg or the pelvis and carried in the bloodstream through the heart to the pulmonary vessels. The subsequent cardiopulmonary effects depend on the size and location of the thrombi in the lung tissue. It occurs as a complication of surgery and childbirth, and in patients who are immobilized for any reason. It is a rare but significant cause of maternal death.

embolization (em-bo-li-za'shun) The process by which natural or artificial substances in the circulation impede or obstruct blood or lymph flow.

    angiographic e. Procedure for arresting persistent postpartum hemorrhage; pieces of absorbable gelatin sponge or other suitable material are injected into a damaged pelvic or uterine blood vessel under fluoroscopic viewing; if the bleeding site cannot be located, the sponge is introduced into the internal iliac vessels.

    hypogastric e. Embolization of an internal iliac artery to control pelvic bleeding; clotting material (blood and tissues from the patient or absorbable gelatin sponge) is introduced into the bleeding artery via the internal iliac artery of the opposite side, under fluoroscopic visualization.

    percutaneous transcatheter e. The deliberate obstruction of a blood vessel with any of a variety of materials; usually performed to stop uncontrollable internal bleeding or to cut off the blood supply of a vascular tumor which is difficult to remove (thereby shrinking the tumor).

    trophoblastic e. Deposition of variable amounts of trophoblast within small pulmonary veins; occurs as a complication of mole pregnancies; the trophoblast is carried in the circulation to the lungs, where it becomes lodged in small arteries, causing respiratory complications, including (when the volume of deposits is large) signs and symptoms of acute pulmonary embolism; rarely, it may have a

fatal outcome. Also called trophoblastic deportation.

embolus (em'bo-lus) A plug within a vessel (e.g., a blood clot, air bubble, fat, or tumor mass) that is carried in the bloodstream from another site until it lodges and becomes an obstruction to the blood circulation.

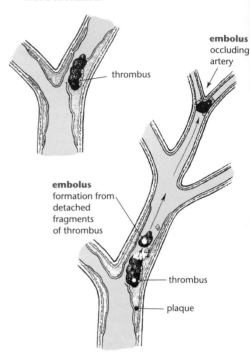

embryo (em'bre-o) An organism in its earliest stage of development; in humans, from conception to the end of the eighth week, at which time it is 2.1 to 2.5 cm long and weighs 1 gram; the head constitutes about half the bulk; the lobes of the liver may be recognized; the kidneys are forming; red blood cells containing hemoglobin are forming in the yolk sac and liver; the heart is functionally complete, with a rate of over 80 beats per minute; the hands and feet are formed and distinctly human.

    presomite e. An embryo before the appearance of the first pair of somites, approximately 20 to 21 days after fertilization.

    previllous e. An embryo before the formation of chorionic villi.

embryoblast (em'bre-o-blast) An aggregation of cells forming the portion of the blastocyst from which the embryo itself develops (i.e., excluding the placenta and other extraembryonic structures). Also called inner cell mass.

embryogenesis (em-bre-o-jen'ĕ-sis) The

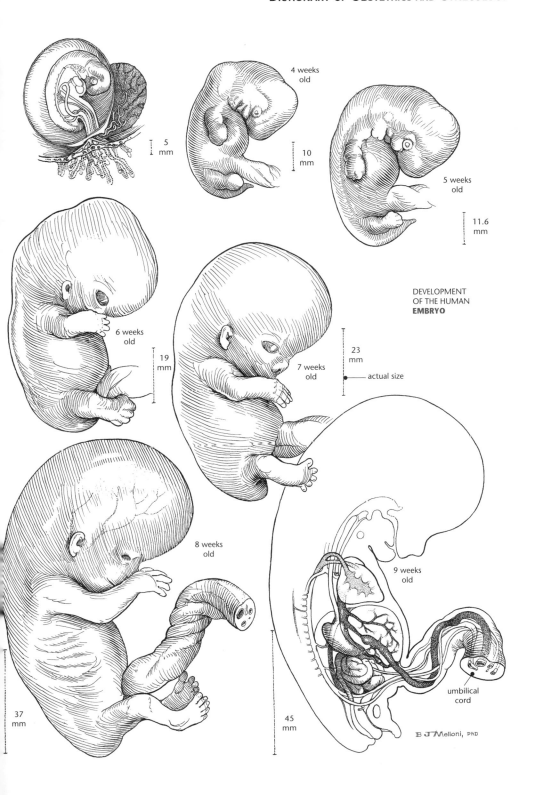

5 mm

4 weeks old

10 mm

5 weeks old

11.6 mm

6 weeks old

19 mm

7 weeks old

23 mm

actual size

DEVELOPMENT OF THE HUMAN **EMBRYO**

8 weeks old

9 weeks old

umbilical cord

37 mm

45 mm

B.J.Melloni, PhD

development of the embryo from the fertilized egg.

embryogenic (em-bre-o-jen'ik) **1.** Relating to the development of an embryo. **2.** Producing an embryo.

embryogeny (em-bre-oj'ĕ-ne) The formation of the embryo.

embryology (em-bre-ol'ŏ-je) The science concerned with living organisms from fertilization of the ovum until birth; the study of the development of the ovum. Also called developmental anatomy.

embryoma (em-bre-o'mă) See embryonal tumor, under tumor.

embryomorphous (em-bre-o-mor'fus) Resembling an embryo or embryonic tissue in form or development; applied to certain abnormal adult tissues or cells.

embryonal (em'bre-o-nal) Relating to an embryo.

embryonate (em'bre-o-nāt) Containing an embryo.

embryonic (em-bre-on'ik) Relating to an embryo.

embryonization (em-bre-o-nĭ-za'shun) The reversion of cells or tissues to a primitive form.

embryopathy (em-bre-op'ă-the) An abnormal condition in an embryo.

embryotomy (em-bre-ot'ŏ-me) The mechanical destruction of a fetus to facilitate its removal through the birth canal when delivery is not otherwise possible.

eminence (em'ĭ-nens) A rounded prominence; a raised area, especially on the surface of a bone.

    iliopectineal e. See iliopubic eminence.

    iliopubic e. The rounded elevation on the medial border of the hipbone that marks the union of the superior ramus of the pubic bone with the body of the ilium. Also called iliopectineal eminence.

    parietal e. The most prominent part of the parietal bone on either side of the skull, just above the superior temporal line; it indicates the site where ossification of the parietal bone first occurred. Also called parietal protuberance.

emmenagogic (e-men-ă-goj'ik) Inducing the menstrual flow.

emmenagogue (e-men'ă-gog) Denoting an agent that induces menstruation.

    direct e. Any agent or procedure that acts on the organs involved in the menstrual cycle to induce menstruation.

    indirect e. Any agent that induces or increases the menstrual flow by relieving another condition causing amenorrhea or scant menstruation.

emmenia (e-me'ne-ă) Menses.

encephalitis (en-sef-ă-li'tis), pl. encephalitides Inflammation of the brain; may result from bacterial, viral, or fungal infection; initial symptoms include headache, nausea, vomiting, fever, and lethargy.

encephalo-, encephal- Combining forms meaning brain.

encephalocele (en-sef'ă-lo-sēl) Protrusion of brain tissue through a congenital or traumatic opening in the skull. Also called craniocele.

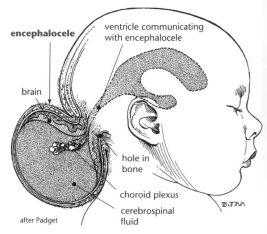

encephalocele — ventricle communicating with encephalocele

brain

hole in bone

choroid plexus

cerebrospinal fluid

after Padget

B.JAA

encephalon (en-sef'a-lon) See brain.

encephalopathy (en-sef-ă-lop'ă-the) Any disease or dysfunction of the brain.

    neonatal e. Encephalopathy of the newborn infant; classified as *mild*, characterized by hyperalertness, irritability, jitteriness, and alternating episodes of excessive and reduced muscle tone; *moderate*, marked by lethargy, severely increased muscle tone, and occasional seizures; *severe*, characterized by coma, apnea, and numerous seizures.

endo-, end- Prefixes meaning within.

endocarditis (en-do-kar-di'tis) Inflammation of the lining membrane of the heart chambers.

    bacterial e. See infective endocarditis.

    infective e. (IE) Endocarditis caused by colonization of the heart valves with blood-borne microorganisms (e.g., *Streptococcus viridans* and *Neisseria gonorrhoeae*), leading to the formation of infected vegetations and deformation of the valve leaflets; may be acute or subacute; predisposing conditions include congenital heart defects and may be associated with certain surgical procedures and with intravenous drug abuse. Also called bacterial endocarditis.

endocervical (en-do-ser'vĭ-kal) Within the uterine cervix. Also called intracervical.

endocervicitis (en-do-ser-vĭ-si'tis) Inflammation of the lining of the uterine cervix.

endoderm (en'do-derm) The innermost of the three germ layers of the embryo; it gives rise to the lining of the gastrointestinal tract from the pharynx to the rectum and to neighboring glands (e.g., liver, pancreas, thyroid). Also called entoderm.

endometrial (en-do-me'tre-al) Relating to the inner lining of the uterus (endometrium).

endometrioid (en-do-me'tre-oid) Microscopically resembling the lining (endometrium) of the uterus.

endometrioma (en-do-me-tre-o'mă) See chocolate cyst, under cyst.

endometriosis (en-do-me-tre-o'sis) Disorder in which abnormal growths of tissue, microscopically resembling the uterine lining membrane (endometrium), are present in locations other than the inner surface of the uterus, most commonly over pelvic organs; growths vary from microscopic to large masses invading underlying organs; may be asymptomatic or cause intense pain and infertility; seen almost exclusively in women of reproductive age but may occasionally occur in postmenopausal women.

    e. interna See adenomyosis.

endometritis (en-do-me-tri'tis) Inflammation of the uterine lining (endometrium).

    postpartum e. See puerperal endometritis.

    puerperal e. Endometritis occurring after childbirth. Also called postpartum endometritis.

endometrium (en-do-me'tre-um) The velvety mucous membrane lining the interior of the uterus; it consists of a surface epithelium and a subepithelial layer containing blood vessels,

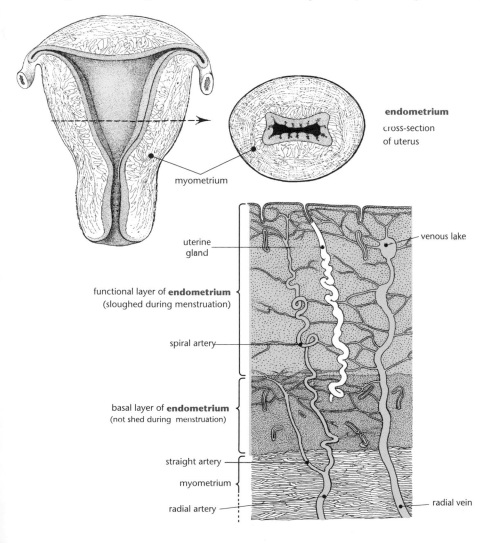

endometrium
cross-section
of uterus

myometrium

uterine gland

venous lake

functional layer of **endometrium**
(sloughed during menstruation)

spiral artery

basal layer of **endometrium**
(not shed during menstruation)

straight artery

myometrium

radial artery

radial vein

lymphatic spaces, and tubular glands that extend through the whole thickness of the endometrium and open into the uterine cavity; its structure changes with age and with the menstrual cycle.

Swiss cheese e. Cystic hyperplasia of the tube-like endometrial glands, which give the appearance of Swiss cheese to histologic sections.

endonuclease (en-do-nu'kle-ās) Any enzyme that promotes the breaking of interior chemical bonds of DNA and RNA chains, producing fragments of short (oligo-) or long (poly-) nucleotides.

restrictive e. One of many endonucleases isolated from bacteria that act as molecular scissors to cut DNA molecules at specific locations, thus inactivating a foreign DNA (e.g., from a virus) and restricting its activity; used extensively as a laboratory tool. Also called restrictive enzyme; commonly called chemical knife.

endorphin (en-dor'fin) One of a group of low-molecular weight peptides normally found in the brain and other parts of the body; capable of producing effects similar to those of opiates.

endosalpinx (en-do-sal'pinks) The mucous membrane lining the interior of a fallopian (uterine) tube.

endoscope (en'do-skōp) A tubular instrument with lenses and a light source attached for viewing the interior of a hollow organ, tubular structure, or body cavity; may be used with a camera or video recorder.

endoscopy (en-dos'kŏ-pe) Inspection of a body cavity or organ with an endoscope.

peritoneal e. See laparoscopy.

endothelin (en-do-thēl'in) Polypeptide that is one of the most potent constrictors of vascular smooth muscle, derived from the inner lining of blood vessels; it is released in response to stretching of blood vessels; there are three forms encoded by three different genes and designated *endothelin 1, endothelin 2,* and *endothelin 3.*

enema (en'ĕ-mă) **1.** Infusion of a fluid into the rectum for therapeutic or diagnostic purposes. **2.** The liquid so infused.

barium e. Installation of the radiopaque medium barium sulfate in solution prior to x-ray examination of the bowel.

contrast e. Enema using any radiopaque medium.

enflurane (en'floo-rān) An inhalation anesthetic that is neither flammable nor explosive; used in obstetrics in subanesthetic concentrations for normal vaginal deliveries; it has no detectable toxicity in mothers or newborns.

engagement (en-gāj'ment) A cardinal movement of labor during which the biparietal plane of the fetal head descends to a level below that of the pelvic inlet.

engineering (en-jin-er'ing) The practical application of the principles of mathematics and the physical sciences.

biomedical e. Application of engineering principles to solve medical problems in research and practice. It includes development of such devices as prostheses (e.g., artificial limbs and heart valves) and electrical devices (e.g., pacemakers). Also called bioengineering.

genetic e. Directed alteration of the genetic material of a living organism to study genetic processes, to modify heredity, to produce hormones or proteins, and potentially to correct genetic defects.

engorgement (en-gorj'ment) The condition of being distended to excess due to accumulation of a fluid, usually blood or lymph.

postpartum breast e. Condition of the breasts, occurring during the first week after childbirth, in which the breasts become extremely distended, firm, warm, and nodular, accompanied by pain and (when severe) slight fever; caused by excessive accumulation of lymph and venous blood. Popularly called caked breasts.

enhancer (en-hans'er) The specific DNA sequence that increases the expressivity of a gene; it initiates DNA action and is activated upon binding by regulatory proteins.

enkephalins (en-kef'ă-lins) A group of pentapeptides, or any of their synthetic derivatives, that mimic the action of morphine in the nervous system; found primarily in the brain and pituitary; also found in nerve endings throughout the body.

enkephalinase (en-kef'ă-lin-ās) Enzyme that promotes the decomposition of enkephalin; found especially abundantly in the chorion laeve (the avascular membrane that forms the greater part of the amnion).

enteral (en'ter-al) Within the intestine or by way of the gastrointestinal tract (e.g., administration of drugs or nutrients).

enteric (en-ter'ik) Relating to the intestines.

enteritis (en-ter-i'tis) Inflammation of the intestines.

regional e. See Crohn's disease, under disease.

enterobiasis (en-ter-o-bi'ă-sis) Intestinal infection with *Enterobius vermicularis*, a short roundworm commonly called pinworm.

Enterobius (en-ter-o'be-us) A genus of

roundworms found in the large intestines of humans and primates.

E. vermicularis The pinworm.

enterocele (en'ter-o-sēl) A herniation of Douglas' pouch (rectouterine pouch) that may protrude *(a)* anteriorly into the rectovaginal septum forming a bulge in the posterior vaginal wall, *(b)* posteriorly into the anal canal simulating a prolapsed rectum, or *(c)* (rarely) in both directions, out through the vagina and through the anal canal as a 'saddle hernia'; usually seen in menopausal or postmenopausal women who have borne more than one child; it is almost always associated with other musculofascial weakness (e.g., cystocele, rectocele, uterine prolapse). Also called posterior vaginal hernia; cul-de-sac hernia; Douglas' pouch hernia.

saddle e. See saddle hernia, under hernia.

enterocolitis (en-ter-o-ko-li'tis) Inflammation of the intestinal mucous membrane.

chronic radiation e. Enterocolitis resulting from pelvic irradiation for malignancies of the genitourinary organs; it usually involves the terminal ileum, cecum, sigmoid portion of the colon, and rectum.

necrotizing e. (NEC) An acquired disease of newborn infants, resulting from vascular and mucosal damage of the intestinal wall, which allows bacterial/viral invasion and gangrenous deterioration of the bowel; clinical findings usually include abdominal distention, ileus, and bloody stools, along with radiologic evidence of pneumatosis intestinalis caused by intestinal wall gas of bacterial origin. It usually occurs in premature infants within the first week of life and 3 to 7 days after institution of feeding through a tube inserted into the stomach (enteral nutrition). Several bacteria and viruses have been implicated (e.g., *Escherichia coli*, enterobacter, salmonella, coronoviruses, rotaviruses, and enteroviruses), as well as certain medications (e.g., indomethacin).

pseudomembranous e. A severe form of colitis with formation, and passage in the feces, of a membrane-resembling material or plaques containing bits of intestinal mucosa; associated with prolonged antibiotic therapy.

ento-, ent- Prefixes meaning inside.

entoderm (en'to-derm) See endoderm.

enuresis (en-u-re'sis) Involuntary release of urine.

enzymatic (en-zī-mat'ik) Relating to an enzyme. Also called enzymic.

enzyme (en'zīm) A protein that acts as a catalyst, regulating the rate of chemical reactions of other body substances while remaining unchanged in the process.

respiratory e. Enzyme that takes part in oxidation–reduction processes.

restrictive e. See restrictive endonuclease, under endonuclease.

enzymic (en-zim'ik) See enzymatic.

epididymis (ep-ĭ-did'ĭ-mis) The tortuous, cordlike excretory duct connected to the posterior border of the testis that provides storage, transit, and maturation of the spermatozoa; it consists of a head (15–20 coiled tubules), a body, and a tail (single convoluted duct continuous with the deferent duct).

epilepsy (ep'ĭ-lep-se) A chronic disorder, or group of disorders, characterized by recurrent, unpredictable seizures occurring spontaneously without consistent provoking factors; the seizures reflect a temporary physiologic dysfunction of the brain in which nerve cells (neurons) in the cerebral cortex produce excessive electrical discharges.

absence e. Epilepsy characterized by absence seizures; sudden, transient (10 to 30 s) breaks of consciousness of thought or activity, sometimes accompanied by rapid eyelid flutterings. Also called petit mal epilepsy.

focal e. Epilepsy characterized by minor seizures restricted to isolated areas of the body, arising in a localized area of a cerebral hemisphere. Also called partial epilepsy, local epilepsy.

generalized e. Epilepsy characterized by seizures that result from involvement of both cerebral hemispheres; may range from minor (absence seizures) to major (tonic–clonic seizures).

generalized tonic–clonic e. Epilepsy marked by loss of consciousness and stiffness of the entire body (i.e., sustained [tonic]) muscular contractions), followed by jerking (clonic) movements. Also called grand mal epilepsy; major epilepsy; falling sickness.

grand mal e. See generalized tonic–clonic epilepsy.

jacksonian e. Focal epilepsy in which the seizure arises in a localized area of the motor cortex and spreads to adjacent areas, manifested by a twitching beginning at the periphery of a structure, progressing to involve the entire musculature of one side.

local e. See focal epilepsy.

major e. See generalized tonic–clonic epilepsy.

nocturnal e. Epilepsy in which the attacks occur mainly at night, while the person sleeps.

partial e. See focal epilepsy.

petit mal e. See absence epilepsy.

post-traumatic e. Epilepsy caused by brain damage incurred in a head injury. Most frequently seen in penetrating brain injuries and in depressed skull fractures with injury to underlying brain; it occurs also in closed head trauma.

temporal lobe e. A type of focal epilepsy in which the seizure arises from all or part of the temporal lobe, often producing auditory, olfactory, or gustatory hallucinations, as well as bizarre activity and behavior; it often arises after injury to the temporal lobe.

uncinate e. A type of temporal lobe epilepsy in which the seizure arises from the anteromedial aspect of the temporal lobe, causing impairment of consciousness and a dreamy state with hallucinations of smell and taste; usually caused by a medial temporal lesion.

epileptic (ep-ĭ-lep'tik) **1.** Relating to epilepsy. **2.** A person who has epilepsy.

epimenorrhea (ep-ĭ-men-o-re'ă) Menstruation occurring at excessively short intervals.

episio- Combining form meaning vulva.

episioperineorrhaphy (ĕ-piz-e-o-per-ĭ-ne-or'ă-fe) Surgical repair of a lacerated vulva and adjoining musculofibrous tissues (perineum).

episioplaste (ĕ-piz-e-o-plas'te) Surgical repair of a defect of the vulva.

episiotomy (ĕ-piz-e-ot'o-me) Incision of the perineum for controlled enlargement of the introital opening at the time of emergence of the presenting fetal part from the birth canal; performed to prevent vaginal, vulvar, or perineal tears, to shorten the second stage of labor, and to prevent undue pressure on the fetal skull during childbirth. The two most common incisions are median and mediolateral. Also called perineotomy.

epistasis (ĕ-pis'tă-sis) **1.** The suppressive action of one gene over another. **2.** A surface film formed on standing urine.

epithelial (ep-ĭ-the'le-al) Relating to the outermost layer (epithelium) covering all body surfaces.

epithelioid (ep-ĭ-the'le-oid) Resembling the outermost layer (epithelium) of skin or mucous membranes.

epithelioma (ep-ĭ-the-le-o'mă) Malignant tumor of the skin or mucous membrane.

chorionic e. See choriocarcinoma (1).

epithelium (ep-ĭ-the'le-um) The nonvascular, closely-packed cellular layer that covers the external surface and the mucous membrane of the entire body; functions as a selective barrier, capable of facilitating or preventing the passage of substances across the surfaces which it covers; classified as simple (one-layered) and stratified (multilayered).

germinal e. Specialized covering of the free surface of the ovary; in the young female it is composed of cuboidal cells, in older adults the cells are flattened.

epitope (ep'ĭ-tōp) See antigenic determinant, under determinant.

epoophoron (ep-o-of'ŏ-ron) Vestiges of the embryonic mesonephros (wolffian body) consisting of rudimentary tubules located in the mesosalpinx between the ovary and ovarian tube. Also called organ of Rosenmüller.

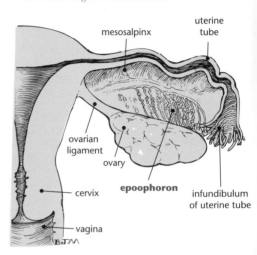

epostane (e'pos-tān) A 3-beta-hydroxysteroid dehydrogenase inhibitor; it blocks progesterone production, thus preventing implantation of a fertilized ovum; it is also effective in inducing abortion when taken within 4 weeks of the last menstrual period.

epsilon-aminocaproic acid (ep'sĭ-lon ă-me-no-kă-pro'ik as'id) (EACP) A compound that inhibits dissolution of fibrin in the blood; used to prevent abnormal bleeding, such as excessive and prolonged menstruation (menorrhagia); used as an adjunct in the treatment of bleeding tendencies associated with certain types of hemophilia.

epulis (ĕ-pu'lis) A tumor of the gums.

e. gravidarum See epulis of pregnancy.

e. of pregnancy Benign tumor of the gums typically occurring during pregnancy and regressing after childbirth. Also called epulis gravidarum.

equation (e-kwa'zhun) A mathematical or chemical representation as a linear array of symbols expressing the quality of two things, separated into left and right sides by an equal sign.

Hasselbalch's e. See Henderson–Hasselbalch equation.

Henderson–Hasselbalch e. An equation for determining the pH of a buffer solution such as blood plasma; $pH = pK + \log (HCO_3^-/CO_2)$. Also caled Hasselbalch's equation.

erectile (ĕ-rek'til) Capable of becoming turgid.

erogenous (ĕ-roj'e-nus) Producing sexual desire. Also called erotogenic.

erosion (e-ro'zhun) A gradual wearing away.

cervical e. Red, velvety, noninflammatory lesions extending from the external os (to various degrees) outward on the cervical surface epithelium; it is a common occurrence during pregnancy; also seen as a complication of the late postpartum period.

erotic (ĕ-rot'ik) Relating to sexual arousal.

eroticism (ĕ-rot'ĭ-sizm) A state of sexual excitement.

erotogenic (ĕ-rot-o-jen'ik) See erogenous.

error (er'or) Defect.

inborn e. of metabolism Inherited disorders caused by a gene-determined defect; each involves a single enzyme; manifestations may be the result of accumulation of the substance upon which the enzyme acts (substrate), a deficiency of the product of the enzyme, or the result of forcing metabolism through an auxiliary path.

eruption (e-rup'shun) **1.** The process of breaking out with skin lesions. **2.** Skin lesions; a rash.

papular e. The appearance of multiple solid elevations on the skin.

erysipelas (er-ĭ-sip'ĕ-las) Acute, contagious skin disease with involvement of cutaneous lymphatic vessels; caused by group A streptococcus organisms; marked by a rapidly spreading reddish rash with sharp borders (chiefly on the face), with fever, chills, and vomiting.

e. internum Erysipelas occurring in the vagina, uterus, and peritoneum.

surgical e. Erysipelas occurring after a surgical procedure; seen occasionally on the vulva, accompanied by fever, chills, and malaise.

erysipeloid (er-ĭ-sip'ĕ-loid) Infection of the hands with the bacillus *Erysipelothrix rhusiopathiae*; marked by a self-limiting reddish eruption at a site of injury; seen in animal handlers (butchers, fishermen, veterinarians).

erysipelotoxin (er-ĭ-sip-ĕ-lo-tok'sin) Toxin produced by group A hemolytic streptococci bacteria; present in erysipelas.

erythema (er-ĭ-the'mă) Redness of the skin.

e. chronicum migrans The characteristic lesion of Lyme disease; an oval, peripherally expanding red eruption, with a central clearing at the site of an infected tick's bite. See also Lyme disease, under disease.

e. induratum Inflammation of subcutaneous fat (panniculitis) typically affecting adolescents and menopausal women; marked by formation of nodules, especially on the legs, which eventually ulcerate. Cause is unknown.

e. infectiosum A mild viral infection caused by human parvovirus B19, most commonly seen in school-aged children; marked by a red lacelike skin rash on the cheeks, producing a 'slapped cheek' appearance; it is sometimes accompanied by joint pains and, in adults, it may be asymptomatic; occasionally, infection in a pregnant woman is associated with deleterious pregnancy outcomes, including abortion and fetal death. Also called fifth disease; slapped-cheek disease; slapped-cheek measles.

e. multiforme Eruption of skin lesions occurring in a variety of forms, most commonly red papules and vesicles, often circular with a dark necrotizing center (target or iris lesion); most common causes include reactions to drugs or to concurrent infections (e.g., herpes simplex and mycoplasma infections).

e. nodosum Inflammation of subcutaneous fat (panniculitis) typically of abrupt onset, occurring as a hypersensitive reaction to a drug (e.g., birth control pills) or in association with infections, inflammatory bowel disease, sarcoidosis, or internal organ cancer; characterized by bright red, painful nodules on the shins, frequently on the anterior thighs and extensor surfaces of the forearms. Also called nodal fever.

palmar e. Erythema on the palms of the hands, seen in patients with liver disease; also seen frequently in normal pregnant women probably as a result of increased circulating estrogens; it disappears after childbirth.

e. toxicum Diffuse skin rash occurring as an allergic reaction to a toxic substance. A form of erythema toxicum frequently seen in newborn infants (50%), usually at 24 to 48 hours of age, is characterized by blotches of reddish macules 2 to 3 cm in diameter anywhere on the body but most prominently on the chest; lesions usually fade within 48 hours.

erythro-, erythr- Combining forms meaning red.

erythroblastosis (ĕ-rith-ro-blas-to'sis) Abnormally large number of immature red blood cells (erythroblasts) in the blood.

 e. fetalis, fetal e. See hemolytic disease of the newborn, under disease.

erythrocyte (e-rith'ro-sīt) A mature red blood cell; it has a life span of about 120 days.

erythrogenesis imperfecta (ĕ-rith-ro-gen'ĕ-sis im-per-fek'tă) See congenital hypoplastic anemia, under anemia.

escutcheon (es-kuch'an) The characteristic distribution of pubic hair over the mons pubis in the female; it has a triangular shape with the base at the upper margin of the pubic symphysis.

-esis Suffix meaning a process (e.g., amniocentesis).

esophagitis (ĕ-sof-ă-ji'tis) Inflammation of the esophagus; may be acute or chronic, and caused by bacteria, viruses, chemicals, or trauma.

 Candida e. Esophagitis caused by infection with *Candida* organisms; predisposing factors include deficiency of immune system (e.g., in AIDS), diabetes, malignancy, and corrosive injuries; symptoms include painful, difficult swallowing and oral thrush.

 herpes e. Esophagitis caused by herpes I or II, varicella-zoster virus, or cytomegalovirus, which produce painful, difficult swallowing, fever, and bleeding.

 peptic e. See reflux esophagitis.

 reflux e. Diffuse inflammation of the distal esophagus caused by habitual regurgitation of gastric juice and/or other stomach contents through an incompetent lower esophageal sphincter muscle; frequently associated with a hiatal hernia or a duodenal ulcer; it is also a common occurrence in late pregnancy. Also called peptic esophagitis.

esophagus (ĕ-sof'ă-gus) The part of the digestive tract consisting of a musculomembranous tube that extends downward from the pharynx to the uppermost part (cardia) of the stomach, just below the diaphragm.

estradiol (es-tră-di'ol) An estrogenic hormone of ovarian and placental origin; it prepares the endometrium for implantation of the fertilized ovum, and it is essential for the development and functioning of female reproductive organs; a synthetic preparation is used in estrogen replacement therapy.

 ethinyl e. A semisynthetic derivative of estradiol; used as a component of many oral contraceptives.

estriol (es'tre-ol) An abundant but relatively weak estrogenic hormone; a major metabolic product of the hormones estradiol and estrone; found in urine.

estrogen (es'tro-jen) General term for the group of female sex hormones, responsible for stimulating the development and maintenance of female secondary sex characteristics; formed in the ovary, placenta, testis, adrenal cortex, and some plants; therapeutic uses (with natural or synthetic preparations) include the relief of menopausal symptoms and amelioration of cancer of the prostate.

 conjugated e. A buff-colored powder, a mixture of the sodium salts of the sulfate esters of estrogenic hormones (chiefly estrone and equilin, the types excreted by pregnant mares).

estrone (es'trōn) An estrogenic hormone found in the ovary and in the urine of pregnant mares.

ethical (eth'ĭ-kal) **1.** Relating to ethics. **2.** In conformity with professionally accepted principles.

ethics (eth'iks) Standards of conduct governing an individual or a profession.

 medical e. A code of behavior that governs professional relationships between physician and patient and the patient's family, and among physicians.

ethynodiol diacetate (ĕ-thi-no-di'ol di-as'ĕ-tāt) A progestin used in combination with an estrogen in oral contraceptives. May cause fetal malformations. Recent studies suggest that there are no teratogenic effects insofar as cardiac anomalies and limb reduction defects are concerned when oral contraceptives are taken inadvertently during early pregnancy.

etio- Combining form meaning cause.

etiocholanolone (e-te-o-ko-lan'o-lōn) Product of metabolism of hormones from the adrenal cortex and the testis; excreted in the urine.

etiology (e-te-ŏl'o-je) Study of the causes of disease and their mechanism of action.

etoposide (e-tŏ-po'sīd) A semisynthetic derivative of podophyllotoxin that inhibits cell division, decreases DNA production, and is effective against certain tumors. Adverse effects may include nausea and vomiting, fever and chills, bone marrow depression, and kidney damage.

eukaryote (u-kar'e-ōt) Organism with cells that have a well defined nucleus (containing chromosomes and enclosed by a nuclear membrane) and a mitotic cycle.

euploidy (u-ploi'de) The state of having the normal number of chromosomes.

eury- Combining form meaning wide.

euryon (u're-on) A point on the right and the left sides of the head (on each parietal bone) marking the longest transverse diameter of the head.

eutonic (u-ton'ik) See normotonic.

evacuation (e-vak-u-a'shun) **1.** The process of emptying or removing. **2.** The material discharged from the bowels.

    fimbrial e. The aspiration of an ectopic embryo located in the distal end of a fallopian (uterine) tube.

evaluation (e-val-u-a'shun) Examination and judgment of the significance of something.

    clinical e. Evaluation based on direct observation of a patient.

    vaginal smear e. Laboratory test performed as an aid in assessing the estrogenic status of a patient; scrapings from the lateral vaginal wall are examined and, using the pyknotic index, the estrogenic effect is assessed by determining the percentage of superficial and intermediate squamous cells with fatty pyknotic nuclei. See also Pap test, under test.

evisceration (e-vis-er-a'shun) **1.** Removal of an organ. **2.** Extrusion of an internal organ. **3.** A critical postoperative complication involving an abdominal wall incision in which all layers of the wound separate, allowing intestinal protrusion through the opening. Also called burst abdomen. Compare with dehiscence.

ex- Prefix meaning out of, from.

examination (eg-zam-ĭ-na'shun) An investigation conducted as a means of arriving at diagnosis or assessing a therapy.

    bimanual pelvic e. Palpation conducted with the index and middle fingers of one hand in the vagina and the flat surface of the other hand on the lower abdominal wall; performed to assess the position, size, consistency, shape, and mobility of the uterus and adjacent structures.

    cytologic e. Microscopic examination of cells.

    gynecologic e. Examination that includes pelvic, bimanual pelvic, vaginal, rectovaginal, and breast examinations.

    Papanicolaou e. See Pap test, under test.

    pelvic e. An examination that includes vaginal, bimanual pelvic, and rectovaginal examinations in addition to inspection of the genital area to note pubic hair distribution, clitoris size, vulvar lesions or masses, patency of hymenal orifice, discharge, and inflammation or discoloration of the vaginal and urethral openings.

    rectovaginal e. Palpation conducted by gently inserting the middle finger into the rectum and the index finger of the same hand in the vagina, and raising the cervix toward the abdominal wall; performed to detect masses, tenderness or abnormalities in the lower rectum and the posterior vaginal wall and fornix, and to obtain a histologic sample from the rectum.

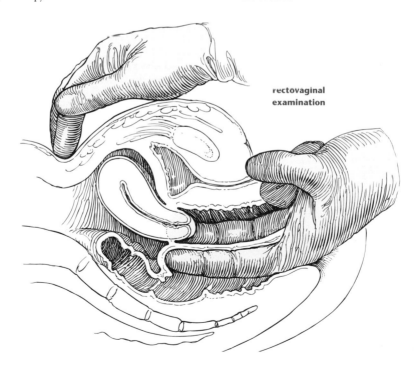

rectovaginal
examination

self-breast e. Inspection of her own breasts by a woman to detect lumps, asymmetry of the breasts (considered unusual for the individual), and slight dimpling of the skin; first, while standing in front of a mirror, the person looks for changes on her breasts as she places her hands on her sides, as she elevates her hands over her head, and as she places them on her hips and presses firmly to contract the pectoral muscles; second, in a supine position, she palpates each breast with the hand of the opposite side.

ultrasound e. See ultrasonography.

vaginal e. (1) *Routine vaginal e.*: Examination that consists of inspection of the vagina with a speculum for visual detection of abnormalities and to obtain a smear for cytologic examination; palpation of the vaginal walls with the index and middle fingers to detect the presence of a cystocele, rectocele, or any other masses. This routine is modified accordingly when examining a child. (2) *Vaginal e. during labor:* Examination that consists of inspection of the posterior vaginal fornix to detect the presence of amniotic fluid and (if present) to collect a sample for detection of meconium, or vernix caseosa or for certain biochemical or bacteriologic studies; palpation of the cervix for assessment of softness, degree of cervical effacement, extent of cervical dilatation, detection of fetal membranes, position of cervical os in relation to the fetal head (i.e., posterior, midposition, anterior), and the fetal station (i.e., the degree of descent of the presenting part into the birth canal); palpation of the presenting part to determine its nature (e.g., vertex, face, breech), its position (e.g., in vertex presentation, by locating the fontanels and, in frank breech, by locating the fetal ischial tuberosities); examination of the pelvic architecture for re-evaluation of the diagonal conjugate, ischial spines, and sacrum.

excess (ek'ses) An amount that exceeds that which is usual or sufficient.

base e. The amount of acid or base that would restore 1 liter of whole blood to normal acid–base composition at a P_{CO_2} of 40 mmHg at 37°C. The value is positive in metabolic alkalosis and negative in metabolic acidosis.

excision (ek-sizh'un) The surgical removal of tissues or organs.

wide e. Complete removal of a lesion or tumor, including a margin of healthy tissue.

exenteration (ek-sen-ter-a'shun) Removal of internal organs and tissues from a body cavity; the term denotes an extensive operation.

pelvic e. Removal of organs and tissues from the pelvic cavity for the treatment of advanced and recurrent pelvic cancer. Designated: *Anterior pelvic e.*, when the excision includes the bladder, lower portion of the ureters, and urethra in addition to the uterus, vagina, adnexa, and lymph nodes; the rectosigmoid portion of the bowel is left in place; the urinary stream is diverted into an ileal or sigmoid conduit. *Posterior pelvic e.*, when the excision includes the rectosigmoid bowel in addition to the uterus, vagina, adnexa, and lymph nodes; the bladder, ureters, and urethra are left in place; fecal contents are diverted through a colostomy. *Total pelvic e.*, when all pelvic organs are removed *en bloc*, including the bladder, lower ureters, urethra, and rectosigmoid bowel; the urinary stream is diverted via an ileal conduit and fecal contents through a colostomy.

exercise (ek'ser-sīz) Repetitive activity that has, or is intended to have, a long-range effect in improving, maintaining, or restoring health or skill, or that is used for diagnosis.

Kegel e. Contraction of the levator ani and perineal muscles to strengthen the pelvic floor in the perinatal and postpartum periods or for the management of urinary stress incontinence.

exo- Prefix meaning outside.

exomphalos (eks-om'fă-los) See omphalocele.

exophytic (ek-so-fit'ik) Tending to grow outward; in oncology, applied to a lesion or tumor that arises on the surface of an organ or tissue (e.g., within the cervical epithelium) and grows outward.

exploration (eks-plo-ra'shun) A diagnostic search; may be a digital, instrumental, or surgical examination of tissues or organs.

uterine e. Exploration of the cavity of the uterus to detect defects in the uterine walls; usually performed after vaginal delivery in a woman who had a previous cesarean section.

expressivity (eks-pres-siv'ĭ-te) The variation (i.e., different phenotypes) with which a gene expresses itself (e.g., myotonic dystrophy and neurofibromatosis). Compare with penetrance.

exstrophy (ek'stro-fe) Congenital turning inside-out of a hollow organ.

e. of bladder Malformation consisting of a gap in the lower abdominal wall and absence of the anterior bladder wall; the posterior bladder wall may extrude through the opening or lie exposed as an open sac; defect occurs in varying degrees of severity. Also called ectopia vesicae.

extocervix (eks-to-ser'viks) See portio vaginalis, under portio.

extra- Prefix meaning beyond, outside of, in addition.

extracorporeal (eks-tra-kor-po're-al) Outside the body.

extraction (eks-trak'shun) The act of moving or drawing out, such as the removal of a fetus from the birth canal either manually or with instruments.

assisted breech e. See partial breech extraction.

breech e. Extraction of the infant from the birth canal by its buttocks or lower limbs.

menstrual e. See menstrual aspiration, under aspiration.

partial breech e. An operation for the delivery of a fetus presenting in the breech position during which the infant is allowed to spontaneously deliver to the level of its umbilicus whence the operator, through a series of maneuvers (rotation, traction, etc.), assists in delivery of the shoulders, arms, and head. Also called assisted breech extraction.

total breech e. Procedure in which the infant's whole body is manually delivered by the operator. The procedure is only rarely performed; in most instances cesarean section is the preferred method of delivery.

extractor (eks-trak'tor) Any instrument or device used in drawing out or pulling out.

Malstrom vacuum e. Vacuum extractor consisting basically of a metal cap connected to a suction pump through a hose, and a chain attached to the metal cap to apply traction.

Mityvac vacuum e. Vacuum extractor with a disposable soft cup measuring 60 mm in diameter.

Silastic cup e. Vacuum extractor with a soft reusable cup measuring 65 mm in diameter.

vacuum e. Any traction device attached by suction to the scalp of a fetus to apply traction on the fetal head; the device is applied after the head has engaged (i.e., after it has passed through the pelvic inlet). Also called vacuum forceps.

extrauterine (eks-tra-u'ter-in) Outside the uterus.

extraversion (eks-tra-ver'zhun) See extroversion.

extremity (eks-trem'ĭ-te) A limb; an arm or a leg.

extroversion (eks-tro-ver'zhun) A turning inside-out of a hollow organ (e.g., of the uterus).

extubation (eks-tu-ba'shun) The process of withdrawing a tube from a cavity of the body.

ex vivo (eks ve'vo) Outside the living body.

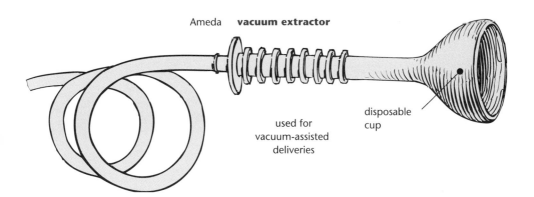

Ameda **vacuum extractor**

used for vacuum-assisted deliveries

disposable cup

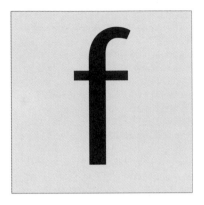

factor (fak'tor) (F) A substance, circumstance, or influence that contributes to an action, process, or result such as blood clotting or the growth process. The term is generally used when the nature or mechanism of action of a substance is unknown; when those properties become known, factors are redesignated, frequently as hormones.

bifidus f. A nitrogen-containing carbohydrate found in the intestinal flora of breast-fed infants; thought to enhance the infant's defenses against infection.

clotting f., coagulation f. Any of the substances in the blood that are essential for blood clotting; some are designated by Roman numerals, others by Arabic numerals.

colony-stimulating f. (CSF) A polypeptide that promotes restoration of blood-forming function (e.g., after bone marrow suppression in chemotherapy).

insulin-like growth f.'s (IGF) Serum peptides resembling insulin in structure and biologic activities; formed primarily in the liver and ovary; they are important as mediators of growth hormone; two forms have been isolated: *IGF-I*, active in embryonic development, and *IGF-II*, active postnatally. Formerly called somatomedins.

luteinizing hormone-releasing f. (LHF) See luteinizing hormone-releasing hormone, under hormone.

macrophage-activating f. (MAF) A group of soluble substances (products of lymphocytes) that participate in inducing immunologic responses. Interferon-gamma (INF-γ) is a major type.

prolactin-inhibiting f. (PIF) See prolactin-inhibiting hormone, under hormone.

prolactin-releasing f. (PRF) See prolactin-releasing hormone, under hormone.

testis-determining f. (TDF) A factor, encoded by a gene present on the short arm of the Y chromosome, which initiates the differentiation of the gonad into a testis.

transfer f. (TF) (1) A genetic particle in bacterial cells that is transferred from one bacterium to another. (2) A substance, free of nucleic acid and antibody, capable of transferring antigen-specific cell-mediated immunity from donor to recipient.

tumor-angiogenesis f. (TAF) A substance that stimulates rapid formation of new blood vessels; secreted by malignant tumors and not found in normal tissues except the placenta.

tumor necrosis f. (TNF) A hormone-like chemical messenger that affects the immune response; it is secreted by certain activated cells (monocytes and lymphocytes) and can induce hemorrhagic destruction of tumors.

X f. Designation for a set of conditions (e.g., first pregnancy in an elderly woman, ruptured membranes without labor, and diabetes) that would have to be present with another condition (e.g., postmaturity) to warrant the performance of a cesarean section (i.e., X factor alone would not be a sufficient reason for that form of delivery).

failure (fāl'yer) **1.** The condition of being insufficient. **2.** A cessation of normal functioning.

acute renal f. (ARF) Condition in which the filtration rate within the kidneys is abruptly reduced, causing a sudden retention of metabolism products that are normally cleared by the kidneys, such as urea, potassium, phosphate, sulfate, and creatinine.

f. to progress A vague term applied when labor stops before full dilatation of the cervix is attained and no change is noted for 2 or 3 hours; causes may range from inertia to cephalopelvic disproportion.

renal f. Cessation or diminution of kidney function.

falling of the womb See prolapse of uterus, under prolapse.

falloposcopy (fă-lo-pos'kŏ-pe) Endoscopic examination of the lumen of a fallopian (uterine) tube with the aid of a self-seeking guidewire introduced through the uterine cavity. Also called tuboscopy.

false-negative (fawls' neg'ă-tiv) Denoting a test result that wrongly indicates that a person does not have the attribute or disease for which the test is conducted.

false-positive (fawls' pos'ĭ-tiv) Denoting a test result that wrongly indicates that a person has the attribute or disease for which the test is conducted.

falx (falks) A sickle-shaped structure.

inguinal f. See conjoined tendon, under tendon.

fascia (fash'c-ă) An aggregation of connective tissue that lies just under the skin or forms a covering for muscles and various organs.

f. of abdominal wall Fascia of the anterior abdominal wall, divisible into: (1) a thick subcutaneous fascia composed of a superficial fatty layer (Camper's fascia) and a deeper membranous layer (Scarpa's fascia), between which are superficial lymph nodes, vessels, and nerves; (2) a thin, semitransparent fascia (transverse fascia).

anal f. See inferior fascia of pelvic diaphragm.

Camper's f. The thick subcutaneous fatty layer of the superficial fascia of the lower part of the anterior abdominal wall.

f. of clitoris A dense fibrous sheath that encases the two corpora cavernosa of the clitoris; it is continuous with the suspensory ligament of the clitoris.

Colles' f. See superficial fascia of perineum (2).

endopelvic f. See visceral pelvic fascia, under pelvic fascia.

inferior f. of pelvic diaphragm The thin fascia covering the inferior aspect of the levator ani and coccygeus muscles. Also called anal fascia.

inferior f. of urogenital diaphragm The lower layer of fascia of the urogenital diaphragm, stretched across the anterior half of the pelvic outlet (filling the gap of the pubic arch) and between the ischiopubic rami; it covers the underside of the urethral sphincter and deep transverse perineal muscles, in the female, it is penetrated by the urethra and

vagina; in the male, by the urethra and the ducts of the bulbourethral glands. Also called perineal membrane.

obturator f. The portion of the parietal pelvic fascia that covers the pelvic surface of the internal obturator muscle.

pectoral f. Fascia that invests the greater pectoral (pectoralis major) muscle; it is attached to the breastbone (sternum) and collarbone (clavicle) and is continuous with neighboring fascia.

pelvic f. Fascia of the pelvis, composed of two layers: *parietal pelvic f.*, fascial sheaths of the pelvic muscles, above the level of origin of the levator ani muscle; and *visceral pelvic f.*, fascial sheaths from around the pelvic organs and their blood vessels and nerves to the upper surface of the levator ani muscle. Also called endopelvic fascia.

pubovesicocervical f. A formation of endopelvic fascia extending between the bladder and vagina; it stretches from its origin at the pubic symphysis beneath the bladder to blend with fascia that surrounds the cervix.

Scarpa's f. The deep layer of the superficial fascia of the anterior abdominal wall, adhered anteriorly to the linea alba and pubic symphysis; posteriorly, it is continuous with the perineal membrane.

superficial f. of perineum The subcutaneous tissue of the urogenital region, composed of two layers: (1) a superficial fatty layer that is continuous superiorly with Camper's fascia (the superficial fatty layer of the lower abdomen); and (2) a deep membranous layer continuous superiorly with Scarpa's fascia (the deep layer of the superficial abdominal fascia); also called Colles' fascia.

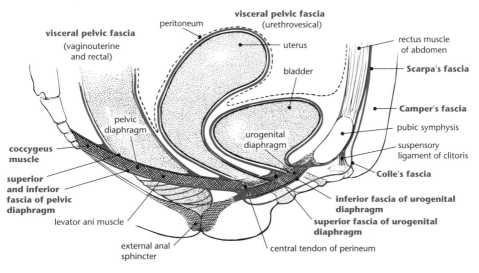

superior f. of pelvic diaphragm The fascia on the superior surface of the pelvic diaphragm (i.e., the levator ani and coccygeus muscles).

superior f. of urogenital diaphragm The fascia on the superior surface of the urogenital diaphragm (i.e., the urethral sphincter and deep transverse perineal muscles); anteriorly, it extends across the pubic arch; posteriorly, it blends with the inferior fascia of the diaphragm, the perineal body, and the membranous layer of the superficial perineal fascia.

transverse f., transversalis f. The fascial lining of the abdominal cavity between the inner surface of the abdominal musculature and the peritoneum.

triangular f. of abdomen See reflex inguinal ligament, under ligament.

fascial (fash'e-al) Relating to fascia.

fasciitis (fas-e-i'tis) Inflammation of a fascia.

necrotizing f. A serious, rapidly progressing inflammation and necrosis of the skin, subcutaneous fat, superficial fascia, and sometimes underlying muscle; caused by mixed aerobic-anaerobic bacteria, although a single pathogen (e.g., group A streptococcus or clostridia) may be isolated. Predisposing conditions include diabetes, obesity, and hypertension.

fecundability (fe-kun-dă-bil'ĭ-te) The probability of becoming pregnant within one menstrual cycle.

fecundate (fe'kun-dāt) To fertilize, to impregnate.

fecundation (fe-kun-da'shun) Fertilization.

fecundity (fĕ-kun'dĭ-te) The ability to produce a live offspring within one menstrual cycle. Distinguished from fertility.

feeding (fēd'ing) The giving or taking of nourishment.

fellatio (fĕ-la'she-o) Oral stimulation of the penis.

feminization (fem-ĭ-nĭ-za'shun) **1.** The development of female characteristics in the male. **2.** Abnormal development of female sexual tissues in the male.

complete testicular f. An X-linked recessive inheritance characterized by the presence of female external genitalia and a rudimentary, short vagina (ending in a blind pouch); the uterus, uterine tubes, and ovaries are absent; testes are typically present (but located within the abdomen or partially descended into the inguinal canal); sperm formation is absent. The condition is caused by lack of androgenic activity in androgen-dependent tissues, due to lack of cellular receptors for testosterone and

dihydrotestosterone. Also called complete androgen insensitivity.

incomplete testicular f. An X-linked recessive inheritance characterized by external genitalia with an abnormally large clitoris and posterior fusion of the labial folds; caused by variable degrees of defective androgenic activity in androgen-dependent tissues. Also called incomplete androgen insensitivity.

ferning (fern'ing) The typical palm-leaf or 'arborization' pattern observed in a dry specimen of endocervical mucus or amniotic fluid; crystallization of the fluid is dependent upon the concentration of electrolytes, particularly sodium chloride; used as an adjunctive test to confirm chorioamnion rupture during pregnancy. Ferning is a normal physiologic phenomenon in a specimen obtained at midmenstrual cycle (i.e., from days 7 to 18, peaking on day 14).

ferning

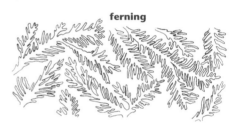

fertile (fer'til) Capable of reproducing.

fertility (fer-til'ĭ-te) The capacity to conceive and bear offspring.

impaired f. See infertility (2).

fertilization (fer-tĭ-lĭ-za'shun) The union of a spermatozoon with an ovum.

in vitro f. (IVF) The process of extracting several oocytes, placing them in a Petri dish containing a culture medium (e.g., blood serum and nutrients) and adding sperm; fertilized eggs are transferred to another Petri dish where they are allowed to grow for 3 to 6 days; the embryos are then transcervically placed within the uterus. Popularly called test-tube fertilization.

test-tube f. See *in vitro* fertilization.

fetal (fe'tal) Relating to the fetus.

fetal loss (fe'tal los) See spontaneous abortion, under abortion.

feticide (fe'tĭ-sīd) Intentional destruction of the embryo or fetus in the uterus.

feto- Combining form meaning fetus.

fetography (fe-tog'ră-fe) Radiography of the fetus in the uterus.

fetology (fe-tol'ŏ-je) The study of the fetus and its diseases.

fertilization

The penetration of sperm through the corona radiata and the zona pellucida is accomplished by the release of acrosomal enzymes (acid phosphatase and acrosomase) by many sperms.

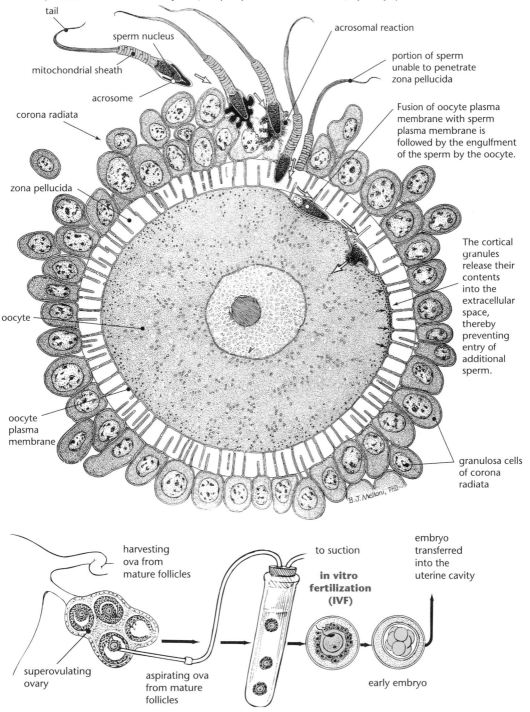

tail

sperm nucleus

acrosomal reaction

mitochondrial sheath

portion of sperm unable to penetrate zona pellucida

acrosome

corona radiata

Fusion of oocyte plasma membrane with sperm plasma membrane is followed by the engulfment of the sperm by the oocyte.

zona pellucida

oocyte

The cortical granules release their contents into the extracellular space, thereby preventing entry of additional sperm.

oocyte plasma membrane

granulosa cells of corona radiata

B.J. Melloni, PhD

harvesting ova from mature follicles

to suction

embryo transferred into the uterine cavity

in vitro fertilization (IVF)

superovulating ovary

aspirating ova from mature follicles

early embryo

fetomaternal (fe-to-mă-ter'nal) Relating to both the fetus and its mother (e.g., hemorrhage).

fetometry (fe-tom'ĕ-tre) Estimation of the size of the fetal head before delivery.

fetopelvic (fe-to-pel'vik) Relating to the fetus and the maternal pelvis (e.g., disproportion).

fetoplacental (fe-to-plă-sen'tal) Relating to the fetus and placenta.

α-fetoprotein (al'fă fe-to-pro'tēn) See alpha-fetoprotein.

fetoscope (fe'to-skōp) Instrument for listening to the fetal heartbeat.

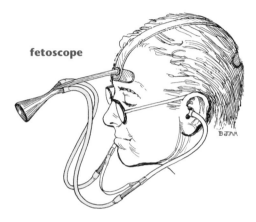

fetoscope

fetotoxic (fe-to-tok'sik) Characterized by fetotoxicity.

fetotoxicity (fe-to-tok-sis'ĭ-te) Injurious alteration of the developmental processes of the fetus caused by maternal exposure to such agents as radiation, viruses, gases, and drugs; effects may include malformations, intrauterine growth retardation, or death.

fetus (fe'tus) The developing young in the uterus from the end of the seventh week of gestation to birth. See also embryo; infant.

   f. compressus See fetus papyraceus.

   f. papyraceus A flattened, partly mummified twin fetus that dies early in pregnancy and remains in the uterus until completion of term, compressed between the uterine wall and the amniotic sac of the living twin; its portion of the placenta becomes pale and atrophic. Also called fetus compressus.

   f. at term A fetus at the completion of 42 weeks of gestation. See also infant.

fever (fe'ver) **1.** A rise in body temperature above the normal range; an early morning temperature of 32.2°C [99.0°F] or greater, or an evening temperature of 37.8°C [100°F] or greater. **2.** Condition in which the body temperature is above the normal. Also called pyrexia.

   childbed f. See puerperal fever.

   enigmatic f. Fever occurring in the absence of clinically apparent illness.

   glandular f. See infectious mononucleosis, under mononucleosis.

   nodal f. See erythema nodosum, under erythema.

   puerperal f. Fever occurring after childbirth; may be due to infection. Popularly called childbed fever.

fibrin (fi'brin) A fibrous, insoluble protein derived from fibrinogen by the action of the enzyme thrombin; it is the basic component of a blood clot; during blood clot formation, blood cells become entangled in the fibrin network.

fibrinogen (fi-brin'o-jen) A protein present in dissolved form in blood plasma; it is converted into a network of delicate elastic filaments (fibrin) by the action of the enzyme thrombin.

fibro-, fibr- Combining forms meaning fiber.

fibroadenoma (fi-bro-ad-ĕ-no'mă) A benign tumor derived from glandular epithelium.

   f. of breast A single, freely movable nodule 1 to 10 cm in diameter; it is the most common benign tumor of the female breast, usually occurring during the reproductive years.

fibrocarcinoma (fi-bro-kar-sĭ-no'mă) See scirrhous carcinoma, under carcinoma.

fibrocystic (fi-bro-sis'tik) Having fibrous and cystic components.

fibroid (fi'broid) **1.** Commonly used term for a usually benign tumor more properly called leiomyoma, since the tumor mass is primarily composed of smooth muscle rather than fibrous tissue. See leiomyoma. **2.** Composed of or resembling fibrous tissue.

fibroma (fi-bro'ma) A benign tumor derived from fibrous tissue.

   ovarian f. A hard, solid, gray-white tumor, usually unilateral and frequently associated with accumulation of noninflammatory fluid around the lungs and in the abdominal cavity.

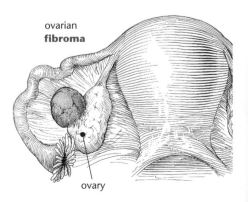

ovarian
fibroma

ovary

fibromatosis (fi-bro-mǎ-to'sis), pl. fibromatoses
1. Any of a group of conditions with abnormal proliferation of fibrous tissue as the common feature (e.g., Dupuytren's contracture, Peyronie's disease). **2.** Condition marked by formation of multiple fibromas.
    aggressive f. See desmoid.
fibromyoma (fi-bro-mi-o'mǎ) See leiomyoma.
fibroplasia (fi-bro-pla'se-ǎ) Abnormal production of fibrous tissue.
    retrolental f. See retinopathy of prematurity, under retinopathy.
fibroplastic (fi-bro-plas'tik) Relating to fibroplasia.
filter (fil'ter) **1.** A porous material for trapping particles suspended in a gas or liquid. **2.** A device that permits passage of rays of certain wavelengths only; used in radiologic diagnosis or treatment. **3.** To pass a substance or rays through such devices.
    bird's nest f. A device placed in the vena cava for the treatment of recurrent pulmonary embolism.
filum (fi'lum), pl. fila A filamentous or threadlike structure or part; Latin for thread.
    f. of spinal dura mater The extension of the dura mater surrounding the spinal cord; it starts from the apex of the dural sac and descends for about 5 cm, and then fuses with the filum terminale before attaching to the periosteum of the coccyx.
    f. terminale The slender threadlike prolongation of the spinal cord, about 20 cm long, consisting mainly of filaments of connective tissue (continuous with the pia mater of the spinal cord); it extends from the conus medullaris of the spinal cord to the apex of the dural sac where it unites with the filum of spinal dura mater before attaching to the periosteum of the coccyx; usually seen from the level of the second lumbar vertebra to the coccyx.
fimbria (fim'bre-ǎ), pl. fimbriae Any fringelike structure.
    f. ovarica See ovarian fimbria.
    ovarian f. The longest and most deeply grooved fimbria of the fallopian (uterine) tube that runs along the lateral border of the mesosalpinx to attach to the tubal end of the ovary. Also called fimbria ovarica.
    fimbriae of uterine tube The numerous diverging fringelike processes on the margins of the distal end of the fallopian (uterine) tube; they are closely applied to the surface of the ovary during ovulation.
fimbriated (fim'bre-at-ed) Having fimbriae.

fimbriectomy (fim-bre-ek'tŏ-me) Surgical removal of the fimbrial end of the fallopian (uterine) tubes for the purpose of sterilization. Also called Kroener's sterilization.

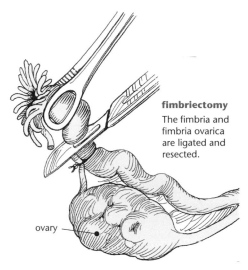

fimbriectomy
The fimbria and fimbria ovarica are ligated and resected.

ovary

fimbrioplasty (fim-bre-o-plas'te) Reconstruction of existing fimbriae in a partially or totally occluded fallopian (uterine) tube.
fissural (fish'u-ral) Relating to a fissure.
fissuration (fish-u-ra'shun) The formation of a fissure.
fissure (fish'ur) A cleft, groove, depression, or slit; a sulcus or deep fold.
    anal f. A painful slit, difficult to heal, in the mucous membrane at the margin of the anus.
    decidual f. A cleft in the decidua basalis of the placenta, as seen toward the end of pregnancy.
    intercotyledonal f.'s Grooves that separate some 15 to 30 lobules (cotyledons) on the maternal side of the placenta.
    pudendal f. See vulval cleft, under cleft.
    urogenital f. See vulval cleft, under cleft.
fistula (fis'tu-lǎ), pl. fistulas An unnatural passage between one organ and another, or between an organ and the surface of the body; usually designated according to the organ with which it communicates.
    anal f. An open channel in the region of the anus, invariably the result of an abscess; the port of entry is generally an anal crypt and from there it could course submucously, subcutaneously, or transsphincterally to the surrounding tissue, exiting to the skin near the anal opening or ascending to open in the rectum.
    anovestibular f. Anal fistula opening into

the posterior vestibule of the vagina.

enterovaginal f. A fistula between the vagina and neighboring intestine, usually associated with intestinal disease, especially diverticulitis.

genitourinary f. An uncommon fistula between the genital and urinary tracts; may occur concomitantly with a malignant tumor or (when multiple) may be the result of radiation therapy.

pilonidal f. See pilonidal sinus, under sinus.

rectovaginal f. A fistulous passage between the rectum and the vagina; may occur as a result of radiation therapy or may be caused by direct surgical trauma.

urachal f. A fistula between the bladder and the umbilicus; a congenital abnormality that occurs when the lumen of the embryonic urachus (which extends from the bladder to the umbilicus) fails to obliterate during intrauterine life and persists over the entire length, allowing urine to seep through the umbilicus. Also called patent urachus; vesicoumbilical fistula.

ureterovaginal f. Fistula between a ureter and the vagina, sometimes occurring after a hysterectomy.

urethrovaginal f. A fistula between the urethra and the vagina; may be due to obstetrical injury or may be congenital.

vesicouterine f. A fistula between the bladder and the uterus, usually caused by cancer of the cervix.

vesicovaginal f. A fistula between the bladder and the vagina, often the result of advanced cancer or traumatic delivery.

vesicoumbilical f. See urachal fistula.

fistulation (fis-tu-la'shun) The formation of a fistula.

fistulatome (fis'tu-lă-tōm) A thin-bladed long knife for cutting open a fistula.

fistulectomy (fis-tu-lek'tŏ-me) Surgical obliteration of a fistula by removal of its walls, thus creating an open wound that heals from within outward.

fistulotomy (fis-tu-lot'ŏ-me) A surgical incision into a fistula.

fistulous (fis'tu-lus) Containing a fistula.

floor (flor) The lower, supporting surface of a cavity or structure.

pelvic f. The broad hammock of muscle and fascia sweeping down from the pelvic brim attaching posteriorly to the sacrum and coccyx, and separating the pelvic cavity (which contains the pelvic viscera) from the perineum (below). See also muscles.

flora (flo'ră) The bacteria or fungi present in or on

an organ or body part; may be either pathogenic or the normal inhabitants of the given area.

flow (flo) **1.** A movement, as of a fluid or gas. **2.** Popular term for the menstrual discharge. See also menstruation; menstrual cycle, under cycle.

fluid (floo'id) **1.** Any nonsolid substance, either liquid or gas. **2.** Capable of flowing.

amniotic f. Fluid within the amnion, the membrane in which the fetus floats; it begins to accumulate from the twelfth day of gestation.

cerebrospinal f. (CSF) The clear fluid within the four ventricles of the brain, the subarachnoid space surrounding the brain and spinal cord, and the central canal of the spinal cord.

extracellular f. (ECF) The body fluid outside the cells; sometimes the term is restricted to the interstitial fluid and blood plasma.

follicular f. An albuminous fluid secreted by the granulosa (follicular) cells in a developing follicle of the ovary. Also called liquor folliculi.

interstitial f. Tissue fluid in spaces between cells.

seminal f. See semen.

fluorometer (floōr-om'ě-ter) Device for the detection and analysis of fluorescence.

fluoroscope (floor'-o-skōp) A type of x-ray apparatus, used in medical diagnosis, in which x-rays passing through the body strike upon a fluorescent screen, which absorbs the radiation and produces a visible image of various densities.

fluoroscopic (floor-o-skŏp'ik) Relating to fluoroscopy.

fluoroscopy (floōr-os'kŏ-pe) Examination of internal structures of the body with a fluoroscope.

fluorosis (floōr-o'sis) Condition characterized by mottling of tooth enamel, caused by excessive intake of fluorides during tooth formation.

fluorouracil (floor-o-ūr'ă-sil) (5-FU) A pyrimidine analog used intravenously for the treatment of cancer (e.g., of the breast, cervix, and gastrointestinal tract); may cause fetal malformations when taken during the first trimester, cyanosis and jerking of the limbs in third-trimester use, and low birth weight when taken anytime during pregnancy.

fluoxetine (floo-ok'sě-tēn) An antidepressant drug used for the treatment of obsessive–compulsive disorder; thought to exert its effect by inhibiting central nervous system uptake of the vasoconstrictor serotonin. The drug is secreted in milk and may affect the breast-fed infant.

foam (fōm) A frothy substance.

contraceptive f. See spermicide.

fold (fōld) **1.** The doubling of a part upon itself. **2.** A thin ridge or margin in soft tissue, usually of the external surface of the body.

Douglas f.'s See rectouterine folds.

medial umbilical f. One of two folds of peritoneum on the inner surface of the abdominal wall that cover the obliterated umbilical arteries as they ascend from the pelvis toward the navel.

median umbilical f. The fold of peritoneum on the inner surface of the anterior abdominal wall that covers the median umbilical ligament; it extends from the apex of the urinary bladder to the navel. Also called fold of urachus.

Rathke f.'s In embryology, two mesodermal folds in the right and left sides of the cloaca of a 5 to 7 week old embryo; together with the Tourneux fold, they form the urogenital fold.

rectouterine f.'s Folds of peritoneum that extend from the uterine cervix on either side of the rectum, to the posterior wall of the pelvis. Also called Douglas folds.

rectovaginal f. A fold of peritoneum extending from the front of the rectum to the back of the posterior fornix of the vagina; it forms the floor of the deep rectovaginal pouch. Also called posterior ligament of uterus.

rectovesical f. See sacrogenital fold.

sacrogenital f. A peritoneal fold extending posteriorly from the sides of the urinary bladder, on either side of the rectum, to the front of the sacrum; it bounds the rectovesical pouch. Also called rectovesical fold.

Tourneux f. In embryology, the mesodermal structure between the allantois and the primitive hindgut; it fuses with the two Rathke folds to form the urorectal septum, which divides the cloaca into the urogenital sinus and rectum.

tubal f.'s of uterine tube A series of major plicated folds of mucous membrane projecting into the lumen of the fallopian (uterine) tube; especially well developed in the ampulla of the tube.

f. of urachus See median umbilical fold.

uterovesical f. A fold of peritoneum extending from the front of the uterus to the upper surface of the urinary bladder. Also called anterior ligament of uterus.

vaginal f.'s See rugae of vagina, under ruga.

folic acid (fo'lik as'id) A constituent of the vitamin B complex; essential for production of red blood cells in bone marrow; deficiency may occur in malnourished people, alcoholics, and in malabsorption states, and results in megaloblastic anemia; deficiency occurring in the pregnant state may result in fetal anomalies.

folinic acid (fo-lin'ik as'id) A reduced form of folic acid. Also called leukovorin.

follicle (fol'lĕ-kl) **1.** A somewhat spherical mass of cells usually containing a cavity. **2.** A small crypt, such as the depression in the skin from which the hair emerges. **3.** A small circumscribed body.

atretic ovarian f. A follicle in the ovary that degenerates before reaching maturity, or one that enlarges but fails to ovulate.

dominant f. The single ovarian follicle that starts to grow rapidly approximately on the sixth day of the menstrual cycle and develops into the vesicular ovarian follicle.

graafian f. See vesicular ovarian follicle.

mature ovarian f. See vesicular ovarian follicle.

Montgomery f.'s See areolar glands, under gland.

multilaminar primary ovarian f. A primary ovarian follicle in which the flattened follicular cells of a single layer become cuboidal and proliferate to form a stratified epithelium; it has a distinct basement membrane.

nabothian f. See nabothian cyst, under cyst.

ovarian f. The ovum together with its surrounding cells, at any stage of development.

primary ovarian f. A developing follicle in the ovary before the appearance of a fluid-filled antrum; it is composed of a growing oocyte and a single layer of flattened follicular cells surrounded by a sheath of stroma (theca); it usually develops during adolescence. Also called unilaminar primary ovarian follicle.

primordial f. The earliest and most immature ovarian follicle consisting of the original primordial germ cell, the oogonium, and a thin single layer of squamous (flattened) follicular cells; at birth, there are about 400,000 primordial follicles in each ovary; most undergo atresia, and at the time of puberty there are about 200,000 left; they continue to decline in number throughout reproductive life. Also called unilaminar follicle.

secondary ovarian f. A growing ovarian follicle in which the follicular cells have proliferated into 7 to 12 layers, surrounded by developing follicular theca cells; small lakes of follicular fluid appear in the follicle. Also called solid secondary ovarian follicle.

solid secondary ovarian f. See secondary ovarian follicle.

tertiary ovarian f. See vesicular ovarian follicle.

    unilaminar f. See primordial follicle.

    unilaminar primary ovarian f. See primary ovarian follicle.

    vesicular ovarian f. A large mature follicle in the ovary in which the accumulations of lakes of follicular fluid enlarge and coalesce to form a fluid-filled cavity (antrum); the fluid, liquor folliculi, is rich in hyaluronic acid; when the cavity is completely formed the eccentric oocyte attains full size (about four times that of the primordial germ cell, from 120 to 150 μm in humans); at this stage of development, the follicle migrates toward the surface of the ovary, causing a preovulatory swelling. Also called graafian follicle; mature ovarian follicle; tertiary ovarian follicle.

folliculitis (fo-lik-u-li'tis) Inflammation of hair follicles.

    vulvar f. Folliculitis caused by staphylococcal infection of the pubic hair follicles.

follicular (fo-lik'u-lar) Relating to a follicle.

folliculoma (fo-lik-u-lo'mă) See granulosa cell tumor, under tumor.

fontanel, fontanelle (fon-tă-nel') Any of the normally six unossified spaces in the fetal and infant skull, covered by a fibrous membrane. Commonly called soft spot.

    anterior f. The largest of the six fontanels; it is diamond-shaped and located at the junction of the frontal, sagittal, and coronal sutures; it normally ossifies within 18 months of birth. Also called frontal fontanel, bregmatic fontanel.

    anterolateral f. See sphenoidal fontanel.

    bregmatic f. See anterior fontanel.

    frontal f. See anterior fontanel.

    lateral f.'s The mastoid and sphenoidal fontanels.

    mastoid f. An irregularly shaped, small fontanel on either side of the skull, between the adjacent edges of the parietal, temporal, and occipital bones; ossification generally occurs by the first year after birth. Also called posterolateral fontanel.

    occipital f. See posterior fontanel.

    posterior f. A triangular fontanel located at the junction of the sagittal and lambdoid sutures; it generally ossifies within two or three months of birth. Also called occipital fontanel.

    posterolateral f. See mastoid fontanel.

    sphenoidal f. An irregularly shaped, small fontanel located on either side of the skull at the junction of the frontal, parietal, temporal, and sphenoid bones; it generally ossifies within 2 or 3 months of birth. Also called anterolateral fontanel.

foramen (fo-ra'men), pl. foramina A natural opening through a bone or a membranous structure.

    interventricular f. An oval channel between the lateral and third ventricles of the brain, permitting circulation of cerebrospinal fluid. Also called foramen of Monro.

    f. of Luschka See lateral aperture of fourth ventricle, under aperture.

    f. of Magendie See medial aperture of fourth ventricle, under aperture.

    f. magnum The large median opening on the occipital bone at the base of the skull; it is the opening through which the medulla oblongata extends caudally as the spinal cord; it also transmits the vertebral arteries and the spinal roots of the accessory (11th cranial) nerve.

    f. of Monro See interventricular foramen.

    obturator f. The large opening in the hipbone (large and oval in males and smaller and nearly triangular in females); it is bounded by the pubic bone and ischium and is almost completely covered by a fibrous sheet (obturator membrane) except the upper area, where a small gap (obturator canal) permits direct communication between the pelvis and the thigh; it transmits the obturator nerve and vessels.

    vertebral f. The large enclosed space within a vertebra, between the neural arch (posterior aspect) and the body (anterior aspect); it is occupied by the spinal cord, filaments of dorsal and ventral roots, associated vessels, and adipose tissue.

foramina (fo-ram'ĭ-na) Plural of foramen.

forceps (for'seps) An instrument resembling a pair of tongs or pincers with blades used for grasping, compressing, manipulating, applying traction, cutting, crushing, or extracting.

    axis-traction f. A specially jointed obstetrical forceps by which traction on the fetal head can be exerted in the axis corresponding to the curvature of the birth canal.

    Bailey-Williamson f. A long-shank instrument with a fenestrated blade, round cephalic curve, and an English lock; designed for midstation application.

    Barton f. Instrument with a fixed curved blade and a hinged anterior blade, used when the fetal head is arrested in transverse and posterior positions.

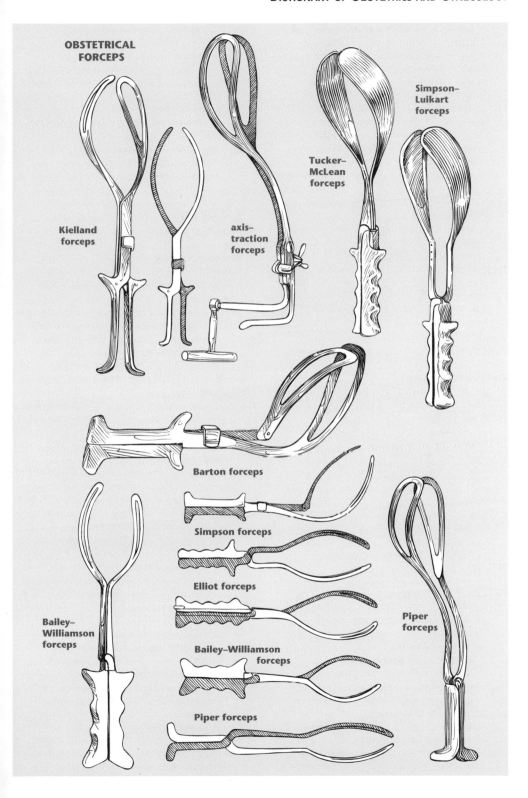

OBSTETRICAL FORCEPS

Simpson–Luikart forceps

Tucker–McLean forceps

Kielland forceps

axis–traction forceps

Barton forceps

Simpson forceps

Elliot forceps

Bailey–Williamson forceps

Bailey–Williamson forceps

Piper forceps

Piper forceps

bulldog f. See bulldog clamp, under clamp.

Elliot f. Instrument with a short straight shank suitable for delivery of the head in cesarean section.

high f. See high forceps delivery, under delivery.

Kielland f. A light-weight forceps with a sliding lock, a greatly diminished or no pelvic curve, and a pronounced cephalic curvature; used when the fetal head is arrested in a deep transverse position.

Kocher-Ochsner f. A commonly used sponge forceps.

low f. See low forceps delivery, under delivery.

obstetrical f. Instrument designed to assist the passage of the fetal head through the birth canal; its primary functions are traction and rotation; consists of two matching units, each composed of four parts: blade, shank, lock, and handle; the blade has a cephalic curve to fit around the fetal head and a pelvic curve to fit the curvature of the maternal pelvis.

outlet f. See outlet forceps delivery, under delivery.

Piper f. Forceps for delivering the aftercoming head in breech extraction; it has fenestrated blades, a flattened pelvic curve, long arched shank, and depressed handles.

prophylactic f. See prophylactic forceps delivery, under delivery.

punch f. A forceps with sharp cutting edges at the tip of the blades which, when closed, cut out a small piece of tissue for examination under the microscope (e.g., Tischler and Younge-Kevorkian cervical biopsy forceps).

Simpson f. Forceps with a short shank and a pelvic curve to fit the curvature of the maternal pelvis; it is the most commonly used instrument for low forceps delivery and is suited for fitting on a fetus with marked elongation (molding) of the head.

sponge holding f. A hemostat-like forceps with straight, curved, or ringed blades, with tips that are either smooth or serrated; has multiple uses in addition to facilitating the operative use of sponges (e.g., securing the ovary during surgery).

trial f. See trial forceps delivery, under delivery.

towel f. See towel clip, under clip.

Tucker-McLane f. Forceps with smooth solid blades, which reduce the likelihood of soft tissue injury; used for low forceps delivery when no significant traction is needed, and when the head of the fetus is not elongated (molded).

uterine f. Any forceps designed for surgery on the uterus, including single-toothed tenaculum, double-toothed tenaculum and quadruple-toothed tenaculum; the selected forceps depends upon the size of the uterus and the available exposure of the operative field.

vacuum f. See vacuum extractor, under extractor.

forebag, foresac, forewaters (for'bag, for'sak, for'wŏt-erz) The portion of fluid-filled amniotic sac that bulges into the cervical canal in front of the fetal head or any other presenting part of the fetus during the second stage of labor.

foremilk (for'milk) Popular name for colostrum.

foreplay (for'pla) Sexual stimulation leading to sexual intercourse.

foreskin (for'skin) See prepuce.

fornix (for'niks), pl. fornices **1.** Any arched structure. **2.** Any space created by such a structure.

    f. of vagina The space at the upper end of the vagina between the vaginal wall and the uterine cervix; it extends higher on the posterior than the anterior surface of the cervix. Also called fundus of vagina.

fossa (fos'ă), pl. **fossae** A pit, hollow, or depression.

    f. of vestibule of vagina The fossa between the vaginal opening and the frenulum of the labia minora.

fourchette (foor-shet') See frenulum of labia minora.

fractionation (frak-shun-a'shun) In radiation therapy, division of the total dose of a therapeutic dose of radiation into small doses of low intensity administered over a period of time, usually at daily or alternate day intervals.

fracture (frak'chur) (fx) The breaking of a bone or cartilage.

    pathologic f. Bone fracture through an area of bone weakened by preexisting disease (e.g., malignant tumor or osteoporosis) and inflicted by relatively minor trauma, or occurring with no trauma at all.

    ping-pong f. A circular fracture of the skull, so called because it resembles a ping-pong ball that has been pushed in with a finger; it can occur on the fetal skull delivered by cesarean section as the head is lifted out of the pelvis, or pushed out from below. Also called pond fracture.

    pond f. See ping-pong fracture.

frambesia (fram-be'ze-ă) See yaws.

frenulum (fren'u-lum) A small fold of mucous membrane that restrains the movements of an

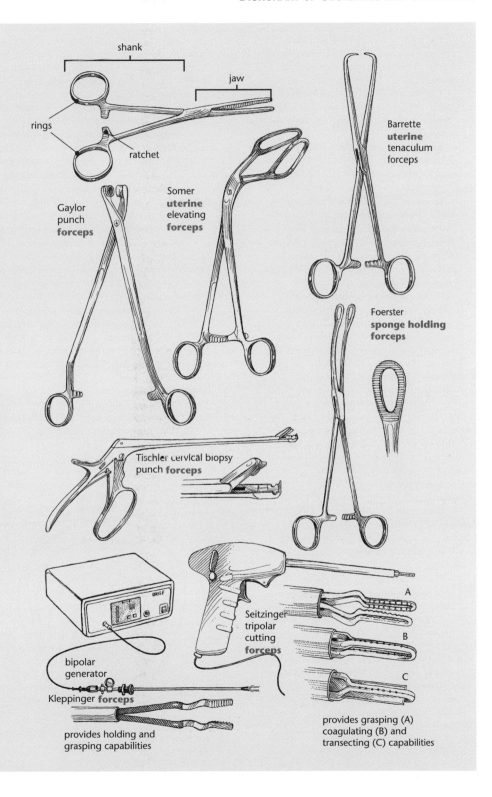

shank

jaw

rings

ratchet

Gaylor punch **forceps**

Somer **uterine** elevating **forceps**

Barrette **uterine** tenaculum forceps

Foerster **sponge holding forceps**

Tischler cervical biopsy punch **forceps**

Seitzinger tripolar cutting **forceps**

bipolar generator

Kleppinger **forceps**

provides holding and grasping capabilities

A

B

C

provides grasping (A) coagulating (B) and transecting (C) capabilities organ or movable part. Also called frenum.

f. of clitoris A suspensory fold connecting the undersurface of the clitoris with the labia minora; homologous with the frenulum of the prepuce.

f. of labia minora The posterior union of the two labia minora. Also called fourchette, frenulum of pudendal labia, frenulum of pudendal lips.

f. of pudendal labia, f. of pudendal lips See frenulum of labia.

frequency (freʹkwen-se) The number of recurrences of an event per unit time.

urinary f. The condition of urinating more frequently than usual for a given person; in severe cases, the desire to urinate may become constant, with each voiding producing only a few cubic centimeters of urine; causes are varied; they include infection of the bladder, stones, tumors, radiation cystitis, and tuberculosis. It is a natural condition in pregnancy due to blood vessel engorgement, hormonal changes that alter bladder function and, in late pregnancy, decreased bladder capacity due to pressure from the enlarging uterus. Distinguished from polyuria.

frigid (frijʹid) **1.** Very cold. **2.** Abnormally lacking the desire for sexual intercourse or unable to achieve orgasm during intercourse; applied chiefly to women.

frigidity (frĭ-jidʹĭ-te) The state of being frigid.

function (funkʹshun) **1.** The natural or special type of activity that is proper for an organ or body part. **2.** To perform such an action.

ventricular f. The performance of the ventricles of the heart in relation to size, volume, or pressure at the end of diastole.

fundal (funʹdal) Relating to a fundus.

fundus (funʹdus), pl. fundi The portion of a hollow organ that is farthest from, or opposite its opening.

f. of uterus The rounded portion of the uterus, above the orifices of the fallopian (uterine) tubes.

f. of vagina See fornix of vagina, under fornix.

funguria (fung-uʹre-a) Urinary tract infection with a fungus-like yeast (e.g., *Candida albicans* and *Torulopsis glabrata*); usually seen in patients with indwelling urinary catheters, and those undergoing anticancer and immunosuppressive therapy.

fungus (fungʹgus), pl. fungi General term for a large group of spore-bearing forms of the kingdom Protista; characterized by lack of chlorophyll, asexual reproduction, and parasitic

qualities; some cause disease in humans.

thrush f. See *Candida albicans*, under *Candida*.

funic (fuʹnik) Relating to the umbilical cord. See also funic presentation, under presentation.

funis (fuʹnis) **1.** The umbilical cord. **2.** Any cordlike structure.

funneling (funʹel-ing) The act or process of assuming a conical shape.

cervical f. In obstetrics, descriptive term indicating the assumption of a conical shape by the cervical canal due to opening of the internal os, which allows protrusion of the amniotic sac into the canal.

furrow (furʹo) A groove, generally long, narrow, and shallow.

nympholabial f.'s The grooves separating the labia majora from the labia minora.

gluteal f. The groove between the buttocks.

Fusobacterium (fu-zo-bak-terʹe-um) Genus of Gram-negative, anaerobic organisms; some members are natural inhabitants of body cavities of humans and other mammals, others are pathogenic; some species are commonly found in amniotic fluid during a preterm labor; others are associated with intrauterine infections and are present in the amnion and the Wharton jelly of the umbilical cord.

fusobacteria (fu-zo-bak-terʹe-ă) Any member of the genus *Fusobacterium*.

fusospirochetal (fu-so-spi-ro-keʹtal) Relating to a mixed infection with fusiform and spirochetal microorganisms.

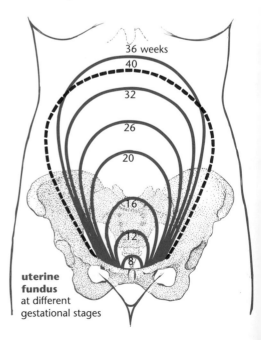

36 weeks
40
32
26
20
16
12
8

uterine fundus at different gestational stages

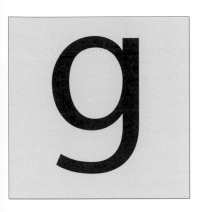

galactacrasia (gal-ak-tă-kra'se-ă) Abnormal composition of human milk.

galactagogue (gă-lak'tă-gog) Any agent that promotes the flow of milk. Also called lactagogue.

galactic (gă-lak'tik) Relating to milk.

galactischia (gal-ak-tisk'e-ă) Suppression of the secretion of milk.

galacto-, galact- Combining forms meaning milk.

galactoblast (gă-lak'to-blast) See colostral corpuscle, under corpuscle.

galactocele (gă-lak'to-sēl) See milk-retention cyst, under cyst.

galactophore (gă-lak'to-for) A milk duct.

galactophorous (gal-ak-tof'o-rus) Conveying milk.

galactophygous (gal-ak-tof'ĭ-gus) Arresting the flow of milk.

galactopoiesis (gă-lak-to-poi-e'sis) Secretion of milk.

galactopoietic (gă-lak-to-poi-et'ik) Relating to milk secretion.

galactorrhea (gă-lak-to-re'ă) 1. Profuse discharge of milk from the breasts after the child has been weaned. 2. A milky discharge from the breasts due to a pathologic condition unrelated to pregnancy.

galactosis (gal-ak-to'sis) The formation of milk.

gamete (gam'et) In embryology, either of the two reproductive cells (ovum or spermatozoon); it contains only one member of each chromosome pair (haploid chromosome number) and combines with the other reproductive cell to form a zygote, from which a new organism develops.

gameto- Combining form meaning gamete.

gametocide (gă-me'to-sīd) Any agent destructive to gametes.

gametocyte (gă-me'to-sīt) A cell (either spermatocyte or oocyte) from which gametes are produced by cell division.

gametogenesis (gam-e-to-jen'ĕ-sis) The production of gametes (ova or spermatozoa).

gamma-aminobutyric acid (gam'ă a-me-no-bu-ter'ik as'id) (GABA, g-Abu) An amino acid neurotransmitter present in brain tissue, especially in the basal ganglia, which inhibits nerve impulses.

ganciclovir (gan-si'klo-vir) Antiviral agent used in the treatment of cytomegalovirus (CMV) infections.

ganglion (gang'gle-on), pl. ganglia, ganglions A collection of nerve cell bodies located outside the brain and spinal cord.

    autonomic g. Any ganglion of the sympathetic and parasympathetic nervous systems.

Gardnerella vaginalis (gard-ner-el'ă vaj-ĭ-na'lis) A nonmotile, Gram-negative bacterium (genus *Gardnerella*) that is a major cause of vaginitis, transmitted by sexual contact; may occasionally cause bacteremia in women after childbirth; has been isolated also from the genital tract of healthy women.

gas (gas) 1. An airlike state of matter with freely moving molecules, capable of expanding and contracting with changes in temperature and pressure. 2. Popular name for inhalation anesthesia.

    alveolar g. The gas in the air sacs (alveoli) of the lungs.

    blood g.'s Term used to express the determination of partial pressures of oxygen and carbon dioxide in the blood.

gastro-, gastr- Combining forms meaning stomach.

gastroschisis (gas-tros'kĭ-sis) In newborn infants, a full-thickness defect of the abdominal wall located just to the right of the intact umbilical cord; consists of an opening 2 to 4 cm in diameter through which protrudes an exposed loop of intestine (without a protective covering sac).

gastrula (gas'troo-lă) An early embryo at about the third week of gestation, following the blastula; consists of a trilaminar disk composed of ectoderm, mesoderm, and endoderm.

gastrulation (gas-troo-la'shun) In embryology, the formation of a gastrula; the stage of development when the three germ layers (ectoderm, mesoderm, endoderm) begin to form.

gemellology (jem-ĕl-ol'ŏ-je) The study of twins and twinning.

geminate (jem'ĭ-nāt) Occurring in pairs.

-gen Combining form meaning something that produces; something produced (e.g., pathogen;

chromogen).

gender (jen'der) (g) Sex category.

gene (jēn) The hereditary unit occupying a fixed position (locus) in the chromosome, capable of reproducing itself at each cell division and of directing the formation of proteins. In molecular terms, it is a segment of the DNA molecule containing the code for a specific function.

    fibrillin g. A gene located on chromosome 15q. Abnormality of this gene is associated with Marfan syndrome.

    holandric g. A gene occurring only in the male of the species, located on the nonhomologous portion of a Y (male) chromosome. Also called Y-linked gene.

    PIG-A g. Phosphatidylinositol glycan class A gene; a gene located on the X chromosome, responsible for paroxysmal nocturnal hemoglobinuria.

    retinoblastoma g., RB g. A recessive mutation of a tumor-suppressor gene that leads to tumor formation.

    sex-linked g. A gene located on a sex (X or Y) chromosome.

    tumor-supressor g. A normal gene involved in the regulation of cell growth and in the inactivation or deletion of tumor cells.

    X-linked g. A gene carried on an X (female) chromosome.

    Y-linked g. See holandric gene.

generative (jen'er-ă-tiv) Relating to reproduction.

genetic (jĕ-net'ik) **1.** Relating to the study of heredity. **2.** Determined by genes (distinguished from congenital).

genetics (je-net'iks) The science of heredity; the study of the way in which particular qualities or traits are transmitted from parents to offspring.

    medical g. The study of the causes, symptoms, treatment, and prevention of genetic disorders.

    reverse g. Indirect investigation of a genetic disorder by identifying the location of the responsible gene on a given chromosome, then cloning and translating its DNA, and comparing the gene's protein product with the product of the normal allele.

-genic Combining form meaning producing; formed by (e.g., oncogenic).

genic (jen'ik) Relating to genes.

genital (jen'ĭ-tal) **1.** Relating to the genitals. **2.** Relating to reproduction.

genitalia (jen-ĭ-ta'le-ă) The genitals.

genitals (jen'ĭ-tals) The organs of reproduction, male and female.

genitourinary (jen-ĭ-to-u'rĭ-nar-e) (GU) Relating to the organs of reproduction and the urinary

tract. Also called urogenital.

genodermatosis (jen-o-der-mă-to'sis) A genetically determined condition of the skin.

genome (je'nōm) The total genetic information packed in a chromosome.

genotype (jen'o-tīp) The full set of genes carried by an individual, including those that are not obviously expressed.

genotypical (jen-o-tĭ'pik-al) Relating to a genotype.

gentamicin (jen-tă-mi'sin) An aminoglycoside antibiotic useful in the treatment of serious Gram-negative bacillary infections; serious side-effects include kidney damage and irreversible damage to the eighth cranial nerve.

germ (jerm) **1.** A disease-causing microorganism; a pathogen. **2.** An embryonic structure; a primordium.

gestagen (jes'tă-jen) A class of steroids having progestational activity (i.e., they are conducive to pregnancy).

gestagenic (jes-tă-jen'ik) Inducing prostagenic changes in the uterus.

gestation (jes-ta'shun) Development of the young in the uterus from the time of fertilization of the ovum to birth. See also pregnancy.

    multifetal g. Intrauterine development of more than one fetus.

girdle (ger'dl) An encircling band, structure, region, or zone.

    pelvic g. The bony ring formed by the sacrum and two hipbones. See also pelvis; sacrum; hipbone.

glabella (glă-bel'ă) The most prominent point between the eyebrows; a craniometric point.

gland (gland) An organized aggregation of epithelial cells that elaborate secretions or excretions.

    adrenal g.'s A pair of flattened endocrine glands positioned at the upper pole of each kidney; the shape of the right adrenal gland is somewhat triangular, while the left one is crescent-shaped; their cortex produces steroid hormones (aldosterone, androgens, glucocorticoids, progestins, and estrogens); their medulla produces epinephrine and norepinephrine. Also called suprarenal glands.

    areolar g.'s A group of small sebaceous glands in the skin of the areola appearing as small nodules, which provide lubrication for the nipple; they enlarge markedly during the third trimester of pregnancy. Also called Montgomery glands; Montgomery follicles.

    Bartholin's g.'s See greater vestibular glands.

    greater vestibular g.'s Two small glands

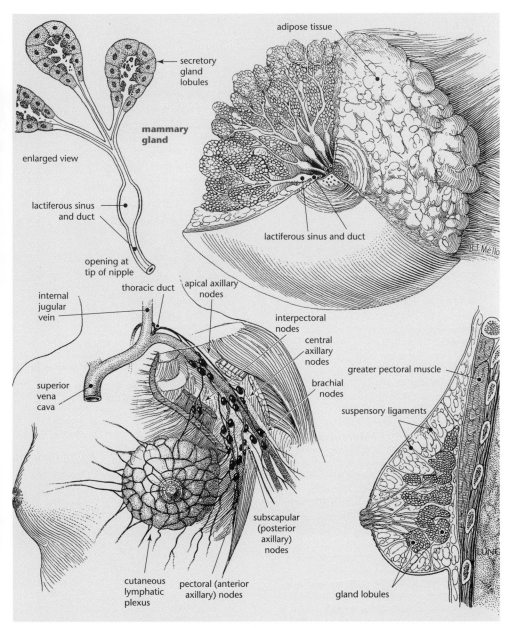

secretory gland lobules

adipose tissue

mammary gland

enlarged view

lactiferous sinus and duct

lactiferous sinus and duct

opening at tip of nipple

internal jugular vein

thoracic duct

apical axillary nodes

interpectoral nodes

central axillary nodes

greater pectoral muscle

brachial nodes

suspensory ligaments

superior vena cava

subscapular (posterior axillary) nodes

cutaneous lymphatic plexus

pectoral (anterior axillary) nodes

gland lobules

LUNG

B.J. Mello

(about 0.5–1 cm in diameter) located on either side of the vaginal orifice (introitus), under the constrictor muscle of the vagina; each has a duct opening between the hymen and the labia minus; their major function is the production of a mucoid material for lubrication of the introitus. Also called Bartholin's glands; vulvovaginal glands.

lactiferous g. See mammary gland.

lesser vestibular g.'s The minute glands within the mucous membrane of the vestibule; their openings are located between the urethral and vaginal orifices.

mammary g. Either of two compound milk-producing glands that form the major part of the female breast during the childbearing age; the adult gland consists of 15 to 20 lobes, each composed of many lobules; each lobe has a separate lactiferous duct opening at the apex of the nipple; the mammary gland reaches functional maturity after childbirth. Also called lactiferous gland; milk gland. See also breast.

milk g. See mammary gland.

Montgomery g.'s See areolar glands.

pituitary g. See hypophysis.

sebaceous g. A simple branched holocrine gland in the dermis of the skin that usually opens into the distal part of the hair follicle and secretes an oily substance (sebum).

Skene's g.'s See urethral glands of female urethra.

suprarenal g.'s See adrenal glands.

urethral g.'s of female urethra Numerous small glands in the mucous membrane of the urethra; some empty directly onto the urethral surface, others are grouped along the side and drain through a common duct.

uterine g.'s The numerous tubular glands extending through the whole thickness of the endometrium and opening into the cavity of the uterus; they secrete a fluid that keeps the interior of the uterus moist.

vulvovaginal g.'s See greater vestibular glands.

glans (glanz), pl. glandes A small glandlike structure.

g. clitoridis, g. of clitoris The small rounded tip of the body of the clitoris.

globulin (glob'u-lin) Any of a category of simple proteins that are insoluble in water, soluble in saline solutions, and coagulable by heat; found in blood and cerebrospinal fluid; human serum globulin is divided into alpha, beta, and gamma fractions on the basis of electrophoretic mobility.

gamma g.'s, γ-g.'s Serum proteins that constitute the majority of immunoglobulins and antibodies; used in the prevention of numerous diseases, including measles and certain types of hepatitis.

hepatitis B immune g. Immune globulin derived from donors carrying antibodies against B surface antigen (HBsAg); used as a postexposure preventive measure and given to infants born to mothers with hepatitis B.

immune serum g. A sterile preparation containing a number of antibodies that are normally present in adult human blood; used as an immunizing agent.

Rh₀ immune g., D immune g. A preparation of antibody specific against the Rh₀ antigen (D antigen); administered to an Rh-negative woman within 72 hours after delivery of her first Rh-positive child, or following an abortion, to prevent the deleterious effects of Rh sensitization. See also Rh isoimmunization,

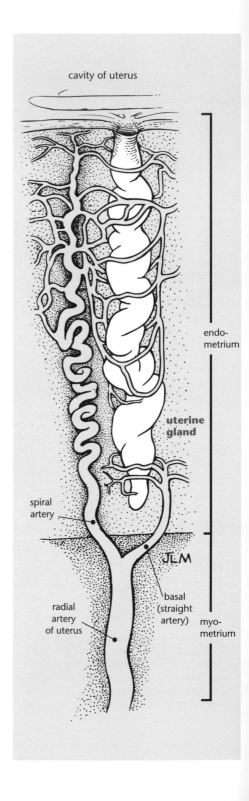

cavity of uterus

endo-
metrium

uterine
gland

spiral
artery

radial
artery
of uterus

basal
(straight
artery)

myo-
metrium

JLM

under isoimmunization.

thyroxine-binding g. (TBG) An alpha globulin with a strong affinity for the hormone thyroxine; it acts as a carrier of thyroxine in the blood; significant changes in the levels of TBG may alter measured thyroxine levels.

glomeruloendotheliosis (glo-mer-u-lo-en-do-the-le-o'sis) A lesion characteristic of pre-eclampsia, consisting of a swelling of the glomerular capillary endothelium that causes decreased glomerular perfusion and glomerular filtration rate. Also called glomerular capillary endotheliosis.

glomerulonephritis (glo-mer-u-lo-ně-fri'tis) (GN) Kidney disease characterized by changes in the structure of the filtering units (glomeruli) within the kidney; basically, it may be acute, subacute, or chronic. Pregnant women affected by the disease experience complications, sometimes severe, depending on the degree of kidney function impairment.

glucocorticoid (gloo-ko-kor'tǐ-koid) Any of a class of steroid hormones produced by the adrenal cortex (or synthetically) that regulate carbohydrate, protein, and lipid metabolism; other properties include anti-inflammatory activity and ability to suppress the synthesis of ACTH (adrenocorticotropic hormone) and MSH (melanocyte-stimulating hormone).

glycoprotein (gli-ko-pro'tēn) Any of several protein–carbohydrate compounds (conjugated proteins); they include the mucins, the mucoids, and the chondroproteins.

pregnancy-specific beta 1-g. A glycoprotein present in the plasma of a pregnant woman; it is produced by the trophoblast of the placenta and passed into the maternal bloodstream; can be detected 18 days after ovulation.

gonad (go'nad) A sexual gland.

female g. An ovary.

indifferent g. The embryonic gonad at a stage before it differentiates into an ovary or a testis.

male g. A testis.

streak g. A cord usually found in the broad ligament, parallel to a fallopian (uterine) tube; composed of connective tissue stroma and undeveloped gonadal structures but lacking germ cells; frequently occurs in individuals afflicted with Turner's syndrome.

gonadal (go-nad'al) Relating to the ovaries or the testes.

gonadectomy (go-nă-dek'tǒ-me) Removal of an ovary or a testis.

gonado-, gonad- Combining forms relating to the ovaries or testes.

gonadoblastoma (gon-ă-do-blas-to'mă) An uncommon benign tumor of the ovary, often bilateral, composed of germ-cell and gonadal stroma derivatives; may give rise to malignant growths.

gonadopathy (gon-ă-dop'ă-the) Any disease of a gonad.

gonadogenesis (gon-ă-do-jen'ě-sis) The development of the embryonic gonads.

gonadoinhibitory (gon-ă-do-in-hib'ǐ-to-re)

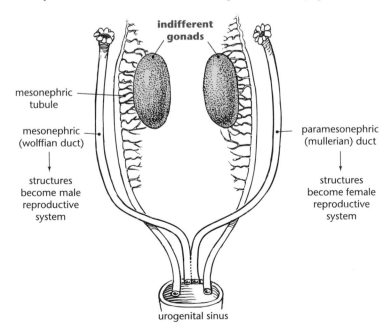

indifferent gonads

mesonephric tubule

mesonephric (wolffian duct)

↓

structures become male reproductive system

paramesonephric (mullerian) duct

↓

structures become female reproductive system

urogenital sinus

Preventing or reducing the physiologic activity of the gonads.

gonadokinetic (gon-ă-do-kĭ-net'ik) Stimulating the physiologic activity of the gonads.

gonadopause (go-nad'o-paws) The normal loss of gonadal activity resulting from the aging process.

gonadotrophic (gon-ă-do-trof'ik) See gonadotropic.

gonadotropic (gon-ă-do-trop'ik) Influencing the gonads (e.g., hormones produced by the adenohypophysis, which stimulate the ovaries or testes). Also called gonadotrophic.

gonadotropin (gon-ă-do-tro'pin) Any hormone that stimulates the ovaries or testes.

   chorionic g. (CG) See human chorionic gonadotropin.

   human chorionic g. (hCG) A protein hormone produced by trophoblastic cells that enter into formation of the early placenta (i.e., the syncytiotrophoblast); its secretion begins soon after implantation of the fertilized ovum, with concentration peaking at 60 to 95 days; also produced by abnormal chorionic epithelial tissue such as hydatidiform moles, chorioadenoma destruens, and choriocarcinoma; used in diagnostic tests.

   human menopausal g. (hMG) An extract of gonadotropins obtained from the urine of postmenopausal women that stimulates growth and maturation of ovarian follicles; used to induce ovulation in the treatment of female infertility.

gonococcal (gon-o-kok'al) Relating to gonococci.

gonococcemia (gon-o-kok-se'me-ă) The presence of gonococci in the blood.

gonococcic (gon-o-kok'sik) Gonococcal.

gonococcus (gon-o-kok'us), pl. gonococci The bacterium that causes gonorrhea, a member of the genus *Neisseria gonorrhoeae.*

gonocyte (gon'o-sīt) A primitive reproductive cell.

gonorrhea (gon-o-re'ă) A common contagious disease caused by *Neisseria gonorrhoeae,* transmitted chiefly by sexual intercourse; incubation period 2 to 5 days; characterized by inflammation of the mucous membrane of the genital tract, purulent discharge and painful, frequent urination; if untreated may lead to complications such as epididymitis, prostatitis, tenosynovitis, arthritis, and endocarditis; in females it may lead to sterility, and in males to urethral stricture.

   pharyngeal g. See gonococcal pharyngitis, under pharyngitis.

   rectal g. Gonorrhea of the rectum; may be asymptomatic or cause a purulent discharge,

swelling, and pain.

gonorrheal (gon-o-re'al) Relating to gonorrhea.

gossypol (gos'ĭ-pol) A cottonseed oil derivative at one time considered a potential male contraceptive; however, its clinical usefulness is precluded by a high incidence of unacceptable side-effects.

grading (grād'ing) A histologic method of providing an estimate of the gravity of a cancerous tumor, based on the degree of cell differentiation and the number of cell divisions within the tumor.

graft (graft) **1.** Any tissue transplanted into a body. **2.** To insert such a tissue.

granulation (gran-u-la'shun) **1.** The formation of small red, moist masses on the surface of an ulcer or wound during the healing process. **2.** The masses so formed. **3.** A mass of numerous tiny blood vessels.

granuloma (gran-u-lo'mă) A tumor composed chiefly of granulation tissue; characteristic of certain diseases that may be caused either by infectious microorganisms (e.g., tuberculosis), mineral dust (e.g., silicosis), or due to unknown causes (e.g., sarcoidosis).

   g. gravidarum A suppurating granuloma of the gums (gingiva) occurring during pregnancy; thought to be due to hormonal activity.

   g. inguinale A sexually transmitted chronic infection of the skin and subcutaneous tissues,

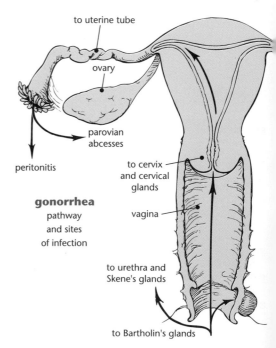

to uterine tube

ovary

parovian abcesses

peritonitis

to cervix and cervical glands

gonorrhea
pathway
and sites
of infection

vagina

to urethra and Skene's glands

to Bartholin's glands

characterized by ulcerations in the groin, perineum, and the genitals; caused by infection with the bacterium *Calymmatobacterium granulomatis*; incubation period 2 to 3 months; may cause lymphatic obstruction and elephantiasis.

graph (graf) Any pictorial device depicting a relationship of values.

   Liley g. A pictorial means of assessing the degree of fetal jeopardy secondary to the hemolysis of isoimmunization. It correlates the intensity of amniotic fluid optical density at 450 mμ from 28 to 40 weeks of gestation with the risk of fetal morbidity.

gram (gram) (g) Metric unit of mass or weight equal to 0.001 kilogram.

gravid (grav'id) Pregnant.

gravida (grav'ĭ-dă) A pregnant woman. A Roman numeral designates the number of pregnancies (e.g., gravida I is a woman in her first pregnancy, gravida II in her second, etc.).

gravidity (gră-vid'ĭ-te) The total number of pregnancies including abortions, ectopic pregnancies, hydatidiform moles, and normal intrauterine pregnancies.

gray (gra) (Gy) The unit of absorbed dose of ionizing radiation in the International System of Units (SI); 1 Gy = 100 rad; equivalent to 1 joule per kilogram of tissue.

groove (grōōv) A narrow, elongated depression; a sulcus, a furrow, a niche.

   medullary g. See neural groove.

   neural g. The transitory groove on the dorsal surface of the young embryo produced by the thickened ectoderm (neural plate), as it begins to close to form a tubular structure (neural tube). Also called medullary groove.

   primitive g. In embryology, the median furrow extending lengthwise in the primitive streak of the embryo.

growth (grōth) **1.** A progressive development or increase in size of an organism. **2.** A tumor.

gumma (gum'ă), pl. gummas, gummata A soft, gummy, infectious tumor usually seen in the third stage of syphilis.

gummatous (gum'ătus) Relating to a gumma.

gut (gut) The intestine.

   primary g. See archenteron.

   surgical g. See catgut.

gyn-, gyneco-, gyno- Combining forms meaning woman.

gynandroid (jĭ-nan'droid) A female pseudohermaphrodite.

gynandromorphous (jĭ-nan-dro-mor'fus) Having both male and female characteristics.

gynatresia (jin-ă-tre'ze-ă) Occlusion of a portion of the female genital tract.

gynecic (jĭ-nes'ik) Relating to women.

gynecoid (jin'ĕ-koid) Resembling a female.

gynecologic (gi-nĕ-kŏ-loj'ik) Relating to gynecology.

gynecologist (gi-nĕ-kol'ŏ-jist) A specialist in gynecology.

gynecology (gi-nĕ-kol'ŏ-je) (GYN) The medical-surgical specialty concerned with disorders of the female endocrinology and reproductive physiology; for the most part it is not concerned with the pregnant state.

gynecomania (jin-ĕ-ko-ma'ne-ă) Insatiable sexual desire for women.

gynecomastia (jin-ĕ-ko-mas'te-ă) Abnormal overdevelopment of the mammary glands in the male.

gynecophobia (jin-ĕ-ko-fo'be-ă) Abnormal fear of or aversion to women.

gynecoplasty (jin-ĕ-ko-plas'te) Reparative surgery of the female genitals.

gynopathy (jin-op'ă-the) Any disease of the female organs.

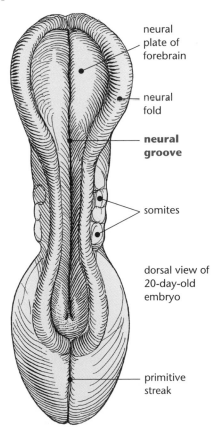

neural plate of forebrain

neural fold

neural groove

somites

dorsal view of 20-day-old embryo

primitive streak

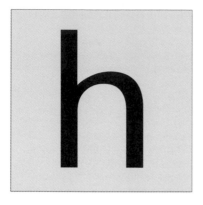

habitus (hab'ĭ-tus) **1.** Physical and constitutional characteristics of a person, especially in relation to susceptibility to disease. **2.** Position of the body; posture.

    fetal h. See fetal attitude, under attitude.

Haemophilus (he-mof'ĭ-lus) A genus of Gram-negative bacteria that require blood components for growth; some cause disease in humans. Also spelled *Hemophilus.*

    H. ducreyi A species that causes chancroid (soft chancre) on the genitals of humans. Also called Ducrey's bacillus.

hair (hār) One of the long threadlike skin appendages covering almost the entire surface of the human body; consists of a root implanted in the skin within a flasklike pit (follicle) and a portion projecting from the surface (shaft); during pregnancy, hair growth accelerates until the time of delivery; then, about 4 weeks after, there is an increase in the hair loss rate, becoming normal again about 2 to 6 months later. See also hirsutism.

    primary h. See lanugo.

    pubic h.'s Thick terminal hairs of the pubic region; their development and growth are under hormonal control.

    secondary h. See vellus.

    terminal h. Coarse hair that replaces secondary hair (vellus) in various areas of the body during adult years, including eyebrow, axillary, scalp, and pubic hairs, as well as those hairs in the nose and ears and on the face and chest in the male.

    vellus h. See vellus.

Hantavirus (han-tă-vi'rus) A genus of RNA viruses of the family Bunyaviridae that cause hemorrhagic fever and pneumonia.

haploid (hap'loid) The chromosome number contained in a normal sex cell (sperm or egg cell); it is half the usual number of chromosomes, that is, with only one member of each

chromosome pair contained in the rest of the body cells. In humans, the haploid number is 23.

head (hed) **1.** The upper or anterior end of the body. **2.** The end of a bone or organ (e.g., pancreas) that is nearest the vertebral column; the proximal end.

    trapped h. An aftercoming head in a breech delivery that is unable to pass through an incompletely dilated cervix.

headache (hed'āk) Pain in the head. Also called cephalalgia.

    lumbar puncture h. Headache on the frontal and occipital areas, exacerbated in the sitting and standing positions and diminished when lying down; it usually begins 1 or 2 days after performance of a lumbar puncture and lasts 3 to 4 days; thought to be caused by leakage of cerebrospinal fluid through the puncture site to extradural areas. Also called spinal headache, postpuncture headache.

    postpartum h. Headache experienced any time during the first 6 weeks after delivery; may be due to a variety of causes.

    postpuncture h. See lumbar puncture headache.

    spinal h. See lumbar puncture headache.

healing (hēl'ing) The process of restoring to health.

    h. by first intention A relatively rapid healing of wounds when the edges are in close apposition and there is no suppuration. New connective tissue may form an almost imperceptible, temporary scar. Also called primary adhesion.

    h. by second intention A delayed process occurring when the edges of a wound are not in close approximation; granulation tissue develops to unite the wound edges, after some suppuration has occurred, generally leaving a visible scar. Also called secondary adhesion.

    h. by third intention The slow process of filling the gap of a wound or ulcer with granulations, which leaves a scar of tough fibrous tissue.

heartburn (hart'bern) A burning sensation felt in the lower chest, which may extend from the tip of the breastbone to the throat, caused by irritation of the esophagus; occurs when stomach acid flows back into the esophagus, usually due to a relaxed condition of the lower esophageal sphincter muscle. It frequently occurs in late pregnancy, possibly facilitated by the upward displacement of the stomach by the uterus. Also called pyrosis.

height (hīt) A vertical measurement.

    fundal h. A measurement of the pregnant

uterus, obtained with a centimeter measuring tape, from the pubic symphysis to the top of the uterine mass over the curve of the abdominal surface.

Helicobacter (hel-ĭ-ko-bak'ter) Genus of motile, spiral, Gram-negative bacteria found in the intestinal tract and reproductive organs of animals and the intestinal tract of humans. Some species cause disease, which may be exacerbated by pregnancy in some patients.

H. pylori A species causing active chronic inflammation of the stomach (type B gastritis); found in more than 90% of patients with duodenal ulcers and believed to play a central role in development of this condition. The organism has been implicated as a cause of stomach cancer. Formerly called *Campylobacter pyloris*.

helix (he'liks) 1. The folded skin-covered cartilage forming the margin of the outer ear (auricle). 2. A coiled structure.

DNA h. See double helix.

double h. The spiral structure formed by two strands of DNA (ribonucleic acid) held together by hydrogen bonds between pairs of bases projecting from each strand. Also called DNA helix; twin helix; Watson-Crick helix.

twin h. See double helix.

Watson–Crick h. See double helix.

hemagogue, hemagog (hem'ă-gog) Any agent that stimulates blood flow, particularly during menstruation.

hemangioma (he-man-je-o'mă) A benign lesion formed of blood vessels, usually present at birth and occurring in the skin, mucous membranes, or some organs (e.g., brain and liver); composed of small superficial capillaries or deeper thin-walled channels, or both.

port-wine h. See nevus flammeus, under nevus.

strawberry h. A well-demarcated capillary hemangioma present at birth and growing rapidly into a red, rough, elevated lesion; it usually peaks in 1 to 3 years and gradually disappears without treatment by age 5 to 7. Also called nevus vasculosus; nevus vascularis.

hemangiosarcoma (he-man-je-o-sar-ko'mă) See angiosarcoma.

hematocrit (he-mat'o-krit) (HCT) 1. The volume percentage of packed red blood cells in a whole blood sample. 2. A small centrifuge for separating the cellular constituents of blood from the plasma.

hematoma (he-mă-to'mă) A mass of blood accumulated outside a blood vessel, often found in a partly clotted state, usually developed after

injury to the vessel and without laceration of superficial tissues.

broad ligament h. Hematoma developed between the folds of the broad ligament; it sometimes ruptures, causing shock; may be formed after an ectopic intraligamentous pregnancy ends in fetal death; may also be formed from a slow leakage of blood from an incomplete rupture of the uterus.

hepatic h. Hematoma occurring as a result of liver damage caused by severe pre-eclampsia and eclampsia; most commonly develops along the upper right side of the liver just within its capsule or, less frequently, within the liver substance; causes upper abdominal pain and tenderness.

intramural h. Hematoma developed within the wall of a structure (e.g., of the vagina, bowel, and bladder).

paravaginal h. Hematoma developed within the tissues surrounding the vagina, forming a fluctuant mass and frequently causing fever and unexplained anemia; may develop during childbirth but remain undetected until the 6-week postpartum examination is performed. Paravaginal hematomas may also develop in victims of sexual abuse.

pelvic h. Any hematoma formed in or around structures of the pelvis; classified as vulvar, paravaginal, broad ligament, and retroperitoneal hematomas according to their location, which is determined by the fascial planes forming boundaries around the bleeding vessel.

puerperal h., postpartum h. Any type of pelvic hematoma occurring after vaginal delivery (immediately after or within 6 weeks following delivery) and after either spontaneous or operative delivery.

retroperitoneal space h. Hematoma behind the peritoneum, caused by blood leakage from a hematoma at the base of the broad ligament; occasionally may extend up to the level of the kidneys, or even the lower margin of the diaphragm.

retroplacental h. Accumulation of blood between the placenta and the uterine wall occurring normally during the third stage of labor (i.e., expulsion of the placenta); as the central portion of the placenta begins to separate from the uterine wall, blood accumulates in the space thus created; the weight of the hematoma is thought to help the process of placental extrusion. See also abruptio placentae.

umbilical cord h. Hematoma formed in the

umbilical cord, usually caused by rupture of a varicose umbilical vein; may also develop after umbilical vessel venipuncture directed by ultrasound to obtain a fetal blood sample.

vulvar h. A painful fluctuant hematoma just beneath the skin of the vulva with discoloration of the overlying skin; caused by rupture of blood vessels below the levator ani muscles; sometimes seen as a consequence of sexual assault; the increased vascularity associated with pregnancy predisposes to its formation from accidental trauma, or its development during natural or operative vaginal delivery.

wound h. Collection of blood and blood clots in a surgical wound due to imperfect hemostasis; episiotomy incisions are common sites and vigorous coughing immediately after delivery is a frequent contributing factor.

hematopoiesis (he-mă-to-poi-e'sis) The process by which blood components are formed.

hematosalpinx (he-mă-to-sal'pinx) Distention of a fallopian (uterine) tube with accumulated blood. Also called hemosalpinx.

hemi- Combining form meaning one-half.

hemiplegia (hem-ĕ-ple'je-ă) Paralysis of one side of the body.

hemivertebra (hem-ĕ-ver'te-bră) Developmental defect in which one side of a vertebra fails to develop.

hemo-, hem- Combining forms meaning blood.

hemodilution (he-mo-di-lu'shun) Increased plasma content of the blood with consequent decreased concentration of red blood cells and hemoglobin.

hemoglobin (he-mo-glo-bin) The oxygen-carrying pigment of red blood cells.

glycosylated h. A minor component of hemoglobin A (sometimes designated hemoglobin A_{1c}); useful in the management of diabetes mellitus because it reflects plasma glucose levels over the preceding 6- to 12-week period.

hemoglobinuria (he-mo-glo-bĭ-nu're-ă) The presence of free hemoglobin in the urine, an indication of recent injury or destruction of red blood cells of at least moderate severity.

paroxysmal nocturnal h. (PNH) An uncommon disease of circulating red blood cells characterized by increased sensitivity of the cell membranes to complement, with resulting destruction of the cells.

hemophilia (he-mo-fil'e-ă) An inherited disorder caused by deficiency of a specific blood-clotting factor; occurs in two main forms, hemophilia A and hemophilia B.

h. A The most common form of hemophilia, transmitted as an X-linked recessive inheritance; characterized by prolonged clotting time, easy bruising, and bleeding into joints and muscles; caused by a reduced amount or activity of factor VIII, a component of the blood-clotting process. The defective gene is transmitted by female carriers who (except in rare occasions) are asymptomatic. Also called classic hemophilia.

h. B A form of hemophilia, caused by deficiency of factor IX, that has clinical and laboratory features similar to those of hemophilia A; transmitted as an X-linked recessive inheritance. Also called Christmas disease (after a man named Christmas, the first patient in whom the disease was shown to be distinct from hemophilia A).

classic h. See hemophilia A.

Hemophilus (he-mof'ĭ-lus) See *Haemophilus*.

hemorrhage (hem'ŏ-rij) Bleeding, especially profuse.

antepartum h. Excessive bleeding occurring at the onset of labor, as seen in premature separation of a placenta previa.

accidental h. See abruptio placentae.

dysfunctional uterine h. Abnormal bleeding from the uterus in the absence of organic disease or lesion.

fetomaternal h. The leakage of red blood cells from the fetal to the maternal circulation.

intraventricular h. Extravasation of blood into the ventricles of the brain, usually occurring in preterm infants within 72 hours of birth.

postpartum h. Excessive bleeding (in excess of 500 ml) following vaginal delivery; designated *early* when it occurs within 24 hours after delivery, and *late* when it occurs between 24 hours and 6 weeks after delivery.

subgaleal h. Hemorrhage under the scalp of a newborn infant caused by trauma to the head as it is forced against the uterine cervix during birth.

third-trimester h. Hemorrhage occurring during late pregnancy; may be due to non-obstetric conditions (including invasive carcinoma of the cervix), or to obstetric causes (e.g., premature separation of the placenta, placenta previa, or extrusion of the cervical plug).

hemorrhagenic (hem-o-ră-jen'ik) Causing hemorrhage.

hemorrhoids (hem'ŏ-roids) A varicose distention of superficial veins at or within the anus; may become strangulated, ulcerated, or fissured;

generally associated with recurrent constipation, pregnancy (due to pressure against the veins) or, occasionally, portal hypertension.

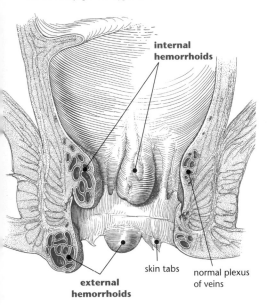

internal hemorrhoids

skin tabs normal plexus of veins

external hemorrhoids

hemosalpinx (he-mo-sal'pinks) See hematosalpinx.

hemostasis (he-mo-sta'sis) The arrest of bleeding.

hepatitis (hep-ă-ti'tis) Inflammation of the liver.

h. A Hepatitis caused by the hepatitis A virus (HAV), an RNA virus transmitted through fecal contamination of food and water (fecal–oral route); it has a 15- to 45-day incubation period; may occur sporadically or in epidemics; it does not produce a chronic disease or a carrier state; in pregnancy, the infection increases only slightly the risk of a preterm delivery; the infection is not usually transmitted to the offspring. Formerly called infectious hepatitis.

h. B Hepatitis caused by the hepatitis B virus (HBV), a bloodborne DNA virus transmitted via transfusion of infected blood or blood products, through the use of contaminated needles (by intravenous drug abusers), by needle-prick accidents (in health care personnel), via the sexual route (through saliva, vaginal secretions, and semen), or from mother to newborn or older infant (by ingestion of infected material during delivery or through breast-feeding); infection during pregnancy increases the risk of preterm delivery; incubation period is 4 to 26 weeks (typically 6–8 weeks); it produces an

asymptomatic carrier state and plays a significant role in development of cancer of the liver (hepatocellular carcinoma). Formerly called serum hepatitis.

h. C Hepatitis caused by the hepatitis C virus (HCV), a bloodborne RNA virus transmitted via transfusion of infected blood or blood products, the use of contaminated needles, needle-prick accidents, the sexual route, and from mother to newborn (predominantly with HIV coinfection); often causes chronic hepatitis, possibly with highest incidence in newborns, leading to cirrhosis; incubation period is 8 to 12 weeks. Formerly called transfusion-associated non-A, non-B hepatitis.

h. D Hepatitis caused by the hepatitis D virus (HDV), an RNA virus developed only in the presence of hepatitis B virus (HBV); may occur when transfused blood contains both viruses (coinfection), or as an additional infection of a chronic HBV carrier (superinfection); it has reportedly been transmitted from mother to newborn; incubation period is 30 to 120 days (typically 60 days). Also called delta hepatitis, delta agent hepatitis.

delta h., delta agent h. See hepatitis D.

h. E Self-limited hepatitis (with a high mortality rate in pregnant women) caused by the hepatitis E virus (HEV), an RNA virus transmitted through fecally contaminated food and water (fecal–oral route); may occur in waterborne epidemics; incubation period is 14 to 60 days (typically 40 days); it does not produce a chronic state. Formerly called non-A, non-B hepatitis.

infectious h. See hepatitis A.

neonatal h. General term for a variety of disorders of newborn infants, involving injury to liver cells and tissues and causing hyperbilirubinemia and jaundice; cause is unknown; may be associated with hepatitis B.

non-A, non-B (NANB) h. See hepatitis C and E.

serum h. (SH) See hepatitis B.

transfusion-associated non-A, non-B h. See hepatitis C.

viral h. Hepatitis caused by a virus; unless otherwise specified, the term refers to infection of the liver by a small group of viruses (A, B, C, D, and E viruses) that have an affinity for the liver and produce similar patterns of clinical and morphologic acute hepatitis, but vary in their potential to induce chronic or fulminant hepatitis or the carrier state of the disease.

heparin (hep′ă-rin) An anticoagulant compound used in the prevention and treatment of abnormal blood clot formation (thrombosis); administered subcutaneously to high risk patients before and after surgery (e.g., those with an abnormally high tendency to form clots).

hepato-, hepat- Combining forms meaning liver.

hepatoma (hep-ă-to′mă) Malignant tumor of the liver originating in the parenchymal cells; commonly arises in the presence of chronic hepatitis often associated with an increase in the blood level of alpha-fetoprotein. Also called hepatocellular carcinoma.

hermaphrodite (her-maf′ro-dīt) An individual possessing the characteristics of hermaphroditism.

> **true h.** An individual who has both ovarian and testicular tissues, either combined in one gonad (ovotestes) or with a different gonad on each side. See also pseudohermaphrodite.
>
> **female h.** See pseudohermaphrodite.
>
> **male h.** See pseudohermaphrodite.

hermaphroditism (her-maf′ro-dī-tizm) The presence of both ovarian and testicular tissues in one individual. Also called intersexuality. See also pseudohermaphroditism.

hernia (her′ne-ă) Protrusion of part of an organ through an abnormal opening in its surrounding tissues.

> **congenital diaphragmatic h.** Protrusion of abdominal organs into the chest cavity through a developmental defect in the diaphragm (usually a large posterolateral opening or through an enlarged foramen of Morgagni). Also called diaphragmatic hernia.
>
> **cul-de-sac h.** See enterocele.
>
> **diaphragmatic h.** See congenital diaphragmatic hernia.
>
> **Douglas pouch h.** See enterocele.
>
> **femoral h.** Protrusion of a sac-enclosed loop of intestine through the femoral ring and into the femoral canal. The hernia may be one of two types: *incomplete femoral h.*, if it remains in

the canal as far as the saphenous opening; or *complete femoral h.*, if it passes through the opening and into the loose tissues of the groin; seen most frequently in women, especially those who have borne several children.

> **incisional h.** Hernia through a surgical incision, occurring almost exclusively in the abdominal wall; factors most commonly responsible include poor suturing technique, type of incision made, postoperative wound infection, placement of drains in the primary incision, postoperative pulmonary complications that produce forceful coughing, obesity, advanced age, and general debility of the patient.
>
> **posterior vaginal h.** See enterocele.
>
> **rectovaginal h.** See rectocele.
>
> **saddle h.** An uncommon hernia formed by an extremely large herniation of the rectouterine pouch that extends anteriorly through the vaginal opening and posteriorly through the anal canal. Also called saddle enterocele.
>
> **umbilical h.** Hernia in which part of the intestine protrudes through the umbilical ring; it usually results from a fascial and muscular defect with failure of the umbilical ring to close.

heroin (her′o-in) A highly addictive narcotic compound prepared from morphine by acetylation. Prolonged high-dose use of heroin during pregnancy may have deleterious effects on the fetus or newborn infant (e.g., fetal growth retardation, respiratory distress syndrome, jaundice, low Apgar scores, withdrawal symptoms, and increased perinatal death). Also called diacetylmorphine.

herpes (her′pēz) Inflammatory eruption of a cluster of deep-seated vesicles caused by a herpesvirus.

> **genital h., h. genitalis** Sexually transmitted herpes simplex of the genital organs (including the cervix and vagina), usually caused by human herpesvirus 2 (HHV-2);

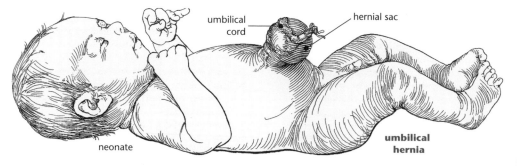

neonate

umbilical cord

hernial sac

umbilical hernia

blisters appear from 2 to 12 days after contact with a person who has active lesions; ulcerations heal within 2 weeks; initial (primary) infection in a pregnant woman may be transmitted to the fetus through the placenta; if the mother has an active eruption at the time of delivery, the newborn may become infected during its passage through the birth canal. An HHV-2 infection is frequently associated with other sexually transmitted diseases.

h. gestationis An eruption of reddish plaques and vesicles, usually in the arm and legs, occurring during the second or third trimester of pregnancy; despite its name, the condition is not caused by a herpesvirus; cause is unknown. Also called hydroa gestationis.

neonatal h. Infection of the newborn with human herpesvirus 2 (HHV-2); a potentially fatal infection (60% mortality rate), acquired during one of three periods: intrauterine through the placenta; during birth as an ascending infection through ruptured membranes (80%), or by delivery through an infected cervix and vagina; or after birth. The infant appears healthy at birth, becoming symptomatic at 1 to 4 weeks of age; infection may be localized (causing lesions in the skin, eyes, or oral cavity), may involve the brain (causing encephalitis, seizures, lethargy, tremors, temperature instability, a bulging fontanel), or may be disseminated (producing a variety of symptoms and signs, such as jaundice, low blood pressure, disseminated intravascular coagulation, respiratory distress, bleeding, shock).

h. simplex An acute eruption of painful blisters caused by human herpesvirus 1 and 2 (HHV-1, HHV-2); once established, the infection remains in the body and recurs at intervals with complete healing of the eruption between episodes; reappearance may be precipitated by emotional stress, febrile disease, local trauma, or menstruation.

herpesvirus (her-pēz-vi'rus) Any of a group of viruses that share the following features: they contain double-stranded DNA, replicate in the cell nucleus, accumulate between inner and outer layers of nuclear membrane and in the cisterna of endoplasmic reticulum, are transported to the cell surface through modified endoplasmic reticulum, and may remain latent in their host for several years or the lifetime of the host.

human h. 1 (HHV-1) Herpes simplex 1; the virus causing herpes simplex 1, responsible for most cases of nongenital herpes. The organism enters the cell through the fibroblast growth factor receptor on the cell membrane.

human h. 2 (HHV-2) Herpes simplex 2; the herpesvirus infecting primarily the genital organs of both male and female (including the cervix and vagina), and the anal and perianal areas of homosexual men; the organism has been recovered from the urethra and prostate of asymptomatic men; extragenital involvement (e.g., of the eyes and fingers) usually occurs through self-infection; infection of the newborn is associated with a high mortality rate (about 60%), and about half of the survivors have serious neurological or eye complications. An HHV-2 infection is frequently associated with other sexually transmitted diseases.

human h. 3 (HHV-3) Herpes varicella-zoster virus; the organism causing two clinical forms of infection: acute HHV-3 (varicella, commonly called chickenpox) and chronic HHV-3 (herpes zoster, commonly called shingles).

human h. 4 (HHV-4) The Epstein-Barr virus (EBV), with specificity for B cells (B lymphocytes); the cause of infectious mononucleosis, transmitted by saliva; associated with malignancies such as Burkitt's lymphoma, anaplastic nasopharyngeal cancer, and B-cell lymphomas in immunosuppressed patients (e.g., organ transplants and AIDS).

human h. 5 (HHV-5) See cytomegalovirus.

human h. 6 (HHV-6) A herpesvirus with affinity for B cells (B lymphocytes), occurring frequently as a coinfection with human immunodeficiency virus (HIV). An initial (primary) infection with HHV-6 is a frequent cause of exanthem subitum, an acute febrile illness in infants and young children, usually associated with a variety of clinical manifestations; it is also associated with syndromes resembling infectious mononucleosis.

human h. 7 (HHV-7) A herpesvirus isolated from activated, CD4-positive T lymphocytes obtained from the blood of healthy people.

herpetic (her-pet'ik) Relating to herpes or herpesvirus.

herpetiform (her-pet'ĭ-form) Resembling herpes.

hesitancy (hez'ĭ-tan-se) A delay.

urinary h. An abnormal delay in starting the urinary stream.

hetero- Combining form meaning other; different.

heteroerotic (het-er-o-er-ot'ik) Denoting sexual

feelings for another person.

heterogeneity (het-er-o-jě-ne'ĭ-te) In genetics, production of the same observable characteristic either from mutations at different loci in the chromosome, or the same locus, or from different genetic mechanisms.

heterosexuality (het-er-o-sek-shoo-al'ĭ-te) The state of having one's sexual interests directed toward a member of the opposite sex; opposite of homosexuality.

hexachlorophene (hek-să-klo'ro-fēn) An antibacterial compound used as a local antiseptic in soaps and detergents; associated with toxicity of the nervous system, especially in newborns; excessive use during the first trimester of pregnancy results in increased risk of fetal abnormalities.

hexamethylmelamine (hek-se-mě-thil-mel'ă-mīn) An antineoplastic agent used to treat ovarian epithelial cancer. It is potentially hazardous to the fetus, especially if used during the first trimester of pregnancy.

hilar (hi'lar) Relating to a hilum.

hilum (hi'lum), pl. hila The point or depression at which nerves, vessels, or ducts enter and leave an organ. Also called hilus.

    h. of ovary The slight indentation on the straight mesovarian border of the ovary where the blood vessels and nerves enter and leave.

hilus (hi'lus) See hilum.

hipbone (hip'bōn) One of the two large, flattened bones enclosing the pelvic cavity; formed by the fusion of three bones (ilium, ischium, pubis). Formerly called innominate bone.

hirsute (hir'soot) 1. Relating to hair or to hirsutism. 2. Hairy.

hirsutism (hir-soot'izm) Excessive growth of androgen-dependent hair especially on the face and chest of women; may be due to hormonal imbalance originating from the ovaries or adrenal (suprarenal) glands, or both. Mild hirsutism frequently develops in the pregnant state. Also called pilosis.

    constitutional h. See idiopathic hirsutism.

    idiopathic h. Hirsutism occurring without a known cause (i.e., in the absence of adrenal or ovarian dysfunction or without intake of steroid hormones). Also called constitutional hirsutism.

histamine (his'tă-mēn) A bioactive amine occurring in all animal and plant tissue; it causes contraction of bronchioles and small blood vessels, increased permeability of capillaries, increased secretion of nasal and bronchial mucous glands, and a fall in blood pressure.

histology (his-tol'o-je) The branch of anatomy concerned with the microscopic structure and function of tissues. Also called microscopic anatomy.

history (his'tŏ-re) A chronologic account of related events.

    medical h. Documentation of a patient's previous health care, illnesses, treatments, etc., that becomes part of that patient's medical record.

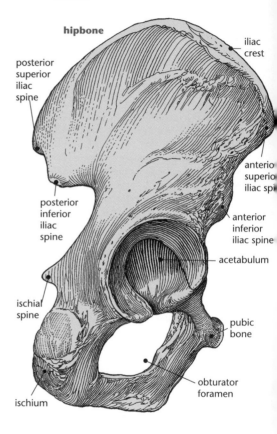

hipbone

iliac crest

posterior superior iliac spine

anterior superior iliac spine

posterior inferior iliac spine

anterior inferior iliac spine

acetabulum

ischial spine

pubic bone

ischium

obturator foramen

holandric (hol-an'drik) Relating to males only or to a gene on the Y chromosome (e.g., a pattern of inheritance of genes on the Y chromosome from a father to his sons, not to his daughters).

holoprosencephaly (hōl-o-pros-en-sef'ă-le) A craniofacial malformation of several types that can include: presence of a single orbit (cyclopia), abnormally close orbits (hypotelorism), absence of the nose, presence of a tubular appendage (proboscis), cleft lip, and cleft palate. It may be associated with chromosomal abnormalities such as the presence of an extra chromosome 13 (trisomy 13).

homo- Combining form meaning the same; alike.

homoeroticism (ho-mo-ě-rot'ĭ-sizm)

Homosexuality.

homogametic (ho-mo-gă-met'ik) Producing only one kind of germ cell in terms of the sex chromosomes it contains; such as the human female, whose ova contain only X chromosomes. Also called monogametic.

homosexual (ho-mo-sek'shoo-al) **1.** Relating to homosexuality. **2.** Characterized by homosexuality.

homosexuality (ho-mo-sek-shoo-al'ĭ-te) Sexual interest in, or sexual relationship with, members of one's own sex.

homozygosis (ho-mo-zi-go'sis) The formation of a zygote by the union of genetically identical gametes.

homozygosity (ho-mo-zi-gos'ĭ-te) The state of being homozygous.

homozygote (ho-mo-zi'gōt) A homozygous individual.

homozygous (ho-mo-zi'gus) Characterized by having two corresponding genes that are identical (i.e., having identical genes at a given locus of homologous chromosomes).

hood (hood) A pliable cover.

    vaginal h. A deformity of the vagina occurring in a young woman whose mother was treated with diethylstilbestrol (DES) in early pregnancy; consists of a fold of mucous membrane surrounding the vaginal opening of the cervix (external os).

hookworm (hook'werm) Any parasitic, bloodsucking roundworm, especially of the genera *Ancylostoma* and *Necator.*

hormonal (hor-mo'nal) Relating to a hormone.

hormone (hor'mōn) Any chemical substance elaborated and secreted into the bloodstream by specialized cells; they are carried by the blood to specific target organs or tissues elsewhere in the body, where they produce a particular effect (either stimulate or retard function).

    adrenal androgen-stimulating h. (AASH) A pituitary hormone, as yet un-isolated, which may be responsible for increased secretion of androgen at the time of puberty (adrenarche).

    adrenocorticotropic h. (ACTH) Hormone produced by the anterior lobe of the pituitary; its primary action is to stimulate the adrenal cortex to functional activity (i.e., production and secretion of corticosteroids and androgens). Also called adrenocorticotropin; corticotropin; corticotropic hormone.

    androgenic h. Any of the masculinizing hormones including testosterone, the most potent one.

    antimullerian h. (AMH) See mullerian-inhibiting substance, under substance.

    corticotropic h. See adrenocorticotropic hormone.

    follicle-stimulating h. (FSH) A glycoprotein hormone of the anterior lobe of the pituitary that stimulates normal cyclic growth of the ovarian follicle in females and stimulates the seminiferous tubules to produce spermatozoa in males.

    follicle-stimulating hormone-releasing h. (FSH-RH) A hypothalamic hormone capable of accelerating pituitary secretion of follicle-stimulating hormone.

    gonadotropin-releasing h. (GnRH) A decapeptide secreted by the hypothalamus that stimulates the pituitary to produce luteinizing hormone and follicle-stimulating hormone.

    growth h. (GH) Hormone secreted by the anterior lobe of the pituitary of the brain; it promotes fat mobilization, affects the rate of skeletal growth, and inhibits utilization of sugar (glucose); can produce diabetes when present in excess. Also called somatotropin.

    growth hormone-releasing h. (GRH, GH-RH) A peptide hormone produced primarily in the arcuate nucleus of the hypothalamus; it stimulates the release of growth hormone.

    luteinizing h. (LH) A glycoprotein hormone of the anterior pituitary that stimulates secretion of estrogen and progesterone from the ovary; it promotes maturation of an ovarian follicle and its rupture to release the egg, and the subsequent conversion of the ruptured follicle into the corpus luteum; continued release of LH stimulates secretion of progesterone. Also called lutein-stimulating hormone (LSH).

    luteinizing hormone-releasing h. (LH-RH, LRH) Hypothalamic hormone capable of accelerating pituitary secretion of luteinizing hormone. Formerly called luteinizing hormone-releasing factor.

    lutein-stimulating h. (LSH) See luteinizing hormone.

    ovarian h.'s Hormones secreted by the human ovary including estradiol, estrone, estriol, and progesterone.

    placental h. Any of the hormones secreted by the placenta, namely human chorionic gonadotropin, estrogen, progesterone, and human placental lactogen.

    progestational h. Progesterone.

    prolactin-inhibiting h. (PIH) Hormone of hypothalamic origin that inhibits elaboration and release of prolactin by the anterior pituitary (adenohypophysis).

    prolactin-releasing h. (PRH) A hypothalamic

hormone that stimulates elaboration and release of prolactin by the anterior pituitary (adenohypophysis).

sex h.'s Estrogens (female sex hormones) and androgens (male sex hormones) formed by ovarian, testicular, and adrenocortical tissues.

somatotrophic h. See growth hormone.

thyroid h. A term that commonly refers to thyroxine, but may also include triiodothyronine.

thyroid-stimulating h. (TSH) See thyrotropin.

thyrotropic h. See thyrotropin.

thyrotropin-releasing h. (TRH) A tripeptide hormone from the hypothalamus that stimulates pituitary secretion of thyrotropin.

horn (horn) Any anatomic structure projecting from a base and suggestive of a horn. Also called cornu.

coccygeal h.'s See coccygeal cornua, under cornu.

lateral h.'s of uterus The hornlike extensions of the body of the uterus to the upper right and left lateral borders where the fallopian (uterine) tubes join the uterus. Also called uterine horns, uterine cornua.

rudimentary h. An underdeveloped uterine lateral horn that remains attached to the lower portion of the remaining unicornuate uterus; it may or may not contain an endometrial cavity; when present, the cavity may or may not communicate with that of the unicornuate uterus. Undetected pregnancy in a non-communicating rudimentary horn may lead to rupture, usually before 20 weeks of gestation, causing life-threatening maternal hemorrhage.

sacral h.'s See sacral cornua, under cornu.

uterine h.'s See lateral horns of uterus.

hump (hump) A rounded protuberance or mass.

buffalo h. A soft tissue protuberance of the upper back and shoulder associated with hypercortisolism (e.g., Cushing's syndrome).

dowager's h. Popular term for a protuberance on the upper back, caused by osteoporosis of the spine.

hydramnios, hydramnion (hi-dram'ne-os, hi-dram'ne-on) See polyhydramnios.

hydranencephaly (hi-dran-en-sef'ă-le) Congenital absence of most of the cerebral hemispheres, the space being filled with cerebrospinal fluid; the skull is intact and usually enlarged, but often of normal size and shape; initially the newborn infant sucks without difficulty and abnormal neurological signs are not originally obvious.

hydro-, hydr- Combining forms meaning water; hydrogen.

hydroa (hid-ro'ă) Any eruption of vesicles on the skin.

h. gestationis See herpes gestationis, under herpes.

hydrocephalus (hi-dro-sef'ă-lus) An abnormal increase in the amount of cerebrospinal fluid (CSF) within the ventricles of the brain due to blockage of the CSF flow, causing compression of brain tissue and, in infants, abnormal enlargement of the head. Popularly called water-on-the-brain.

hydrocolpocele, hydrocolpos (hi-dro-kol'po-sēl, hi-dro-kol'pos) Accumulation of fluid in the vagina.

hydrolase (hi'dro-lās) Enzyme that precipitates the breakdown of compounds by hydrolysis.

hydrometra (hi-dro-me'tră) Abnormal accumulation of a fluid in the uterus.

hydrometrocolpos (hi-dro-me-tro-kol'pos) Abnormal accumulation of a fluid in the uterus and vagina.

hydronephrosis (hi-dro-nĕ-fro'sis) Distention of the pelvis and calices of one or both kidneys with urine, associated with progressive atrophy of the kidney, caused by obstruction to the outflow of urine.

hydrophthalmos (hi-drof-thal'mos) See buphthalmos.

hydrops (hi'drops) Abnormal accumulation of clear fluid in body cavities or tissues. Formerly called dropsy.

h. fetalis, fetal h. Hydrops of the fetus, as seen in severe hemolytic disease.

h. tubae profluens See intermittent hydrosalpinx, under hydrosalpinx.

hydrorrhea (hi-dro-re'ă) A profuse watery secretion.

h. gravidarum An uncommon condition in which a pregnant woman passes a clear fluid from the vagina; usually a scant amount throughout the pregnancy, occasionally as much as 500 ml as a one-time occurrence; cause is not known.

hydrosalpinx (hi-dro-sal'pinks) Accumulation of serous fluid in a fallopian (uterine) tube.

intermittent h. Periodic hydrosalpinx characterized by closure of the fimbriated opening of a uterine tube, causing a serosanguinous discharge through the uterus, sometimes accompanied by a colicky lower abdominal pain; sometimes associated with malignancy of the uterine tube. Also called hydrops tubae profluens.

hymen (hi'men) The thin fold of mucous

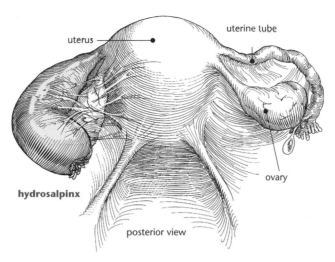

membrane that partially or entirely closes the vaginal orifice in the virgin; it varies much in shape and extent, and occasionally may be absent. Also called virginal membrane.

circular h. A hymen with a small round opening.

cribriform h. A hymen with a number of small perforations. Also called fenestrated hymen; microperforate hymen.

denticular h. A hymen in which the opening has serrated edges.

falciform h. A crescentic-shaped hymen.

fenestrated h. See cribriform hymen.

imperforate h. A hymen which completely closes the vaginal orifice.

infundibuliform h. A protruding hymen with a central opening.

microperforate h. See cribriform hymen.

ruptured h. A hymen that has been forcibly disrupted as a result of injury or coitus.

septate h. A hymen in which the opening is divided by a narrow band of tissue (septum).

hymenal (hi'men-al) Relating to the hymen.

hymenectomy (hi-men-ek'tŏ-me) Excision of the hymen.

hymenorrhaphy (hi-men-or'ă-fe) **1.** Closing of the vagina by suturing the hymen. **2.** Suture of any membrane.

hymenotomy (hi-men-ot'ŏ-me) Surgical cut through the hymen, especially an imperforate hymen.

hypamnios, hypamnion (hi-pam'ne-os, hi-pam'ne-on) The presence of a smaller than usual amount of amniotic fluid in the amniotic sac.

hyper- Prefix meaning over; above; excessive; increased; above normal.

hyperbilirubinemia (hi-per-bil-ĭ-roo-bĭ-ne'me-ă) The presence of abnormally high levels of bilirubin in the blood.

hypercalcemia (hi-per-kal-se'me-ă) An abnormally high concentration of calcium in the blood. Symptoms of severe hypercalcemia include headache, constipation and renal

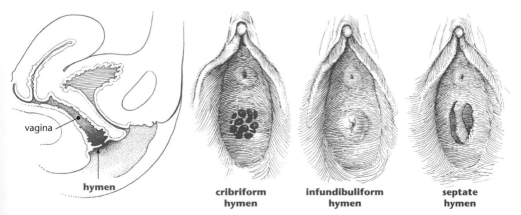

cribriform hymen

infundibuliform hymen

septate hymen

impairment. Causes include hyperparathyroidism, sarcoidosis, bone tumors, and vitamin D intoxication.

hypercoagulable (hi-per-ko-ag'u-lă-bl) Characterized by an abnormally high tendency to form clots.

hypercortisolism (hi-per-kor'tĭ-sol-izm) See Cushing's disease, under disease.

hyperemesis (hi-per-em'ĕ-sis) Excessive vomiting.

> **h. gravidarum** Severe and prolonged vomiting occurring in pregnancy, usually associated with dehydration and ketonuria.

hypergenitalism (hi-per-jen'ĭ-tal-izm) Overdeveloped genital organs for age of the individual.

hyperglycemia (hi-per-gli-se'me-ă) Abnormally high level of sugar (glucose) in the blood.

hypergonadism (hi-per-go'nad-izm) Abnormally increased physiologic activity of the gonads (testes or ovaries), with secretion of gonadal hormones, marked by rapid growth and precocious sexual development.

hyperlactation (hi-per-lak-ta'shun) Excessive or prolonged secretion of milk.

hyperlipidemia (hi-per-lip-ĭ-de'me-ă) High levels of any kind of lipoprotein in blood plasma. Also called lipemia; lipidemia.

hypermagnesemia (hi-per-mag-ne-se'me-ă) Abnormally high levels of magnesium in blood serum. Seen in patients with renal failure who have ingested magnesium-containing antacids. In the newborn, it is most commonly caused by therapeutic administration of magnesium sulfate to the mother during pregnancy.

hypermotility (hi-per-mo-til'ĭ-te) In fertilization, the exaggerated vigorous movements of the spermatozoon, especially in the vicinity of the ovum, which cause it to move in circles rather than in the usual forward direction; considered part of the fertilization process.

hypernephroma (hi-per-ne-fro'mă) See renal adenocarcinoma, under adenocarcinoma.

hyperparathyroidism (hi-per-par-ă-thi'roid-izm) Excessive secretion of parathyroid hormone.

> **primary h.** Hyperparathyoidism resulting from an adenoma or chief cell hyperplasia of one or more parathyroid glands, or rarely from a parathyroid carcinoma; the classic laboratory findings are high serum calcium and low serum phosphate.

> **secondary h.** Hyperplasia of the parathyroid glands and increased secretion of parathyroid hormone secondary to abnormal calcium and phosphorus metabolism in chronic renal disease.

hyperpigmentation (hi-per-pig-men-ta'shun) Increased pigmentation of the skin during pregnancy, especially in such areas as the areolae, linea alba, perineum, and the navel.

hyperplasia (hi-per-pla'ze-ă) Excessive but regulated increase in the number of cells of an organ or body part, usually accompanied by increase in size. Compare with hypertrophy.

> **adenomatous h.** See endometrial hyperplasia.

> **congenital adrenal h.** (CAH) Inherited condition characterized by hyperplasia of the adrenal cortex and excessive secretion of androgens resulting from enzymatic defects in the biosynthesis of corticosteroids; there are four major types: a virilizing form; a sodium-losing form; one causing high blood pressure; and a 3-beta-hydroxysteroid dehydrogenase defect that may produce feminization of male genitals.

> **cystic h. of breast** See fibrocystic change of breast, under change.

> **endocervical h.** The development of small groups of benign, proliferating submucosal glands in the uterine cervix, usually occurring in women taking progesterone-containing oral contraceptives.

> **endometrial h.** Hyperplasia of the uterine lining (endometrium), usually due to excessive estrogenic stimulation, especially when not opposed by progesterone secretion, causing irregular, often profuse uterine bleeding. When there is no evidence of atypical changes in the glandular epithelium (the lining cells of the uterine glands), the condition is considered benign and, depending on the degree of glandular crowding and disordered growth pattern, it may be called *simple h.* or *complex h.*; when the glandular epithelium of the hyperplastic glands exhibits cellular atypia, the condition is designated *atypical h.* and is considered premalignant, classified as *mild atypical h.*, *moderate atypical h.*, and *severe atypical h.* Also called adenomatous hyperplasia; glandular hyperplasia.

> **glandular h.** See endometrial hyperplasia.

hyperplastic (hi-per-plas'tik) Relating to hyperplasia.

hyperprolactinemia (hi-per-pro-lak-tin-e´me-ă) Increased amounts of the hormone prolactin in the blood; normal only during lactation; may be caused by certain medicinal drugs or by a pituitary tumor.

hyperreflexia (hi-per-re-flek'se-ă) Augmentation or exaggeration of reflexes.

> **detrusor h.** See detrusor instability, under instability.

hypersomia (hi-per-so'me-ă) See macrosomia.

hyperspermia (hi-per-sper'me-ă) A high sperm count, more than 200 million per milliliter of semen; sometimes paradoxically associated with (not necessarily the cause of) male infertility.

hypertension (hi-per-ten'shun) High blood pressure, usually described as a blood pressure greater than two standard deviations above normal values for the age and weight of the individual. In general, blood pressure exceeding 140 mmHg systolic and 90 mmHg diastolic pressure (140/90 mmHg).

    benign intracranial h. See pseudotumor cerebri, under pseudotumor.

    essential h. Hypertension occurring without a known cause. Also called idiopathic hypertension; primary hypertension.

    gestational h. Hypertension developed during, and restricted to, the pregnant state (in the absence of pre-eclampsia); usually seen in overweight women and in women with a family history of the disease; there is a high incidence of chronic essential hypertension later in life.

    idiopathic h. See essential hypertension.

    pregnancy-induced h. An increase in blood pressure, usually to greater than 140/90 mmHg, which develops as a consequence of pregnancy and regresses postpartum. See also pre-eclampsia and eclampsia.

    primary h. See essential hypertension.

    persistent pulmonary h. of newborn (PPHN) Pulmonary hypertension in a newborn infant resulting from constriction of the blood vessels in the lungs, which in turn causes a right-to-left shunt (diversion of circulation) through the ductus arteriosus and foramen ovale.

    pulmonary h. Hypertension in the blood circulation of the lungs resulting from primary lung disease (e.g., pulmonary emboli, pulmonary fibrosis) or from heart disease (e.g., left ventricular failure, mitral stenosis).

hypertensive (hi-per-ten'siv) **1.** Relating to hypertension. **2.** Denoting a person afflicted with hypertension.

hyperthecosis (hi-per-the-ko'sis) Hyperplasia of the theca cells of the vesicular ovarian follicles.

    stromal h. The presence of luteinized cells in the stromal layer of the ovary; the condition is usually bilateral.

hyperthelia (hi-per-the'le-ă) See polythelia.

hyperthermia (hi-per-ther'me-ă) Extremely high body temperature.

    malignant h. A rapid rise in body temperature to potentially fatal levels accompanied by muscular rigidity, brought on by general anesthesia; occurs in genetically susceptible individuals (either as an autosomal dominant or recessive inheritance) and, occasionally, in some people afflicted with certain muscular disorders.

hyperthyroidism (hi-per-thi'roi-dizm) Condition caused by excessive production or administration of thyroid hormone; most common symptoms include weight loss, increased appetite, rapid heart rate, tremor, and fatigue; when protrusion of the eyeballs (exophthalmos) is present, the disease is called exophthalmic goiter.

    congenital h. Excessive thyroid hormone present at birth; affected infants usually are born to mothers afflicted with Graves' disease during pregnancy.

    primary h. A form originating from a disorder of the thyroid gland itself.

    secondary h. A form caused by abnormal stimulation of thyroid gland activity by pituitary hormones due to a disorder of the pituitary.

hypertonic (hi-per-ton'ik) **1.** Characterized by excessive tension. **2.** See hypertonic solution, under solution.

hypertonicity (hi-per-to-nis'ĭ-te) The state of being hypertonic.

hypertrophy (hi-per'tro-fe) The enlargement of an organ or part due to the increase in size of the cells composing it; the overgrowth meets a demand for increased functional activity (e.g., in muscle building exercises or in the heart muscle due to heart disease), or it responds to hormonal stimulation (e.g., in the pregnant uterus). Compare with hyperplasia.

    physiologic h. Temporary hypertrophy of an organ in order to meet the demand of a natural increase in functional activity (e.g., in the female breast during pregnancy and lactation).

hypo- Prefix meaning below normal; deficient; diminished; under.

hypoadrenalism (hi-po-ă-dre'nal-izm) Deficient function of the adrenal cortex, with diminished production of steroid hormones. See also Addison's disease, under disease.

hypoestrogenemia (hi-po-es-tro-gĕ-ne'me-ă) Low levels of estrogen in the blood.

hypofibrinogenemia (hi-po-fi-brin-o-je-ne'me-ă) Deficiency of the protein fibrinogen in the blood; seen in pregnant women with a retained dead fetus, 4 to 5 weeks after intrauterine fetal death; may also occur in amniotic fluid embolism, abruptio placenta and, occasionally, in intra-amniotic instillation of hypertonic saline. See also defibrination syndrome, under syndrome.

hypofunction (hi-po-funk'shun) Diminished or

inadequate function of an organ or part.

hypogastric (hi-po-gas'trik) Relating to the hypogastrium.

hypogastrium (hi-po-gas'tre-um) The middle region of the lower abdomen; the pubic region.

hypogenitalism (hi-po-jen'ĭ-tal-izm) Underdevelopment of the genitals.

hypoglycemia (hi-po-gli-se'me-ă) A lower than normal level of sugar (glucose) in the blood; may cause one or several of the following symptoms: sweating, trembling, palpitation, hunger, weakness, lightheadedness, or double vision; symptoms may vary in duration and often disappear after eating a sweet snack. The condition may result from excessive production of insulin by the pancreas (e.g., due to the presence of a tumor); or it may occur in a diabetic person who has either taken too large a dose of insulin or an oral hypoglycemic drug, or who misses a meal or fails to eat enough food after taking an insulin dose, or who exercises too much without taking precautionary measures.

hypogonadism (hi-po-go'nad-izm) Decreased physical development of an individual's sexual characteristics, resulting from insufficient hormone secretion or from defective response to hormonal activity by the target tissues.

> **hypergonadotropic h.** Hypogonadism occurring in spite of the presence of elevated levels of gonadotropins; may be due to defective steroid receptors in target tissues.

> **hypogonadotropic h.** Hypogonadism resulting from insufficient pituitary secretion of gonadotropins.

hypomastia (hi-po-mas'te-ă) Abnormally small size of the female breasts.

hypomenorrhea (hi-po-men-o-re'ă) Scanty menstrual flow, sometimes consisting of only 'spotting'. See also cryptomenorrhea.

hypo-ovarianism (hi-po o-va're-an-izm) Insufficient secretion of hormones from the ovaries.

hypoparathyroidism (hi-po-par-ă-thi'roid-izm) Condition resulting either from lack of hormone secretion by the parathyroid glands, secretion of an inactive form of the hormone, or from target-organ resistance to the hormone; signs and symptoms include reduced plasma calcium level and increased plasma phosphate level, neuromuscular excitability, high intracranial pressure, abnormalities in the conduction system of the heart, and cataracts.

hypophysis (hi-pof'ĭ-sis) An ovoid structure located at the base of the skull in the hypophyseal fossa of the sphenoid bone, attached to the brain by a short stalk (infundibulum); it consists of two

main parts: an anterior part composed of the adenohypophysis and a slender portion of the infundibulum, and a posterior part composed of the neurohypophysis and the major portion of the infundibulum; between them there is a narrow, relatively avascular intermediate zone. Also called pituitary gland; pituitary.

hypoplasia (hi-po-pla'ze-ă) Defective or incomplete development of a body part.

> **vaginal h.** Incomplete development of the vagina.

hypospadias (hi-po-spa'de-as) A congenital defect in which the urethra abnormally opens on the undersurface of the penis in the male or in the vagina in the female.

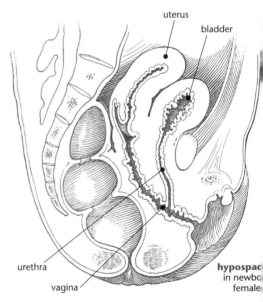

hypothesis (hi-poth'ĕ-sis) A tentative theory subject to verification.

> **cell-kill h.** The concept that the proportion of tumor cells killed by chemotherapy is a constant percentage of the total number of cells present.

> **Goldie-Coldman h.** A hypothesis suggesting that most malignant cells begin with intrinsic sensitivity to chemotherapeutic agents but develop spontaneous resistance at variable rates.

> **Pedersen h.** The assumption that an abnormally large size of the fetus (macrosomia) is due to inadequate management of maternal diabetes mellitus during pregnancy.

hysteralgia (his-ter-al'je-ă) Pain or discomfort in the uterus. Also called hysterodynia.

hysteratresia (his-ter-ă-tre'ze-ă) Abnormal closure of the uterine cavity.

hysterectomy (his-ter-ek'tō-me) Removal of the uterus.

    abdominal h. Removal of the uterus through an incision in the abdominal wall. Also called laparohysterectomy.

    cesarean h. Delivery of a baby through an abdominal and uterine incision, followed by removal of the uterus through the same abdominal incision.

    extended h. Hysterectomy classified into five progressively expanding procedures: *class I, extrafascial h.*, removal of all cervical tissue; *class II*, includes removal of the medial half of the cardinal and uterosacral ligaments, and the upper third of the vagina; *class III*, includes removal of the entire cardinal and uterosacral ligaments, and the upper third of the vagina; *class IV*, includes removal of all connective tissue adjacent to the ureters, the superior vesical artery, and three fourths of the vagina; *class V*, includes removal of the bladder and distal portions of the ureters.

    extrafascial h. See extended hysterectomy, class I.

    laparoscopically assisted vaginal h. (LAVH) An operation devised to reduce the morbidity of major gynecologic surgery by converting an abdominal procedure into a vaginal one. The hysterectomy is begun with an evaluation of the pelvic viscera through the laparoscope to treat conditions that would have precluded the vaginal approach. Once this has been done, the hysterectomy is completed vaginally.

    Meigs h. See modified radical hysterectomy.

    modified radical h. Procedure for early cervical cancer with minimal stromal involvement (i.e., less than 3 mm deep); the extent of tissue removal is tailored to the specific condition of the patient; in general, it usually includes removal of the uterus, the vaginal cuff (which additionally may include the upper portion of the vagina), the medial half of the uterosacral ligaments, and the pelvic lymph nodes below the level of the ovaries; the ovaries and fallopian (uterine) tubes may or may not be removed. Also called Meigs hysterectomy; Okabayashi hysterectomy; Wertheim hysterectomy.

    Okabayashi h. See modified radical hysterectomy.

    radical h. Removal of the uterus, upper third of the vagina, entire uterosacral and uterovesical ligaments, connective tissue surrounding the uterus, fallopian (uterine) tubes, ovaries, and all pelvic lymph nodes.

    subtotal h. See supracervical hysterectomy.

    supracervical h. Operation in which only the main body of the uterus (the fundus) is removed, to the level of the internal os, leaving the cervix in place. Also called subtotal hysterectomy.

    total h. Removal of the entire uterus, including the cervix, leaving in place the ovaries and fallopian (uterine) tubes. Usually simply called hysterectomy.

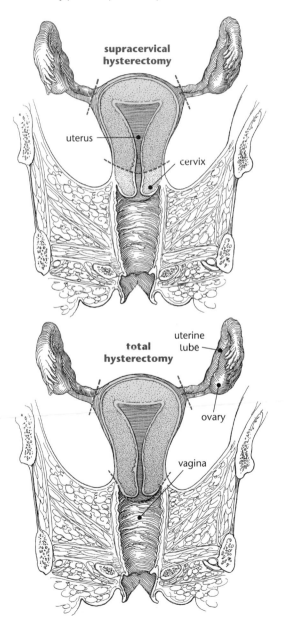

supracervical
hysterectomy

uterus

cervix

total
hysterectomy

uterine
tube

ovary

vagina

vaginal h. Removal of the uterus through the vagina; usually performed in benign conditions when the uterus is not greatly enlarged, or when other repairs are also performed (e.g., for a cystocele or a rectocele). Also called colpohysterectomy; vaginohysterectomy.

Wertheim h. See modified radical hysterectomy.

hystero- Combining form meaning uterus; hysteria.

hysterocolposcope (his-ter-o-kol'po-skōp) Instrument for inspecting the uterine cavity and vagina.

hysterodynia (his-ter-o-din'e-ă) See hysteralgia.

hysterogram (his'ter-o-gram) An x-ray picture of the uterus obtained after filling its cavity with a radiopaque material.

hysterography (his-ter-og'ră-fe) The making of a hysterogram.

hysterolith (his'ter-o-lith) A concretion or calculus in the uterus.

hysterometer (his-tě-rom'ě-ter) A graduated instrument for measuring the depth of the uterine cavity.

hysterometry (his-tě-rom'ě-tre) The process of measuring the dimensions of the uterus.

hysteromyoma (his-ter-o-mi-o'mă) A benign tumor of the uterine wall.

hysteromyomectomy (his-ter-o-mi-o-mek'tŏme) Surgical removal of a myoma from the uterus.

hysteromyotomy (his-ter-o-mi-ot'ŏ-me) A surgical cut into the muscular wall of the uterus.

hystero-oophorectomy (his-ter-o o-of-ŏ-rek'tŏ-me) Removal of the uterus and ovaries.

hysteropathy (his-tě-rop'ă-the) Any disease of the uterus.

hysterorrhaphy (his-ter-or'ă-fe) Surgical repair of a lacerated or ruptured uterus.

hysterorrhexis (his-ter-o-rek'sis) Rupture of the uterus. Also called metrorrhexis.

hysterosalpingectomy (his-ter-o-sal-pin-jek'tŏ-me) Removal of the uterus and at least one fallopian (uterine) tube.

hysterosalpingogram (his-ter-o-sal-pin'gŏ-gram) The graphic record made by hysterosalpingography.

hysterosalpingography (his-ter-o-sal-ping-gog'ră-fe) (HSG) The radiopaque visualization of the cavities of the uterus and fallopian (uterine) tubes after instilling a contrast medium via the cervix; performed as part of an infertility study and as a follow-up to surgery, especially tubal reunification (reanastomosis). Possible complications include perforation of the uterine wall, vasovagal response (i.e., pallor, nausea, rapid fall of blood pressure, sweating), and reaction to the iodinated radiopaque medium.

hysterosalpingo-oophorectomy (his-ter-o-sal-ping'go o-of-ŏ-rek'tŏ-me) Removal of the uterus, fallopian (uterine) tubes and ovaries.

hysterosalpingostomy (his-ter-o-sal-ping-gos'tŏ-me) Operation to restore the patency of an obstructed fallopian (uterine) tube.

hysteroscope (his'ter-o-skōp) An endoscope for direct viewing of the interior of the uterus; consists of a rigid rod equipped with a fiberoptic light source, a channel to introduce a medium to distend the uterus, and a channel through which instruments (e.g., probes, forceps, electrocautery or laser) may be visually manipulated in the uterine cavity. Also called metroscope.

hysteroscopy (his-ter-os'kŏ-pe) Inspection of the interior of the uterus with a hysteroscope.

hysterostomatomy (his-ter-os-tŏ-mat'ŏ-me) See Dührssen's incisions, under incision.

hysterotome (his'ter-o-tōm) Surgical instrument for cutting into the uterus.

hysterotomy (his-ter-ot'ŏ-me) A surgical cut into the uterus. Also called metrotomy; uterotomy; laparohysterotomy.

hysterotrachelectomy (his-ter-o-tra-kel-ek'tŏ-me) See cervical amputation, under amputation.

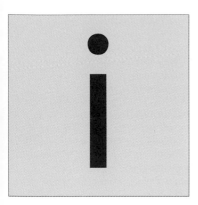

-ia Suffix meaning a state; a condition (e.g., melancholia)

-iasis Suffix meaning disease; infection (e.g., amebiasis)

-iatrics Combining form meaning medical care (e.g., pediatrics).

iatrogenic (i-at-ro-jen'ik) Term currently applied to any result from medical diagnosis and treatment, regardless of whether the condition occurs as a known risk of a procedure or through errors of omission or commission.

I blood group (blud grōōp) A red blood cell antigen expressed in a wide range of strength; it is strongest on fetal and cord red blood cells.

ibuprofen (i-bu-pro'fen) A nonsteroid anti-inflammatory compound, inhibitor of prostaglandin synthetase. When taken during the third trimester of pregnancy, it may cause *in utero* closing of the ductus arteriosus, inhibition of labor, and persistent pulmonary hypertension in the newborn infant.

-ic Suffix meaning relating to (e.g., hypodermic).

ichthyo-, ichthy- Combining forms meaning fish.

ichthyosis (ik-the-o'sis) Disorder characterized by formation of dry, rough, and thick scaling of the skin, caused by a defect of its horny layer; may affect the eyelids, conjunctiva, and cornea. Also called alligator skin; fish skin; sauriasis.

    X-linked i. Recessive inheritance affecting males; characterized by thick, adherent scales on the skin, which may be present at birth or appear in early infancy and usually darken with age; the mother carries the defective gene; both mother and offspring have small cataracts; most patients lack the enzyme steroid sulfatase.

ictal (ik'tal) Relating to convulsion.

icteric (ik-ter'ik) Relating to jaundice.

icterogenic (ik-ter-o-jen'ik) Causing jaundice.

icterus (ik'ter-us) See jaundice.

    i. gravidarum See intrahepatic cholestasis of pregnancy, under cholestasis.

    neonatal i. See physiologic jaundice, under jaundice.

    i. neonatorum See physiologic jaundice, under jaundice.

    physiologic i. See physiologic jaundice, under jaundice.

ictus (ik'tus) A sudden attack or convulsion.

    i. epilepticus An epileptic convulsion.

identity (i-den'tĭ-te) The role of an individual in society and the personal perception of that role.

    gender i. The anatomic-sexual identity of an individual.

idio- Combining form meaning originating from within; one's own; distinctive.

idiogenesis (id-e-o-jen'ĕ-sis) Origin or development without a known cause; applied to an idiopathic disease (i.e., one without a known cause).

idiopathic (id-e-o-path'ik) Of unknown cause; applied to certain diseases.

idiotope (id'ĭ-o-tōp) One of several antigenic determinants in the variable region of an antibody molecule. It can be recognized as antigen by the combining site (receptor) of another antibody in the same species.

idiotype (id'ĭ-o-tīp) The collection of idiotopes in the variable region of an antibody molecule; it gives the variable region its individual antigenic characteristics.

ifosfamide (i-fos'fă-mīd) An alkylating and immunosuppressive agent related to the antineoplastic compound cyclophosphamide; used in treating gynecologic malignancies. Ifosfamide has a risk of causing fetal defects when used during early pregnancy.

ileo- Combining form meaning the ileum.

ileostomy (il-e-os'tŏ-me) Surgical creation of an external opening into the ileum through the abdominal wall for diversion of intestinal contents.

ileum (il'e-um) The longest and most distal of the three portions of the small intestine (the others being duodenum and jejunum); it is continuous proximally with the jejunum and distally with the cecum (the first part of the large intestine).

ileus (il'e-us) Impairment or stoppage of the flow of intestinal contents due either to obstruction or to diminished intestinal motility; depending on the cause, symptoms may include severe colicky pain, abdominal distention, fever, dehydration, and vomiting.

    adynamic i. Ileus resulting from decreased or absent propulsive activity of the intestinal walls, usually causing abdominal distention and vomiting but little or no pain; causes include peritonitis, abdominal surgery, bowel trauma, and damage to mesenteric arteries. Also called paralytic ileus.

meconium i. Ileus occurring in the newborn, caused by obliteration of the bowel lumen by excessively thick meconium; it is frequently the first sign of cystic fibrosis.

obstructive i. Ileus caused by any mechanical reduction or obliteration of the bowel lumen (e.g., by constrictive postoperative adhesions, pressure against the bowel by a tumor, torsion of a bowel segment, or by impaction of any material within the intestine); it is usually associated with persistent vomiting and abdominal cramps.

paralytic i. See adynamic ileus.

i. subparta A mild form of ileus occurring during pregnancy as a result of pressure of the pregnant uterus on the large intestine.

iliac (il'e-ak) Relating to the ilium (one of the bones of the hip).

ilioinguinal (il-e-o-in'gwĭ-nal) Relating to the lateral area of the pelvis and the groin.

iliopectineal (il-e-o-pek-tin'e-al) Relating to the ilium and the pubic bone.

iliosacral (il-e-o-sa'kral) Relating to the ilium and sacrum.

ilium (il'e-um) The superior, broad bone on either side of the pelvis, forming the largest portion of the hipbone; it is surrounded by cartilage in early life and eventually ossifies, fusing with the ischium and pubic bone to form the hipbone; along with the ischium and pubic bone, it contributes to the formation of the acetabulum (the cup-shaped cavity into which the head of the femur fits to form the hip joint). See also pubic bone, under bone; ischium; pelvis.

imaging (im'ă-jing) The process of producing a visual representation.

functional magnetic resonance i. High speed magnetic resonance imaging (MRI) techniques that measure changes in blood volume and flow, thereby producing functional MRI maps of brain activity.

magnetic resonance i. (MRI) A high-resolution *in vivo* diagnostic procedure that provides sectional images of internal structures without the use of radioactive material. Also called nuclear magnetic resonance imaging.

nuclear magnetic resonance (NMR) i. See magnetic resonance imaging.

imbrication (im-brĭ-ka'shun) The turning in of the edges of a surgical wound.

imipramine (im-ip'ră-mēn) A tricyclic compound used for the treatment of depression. Intrauterine exposure may cause fetal malformations and withdrawal symptoms and urine retention in the newborn infant.

immune (ĭ-mūn') **1.** Characterized by a state of being secure against harmful effects from disease-causing agents or influences; having immunity. **2.** Relating to immunity.

immunity (ĭ-mu'nĭ-te) **1.** The physiologic state that enables the body to recognize materials that are not of itself and to neutralize, metabolize, or eliminate them with or without injury to its own tissue. **2.** A conditioning to a specific pathogen; may be natural or inherited.

acquired i. Immunity resulting from exposure to disease after birth; may be active or passive.

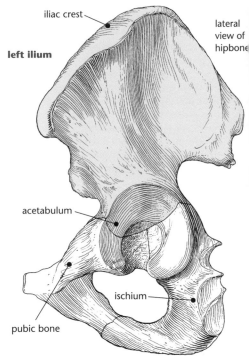

iliac crest

lateral view of hipbone

left ilium

acetabulum

ischium

pubic bone

active i. Immunity resulting from an acquired infection or from vaccination, which triggers the individual's own immune system to produce blood-circulating antibodies directed against the microorganism or its toxins, or it may initiate responses mediated by specifically reactive white blood cells (i.e., lymphocytes or macrophages).

cell-mediated i. (CMI) Immunity in which the participation of certain white blood cells (lymphocytes and macrophages) is predominant.

humoral i. Immunity in which the

involvement of blood-circulating antibodies (immunoglobulins) is predominant.

innate i. Resistance to certain infections that has not been acquired through vaccination or previous infection; it includes species-determined immunity (e.g., resistance of humans to the virus of canine distemper). Also called natural immunity.

natural i. See innate immunity.

neonatal passive i. Passive immunity in a newborn infant acquired as a fetus through transplacental transfer from its mother; it protects the infant from many common infections and lasts about six months.

passive i. Immunity acquired in either of two forms: by means of transferred antibodies either naturally (e.g., from immune mother to fetus), or artificially (e.g., by intentional inoculation with serum); or by means of transferred lymphoid cells from an immune donor.

immunization (im-u-nǐ-za'shun) The act or process of rendering a person or animal resistant to a specific disease.

active i. Administration of antigens (i.e., a modified or killed infectious microorganism or its toxins) to stimulate the subject's immune system into producing a high number of antibodies. The principle is used in many childhood vaccines to provide long-term protection.

combined passive-active i. A simultaneous passive and active immunization undertaken to produce an immediate, transient protection and a slowly durable protection against such diseases as rabies and tetanus.

passive i. Immunization for immediate short-term protection by administration of preformed antibody to a person who has been exposed to an infectious disease. The antibody could be serum from a person who has had the disease (e.g., rubella) or serum from an animal specifically immunized against an antigen (e.g., tetanus toxin).

immunocyte (im-u'no-sīt) A lymphoid cell that, when reacting with antigen, is capable of forming antibodies, or elaborating cells that form antibodies. Also called I cell; immunocompetent cell; antigen-sensitive cell.

immunodeficiency (im-u-no-dě-fish'en-se) Any congenital or acquired impairment of the immune response; may involve the cell-mediated (T-cell) portion of the immune system or the antibody-mediated (B-cell) portion, or both; it may be secondary to a developmental defect, or due to an enzymatic defect, or to unknown

causes; symptoms and signs, in general, are related to the degree of deficiency and the specific body organs that are deficient in function; characteristically, affected persons have a susceptibility to infections. Also called immune deficiency.

immunogen (im-u'no-jen) An antigen stimulating specific immunity.

immunogenic (im-u-no-jen'ik) See antigenic.

immunogenicity (im-u-no-jě-nis'ǐ-te) See antigenicity.

immunoglobulin (im-u-no-glob'u-lin) (Ig) Any of a group of proteins present in serum and tissue fluids of all mammals; five classes of immunoglobulins have been recognized (IgA, IgD, IgE, IgG, IgM), each differing from the others in size, amino acid composition, and carbohydrate content; IgG, the predominant class in serum, is the only one that crosses the placenta, thereby providing the fetus and newborn infant with protection against infection. All antibodies are immunoglobulins; probably all immunoglobulins have antibody activity. See also antibody.

monoclonal i. Immunoglobulin derived from a single clone of plasma cells proliferating abnormally.

Rh$_o$ I. (D) See Rh$_o$ immune globulin, under globulin.

immunoreaction (im-u-no-re-ak'shun) See immune response, under response.

immunosuppression (im-u-no-sǔ-presh'un) Diminution of the body's immune response, either by infection or carried out by any of several means (e.g., drugs, radiation, lymphocyte depletion) as a way to prevent rejection of a transplant.

immunosuppressive (im-u-no-sǔ-pres'iv) Capable of inducing immunosuppression.

immunotherapy (im-u-no-ther'ǎ-pe) **1.** Passive immunization through the use of serum or gamma globulin. **2.** Transplantation of immunocompetent tissues from a donor (e.g., bone marrow, fetal thymus) to an immunodeficient patient. **3.** A therapeutic modality intending to non-specifically induce the immune system of a cancer patient to destroy malignant cells. **4.** Treatment with immunosuppressive drugs or biologic products.

impaction (im-pak'shun) A tight packing or wedging.

fecal i. A mass of compressed, hardened feces retained within the bowel, usually the sigmoid colon or rectum.

imperforate (im-per'fŏ-rāt) Abnormally closed. See also imperforate anus, under anus;

imperforate hymen, under hymen.

implant (im′plant) Any material, object, or device inserted or placed within the body.

> **breast i.** A silicone bag filled with silicone gel, saline, air, or a combination thereof, placed either behind the breast or behind the pectoral muscle to increase breast size (augmentation mammoplasty) or to reconstruct the breast after mastectomy.

> **interstitial i.** In radiation therapy, a radioactive material placed within the tissues (e.g., within the vaginal wall).

> **intracavitary i.** In radiation therapy, a radioactive material placed in a body cavity (e.g., in the vagina or the chest cavity).

> **penile i.** See penile prosthesis, under prosthesis.

> **powder burn i.'s** Descriptive term applied to the characteristic peritoneal lesions of endometriosis; typically, they begin as minute red lesions on the peritoneal surface and grow to about 10 mm in diameter, becoming cystic with scarring and thickening of surrounding tissues, and ranging in color from dark brown or blue to black.

> **subdermal contraceptive i.** A reversible female contraceptive implanted under the skin; effective for an extended period of time (usually 5 years). Trade name: Norplant.

implantation (im-plan-ta′shun) **1.** Attachment of the embryo to the endometrium (the inner layer of the uterine wall); the process begins 5 to 7 days after fertilization of the ovum. **2.** The surgical placement of an implant.

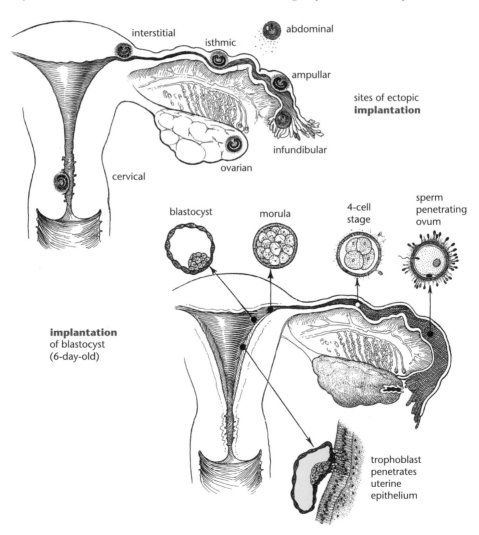

interstitial · isthmic · abdominal · ampullar · infundibular · ovarian · cervical

sites of ectopic **implantation**

implantation of blastocyst (6-day-old)

blastocyst · morula · 4-cell stage · sperm penetrating ovum

trophoblast penetrates uterine epithelium

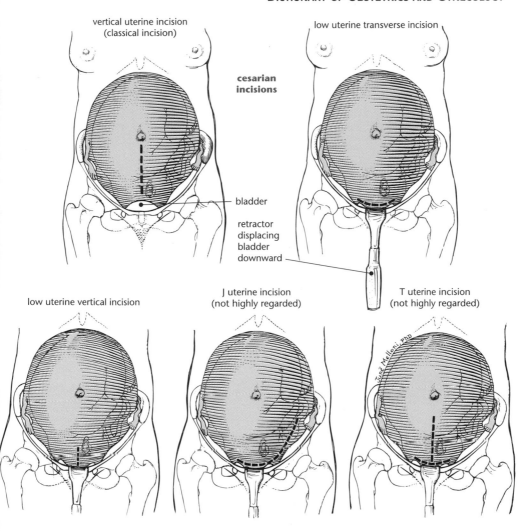

vertical uterine incision
(classical incision)

low uterine transverse incision

cesarian
incisions

bladder

retractor
displacing
bladder
downward

low uterine vertical incision

J uterine incision
(not highly regarded)

T uterine incision
(not highly regarded)

impotence (im'pŏ-tens) Term traditionally used to describe the inability to attain and maintain erection of the penis sufficiently to permit satisfactory sexual intercourse. Currently, the term 'erectile dysfunction' has been suggested as more precise to describe the condition. See erectile dysfunction, under dysfunction.

impregnate (im-preg'nat) **1.** To render pregnant. **2.** To saturate.

in- Prefix meaning in; into; toward; causing to become; becoming; emphasis.

inactivation (in-ak-tĭ-va'shun) Destruction of a biological activity.

    X i. See lyonization.

inborn (in'born) Ambiguous term generally meaning acquired genetically; inherited.

    i. errors of metabolism See under error.

incest (in'sest) Sexual intercourse or sexual activity between persons closely related by blood (e.g., parents and offspring, brothers and sisters).

incestuous (in-ses'chu-us) Relating to incest.

incision (in-sizh'un) **1.** A surgical cut. **2.** The act of cutting.

    Battle's i. A vertical incision along the outer border of the abdominal rectus muscle, with division of the rectus sheath and retraction of the rectus muscle inward. Also called lateral rectus incision.

    bikini i. A horizontal skin incision near the pubic hairline; made to gain access to the uterus (e.g., for an abdominal hysterectomy or cesarean section).

    celiotomy i. An incision through the abdominal wall to gain entry into the peritoneal cavity.

    cesarean i.'s Any incision through the

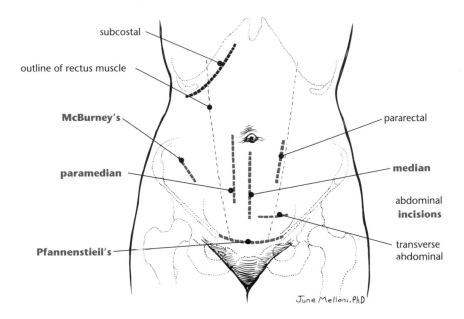

subcostal

outline of rectus muscle

McBurney's

paramedian

Pfannenstieil's

pararectal

median

abdominal **incisions**

transverse abdominal

June Melloni, PhD

anterior abdominal wall and the uterus; made to approach the fetus or fetuses for delivery.

Cherney i. A transverse lower abdominal incision of the skin and subcutaneous tissue in which the rectus muscle is detached at its insertion from the pubic symphysis to gain access to the abdominal parietal peritoneum. See also Maylard incision.

Dührssen's i.'s Two or three longitudinal incisions made in the cervix (when it is fully effaced and more than 7 cm dilated) to facilitate vaginal delivery of the fetal head; performed in current practice only in extreme emergencies (e.g., impaction of an aftercoming head of a premature viable infant in breech presentation). Also called hysterostomatomy.

Kustner i. A variation of the Pfannenstiel incision in which, after separating the skin and subcutaneous tissue, a midline incision of the rectus fascia and peritoneum is made as in the approach of an ordinary midline lower abdominal incision.

lateral rectus i. See Battle's incision.

Maylard i. A transverse lower abdominal incision of the skin and subcutaneous tissue in which the belly of the rectus muscle is transected to gain access to the abdominal parietal peritoneum. See also Cherney incision.

McBurney's i. An oblique abdominal incision, in the right lower quadrant, parallel to the fibers of the external oblique muscle;

located approximately one-third the distance along a line between the anterior superior iliac spine and the navel; commonly used in appendectomy.

median i. A surgical incision in the midline of the anterior abdominal wall; designated *lower median i.* when made below the navel to expose the pelvic organs; or *upper median i.* when made above the navel to expose the stomach and transverse colon. Also called midline incision.

midline i. See median incision.

paramedian i. A vertical incision about 2.5 cm from, and parallel to, the midline of the anterior abdominal wall; it permits the lateral retraction of the abdominal rectus muscle.

Pfannenstiel i. A curved, transverse abdominal incision through the skin and subcutaneous tissue, just above the pubic symphysis; the rectus fascia and peritoneum are subsequently incised transversely.

relief i. A skin incision made away from a wound to relax the tension of the skin so that it can be stretched to cover the wound.

Wiser i. A paramedian incision extending above and below the navel.

inclination (in-klĭ-na'shun) A tilting; a leaning.

pelvic i. The 55-degree angle formed by the horizontal plane and the plane of the pelvic inlet when the individual stands in the erect position.

incompatibility (in-kom-pat-ĭ-bil'ĭ-te) The state of being incompatible.

ABO i. The potential for isoimmunization occurring in about 20% of pregnancies when the mother's major blood group is type O, with anti-A and anti-B in her serum, while the fetal blood group is A, B, or AB. Only 5% of fetuses in such a situation will develop hemolytic disease of the newborn.

incompatible (in-kom-pat′ĭ-bl) Incapable of being mixed or used simultaneously without producing undesirable effects or undergoing chemical changes (e.g., blood which, when administered to someone whose own blood is of a different type triggers harmful immune reactions; or certain drugs whose interactions render them injurious or ineffective).

incompetence (in-kom′pĕ-tens) The state of being insufficient; inability of an organ or part to perform its required function adequately.

   cervical i. Failure of the cervical opening to remain closed during pregnancy due to either an anatomic or a functional defect; it is a frequent cause of second trimester pregnancy loss.

incompetent (in-kom′pĕ-tent) **1.** Characterized by incompetence. **2.** Held to be legally unqualified to make certain kinds of decisions independently, or to participate in a judicial proceeding.

incontinence (in-kon′tĭ-nens) Inability to control the passage of urine or feces.

   anorectal i. Involuntary passage of flatus or feces, which may occur as a complication of operative vaginal delivery; caused by faulty repair or healing of third- and fourth-degree perineal lacerations (which involve the anal sphincter muscles and the lowest portion of the rectum).

   bypass i. Diversion and leakage of urine through an abnormal channel (fistula, ectopic urethral opening, ectopic ureter); may also be the result of an overflow of urine retained within a urethral diverticulum or from pelvic surgery or irradiation.

   overflow i. Transurethral leakage of bladder urine when normal control mechanisms are insufficient to overcome increasing pressure within an overly distending bladder. Commonly associated with a neuropathy.

   stress i. Involuntary passage of urine occurring with physical stress (e.g., coughing, sneezing, or straining). Also called stress urinary incontinence.

   stress urinary i. (SUI) See stress incontinence.

   urge i. Inability to postpone voiding because the urge to urinate is abrupt and uncontrollable.

incontinent (in-kon′tĭ-nent) Characterized by incontinence.

incubation (in-ku-ba′shun) **1.** The phase of an infectious disease from the time the infectious organism enters the body to the appearance of the first symptoms. **2.** The maintenance of the optimal condition of an environment with regard to temperature, humidity, and gas content (e.g., for the care of a premature infant, for maintenance of bacterial cultures, or for the

INCUBATION PERIODS OF VARIOUS DISEASES

disease	incubation periods	rash
diphtheria	2–5 days	—
scarlet fever	1–5 days	1–5 days
measles	10–15 days	10–15 days
rubella	14–21 days	14–21 days
chickenpox	14–21 days	14–21 days
mumps	7–26 days	—
gonorrhea	1–8 days	—
hepatitis A	15–45 days	—
hepatitis B	4–26 weeks (typically 6–8 weeks)	—
hepatitis C	8–12 weeks	—
hepatitis D	30–120 days (typically 60 days)	—
hepatitis E	14–60 days (typically 40 days)	—
syphilis	1–6 weeks	—

preparation of biologic and chemical materials).

index (in'deks), pl. indexes, indices **1.** The forefinger; the second finger of the hand. **2.** A numerical value usually a ratio of one measurement to another.

>**body mass i.** (BMI) The body weight in kilograms divided by the height in meters squared. Also called Quetelet index.

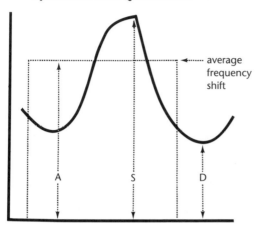

pulsatility index: S–D/A
resistance index: S–D/S
systolic/diastolic ratio = S/D

>**cephalic i.** The ratio of the maximal breadth to the maximal length of the head of a living subject (breadth × 100/length). Also called length–breadth index.

>**chemotherapeutic i.** The ratio of the minimal effective dose of a drug to the maximal tolerated dose.

>**chest i.** See thoracic index.

>**clitoral i.** A ratio of the length to the width of the clitoris expressed in centimeters.

>**fetopelvic i.** A value based on the differences in certain maternal pelvic dimensions, as obtained by x-ray pelvimetry, and certain fetal vertex dimensions obtained by ultrasonography; used to evaluate fetomaternal relationships that may be predictive of a difficult labor (dystocia).

>**hemizona assay i.** (HZI) In testing the functional capacity of sperm: the ratio of the number of zona-bound sperm for the test sample to the number of zona-bound sperm for the fertile donor sample.

>**icterus i.** A value indicating the relative amount of bilirubin in the blood.

>**length-breadth i.** See cephalic index.

>**maturation i.** An index for detecting estrogenic activity by determining the

percentage of mature cells exfoliated from the vagina; the action of estrogen matures the vaginal lining, therefore the higher percentage of mature cells exfoliated suggests increased estrogenic activity.

>**mitotic i.** (MI) The percentage of cells undergoing mitoses in a total cell sample.

>**ponderal i.** (PI) The body weight (or birthweight of a neonate) in grams multiplied by 100, divided by the square of the height (or of the crown–heel length of a neonate) in centimeters.

>**Pourcelot i.** See resistance index.

>**pulsatility i.** Doppler measurements of blood flow in certain maternal and fetal blood vessels, calculated by dividing the difference in systolic (S) and diastolic (D) shifts by the average frequency shift (A).

>**resistance i.** Doppler measurement of the blood flow in certain maternal or fetal blood vessels, calculated by dividing the difference in systolic (S) and diastolic (D) shifts by the systolic value, or (S–D)/S. Also called Pourcelot index.

>**Quetelet i.** See body mass index.

>**thoracic i.** The ratio of the anteroposterior to the transverse diameter of the chest. Also called chest index.

induce (in-doos') To bring about or to effect by stimulation; to cause.

induction (in-duk'shun) The process of inducing.

>**i. of labor** The stimulation of uterine contractions before the spontaneous onset of labor for the purpose of accomplishing delivery.

>**menstrual i.** See menstrual aspiration, under aspiration.

indwelling (in-dwel'ing) Remaining in place; applied to a catheter or drainage tube that is fixed and held in position for a period of time.

inertia (in-er'she-ă) **1.** Resistance offered by a physical mass to a change in its position of rest or motion. **2.** Inability to move unless stimulated by an external force.

>**uterine i.** Absence of effective uterine contractions during labor.

infant (in'fant) An individual from the moment of birth to the end of 1 year of life.

>**appropriate-for-gestational age i., AGA i.** An infant whose weight is between the 10th and 90th percentiles when compared with other infants of the same gestational age.

>**blue on pink i.** A newborn infant whose skin is pink with bluish undertones, or bluish with pink undertones (rather than appearing clearly cyanotic); may indicate inadequate oxygenation, inadequate ventilation, poor perfusion, or polycythemia.

dysmature i. See postmature infant.

excessive-size i. An infant who at the time of birth weighs over 4500 g (9.9 lbs).

extremely low-birthweight i. See very low-birthweight infant.

floppy i. See Werdnig-Hoffmann disease, under disease.

immature i. An infant born between the ages of 20 and 28 weeks of gestation, weighing 500 to 1000 g (1.1–2.2 lbs).

large-for-gestational-age i., LGA i. An infant whose weight is greater than the 90th percentile of that particular gestational age or two standard deviations above the mean weight for gestational age.

live-born i. An infant who, after being expelled or extracted from the mother, breathes or shows other evidence of life (such as beating of the heart, pulsation of the umbilical cord, and definite movements of involuntary muscles) whether or not the umbilical cord has been cut or the placenta has detached.

low-birthweight i., LBW i. An infant weighing 2500 g (5.5 lbs) or less at birth.

mature i. See term infant.

oversize i. Infant weighing over 4000 g (8.8 lbs).

postdates i. See postterm infant.

postmature i. A postterm infant whose placenta has diminished capacity for sufficient exchange, resulting in cutaneous and nutritional changes. Also called dysmature infant. See also postmaturity syndrome, under syndrome.

postterm i. An infant born after 42 or more completed weeks of gestation. Also called postdates infant.

premature i. An infant born between 28 and 38 weeks of gestation, weighing 1000 to 2500 g (2.2–5.5 lbs). Popularly called preemie.

preterm i. General term for an infant born at any time through the 37th week of gestation (259 days).

small-for-gestational-age i., SGA i. An infant whose weight is less than the 10th percentile for all infants at that particular gestational age or more than 2 standard deviations below the mean for gestational age. Also called undergrown infant. See also intrauterine growth retardation, under retardation.

stillborn i. An infant who shows no signs of life at birth.

term i., i. at term An infant born no earlier than 38 weeks but not later than 42 weeks of gestation. Also called mature infant.

undergrown i. See small-for-gestational-age infant.

very low-birthweight i., VLBW i. An infant weighing less than 1000 g (2.2 lbs) at birth. Also called extremely low-birthweight infant.

infanticide (in-fan'tĭ-sīd) The killing of an infant by a willful act of commission or omission.

infarct (in'farkt) An area of dead tissue caused most often by obstruction of its arterial supply or, rarely, by obstruction of venous drainage.

infarction (in-fark'shun) **1.** The formation of an infarct. **2.** An infarct.

myocardial i. (MI) Deterioration and/or death of a portion of the heart muscle as a result of deprivation of its blood supply, usually by occlusion of a coronary artery supplying blood to the area; the occlusion may or may not be due to a blood clot. Popularly called heart attack; coronary.

placental i. Degenerative lesions in the placenta varying in size, location, and degree of degeneration; caused by impairment of the uteroplacental circulation, usually by blood clots obstructing the blood flow through the spiral arteries.

infection (in-fek'shun) A phenomenon characterized by an inflammatory response to the presence of living microorganisms or their invasion of normally sterile tissue.

amniotic fluid i. Infection of the amniotic fluid with any of a variety of microorganisms (e.g., group B streptococci, *Gardnerella vaginalis*, and species of *Mycoplasma* and *Chlamydia*); may follow rupture of the membranes or may occur with intact membranes, leading to preterm labor; clinical symptoms may include fever, uterine tenderness, and a foul-smelling amniotic fluid. Also called intra-amniotic infection.

bacterial i. Infection with any of numerous aerobic and anaerobic bacteria; among those particularly affecting the pregnancy outcome or the newborn infant are species of *Chlamydia*, *Listeria*, *Escherichia*, *Mycoplasma*, *Neisseria*, *Staphylococcus*, and *Streptococcus*. For specific bacterial infections, see the individual disease or bacterium involved.

chlamydial i. Bacterial infection with species of *Chlamydia*, usually *Chlamydia trachomatis*. See also *Chlamydia trachomatis*, under *Chlamydia*; lymphogranuloma venereum.

disseminated gonococcal i. (DGI) A rare but important febrile complication of *Neisseria gonorrhoeae* mucosal infection, characterized by pustular skin lesions in the distal extremities, inflammation of tendon-lining sheaths (tenosynovitis), and arthritis involving multiple joints (polyarthritis). See also Reiter's syndrome, under syndrome.

hospital-acquired i. See nosocomial infection.

inapparent i. The presence of an infection in a person without the occurrence of recognizable clinical manifestations; it is of epidemiological significance because people so infected serve as carriers and spread the infective agent.

intra-amniotic i. See amniotic fluid infection.

latent i. A persistent inapparent infection in which the causative microorganism cannot be detected by currently available methods; the infection may flare up from time to time under certain conditions. Also called subclinical infection.

listerial i. See listeriosis.

MAC i. See *Mycobacterium avium* complex bacteremia, under bacteremia.

mycoplasmal i. Infection with microorganisms of the genus *Mycoplasma*. See also *Mycoplasma*.

nosocomial i. An infection acquired as a result of hospitalization or treatment received at a hospital and that was not present or incubating at the time of exposure to the hospital environment; usually caused by exposure to bacteria or fungi either through diagnostic or therapeutic procedures, or from the natural hospital environment (which harbors a multitude of microorganisms from other patient's infectious diseases), or from the hospital staff; predisposing factors include a patient's susceptible state. Common nosocomial infections include those of the genitourinary tract (e.g., from indwelling catheters), lungs (e.g., from respiratory tract instrumentation), surgical wounds, and newborn infants (e.g., epidemic diarrhea in the nursery). Also called hospital-acquired infection.

opportunistic i. A secondary infection occurring in an individual whose immune system is already debilitated by another prevailing infection (e.g., infections occurring in an AIDS patient).

pelvic i. General term for a variety of infections involving the pelvic organs and adjacent tissues; they include pelvic inflammatory disease, postpartum (puerperal) infections, infections following gynecologic or obstetric surgery, and abortion-associated infections. See also pelvic inflammatory

disease, under disease.

perinatal i. Any infection occurring during the time of life between the completion of 20 weeks of gestation and the first 28 days after birth (i.e., during the perinatal period).

postpartum i., puerperal i. Infection caused by any of a variety of aerobic and anaerobic bacteria that are normal vaginal flora of pregnant and nonpregnant women without causing disease; the infection is thought to be facilitated by the physiologic changes of labor and delivery; typically, it causes a fever of 38°C (100.4°F) or higher on any two successive days after the first 24 hours postpartum and is usually accompanied by chills, headache, malaise, and loss of appetite; it is most commonly seen in those women who have undergone premature rupture of the membranes, prolonged labor, multiple pelvic examinations, and operative delivery.

pyogenic i. A pus-producing infection caused by such bacteria as *Staphylococcus aureus* and *Streptococcus pyogenes*.

retrograde i. An infection of a tubular structure that spreads in a direction opposite to that of the natural flow of secretions.

subclinical i. See latent infection.

urinary tract i. (UTI) Infection of the urinary tract with any of a variety of microorganisms (bacterial, viral, or fungal); the infection may involve the lower urinary tract (urethra, prostate, bladder) or the upper urinary tract (kidneys, ureters), or both, and may be asymptomatic or symptomatic. Pregnancy is a predisposing factor to upper urinary tract infection due to the normal physiologic changes of the pregnant state (e.g., decreased tone and peristaltic activity of the ureters), increasing the risk of premature delivery and death of the newborn infant.

viral i. Infection with any of a variety of viruses; some have deleterious effects on pregnancy and/or the newborn (e.g., cytomegalovirus (CMV), human herpesvirus (HHV), human immunodeficiency virus (HIV), and the virus causing rubella). For specific viral infections, see the individual disease or virus involved.

yeast i. See candidiasis

infectious (in-fek'shus) Capable of being transmitted with or without direct contact.

infecundity (in-fĕ-kun'dĭ-te) A woman's inability to bear children.

infertility (in-fer-til'ĭ-te) **1.** Inability to produce offspring. In males, inability to fertilize the ovum; in females, inability to conceive after 1 year of regular intercourse without use of contraceptives. Infertility may or may not be reversible. Compare with sterility. **2.** Inability of a woman to carry a pregnancy to term. Also called impaired fertility.

infibulation (in-fib-u-la'shun) A form of female circumcision in which the entire clitoris, the whole labia minora, and at least two-thirds of the labia majora are removed, typically performed at the age 7 years. Currently practiced in countries throughout Africa and in the Middle East, and in Muslim populations of Malaysia and Indonesia. Also called pharaonic circumcision.

infiltration (in-fil-tra'shun) **1.** Accumulation of substances that are not ordinarily present in the tissue where they accumulate, or invasion of tissues by cells that are not normal to the site. **2.** Injection of a solution into a tissue (e.g., in local anesthesia).

informed consent (in-form'ed kon-sent') See under consent.

infra- Prefix meaning below, beneath.

infraumbilical (in-fra-um-bil'ĭ-kal) Below the navel.

infundibulum (in-fun-dib'u-lum), pl. infundibula Any funnel-shaped structure or passage; when used alone, the term refers to the infundibulum of the pituitary.

    i. of lung In the embryo, the minute expanded termination of bronchioles from which the air sacs (pulmonary alveoli) develop after the fifth to sixth month of development.

    i. of uterine tube The lateral, funnel-shaped opening of the fallopian (uterine) tube.

inguinal (ing'gwĭ-nal) Relating to the groin.

inheritance (in-her'ĭ-tans) **1.** In genetics, the process of transmitting characters from parent to offspring. **2.** The characters so transmitted.

    autosomal i. The transmission of a character determined by a gene located in any chromosome in the body other than those of the sex cells (sperm and ovum).

    dominant i. An inheritance that is manifest when the individual is heterozygous for the mutant gene (i.e., the individual has one copy of the mutant gene from one parent and one copy of the normal gene from the other parent).

    holandric i. Transmission of a character determined by a gene on the Y chromosome (i.e., occurring only in males).

    hologynic i. Transmission of a character from a mother to all her daughters but not to her sons (i.e., occurring only in females).

    multifactorial i. Inheritance determined by a combination of many factors, both genetic and environmental, each producing a partial

effect. Distinguished from polygenic inheritance.

    polygenic i. Strictly, inheritance determined by a large number of genes located at different sites (loci) on the chromosome and having small additive effects; in this restricted sense, the term may not apply to human disorders but is sometimes used to designate traits caused by multiple genes with no apparent environmental influences. Distinguished from multifactorial inheritance.

    recessive i. An inheritance that is manifest only when an individual is homozygous for the mutant gene (i.e., the individual carries a double dose of the mutant gene, one from each parent).

    sex-linked i. See sex linkage, under linkage.

    X-linked i. See X linkage, under linkage.

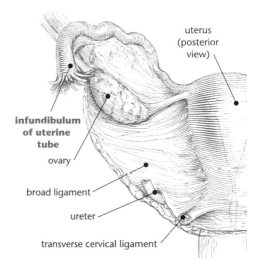

uterus (posterior view)

infundibulum of uterine tube

ovary

broad ligament

ureter

transverse cervical ligament

inhibin (in-hib'in) Either of two glycoproteins, secreted by the Sertoli's cells of the testis and the granulosa cells of the ovary, that inhibit pituitary release of follicle-stimulating hormone (FSH).

inhibitor (in-hib'ĭ-tor) Any agent or nerve that represses or diminishes a physiologic activity.

    ACE i. See angiotensin-converting enzyme inhibitor.

    angiotensin-converting enzyme i. (ACEI) Any of a class of drugs that inhibit the action of the enzyme kininase II, which converts angiotensin I to angiotensin II; used in the treatment of high blood pressure and congestive heart failure. Use of ACEIs during pregnancy increases the risk for fetal death. Also called ACE inhibitor.

    prostaglandin i. An antagonist to the action

of prostaglandins, either by suppressing prostaglandin synthesis or by blocking prostaglandin action on target organs.

initiation (ĭ-nish-e-a'shun) In chemical carcinogenesis, the first stage in the process leading to the development of a cancerous tumor; characterized by irreversible mutagenic changes inflicted upon the DNA of cells by a chemical agent. Affected (initiated) cells do not, at this time, grow and proliferate abnormally; unlike normal cells, however, they give rise to a tumor when subsequently exposed to an appropriate chemical (the promoter). See also promotion.

injection (in-jek'shun) **1.** The act of introducing a fluid into a tissue or body cavity. **2.** The fluid injected. **3.** Popular term for a state of visible congestion or hyperemia (c.g., of blood vessels of the eye).

> **hypodermic i.** See subcutaneous injection.
> **intracytoplasmic sperm i.** (ICSI) An *in vitro* fertilization procedure in which a single sperm is introduced directly into the cytoplasm of the egg. See also insemination.
> **intramuscular (IM) i.** Injection into a muscle.
> **intrathecal i.** Injection into the subarachnoid space (e.g., of an anesthetic solution to induce spinal anesthesia).
> **intravenous (IV) i.** Injection into a vein.
> **subcutaneous i.** Injection into the loose tissue just beneath the skin. Also called hypodermic injection; popularly called hypo.

injury (in'jŭ-re) Damage to any part of the body by any of a wide variety of external means (mechanical, chemical, radiant, electrical, or thermal) and which may or may not cause a disability.

> **birth i.** Damage sustained by an infant during labor and delivery. Usual predisposing conditions include prematurity, prolonged pregnancy, breech birth, an abnormally large fetus, a small maternal pelvic opening, and the use of forceps to extract the infant from the birth canal.
> **irradiation i.** A complication of radiation therapy for the treatment of cancer in which surrounding noncancerous tissues are damaged by radiation exposure; the extent of damage varies, depending on the total dose of radiation used.

inlet (in'let) A passage leading into a cavity.

> **pelvic i.** See pelvic plane of inlet, under plane.

innate (in'nāt) Present at birth.

inotropic (in-o-trop'ik) Affecting muscular contraction.

> **negatively i.** Inhibiting muscular contraction.
> **positively i.** Enhancing muscular contraction

insemination (in-sem-ĭ-na'shun) **1.** Introduction of seminal fluid into the vagina. **2.** Fertilization of an ovum.

> **artificial i.** Deposit of sperm in the vagina, cervix, or within the uterine cavity by means other than sexual intercourse.
> **artificial insemination, donor** (AID) See heterologous insemination.
> **artificial insemination, husband** (AIH) See homologous insemination.
> **direct intraperitoneal i.** (DIPI) Injection of washed, processed sperm into the peritoneal cavity, in the area of the rectouterine pouch, via puncture of the posterior vaginal cul-de-sac; performed at the expected time of ovulation.
> **donor i.** See therapeutic insemination.
> **heterologous i.** Artificial insemination with sperm from a donor other than the woman's husband.
> **homologous i.** Artificial insemination with sperm from the woman's husband.
> **intrauterine i.** (IUI) The direct placement of sperm in the intrauterine cavity using a washed and concentrated specimen (i.e., sperm that has been diluted and centrifuged to remove the prostaglandin-containing seminal fluid); usually performed to bypass the uterine cervix when infertility is due to a cervical condition (i.e., when there are problems with this structure or its secretions). Also called washed intrauterine insemination.
> **subzonal i.** (SUZI) An *in vitro* fertilization technique in which five to ten spermatozoa are injected, with a microneedle, under the zona pellucida of the ovum (i.e., into the perivitelline space); employed in cases of sperm factor infertility. Also called subzonal insertion.
> **therapeutic i.** Procedure in which fresh sperm, either from the husband (TIH) or a donor (TID), is placed in a woman's vagina, cervix, or uterus; performed in the periovulatory part of the menstrual cycle. Also called donor insemination.
> **washed intrauterine i.** See intrauterine insemination (IUI).

insensitivity (in-sen-sĭ-tiv'ĭ-te) Lack of response.

> **complete androgen i.** See complete testicular feminization, under feminization.
> **incomplete androgen i.** See incomplete testicular feminization, under feminization.

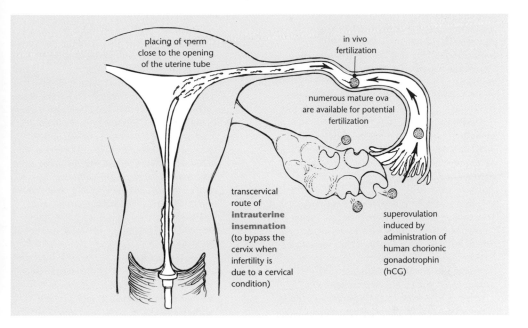

placing of sperm
close to the opening
of the uterine tube

in vivo
fertilization

numerous mature ova
are available for potential
fertilization

transcervical
route of
**intrauterine
insemnation**
(to bypass the
cervix when
infertility is
due to a cervical
condition)

superovulation
induced by
administration of
human chorionic
gonadotrophin
(hCG)

insertion (in-ser'shun) **1.** A place or mode of attachment. **2.** The site of attachment of a muscle to the bone that is most movable during the action of that muscle. **3.** A chromosomal abnormality in which DNA breaks off from one chromosome and is then interposed into a break of a dissimilar chromosome.

> **velamentous cord i.** A type of umbilical cord insertion of practical importance because the umbilical vessels run across the fetal membranes at a distance from the body of the placenta. They are surrounded only by a fold of amnion (devoid of Wharton's jelly); thus they are at risk for rupture and hemorrhage during amniorrhexis. Found most frequently in multiple gestations. See also vasa previa.

> **subzonal i.** See subzonal insemination, under insemination.

in situ (in si'tu) Latin for in place; in its original or normal position. The term is applied especially to an early stage in cancerous tumor development in which abnormal cells are still restricted to the site of origin (i.e., they have not invaded tissues beyond their original confines). Sometimes used synonymously with precancerous.

instability (in-stă-bil'ĭ-te) A lack of physical or emotional stability.

> **detrusor i.** A condition in which uninhibited urinary bladder contractions are associated with urinary incontinence; may be caused by multiple sclerosis or by neurologic lesions, such as those caused by a stroke; commonly no specific cause can be identified. Also called detrusor dyssynergia; detrusor hyperreflexia.

insufficiency (in-sŭ-fish'en-se) Inability to perform a normal function.

> **venous i.** Inadequate drainage of blood from a part resulting from a swollen condition of that part.

insufflation (in-sŭ-fla'shun) The act of blowing a gas, medicated vapor, powder, or anesthetic into a body cavity.

> **tubal i.** The transvaginal introduction of a gas, usually carbon dioxide, into the uterus to determine whether the fallopian (uterine) tubes are free of obstruction. Also called tubal insufflation test; Rubin test.

insulin (in'sŭ-lin) A hormone produced by the beta cells of the islets of Langerhans in the pancreas and secreted in response to increased blood sugar (glucose) levels, vagus nerve stimulation, and other factors; it is concerned with regulating metabolism of carbohydrate, lipid, and protein. Deficiency of insulin results in diabetes mellitus.

intention (in-ten'shun) **1.** A process. **2.** Objective.

> **healing by first i.** See under healing.
> **healing by second i.** See under healing.
> **healing by third i.** See under healing.

inter- Prefix meaning between, among.

intercourse (in'ter-kors) **1.** Interchange or interactions between or among people. **2.** Coitus.

> **sexual i.** Coitus.

interferon (in-ter-fēr'on) (INF) Any of a family of

proteins produced by certain body cells in response to invasion by viruses and other intracellular parasites; it interferes with proliferation of the virus and is effective against such protozoan infections as malaria; may also inhibit growth of cancerous tumors.

i.-gamma, i.-γ (INF-γ) The major interferon produced by T lymphocytes in response to the presence of specific antigen.

interleukin (in-ter-loo'kin) (IL) Any of a group of molecules (IL-1 through IL-7) manufactured by a variety of cells; the molecules mediate cellular activities by acting as messengers transmitting signals between cells.

interleukin-1 A hormone-like molecule (cytokine) that has multiple biologic activities (metabolic, endocrine, immunologic, hematologic), including the ability to induce fever during inflammatory reactions; in the immune system, it acts upon macrophages and monocytes, enhancing their antitumor activities by inducing its own production and the production of other hormone-like substances such as tumor-necrosis factor (TNF) and interleukin-6 (IL-6).

interleukin-2 A glycoprotein that induces proliferation of responsive T lymphocytes; released by certain activated cells.

intermenstrual (in-ter-men'stroo-al) Denoting the interval between two consecutive menstrual periods.

intersex (in'ter-seks) See hermaphrodite.

intersexuality (in-ter-seks-u-al'ĭ-te) See hermaphroditism.

interstitial (in-ter-stish'al) Relating to, occurring, or located within the minute spaces within a tissue.

intertriginous (in-ter-trij'ĭ-nus) Relating to intertrigo.

intertrigo (in-ter-tri'go) Inflammatory skin eruption occurring between two adjacent surfaces (e.g., between the vulva or the scrotum and the thigh).

interval (in'ter-val) **1.** A gap in a continuous process. **2.** A distance between two objects. **3.** The lapse of time between two events or between the recurrence of similar episodes of a disease.

birth i. (1) The lapse of time between the time of sexual intercourse by a woman and the birth of her first child. (2) The lapse of time between successive births.

neonatal i. See neonatal period, under period.

perinatal i. See perinatal period, under period.

intervillous (in-ter-vil'us) Among the minute hairlike projections (villi) on the surface of certain tissues.

intestine (in-tes'tin) The portion of the digestive tract from the pyloric end of the stomach to the anus. Also called bowel.

large i. The sacculated portion of the intestine, extending from the end of the ileum to the anus; subdivided into three parts: cecum (including appendix), colon, and rectum.

small i. The convoluted portion of the intestine, extending from the pyloric end of the stomach to the cecum, where it joins the large intestine; it lies in the central and lower parts of the abdominal cavity and is subdivided into three parts: duodenum, jejunum, and ileum.

intolerance (in-tol'er-ans) Unfavorable reaction to a substance.

lactose i. Intolerance to the milk sugar lactose due to deficiency of the enzyme lactase; characterized by abdominal cramps and diarrhea upon ingestion of milk and milk products.

pregnancy-induced glucose i. See gestational diabetes mellitus, under diabetes.

intra- Prefix meaning within.

intracervical (in-tră-ser've-kal) See endocervical.

intraductal (in-tră-duk'tal) Within a duct.

intraepithelial (in-tră-ep-ĭ-the'le-al) Within the epithelium (i.e., the cells forming the outermost layer of a lining membrane).

intraictal (in-tră-ik'tal) Occurring during a convulsion or seizure.

intraluminal (in-tră-lu'mĭ-nal) Within the lumen of a tubular structure.

intramural (in-tră-mu'ral) Within the walls of an organ, cavity, or any tubular structure.

intraoperative (in-tră-op'er-ă-tiv) Occurring or performed during the actual surgical operation (e.g., ancillary care or procedures, complications).

intrapartum (in-tră-par'tum) Relating to labor and delivery of the child. See also antepartum; postpartum.

intraperitoneal (in-tră-per-ĭ-to-ne'al) (IP) Within the peritoneum-lined cavity (i.e., the abdominopelvic cavity).

intrastromal (in-tră-stro'mal) Within the tissues (e.g., connective tissue) forming the framework of an organ.

intrathecal (in-tră-the'kal) Within a sheath.

intrauterine (in-tră-u'ter-in) Within the uterus.

intravascular (in-tră-vas'ku-lar) Within any blood vessel (vein or artery) or lymphatic vessel.

intravenous (in-tră-ve'nus) (IV) Within a vein.

intro- Prefix meaning into; directed inward.

introitus (in-tro'ĭ-tus) Entrance into a body cavity or hollow organ.

intromission (in-tro-mish'un) Insertion; introduction.

intubate (in'tu-bāt) To perform intubation.

intubation (in-tu-ba'shun) Introduction of a tube into a body cavity, canal, or any other tubular structure. Distinguished from catheterization. See also catheterization.

in utero (in u'ter-o) Latin for within the uterus.

invaginate (in-vaj'ĭ-nāt) To infold; to turn within; to ensheath.

invagination (in-vaj-ĭ-na'shun) **1.** The process of invaginating. **2.** The state of being invaginated.

invasion (in-va'zhun) **1.** The spread of a tumor, usually cancerous, to neighboring tissues. **2.** The beginning of a disease process.

> **stromal i.** Spread of malignant cells into the deeper, connective tissue of an organ (e.g., the spread of carcinoma *in situ* of the cervix, from the epithelium, through and beyond the basement membrane, and into the cervical stroma).

invasive (in-va'siv) **1.** Tending to spread to healthy tissues. **2.** Involving penetration of the skin or any body tissue; applied to certain procedures.

inversion (in-ver'zhun) **1.** A turning inside out. **2.** Any reversal of the normal relation of two organs or structures. **3.** In genetics, a structural abnormality of a chromosome resulting from fragmentation of the chromosome by two breaks, followed by a turning end for end of the fragment and reunification in the same place, so that the gene sequence for the fragment is reversed with regard to the rest of the chromosome.

> **i. of nipple** Failure of the nipple to protrude normally from the breast; it may be a benign congenital anomaly or it may be caused by a cancerous growth within the breast.

> **paracentric i.** Chromosomal inversion that takes place away from the centromere of the chromosome.

> **pericenter i.** Chromosomal inversion involving the centromere of the chromosome.

> **uterine i.** A turning inside out of the uterus; designated *incomplete uterine i.* when the inverted organ collapses into the cervical canal; or *complete uterine i.* when it protrudes into the vagina and, occasionally, through the vaginal opening. Occurs almost always after a vaginal delivery, made worse by excessive pulling of the umbilical cord before the placenta separates, and may be associated with severe postpartum hemorrhage; usually, it is successfully corrected after delivery is

completed. Rarely, the condition is associated with disordered placental implantation (e.g., placenta accreta, increta, or percreta), for which hysterectomy may be necessary.

invert (in'vert) To turn inside out or upside down.

in vitro (in ve'tro) In an environment outside of the body, usually a test tube, Petri dish, or similar artificial environment.

in vivo (in ve'vo) Occurring, or performed, in the living body; applied to biological events, reactions, or procedures.

involution (in-vo-lu'shun) A retrograde process resulting in lessening in the size of a tissue (e.g., the shrinking of body tissues in old age).

> **i. of uterus** The return of the uterus to normal size after childbirth.

involutional (in-vo-lu'shun-al) Relating to involution.

ionization (i-on-ĭ-za'shun) Production of electrically charged atoms or molecules (e.g., by irradiation).

irradiate (i-ra'de-āt) To treat with or to expose to

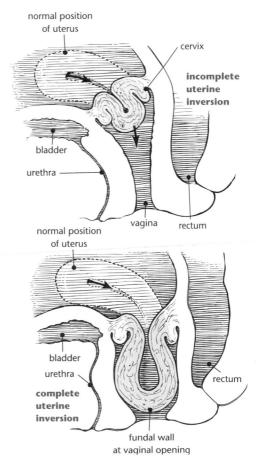

normal position of uterus

cervix

incomplete uterine inversion

bladder

urethra

vagina   rectum

normal position of uterus

bladder

urethra

rectum

complete uterine inversion

fundal wall at vaginal opening

radiation.

irradiation (i-ra-de-a'shun) **1.** Exposure to the action of rays. **2.** The condition resulting from having been subjected to radiation. See also radiation.

> **external i.** See external radiation, under radiation.

> **interstitial i.** See interstitial radiation, under radiation.

> **intracavitary i.** See intracavitary radiation, under radiation.

> **local i.** See local radiation, under radiation.

ischemia (is-ke'me-ă) Lack of blood in a circumscribed area of the body due to mechanical obstruction, or functional constriction of a blood vessel.

ischemic (is-kem'ik) Relating to ischemia.

ischia (is'ke-ă) Plural of ischium.

ischial (is'ke-al) Relating to the ischium.

ischio- Combining form meaning ischium.

ischiopagus (is-ke-op'ă-gus) Conjoined twins joined by the lower back part of the body; they may or may not share a limb.

ischium (is'ke-um), pl. ischia Either of the two bones (right or left) forming the lower, posterior portion of the hipbone; it is surrounded by cartilage in early life and eventually ossifies, fusing with the ilium and pubic bone to form the hipbone; along with the ilium and pubic bone, it contributes to the formation of the acetabulum (the cup-shaped cavity into which the head of the femur fits to form the hip joint); the two ischia are the bones on which the body rests when sitting. See also pubic bone, under bone; ilium; pelvis.

ischuria (is-ku're-ă) Suppression of urine.

iso- Prefix meaning equal; sameness.

isoagglutinin (i-so-ă-gloo'tĭ-nin) An antibody capable of clumping cells of individuals different from the individual from whom it originated, but of the same species. Also called isohemagglutinin.

isoantibody (i-so-an'tĭ-bod-e) An antibody from one individual that reacts with an antigen of another individual of the same species.

isoantigen (i-so-an'tĭ-jen) An antigen (such as a blood group antigen) that is present in some members of the same species and thus induces an immune response when transferred (e.g., by blood transfusion) to those who lack the antigen.

isocarboxasid (i-so-kar-bok'să-zid) Compound used to treat depression. Use during pregnancy has an increased risk of producing fetal malformations.

isogeneic, isogenic (i-so-jĕ-ne'ik, i-so-jen'ik) See syngeneic.

isohemagglutinin (i-so-hem-ă-gloo'tĭ-nin) See isoagglutinin.

isoimmunization (i-so-im-u-nĭ-za'shun) The development of specific antibody following exposure to, and against, an antigen originating in a genetically different individual of the same species.

> **ABO i.** Development of antibodies against major blood group antigens, most often type A and B, in a person of blood type O. When occurring during pregnancy, it can cause a relatively mild hemolytic disease of the newborn that usually is manifest after birth.

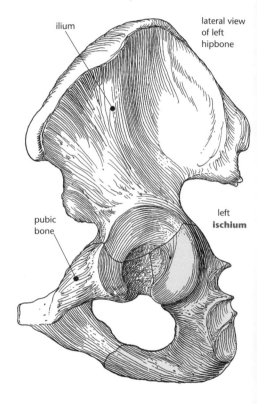

ilium

lateral view of left hipbone

pubic bone

left **ischium**

> **Rh i.** Development of antibodies against Rh antigens, especially the Rh$_0$ antigen (D antigen); may occur in an Rh-negative individual after transfusion of Rh-positive blood; may also occur in an Rh-negative woman pregnant with an Rh-positive fetus when exposed to fetal blood (e.g., during amniocentesis, miscarriage, abortion, or delivery); a subsequent pregnancy with an Rh-positive fetus may result in deleterious conditions in the newborn (e.g., hemolytic disease).

isologous (i-sol'o-gus) See syngeneic.

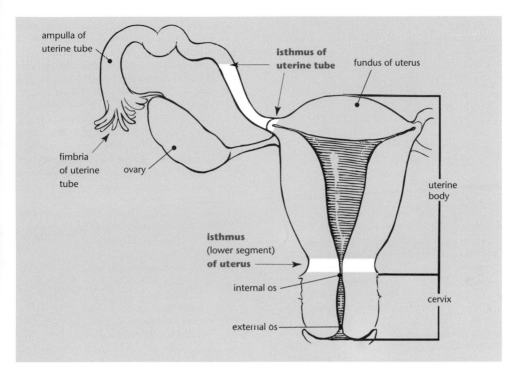

ampulla of
uterine tube

**isthmus of
uterine tube** fundus of uterus

fimbria
of uterine ovary
tube

uterine
body

**isthmus
(lower segment)
of uterus**

internal os

cervix

external os

isoplastic (i-so-plas'tik) See syngeneic.

isosexual (i-so-sek'shoo-al) Having the characteristics of the sex to which the individual belongs.

isosorbide dinitrate (i-so-sor'bīd di-ni'trāt) A vasodilator used for the treatment of cardiac insufficiency and angina pectoris. There is a possible increase of fetal malformations when taken during the first trimester of pregnancy.

Isospora belli (i-sos'pŏ-ră bel'e) A species of bacteria (family Eimeriidae) that is parasitic in human small intestines, sometimes causing mucous diarrhea, especially in children, and a type of diarrhea which is unresponsive to treatment in people with immunosuppressed conditions (e.g., AIDS).

isosporiasis (i-sos-po-ri'ă-sis) Infection with a species of *Isospora*.

isotope (i'so-tōp) One of two or more chemical elements in which all atoms have the same atomic number but varying atomic weights; many are radioactive.

isotretinoin (i-so-tret'ĭ-noin) A retinoid (13-*cis*-retinoic acid) administered systemically to treat cystic acne and other skin conditions. Maternal use during the first trimester of pregnancy produces severe birth defects, including anomalies of the external ear, and the craniofacial, cardiac, and central nervous systems; may also have deleterious effects in a breast-feeding infant when taken by the lactating mother.

isthmus (is'mus), pl. isthmi **1.** A narrow band of tissue connecting two larger parts. **2.** A narrow passage between two larger cavities or tubular structures.

   i. of fallopian tube See isthmus of uterine tube.

   i. of uterine tube The narrowest part of the fallopian (uterine) tube, at its attachment to the uterus. Also called isthmus of fallopian tube.

   i. of uterus The constricted upper third of the uterine cervix, contiguous with the body of the uterus.

-ite Suffix meaning a substance derived from some specified process (e.g., metabolite); a part of the body, especially in a developmental stage (e.g., somite).

-itis pl. -itises, -itides, -ites Word termination meaning inflammation of a specified organ or part (e.g., appendicitis).

-ity Suffix meaning a state; condition (e.g., immunity).

Ixodes (iks-o'dēz) Genus of parasitic ticks (family Ixodidae); some species are vectors of organisms causing human infections.

   I. dammini The deer tick; the chief vector of *Borrelia burgdorferi*, the spirochete causing Lyme disease.

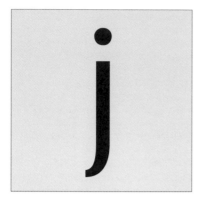

jaundice (jawn'dis) Yellow coloring of the skin and/or sclera resulting from high levels of the bile pigment bilirubin in the blood. Also called icterus.

    breast milk j. Jaundice occurring in some breast-fed newborn infants; usually begins about the fourth day after birth and lasts about 3 or 4 weeks.

    neonatal j. See physiologic jaundice.

    physiologic j. Slight jaundice of the newborn that disappears within 1 week after birth. Also called icterus neonatorum; neonatal icterus; neonatal jaundice; physiologic icterus.

    recurrent j. of pregnancy See intrahepatic cholestasis of pregnancy, under cholestasis.

jejunum (je-joo'num) The middle portion of the small intestine (the others being the duodenum and the ileum).

jelly (jel'e) A semisolid substance with a translucent appearance and resilient consistency.

    contraceptive j. A spermicidal jelly used alone or with a barrier contraceptive device to prevent conception.

    Wharton's j. The soft, homogeneous substance forming the matrix of the umbilical cord; it surrounds and supports the umbilical blood vessels.

jitteriness (jit'ě-re-nes) Condition similar to seizure activity observed in some newborn infants; characterized by abnormal, tremor-like movements of the extremities; unlike the coarse jerky movements of seizures, those of a jittery infant are finer, cease when the child's hands are grasped, and are not accompanied by abnormal eye movements.

joint (joint) The skeletal site at which two or more bones meet; an articulation.

    acromioclavicular j. The articulation between the lateral end of the collarbone (clavicle) and the acromion of the shoulder blade (scapula).

Charcot's j. A swollen, unstable but painless joint; it frequently occurs with destruction of intra-articular ligaments and consequent abnormally increased range of motion; caused by loss of sensory innervation; the lack of sensation deprives the joint of protective reactions to undue stresses. Considered a complication of a neurologic disorder (e.g., tabes dorsalis or diabetic neuropathy). Also called neuropathic joint.

    coccygeal j. See sacrococcygeal joint.

    hip j. The ball-and-socket joint between the head of the femur and the acetabulum of the hipbone.

    lumbosacral j. The joint between the fifth lumbar vertebra and the two articular surfaces of the base of the sacrum.

    neuropathic j. See Charcot's joint.

    sacrococcygeal j. The joint between the sacrum and the tailbone (coccyx). Also called coccygeal joint.

    sacroiliac j. The joint between the vertebral column and the pelvis, specifically between the two auricular surfaces on the upper part of the sacrum and each ilium on the posterior part of the pelvis.

    sternoclavicular j. The joint formed by the medial end of the collarbone (clavicle), the manubrium of the breastbone (sternum), and the cartilage of the first rib.

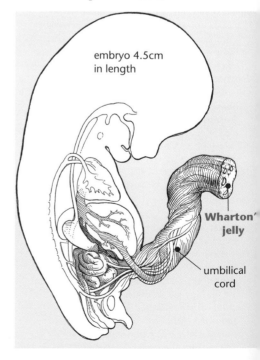

embryo 4.5cm in length

Wharton' jelly

umbilical cord

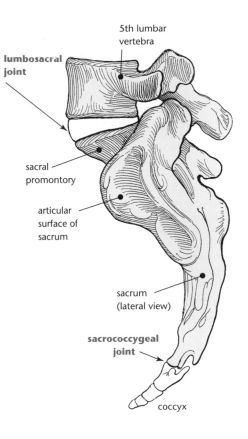

5th lumbar
vertebra

lumbosacral
joint

sacral
promontory

articular
surface of
sacrum

sacrum
(lateral view)

sacrococcygeal
joint

coccyx

joule (jōōl) (J) The unit of energy in the International System of Weights and Measures (SI); the heat generated, or energy expended, when a current of 1 ampere passes through a resistance of 1 ohm for 1 second.

junction (junk'shun) The line of union of two surfaces.

    anorectal j. The area where the rectum ends and the anal canal begins, in front of, and slightly below, the tip of the coccyx.

    gap j.'s Specialized regions of the cell membrane at which aggregates of proteins from adjacent cells interact to form pores permitting the exchange of ions and small metabolites, thereby facilitating their electrical and metabolic coupling.

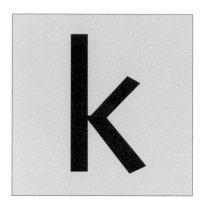

karyokinesis (kar-e-o-kĭ-ne'sis) The division of the nucleus during mitosis. See also mitosis.

karyotype (kar'e-o-tip) **1.** The chromosome constitution of an individual. **2.** A systematized graphic presentation of the whole set of chromosomes present in the nucleus of a single cell, arranged according to the standard classification (i.e., in pairs according to size); the chromosomes are photomicrographed during the metaphase stage of mitosis. **3.** The process of making such an arrangement.

Kell blood group (kel blud grōōp) A blood group of clinical importance because of its immunogenicity; consists of a series of codominant antigens determined by alleles at a site that is thought to be on the short arm of chromosome 2. First detected through antiserum produced by a Mrs. Kell.

kernicterus (ker-nik'ter-us) Deposition of the bile pigment bilirubin in the gray matter of the central nervous system of newborn infants, resulting in severe neurological deficits or death; occurs as a complication of hemolytic disease of the newborn.

ketoacidosis (ke-to-ă-sĭ-do'sis) The presence of an excessive amount of ketone bodies (i.e., acetoacetic acid, beta-hydroxybutyrate, and

1	2	3	4	5	6	7	8	9	10
11	12	13	14	15	16	17	18	19	20
21	22	xx							

individual chromosomes arranged in pairs according to size

karyotype of a normal female

1	2	3	4	5	6	7	8	9	10
11	12	13	14	15	16	17	18	19	20
21	22	xy							

karyotype of a normal male

acetone) in the tissues and body fluids; it occurs in such conditions as diabetes and starvation.

ketoconazole (ke-to-ko'nä-zol) A broad spectrum synthetic antifungal agent that inhibits the growth of certain common infectious fungi and yeasts by impairing the synthesis of ergosterol, a vital component of fungal cell membranes.

ketonemia (ke-to-ne'me-ä) The presence of ketone bodies (i.e., acetoacetic acid, beta-hydroxybutyrate, and acetone) in the blood.

ketones (ke'tōns) See ketone bodies, under body.

ketonuria (ke-to-nu're-ä) The presence of ketone bodies (i.e., acetoacetic acid, beta-hydroxybutyrate, and acetone) in the urine.

Kidd blood group (kid blud grōōp) A blood group consisting of red blood cell antigens determined by the JK gene; the antigens react with anti-JK^a and anti-JK^b antibodies. Named after a Mrs. Kidd in whom the antibodies were first found.

kidney (kid'ne) One of two bean-shaped organs located in the back on either side of the spine and behind the peritoneum; it filters the blood, excretes metabolic wastes in the form of urine, and regulates acid–base concentration and water balance in the tissues. The adult kidney is approximately 11 cm long, 5 cm wide and 2.5 cm thick.

Klebsiella (kleb-se-el'lä) A genus of bacteria (family Enterobacteriaceae) composed of Gram-negative, nonmotile microorganisms; found in the human intestinal tract. Some species cause disease.

   K. pneumoniae Species causing urinary tract infection and bacterial pneumonia.

knot (not) A circumscribed swelling or node.

   primitive k. A knoblike thickening of ectodermal cells at the cranial end of the primitive streak of the embryo from which a strand of cells grows toward the cranium. Also called Hensen's node, primitive node.

koilocytosis (koi-lo-si-to'sis) A condition of superficial or intermediate squamous cells having a large perinuclear cavity ('halo') which is thought to be pathognomonic of human papillomavirus infection.

kraurosis vulvae (kraw-ro'sis vul'vä) See lichen sclerosus of vulva, under lichen.

kyphosis (ki-fo'sis) Excessive backward curvature of the spine, affecting most frequently the upper thoracic and lower cervical vertebrae; may be caused by any of a variety of spinal disorders (e.g., fracture or tumor of the vertebrae); seen frequently in older people, especially women afflicted with osteoporosis, in which case the vertebral bodies collapse upon each other.

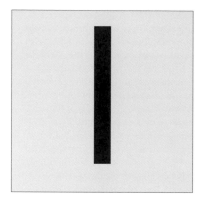

labetalol (lă-bet'ă-lol) A beta-adrenergic drug used to treat chronic hypertension. Intrauterine exposure may cause hypotension and reduced heart rate in the newborn.

labia (la'be-ă) Plural of labium.

labio- Combining form meaning lips.

labium (la'be-um), pl. labia A lip or liplike structure.

  l. anterius The anterior portion of the uterine cervix; it is shorter and thicker than the posterior portion. Also called anterior lip. See also labia uteri.

  labia majora The two prominent mounds of tissue forming the lateral boundaries of the vulva and extending from the mons pubis anteriorly to the perineum posteriorly; embryologically, they correspond to the scrotum of the male. Also called greater lips of pudendum; commonly called major lips.

  labia minora The two narrow folds situated between the labia majora, on either side of the urethral and vaginal openings; anteriorly, each labium minus splits into two folds, the upper ones meet over the free end of the clitoris (forming the prepuce of the clitoris), the lower ones meet under the clitoris (forming the frenulum of the clitoris); posteriorly, each labium minus either blends with its corresponding major lip or, in the virginal state, they join across the midline via a fold of skin (frenulum of labia minora). Also called lesser lips of pudendum; nymphae; commonly called minor lips.

  l. posterius The posterior portion of the uterine cervix; it is longer and thinner than the anterior portion. Also called posterior lip. See also labia uteri.

  labia uteri The portions of the uterine cervix surrounding its vaginal opening (exterior os); most prominently seen in women who have borne children, in whom the originally round opening becomes a transverse slit. See labium anterius; labium posterius.

labor (la'bor) The coordinated sequence of involuntary contractions of the uterus that increase in regularity, intensity, and duration, resulting in effacement and dilatation of the cervix and voluntary bearing-down efforts leading to expulsion of the fetus and placenta via

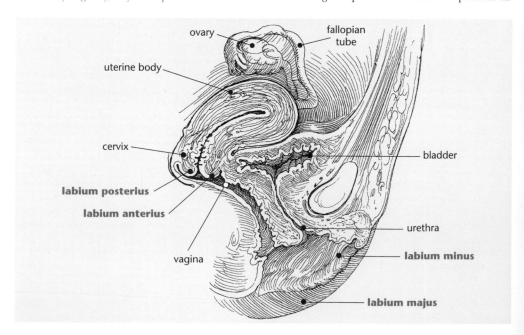

PATTERNS OF DISORDERED LABOR

Labor Pattern	Nullipara	Multipara
Prolonged latent-phase disorder	> 20 hrs	> 14 hrs
Protraction disorders		
Protracted active-phase dilatation	< 1.2 cm/hr	< 1.5 cm/hr
Protracted descent	< 1.0 cm/hr	< 2.0 cm/hr
Arrest disorders		
Prolonged deceleration phase	> 3 hrs	> 1 hr
Secondary arrest of dilatation	> 2 hrs	> 2 hrs
Arrest of descent	> 1 hr	> 1 hr
Failure of descent	no descent in deceleration phase or second stage	no descent in deceleration phase or second phase

the vagina; commonly divided into three stages: *first stage of l.*, begins with the onset of labor to full dilatation of the cervix (10 cm); *second stage of l.*, begins with full dilatation of the cervix and ends with complete delivery (birth) of the baby; *third stage of l.*, *placental stage of l.*, the period from delivery of the infant through delivery of the placenta. Also called true labor.

disordered l. A general term that includes five derangements of labor describing the inefficient progress of labor, occurring secondary to uterine hypofunction, effects of analgesia or anesthesia, fetopelvic disproportion, or other causes.

dry l. Labor occurring after premature rupture of the fetal membranes with loss of amniotic fluid. Also called xerotocia.

false l. Irregular brief uterine contractions occurring in late pregnancy; they are inconsistent in interval, duration, and strength, cause no change in the status of the cervix, and evoke abdominal and/or back pain. See also Braxton Hicks contractions, under contraction.

induced l. Labor brought on by medical or surgical means, usually performed under specific indications (e.g., prolonged pregnancy, premature rupture of membranes, preeclampsia, suspected intrauterine growth retardation).

precipitate l. Labor of unusually short duration, frequently due to abnormally low resistance of maternal soft tissues or abnormally strong contractions of uterine and abdominal muscles.

premature l. See preterm labor.

preterm l. Labor occurring after 20 but before 36 weeks of gestation.

prolonged l. Labor that lasts longer than 18 hours. See also prolonged latent phase of labor, under phase.

prolonged second stage l. In the nulliparous woman, a second stage of labor lasting more than 3 hours with regional analgesia, or more than 2 hours without such analgesia; in the parous woman, one lasting more than 2 hours with regional analgesia, or more than 1 hour without such analgesia.

true l. See labor.

laceration (las-er-a'shun) A superficial tearing of tissue.

obstetric l.'s Lacerations that may occur during the process of vaginal delivery, designated in four degrees: *first degree l.*, involves only vaginal mucous membrane or the skin (or both); *second degree l.*, involves the above tissues plus disruption of the underlying superficial fascia and transverse perineal muscle (excluding the anal sphincter); *third degree l.*, involves all the above structures plus the anal sphincter muscle; *fourth degree l.*, lacerations include all the above structures and extend into the lumen of the rectum, causing profuse bleeding and fecal soiling.

lact-, lacti-, lacto- Combining forms meaning milk.

lactacidemia (lak-tas-ĭ-de'me-ă) See lacticacidemia.

lactagogue (lak'tă-gog) See galactagogue.

lactate (lak'tāt) **1.** To secrete milk. **2.** Any salt or ester of lactic acid.

lactation (lak-ta'shun) The production of milk.

lactic (lak'tik) Relating to milk.

lacticacidemia (lak-tik-as-ĭ-de'me-ă) The presence of lactic acid in the circulating blood. Also called lactacidemia.

lactiferous (lak-tif'er-us) Conveying milk (e.g., ducts).

lactifuge (lak'ti-fuj) An agent that arrests milk secretion.

lactigenous (lak-tij'e-nus) Producing milk.

lactocele (lak'to-sēl) See milk-retention cyst, under cyst.

lactogen (lak'to-jen) Any agent that stimulates milk production.

    human placental l. (hPL) A polypeptide hormone that appears in the blood of pregnant women at about the sixth week of gestation, rises steadily thereafter, and disappears from the blood within 48 hours after childbirth; it is secreted by the placenta and is intimately involved in carbohydrate metabolism of both mother and fetus. It occurs in high concentration in molar pregnancy and in choriocarcinoma.

lactogenic (lak-to-jen'ik) Inducing milk production.

lactorrhea (lak-to-re'ă) See galactorrhea.

lactosuria (lak-to-su're-ă) The presence of lactose in the urine, sometimes occurring in premature newborn infants.

lacuna (lă-ku'nă), pl. lacunae **1.** A small anatomic cavity or depression. **2.** A defect or gap.

    intervillous l. One of numerous spaces filled with maternal blood in the early placenta, formed soon after implantation of the embryo when trophoblasts invade and tap the endometrial blood vessels.

    l. of muscles, l. musculorum A space beneath the inguinal ligament, lateral to the iliopectineal arch, which provides passage for the iliopsoas muscle and the femoral nerve.

    l. of vessels, l. vasorum A space beneath the inguinal ligament, medial to the iliopectineal arch, which provides passage for the femoral vessels.

lambda (lam'dă) (λ) A craniometric point on the back of the skull, at the junction of the sagittal and lambdoid sutures.

lamina (lam'ĭ-nă), pl. laminae A thin layer of cells or soft tissue or a thin plate of bone.

    interpubic fibrocartilaginous l. The fibrocartilaginous disk uniting the articular surfaces of the pubic bones at the symphysis.

    l. of vertebral arch Two broad plates directed dorsally and medially from the right and left pedicles of a vertebra; their posterior midline fusion forms the vertebral arch and completes the vertebral foramen.

Laminaria digitata (lam-ĭ-na're-ă dij-ĭ-tă'tă) A species of seaweed from which tents are made by drying and sterilizing the stems; the dry stem is capable of expanding to about five times its original diameter; used for atraumatic dilatation of the uterine cervix (e.g., as a preoperative procedure in abortion and prior to induction of labor at or near term). See also Laminaria tent, under tent.

lanuginous (lă-noo'jĭ-nus) Covered with fine, downlike hair (lanugo).

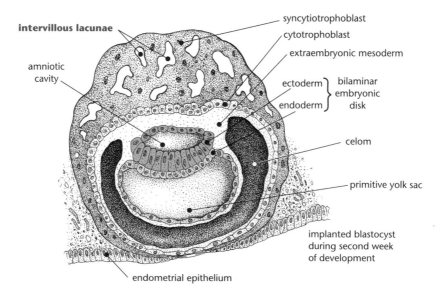

intervillous lacunae

syncytiotrophoblast

cytotrophoblast

extraembryonic mesoderm

amniotic cavity

ectoderm } bilaminar embryonic
endoderm } disk

celom

primitive yolk sac

implanted blastocyst during second week of development

endometrial epithelium

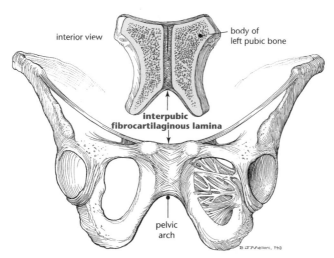

interior view

body of
left pubic bone

interpubic
fibrocartilaginous lamina

pelvic
arch

B. J. Melloni, PhD

lanugo (la-noo'go) The fine soft hairs covering the body of the fetus from the fourth month of pregnancy; they are shed after birth and are replaced by fine hairs (vellus). Also called primary hair.

laparo- Combining form meaning flank or loin; abdominal wall.

laparohysterectomy (lap-ă-ro-his-ter-ek'tŏ-me) See abdominal hysterectomy, under hysterectomy.

laparohysterotomy (lap-ă-ro-his-ter-ot'ŏ-me) See hysterotomy.

laparoscope (lap'ă-ro-skōp) An endoscopic instrument used in laparoscopy.

laparoscopy (lap-ă-ros'kŏ-pe) Visual examination of contents of the abdominal or pelvic cavity by means of a laparoscope introduced through a small incision on the abdominal wall. Also called peritoneoscopy; peritoneal endoscopy.

laparotomy (lap-ă-rot'ŏ-me) A surgical cut into the flank or through any part of the abdominal wall.

    second-look l. Laparotomy performed to determine whether cancer is still present in a patient who has been treated with surgery followed by chemotherapy, and who has no clinical or radiologic evidence of cancer. The term is not applicable to a second operation for persistent disease.

laser (la'zer) A device that transforms high energies into the laser beam, a concentrated narrow beam of monochromatic light (electromagnetic radiation). The laser beam is used as a tool in a variety of surgical and medical procedures. The term is an acronym for light amplification by stimulated emission of radiation.

    argon l. A laser employing argon as the medium; used in eye surgery to repair tears

and stop bleeding of the retina and in plastic surgery to remove certain types of birthmarks.

    carbon-dioxide l. Laser with carbon dioxide as the medium; usually employed in cutting and coalescing of certain tissues, such as vascular anastomoses.

    neodymium: yttrium-aluminum-garnet (Nd:YAG) l. A laser using as a medium a crystal of yttrium, aluminum, and garnet doped with neodymium ions; the beam can be transmitted by a flexible probe through an endoscope to coagulate bleeding sites in deep tissues such as those of the gastrointestinal, urinary, and respiratory tracts.

latent (la'tent) Present but not manifest; concealed.

lateroflexion (lat-er-o-flek'shun) A bending or angulation of an organ (e.g., the uterus) to one side.

lateroversion (lat-er-o-ver'shun) Tilting of an organ (e.g., the uterus) to one side.

lavage (lah-vahzh') The washing out of a body cavity or hollow organ.

    peritoneal l. Lavage of the peritoneal cavity as a means of removing infectious, irritating, or cancerous material, or of identifying intra-abdominal hemorrhage following trauma.

law (law) A principle, rule, or formula expressing a fact based on observed recurrence, order, relationship, or interactions of natural processes or actions.

    Fick's l. The rate of diffusion of a substance through an area depends on the difference in concentration of the substance at two given points.

layer (la'er) **1.** A band of cells or tissue of relatively uniform thickness, especially when part of a larger structure, as in the endometrium, retina,

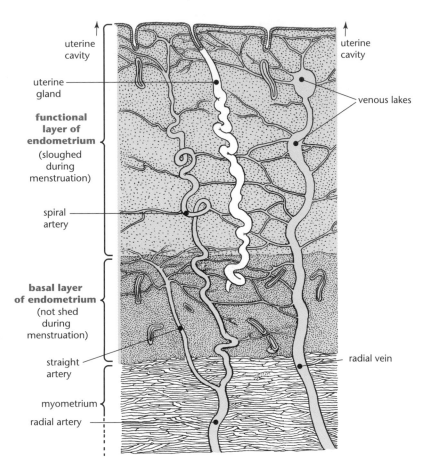

uterine cavity

uterine gland

functional layer of endometrium
(sloughed during menstruation)

spiral artery

basal layer of endometrium
(not shed during menstruation)

straight artery

myometrium

radial artery

uterine cavity

venous lakes

radial vein

cornea, or skin. **2.** A sheetlike coating; a single thickness of tissue covering a surface. Also called lamina.

basal l. of endometrium The deepest layer of the endometrium next to the uterine muscle (myometrium); it accommodates the blind ends of the tubelike uterine glands, which are not shed during menstruation or at parturition and from which the endometrium regenerates. Also called stratum basale; basal zone.

compact l. of endometrium The layer of the endometrium that is shed during menstruation and at parturition; it is nearest the free, luminal surface of the endometrium and contains the neck of the uterine glands, which become filled with secretions during the secretory phase of the menstrual (endometrial) cycle. Together, the spongy and compact layers form the functional layer of the endometrium. Also called stratum compactum; compact zone.

functional l. of endometrium The compact layer of the endometrium along with the spongy layer; during the secretory phase of the endometrial cycle, it becomes tremendously engorged; it is shed during menstruation. Also called stratum functionale; functional zone.

germ l. Any of the three primary layers of cells comprising the early embryo, the ectoderm (outer layer), the mesoderm (middle layer), or the endoderm (inner layer), which give rise to specific tissues of the body.

Nitabuch l. A layer of fibrinoid tissue between the trophoblast and the decidua.

spongy l. of endometrium The middle layer of the endometrium lying between the compact layer on the luminal surface and the basal layer on the myometrial side; seen especially during the late proliferative stage of the menstrual (endometrial) cycle, marked by growth of the stroma and engorged corkscrew convolutions of glands. Also called stratum spongiosum; spongy zone.

lecithin (les′ĭ-thin) (L) See phosphatidylcholine.

leg (leg) The lower limb, between the knee and ankle.

    milk l. See puerperal thrombophlebitis, under thrombophlebitis.

    painful white l. See puerperal thrombophlebitis, under thrombophlebitis.

leiomyofibroma (li-o-mi-o-fi-bro′mǎ) See leiomyoma.

leiomyoma (li-o-mi-o′mǎ) A benign grayish-white tumor composed mostly of smooth muscle cells and varying amounts of collagen; although it may occur in any tissue that has an abundant smooth muscle component, the tumor is seen most frequently in the uterus; may be single or multiple and occur anywhere in the uterine wall; it tends to grow rapidly during pregnancy, sometimes undergoing necrosis with severe abdominal pain; it occasionally diminishes in size after delivery, and usually regresses after menopause. Commonly called fibroid; also called fibroid tumor; fibromyoma; leiomyofibroma; myoma.

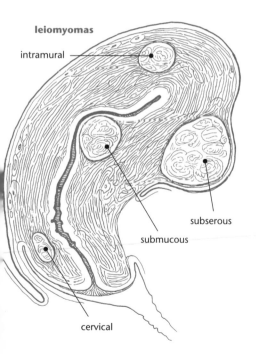

leiomyomas

intramural

subserous

submucous

cervical

leiomyomatosis (li-o-mi-o-mǎ-to′sis) The state of having multiple leiomyomas.

    l. peritonealis disseminata The presence of numerous small, benign tumors throughout the subperitoneum; they are composed of smooth muscle cells and seem to be aggravated by increased estrogenic activity (e.g., during pregnancy and in estrogen replacement therapy).

leiomyosarcoma (li-o-mi-o-sar-ko′mǎ) Malignant tumor of smooth muscle occurring predominantly in the female genital tract, especially the uterus; may occur also in other tissues containing abundant smooth muscle (e.g., intestinal wall, scrotum, nipple).

length (lengkth) Distance between two points.

    crown–heel (C–H) l. The length of an embryo from the top of the head to the heel.

    crown–rump (C–R) l. The length of an embryo from the top of the head to the bottom of the buttocks.

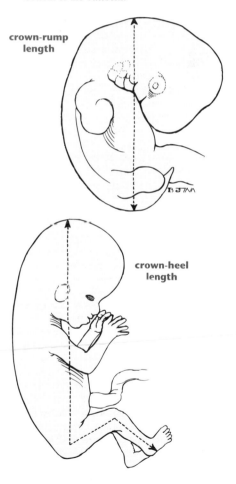

crown-rump length

crown-heel length

lentigo (len-ti′go), pl. lentigines A benign, darkly pigmented flat skin lesion that may be confused with melanoma.

leptotene (lep′to-tēn) In meiosis, a stage in early prophase of the first meiotic division in which chromosomes contract forming slender filaments. See also diplotene; pachytene; zygotene.

lesbian (lez'be-an) **1.** A homosexual female. **2.** Relating to lesbianism.

lesbianism (lez'be-ă-nizm) Female homosexuality.

lesion (le'zhun) General term for any morbid change in the structure or function of tissues due to injury or disease.

    polypoid l. Inflammatory mass arising from the submucosa or muscle layer of a hollow organ and protruding into the lumen.

let-down (let doun) Popular term for the passage of milk from the alveoli of the breasts into the lactiferous ducts in lactating women.

leuko- Combining form meaning white.

leukoderma (loo-ko-der'mă) A benign, localized skin lesion characterized by a loss of pigmentation; may be congenital or become manifest during the healing process following trauma.

leukokraurosis (loo-ko-kraw-ro'sis) See lichen sclerosus of vulva, under lichen.

leukoplakia (loo-ko-pla'ke-ă) A visible white flat lesion occurring in mucous membranes, most commonly of the lips, oral cavity, and the genitals; may be simply an increased thickness of the keratin layer of tissues due to chronic irritation, or it may be precancerous. When it occurs on the lips, it is popularly called smoker's patch.

    atrophic l. See lichen sclerosus of vulva, under lichen.

leukorrhea (loo-ko-re'ă) An abnormal white or yellowish discharge from the vagina containing mucus and pus.

leukovorin (loo-ko-vo'rin) See folinic acid.

Lewis blood group (loo'is blud grōōp) Antigens of red blood cells, saliva, and other body fluids; they are specified by the Le gene and react with the antibodies designated anti-Lea and anti-Leb; named after a Mrs. Lewis in whose blood the antibodies were discovered.

libido (lǐ-be'do, lǐ-bi'do) **1.** The emotional energy associated with primitive biologic impulses. **2.** In psychoanalysis, the term is applied to the motive force of the sexual instinct.

lichen (li'ken) An aggregation of small firm papules occurring on the skin or mucous membranes.

    l. sclerosus (LS) of vulva Chronic disorder of the lining of the vulva, usually occurring in postmenopausal women; characterized by formation of yellowish blue papules or macules that eventually coalesce to form whitish plaques of thin, glistening parchment-like patches. Can be associated with vulvar

malignancy; cause is unknown. Also called kraurosis vulvae; leukokraurosis; atrophic leukoplakia; atrophic vulvitis; leukoplakic vulvitis.

    l. simplex chronicus of vulva Chronic condition of the vulva characterized by circumscribed patches of thickened, furrowed skin; may result from scratching and itching due to a chronic vulvovaginal irritation or infection; may also involve the adjacent inner thigh and perianal and perineal areas. Also called neurodermatitis of vulva.

lie (li) The relation that the long axis of the fetus bears to that of the mother. See also fetal attitude, under attitude; position; presentation.

    longitudinal l. Relationship in which the long axis of the fetus is approximately parallel to the long axis of the mother; noted in about 99% of all labors at term.

    oblique l. Relationship in which the maternal and fetal long axes form a 45-degree angle; it usually becomes either longitudinal or transverse during labor. Also called unstable lie.

    transverse l. Relationship in which the long axis of the fetus is at right angles to that of the mother.

    unstable l. See oblique lie.

ligament (lig'ă-ment) **1.** Any band of thickened white fibrous tissue that connects bones and forms the capsule of joints. **2.** A fold of peritoneum, a fascial condensation, or a cordlike fibrous band that holds an organ in position.

    anococcygeal l. A mass of fibrous and muscular tissue situated between the anal canal and the tip of the coccyx to which some of the fibers of the levator ani muscle are attached.

    anterior l. of uterus See uterovesical fold, under fold.

    arcuate pubic l. A thick arch of ligamentous fibers connecting the lower border of the pubic symphysis, where it intermingles with the interpubic disk of the symphysis; it forms the upper border of the pubic arch.

    broad l. of uterus One of two fibrous folds covered with peritoneum and extending from the lateral surface of the uterus to the lateral pelvic wall, on both sides, and containing the ovary, fallopian (uterine) tube, ligaments, nerves, and vessels.

    Camper's l. See perineal membrane, under membrane.

    cardinal l. See transverse cervical ligament.

    Cooper's l.'s 1. See suspensory ligaments of breast. **2.** See pectineal ligament.

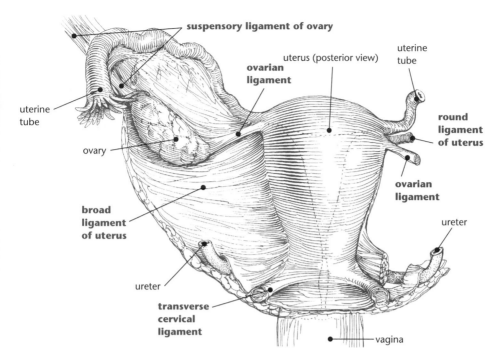

suspensory ligament of ovary

uterus (posterior view)

ovarian
ligament

uterine
tube

uterine
tube

round
ligament
of uterus

ovary

ovarian
ligament

ureter

broad
ligament
of uterus

ureter

transverse
cervical
ligament

vagina

Gimbernat's l. See lacunar ligament.

iliolumbar l.'s Strong bands extending from the transverse processes of the fourth and fifth lumbar vertebrae to the inner lip of the posterior iliac crest and the lateral side of the upper sacrum; they blend below with the ventral sacroiliac ligament.

infundibulopelvic l. See suspensory ligament of ovary.

inguinal l. The thickened upturned lower margin of the aponeurosis of the external oblique muscle, extending from the anterior superior spine of the ilium to the tubercle of the pubic bone. Also called Poupart's ligament.

interfoveolar l. A ligamentous band that connects the lower margin of the transverse abdominal muscle to the superior ramus of the pubic bone; it is inconstant.

lacunar l. A triangular band extending from the medial end of the inguinal ligament to the pectineal line of the pubic bone. Also called Gimbernat's ligament.

lateral umbilical l.'s Obsolete term. See medial umbilical ligaments.

medial umbilical l.'s Two fibrous cords passing along the bladder to the umbilicus; formed by the remains of the obliterated umbilical arteries.

median umbilical l. A fibrous cord

extending on the midline from the apex of the bladder to the umbilicus; formed by the remains of the obliterated urachus. Also called middle umbilical ligament; urachal ligament.

middle umbilical l. See median umbilical ligament.

Mackenrodt's l. See transverse cervical ligament.

ovarian l. A cordlike bundle of fibers between the layers of the broad ligament of the uterus, joining the uterine end of the ovary to the lateral margin of the uterus, immediately behind the attachment of the Fallopian (uterine) tube. Also called utero-ovarian ligament.

pectineal l. A strong fibrous band that extends from the upper border of the pectineal surface of the hipbone to the medial end of the lacunar ligament at the groin, with which it is continuous. Also called Cooper's ligament.

posterior l. of uterus See rectovaginal fold, under fold.

Poupart's l. See inguinal ligament.

pubic l.'s See superior pubic ligament, arcuate pubic ligament.

pubovesical l. A ligament formed by the thickening of the superior fascia of the pelvic diaphragm; it extends laterally from the neck of the bladder to the tendinous arch of the pelvic fascia; medially, it is a continuation of the tendinous arch extending to the pubic bone.

reflex inguinal l. The part of the inguinal ligament that extends from the lateral side of the superficial inguinal ring, and passes upward and medially to interlace at the linea alba with its counterpart from the opposite side of the body. Also called triangular fascia.

round l. of uterus A fibromuscular ligamentous cord extending from the lateral margin of the uterus, on either side; passing between the two layers of the broad ligament of the uterus, it traverses the inguinal canal to become attached to the connective tissue of the labium majus.

sacrococcygeal l.'s The five ligaments uniting the lower portion of the sacrum and the coccyx: *anterior sacrococcygeal, deep posterior sacrococcygeal, superficial posterior sacrococcygeal,* and two *lateral sacrococcygeal l.'s*

sacroiliac l.'s Ligaments that bind the sacrum with the ilium of the hipbone: *Posterior sacroiliac l.,* a set of thick fibrous bands overlying the interosseous sacroiliac ligament, consisting of a lower, superficial group (long posterior sacroiliac ligament) that extends from the posterior superior iliac spine of the hipbone to the transverse tubercles of the third and fourth segments of the sacrum (the bands blend with the sacrotuberous ligament) and an upper, deep group (short posterior sacroiliac ligament) that extends from the posterior inferior iliac spine and adjacent part of the ilium to the back of the sacrum. *Interosseous sacroiliac l.,* short, thick bundles of fibers interconnecting the sacral and iliac tuberosities, posterior to their articular surfaces; one of the strongest ligaments in the body, it serves as the principal bond between the sacrum and ilium. *Anterior sacroiliac l.,* a thin, wide, fibrous layer reinforcing the anterior part of the articular capsule of the sacroiliac joint and stretching from the ala and pelvic surface of the sacrum to the adjoining parts of the ilium.

sacrospinal l. A strong triangular ligament attached by its apex to the spine of the ischium of the hipbone and by its base to the lateral part of the lower sacrum and coccyx.

sacrotuberal l. A long, strong triangular ligament extending from the tuberosity of the ischium of the hipbone to the lateral part of the sacrum and coccyx and to the superior and inferior posterior iliac spines.

superior pubic l. A transverse band that binds the two pubic bones superiorly, and extends as far as the pubic tubercles; it is firmly attached to the interpubic disk at the midline.

suspensory l.'s of breast Coarse connective tissue bands distributed between the lobes of the female breast, extending from the overlying skin to the underlying pectoral fascia. Also called Cooper's ligaments.

suspensory l. of clitoris A fibrous band extending from the fascia of the pubic symphysis to the clitoris.

suspensory l. of ovary The part of the broad ligament of the uterus arising from the tubal side of the ovary and extending upward toward the lateral wall of the pelvis; it contains the ovarian blood vessels, lymphatic vessels, and nerves. Formerly called infundibulopelvic ligament.

transverse cervical l. A fibrous band attached to each side of the uterine cervix and to the lateral fornices of the vagina; it is

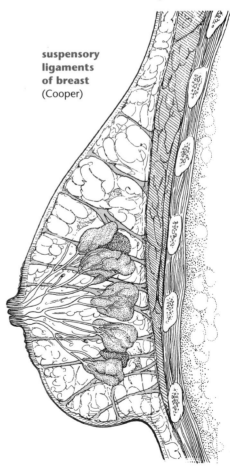

suspensory ligaments of breast (Cooper)

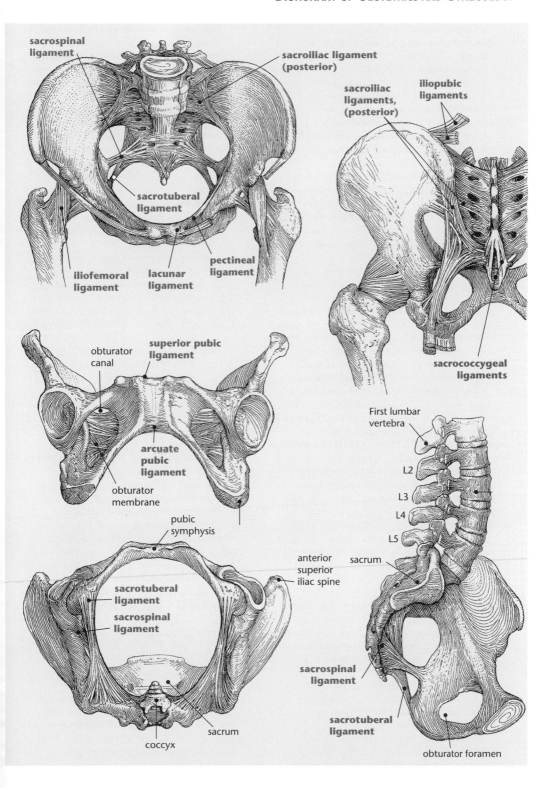

continuous with the tissue surrounding the pelvic blood vessels. Also called cardinal ligament; Mackenrodt's ligament.

urachal l. See median umbilical ligament.

utero-ovarian l. See ovarian ligament.

uterosacral l. Fibromuscular band that extends backward on either side from the uterine cervix, along the lateral wall of the pelvis to the front of the sacrum. It passes by the sides of the rectum and can be palpated on rectal examination.

ligamentum arteriosum (lig-ă-men'tum ar-tĕ-rĭ-o'sum) A short fibromuscular cord extending from the pulmonary trunk to the arch of the aorta, the remains of the ductus arteriosus.

ligate (li'gāt) To constrict a blood vessel, duct, pedicle of a tumor, or any tubular structure, with a firmly tied thread (ligature).

ligation (li-ga'shun) **1.** The act of ligating. **2.** In genetic engineering, the joining of two double-stranded DNA molecules with the enzyme DNA ligase; a step in constructing recombinant DNA.

tubal l. A surgical method of tubal sterilization by interrupting the continuity of the fallopian (uterine) tubes; the approach is either through the abdominal wall or the vagina. See also Irving's, Madlener's, and Pomeroy's operations, under operation; tubal sterilization, under sterilization; fimbriectomy.

ligature (lig'a-chur) Any thread made of synthetic or natural material used in ligation.

lightening (līt'en-ing) The sinking of the fetal head into the pelvic inlet, causing the uterus to descend to a lower level and fall forward, thus relieving pressure on the diaphragm, making breathing easier, and imparting a feeling of 'lightness'.

limbus (lim'bus), pl. limbi A border.

l. foramen ovale The semicircular ridge on the lower border of the fossa ovale, between the two atria of the heart.

linac (lin'ak) See linear accelerator, under accelerator.

line (līn) **1.** A thin area of demarcation designating the junction of two structures. **2.** A thin, continuous strip, mark, or ridge. **3.** A skin crease, a wrinkle. **4.** An imaginary mark connecting, or passing through, two points or landmarks on the body. **5.** A boundary.

gravidic l.'s See striae atrophicae, under stria.

Guaaerin's l. A radiographic finding revealing signs of osteochondritis and an irregular epiphyseal juncture.

iliopectineal l. An oblique ridge on the surface of the ilium and continued on the pelvis, which forms the lower boundary of the

iliac fossa; it separates the true from the false pelvis; it is a posterior continuation of the pectineal line. Also called linea terminalis.

interspinal l. A horizontal line across the abdomen connecting the two anterior superior iliac spines of the hipbones.

mamillary l. An imaginary vertical line on the anterior surface of the body, passing through the nipple of either breast; it corresponds roughly to the vertical line passing through the middle of the collarbone (clavicle). Also called nipple line.

nipple l. See mamillary line.

pectineal l. The sharp edge on the superior ramus of the pubic bone extending from the pubic tubercle anteriorly, to the iliopubic eminence posteriorly.

simian l. See simian crease, under crease.

linea (lin'e-a), pl. lineae A line, strip, or narrow ridge, usually on the surface of a structure; a thin, continuous mark.

l. alba The narrow portion of the anterior aponeurosis extending from the midline of the xiphoid process stretching down to the pubic symphysis, formed by the interlacing aponeurotic fibers of the flat abdominal muscles; the navel is situated slightly below its midpoint.

lineae albicantes See striae atrophicae, under stria.

lineae atrophicae See striae atrophicae, under stria.

lineae gravidarum See striae atrophicae, under stria.

l. nigra A dark streak on the abdomen of some women during the later months of pregnancy, extending from the region of the navel to the pubic symphysis; it is the pigmented linea alba of pregnancy.

linkage (lingk'ij) **1.** In genetics, the relationship between two or more genes on a chromosome whereby they function together as a unit to direct some activity; usually, they are inherited together. **2.** In chemistry, the force that holds together the atoms in a compound.

sex l. Old term for X linkage.

X l. Linkage associated with a gene on the X chromosome.

Y l. Linkage associated with a gene on the Y chromosome.

linoleic acid (lin-o-le'ik as'id) A polyunsaturated fatty acid essential in the human diet; it is a necessary precursor for the biosynthesis of prostaglandins; it strengthens capillary walls, lowers serum cholesterol, and prolongs clotting time.

lip (lip) **1.** One of the two fleshy folds forming the anterior boundary of the mouth. **2.** Any liplike structure.

anterior l. See labium anterius, under labium.

cleft l. A developmental defect of the upper lip; it ranges from a scarlike groove, or a notch on the lip, to a complete cleft extending through the lip into the nasal cavity. Also called cheiloschisis.

greater l.'s of pudendum See labia majora, under labium.

lesser l.'s of pudendum See labia minora, under labium.

major l.'s See labia majora, under labium.

minor l.'s See labia minora, under labium.

posterior l. See labium posterius, under labium.

lipase (lip'ās, li'pās) Any enzyme promoting the breakdown of fat molecules; present in pancreatic juice, blood, and many tissues.

lipemia, lipidemia (lĭ-pe'me-ă, lip-ĭ-de'me-ă) See hyperlipidemia.

liquor (lik'er) **1.** Any fluid. **2.** A body secretion produced by certain tissues.

l. folliculi See follicular fluid, under fluid.

Listeria (lis-te're-ă) Genus of Gram-positive bacteria (family Corynebacteriaceae); found in feces, sewage, and vegetation.

L. monocytogenes A species that has been found in normal gastrointestinal tracts of healthy people without causing ill effects but causing illness under certain conditions (e.g., in pregnancy and deficient immunity states).

listeriosis (lis-ter-e-o'sis) An uncommon but serious food-borne infection caused by *Listeria monocytogenes*, acquired by ingesting raw or undercooked contaminated food, such as poultry, meat, fish, eggs, and cheese, and causing meningitis, septicemia, or abscesses; it is often fatal for persons with weakened immune systems (e.g., by cancer, kidney disease, diabetes, and HIV infection). See also *Listeria monocytogenes*, under *Listeria*.

neonatal l. Listeriosis occurring in the newborn, usually acquired through maternal infection during passage through the birth canal or by aspiration of infected amniotic fluid; occasionally acquired from the hospital nursery; the condition may become evident the first or second day after birth (early onset), or approximately 7 days afterward (late onset); complications include respiratory distress, skin lesions, abscesses in several organs, and meningitis.

pregnancy-associated l. Listeriosis occurring during pregnancy; symptoms may be mild or severe and include fever, backache, muscle ache, diarrhea, abdominal pain, nausea, and vomiting; can cause intrauterine fetal infection, leading to stillbirth, premature delivery, or neonatal complications.

lithium (lith'e-um) A silvery, soft, highly reactive metallic element; symbol Li, atomic number 3, atomic weight 6.9; some of its compounds are used in the treatment of mental disorders, particularly bipolar disorders. Intrauterine exposure during the first trimester may cause cardiac defects, particularly Ebstein's anomaly. Use during pregnancy may be associated with neonatal goiter, depression of central nervous system (CNS), lack of muscle tone, and cardiac murmur.

lithopedion (lith-o-pe'de-on) The calcified remnants of an ectopic pregnancy.

liver (liv'er) The largest glandular organ in the body, situated in the right upper abdomen beneath the diaphragm; it secretes bile and plays an important role in the metabolism of fats, carbohydrates, protein, minerals, and vitamins.

acute fatty l. of pregnancy An uncommon condition usually occurring in late pregnancy (after 35 weeks of gestation); symptoms and signs include lack of appetite, nausea and vomiting, upper abdominal pain, progressive jaundice, edema, and hypertension. May be associated with a genetic defect in the fetus secondary to a trifunctional protein deficiency. Also called acute fatty metamorphosis; acute yellow atrophy.

cirrhotic l. See cirrhosis.

fatty l. An enlarged, yellowish, greasy liver resulting from fatty infiltration and degeneration (fatty metamorphosis); may occur as a complication of any disease involving protein malnutrition; other causes include alcohol abuse, diabetes mellitus, hepatotoxins, drugs, and obesity.

lobe (lōb) **1.** A well defined portion of an organ or gland bounded by structural borders such as fissures, sulci, grooves, or septa. **2.** A rounded, projecting part (e.g., the fatty portion of the external human ear).

anterior l. of pituitary See adenohypophysis.

glandular l. of pituitary See adenohypophysis.

l. of mammary gland Either one of 15 to 20 milk producing lobes of the female breast; each lobe is drained by a lactiferous duct that opens at the nipple.

milk l. One of two ridges on either side of

the ventral surface of the embryo's trunk, extending from the axillary to the inguinal regions; the upper intermediate portion of the ridge thickens to form the mammary primordium, while the rest of the ridge disappears before the end of the embryonic period.

lochia (lo'ke-ă) The discharge from the uterus following childbirth. Initially, it is blood-tinged and includes shreds of tissue (lochia rubra); a few days later, it becomes serous and paler (lochia serosa); during the second week, it becomes thicker, yellowish-white, and mucoid (lochia alba); it ceases by the fifth postpartum week when the placental site heals.

lochiometra (lo-ke-o-me'tră) Distention of the uterus with retained lochia following childbirth due to blocking of the cervical canal with debris from the uterus; associated with inflammation of the uterine lining. Commonly called lochia block.

logipram (loj'ĭ-pram) A form of low molecular weight heparin.

loop (lōōp) A bend in a vessel, cord, or cordlike device.

    detrusor l. A thickening of the urinary bladder base and trigone.

    Lippes l. An intrauterine contraceptive device made of polyethylene impregnated with barium sulfate. It was withdrawn from the market in 1985.

    sentinel l. A radiologic finding in patients with acute appendicitis in which a dilated loop of bowel, secondary to localized inflammation, is present near the cecum.

louse (lous), pl. **lice** Any of various wingless parasitic insects, including the sucking lice (of the order Anoplura) and the biting lice (of the order Mallophaga); some species are vectors of human diseases (e.g., relapsing fever, typhus, and trench fever).

    pubic l. *Phthirus pubis*, a species that infests pubic hair. Popularly called crab; crab louse.

lues (loo'ēz) Syphilis.

luetic (loo-et'ik) Syphilitic

lumbar (lum'bar) Relating to the loins (i.e., the part of the back between the lowest rib and the pelvic bone on either side of the spine).

lumbo- Combining form meaning loins.

lumbosacral (lum-bo-sa'kral) Relating to the lumbar portion of the vertebral column and the sacrum.

lumpectomy (lum-pek'tŏ-me) Surgical removal of a hard mass and a margin of surrounding tissue, especially from the breast.

lung (lung) The paired organ of respiration situated in the chest cavity and enveloped by the pleura; generally the right lung is slightly larger than the left and is divided into three lobes, while the left has but two. The primary purpose of the lungs is the uptake of oxygen from inspired air and the elimination of carbon dioxide from the blood. See also alveolus; pleura; respiration.

    wet l. See transient tachypnea of the newborn, under tachypnea.

lupus (loo'pus) General term used with a qualifying adjective for any of several diseases manifested by characteristic skin lesions.

    systemic l. erythematosus (SLE) A progressive, often severe condition thought to be of autoimmune origin and involving multiple systems (including skin, blood vessels, joints, heart, nervous system, and kidneys); characterized by the presence of antinuclear antibodies (ANA) and other autoantibodies, antibodies producing false positive VDRL (syphilis) tests, antibodies against plasma coagulating protein, and antibodies against antigens on red and white blood cells and platelets, leading to immune destruction of these cells; clinical features are diverse, depending on the location of the immune injury. The disease is associated with an increased risk of preterm births, fetal growth retardation, and the presence of talipes equinovarus in the newborn.

luteal (loo'te-al) Relating to the corpus luteum of the ovary.

lutein (loo'tēn) Yellow pigment present in egg yolk, fat cells, and corpus luteum.

luteinize (loo'te-ĭ-nīz) To form luteal tissue.

luteinization (loo-tēn-ĭ-za'shun) Formation of luteal tissue and the corpus luteum in the ovary after discharge of the ovum.

luteogenic (loo-te-o-jen'ik) Luteinizing; inducing the development of corpora lutea (applied to a hormone or hormone-like substance).

luteolysis (loo-te-ol'ĭ-sis) Degeneration of the corpus luteum.

luteoma (loo-te-o'mă) Noncancerous nodules developed in the ovary, composed of enlarged lutein cells; may be multifocal and bilateral.

    l. of pregnancy Luteoma occurring during pregnancy, usually the last trimester, and regressing after childbirth; the nodules range in size between 5 and 10 cm in diameter.

luteotropic (loo-te-o-trop'ik) Having a stimulating action on the development and function of the corpus luteum.

Lutheran blood group (loo'ther-an blud grōōp) Antigens of red blood cells, specified by the Lu gene, that react with antibodies designated anti-

Lua and anti-Lub; first detected in the serum of an individual who had received many transfusions.

lying-in (li-ing-in') Popular term for the period from childbirth through the first few weeks afterwards.

lymph (limf) The tissue fluids collected by the lymphatic vessels and conveyed to the blood circulation after passing through a filtering system (lymph nodes); composed of a liquid, a number of white blood cells (especially lymphocytes), and a few red blood cells.

 inflammatory l. The slightly yellow fluid collecting on the surface of an acutely inflamed surface wound or membrane.

lymphadeno-, lymphaden- Combining forms meaning lymph node.

lymphadenectomy (lim-fad-ě-nek'tŏ-me) Removal of lymph nodes.

lymphadenography (lim-fad-ě-nog'ră-fe) x-ray examination of a lymph node after injection of a radiopaque substance.

lymphadenopathy (lim-fad-ě-nop'ă-the) Any disorder of the lymph nodes; may be localized, affecting one lymph node group anywhere in the body; or may be generalized, involving several lymph node groups throughout the body, in which case lymphoid tissues or organs (e.g., the spleen) may also be involved.

lymphangioma (lim-fan-je-o'mă) A noncancerous tumor-like mass of dilated lymphatic vessels.

lymphatic (lim fat'ik) Relating to lymph, lymph nodes, or lymph vessels.

lymphedema (lim-fě-de'mă) Progressive swelling, usually of the extremities, caused by obstruction of the lymph flow and consequent accumulation of lymph in tissue spaces.

lymphocele (lim'fo-sēl) A cystic mass containing lymph. Also called lymphocyst.

lymphocyte (lim'fo-sīt) A white blood cell formed in lymphoid tissues; normally constitutes 25–33% of all white blood cells in adult peripheral blood. Also called lymph cell; lymphoid cell.

 B l.'s Lymphocytes, derived from bone marrow, that play an important role in immune regulatory functions; they interact chiefly with the humoral immune system (which involves such substances as antibodies, antigens, and serum complement enzymes in the blood). Also called B cells.

 cytotoxic T l. Lymphocyte that kills target cells (e.g., tumor cells) by releasing a protein (perforin) to perforate the target cell membrane after antibodies have reacted with an antigen on the target cell.

 helper T l. See helper cell, under cell.

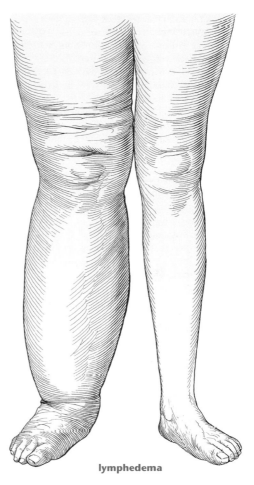

lymphedema

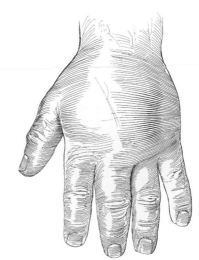

T l.'s Lymphocytes, derived from the thymus, that play an important role in the cellular immune system by responding to antigens and triggering reactions in other cells, such as macrophages. Also called T cells.

    tumor-infiltrating l. (TIL) A lymphocyte that has some antitumor properties.

lymphocyst (lim'fo-sist) An abnormal saclike structure containing lymph.

lymphocytoma (lim-fo-sī-to'mă) A tumor-like mass in a lymph node, chiefly made up of mature lymphocytes.

lymphogranuloma venereum, venereal lymphogranuloma (lim-fo-gran-u-lo'mă ve-ne're-um, ve-ne're-al lim-fo-gran-u-lo'mă) (LGV) A sexually transmitted disease caused by *Chlamydia trachomatis*; characterized by a genital blister or ulcer that heals and disappears in a few days without leaving a scar; may be accompanied by fever, headache, muscle and joint pains, a rash, and inflammation and swelling of lymph nodes in the groin; in females, lymph nodes around the rectum may become involved, causing a stricture. Also called tropical bubo.

lymphostasis (lim-fos'tă-sis) Obstruction to lymph flow.

lyo- Combining form meaning dissolution.

lyonization (li-on-ĭ-za'shun) Random inactivation of one of the two X chromosomes in female somatic cells, occurring early in embryo development. Also called X inactivation.

lysergic acid (li-sur'jik as'id) A crystalline compound derived from ergot.

    l. a. diethylamide (LSD) A hallucinogenic drug derived from lysergic acid; causes chromosomal breakage. It is associated with a higher incidence of spontaneous abortion and fetal anomalies in women who use illicit LSD, but the effects of LSD on the pregnancy and the fetus remain uncertain.

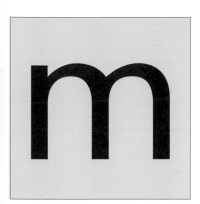

maceration (mas-er-a'shun) The softening and disintegration (without putrefaction) of a dead fetus remaining in the uterus.

macro-, macr- Combining forms meaning large.

macrocephalic (mak-ro-sĕ-fal'ik) Relating to macrocephaly. Also called megacephalic.

macrocephalous (mak-ro-sef'ă-lus) Having an abnormally large head. Also called megacephalous.

macrocephaly (mak-ro-sef'ă-le) Abnormally large head circumference of an infant, i.e., two or more standard deviations above the mean for its age and sex; it may or may not be associated with hydrocephalus; other causes include large cystic defects and slow subdural effusions (usually from trauma). Also called megacephaly.

macrogenitosomia (mak-ro-jen-ĭ-to-so'me-ă) Disorder of the adrenal gland cortex, most commonly affecting male children; characterized by excessive and early development of sexual organs associated with rapid maturation of the musculoskeletal system, resulting in short stature.

macromastia, macromazia (mak-ro-mas'te-ă, mak-ro-ma'ze-ă) Abnormally large size of the breasts.

macrosomia (mak-ro-so'me-ă) Abnormally large size of the body, such as that of a newborn infant of a diabetic mother. Also called hypersomia.

macrosomic (mak-ro-som'ik) Relating to macrosomia.

macula (mak'u-lă), pl. maculae A small area differing in appearance from the surrounding tissue; a circumscribed spot, stain, or tissue thickening. Also called macule.

    m. of follicle A relatively avascular area on the surface of an ovary at which a vesicular ovarian follicle ruptures, forcing the enclosed egg (ovum), cumulus, some detached follicular (granulosa) cells, and follicular fluid out into the peritoneal cavity; usually the rupture point is rapidly sealed off.

    m. of gonorrhea The red, inflamed opening of the duct of the greater vestibular gland, seen in gonorrheal vulvitis.

maculopapular (mak-u-lo-pap'u-lar) An eruption or lesion consisting of spots and elevations (macules and papules).

mal (mahl) French and Spanish for disease.

    grand m. See generalized tonic–clonic epilepsy, under epilepsy.

    petit m. See absence.

malabsorption (mal-ab-sorp'shun) Impaired absorption of dietary nutrients by the intestinal mucosa. Maternal malabsorption may be a predisposing factor in small-for-gestational age infants.

malaise (mal-āz') A vague general discomfort or feeling of illness.

male (māl) One who produces spermatozoa.

    genetic m. An individual with a normal male karyotype, one X and one Y chromosome.

    XX m. A male affected by a chromosomal abnormality characterized by the presence of 46,XX chromosomes, although internal and external sex organs are those of a male; thought to be caused by aberrant exchange of X and Y segments of the chromosomes during meiosis.

malformation (mal-for-ma'shun) A primary structural defect of a body part resulting from a localized developmental error.

    Arnold-Chiari m. Extrusion of brain tissue through the foramen magnum down into the upper cervical canal; the herniated brain structures include the medulla oblongata and fourth ventricle, along with varying portions of the cerebellar vermis.

    Dandy-Walker m. See Dandy-Walker syndrome, under syndrome.

    Ebstein's m. See Ebstein's anomaly, under anomaly.

malignancy (mă-lig'nan-se) The state of being malignant.

malignant (mă-lig'nant) **1.** Tending to become worse and cause death; applied to any disease. **2.** Denoting a tumor that infiltrates adjacent tissues and spreads to other parts of the body with potentially life-threatening results.

malnutrition (mal-noo-trish'un) Faulty nutrition due to inadequate diet (e.g., consuming inadequate amounts or the wrong proportions of nutrients), or to a metabolic abnormality. Maternal malnutrition may be a predisposing factor in small-for-gestational age infants.

malposition (mal-pŏ-zish'un) **1.** An abnormal position. **2.** A position of the fetal vertex other than occiput anterior (e.g., occiput posterior or occiput transverse), which can be responsible for dystocia if persistent during the active phase of labor.

malpractice (mal-prak'tis) Negligence by a professional (e.g., physician, attorney, accountant, etc.).

   medical m. Negligence by a health care professional; specifically, medical care provided to a patient that falls below the accepted standards of medical practice, thereby exposing the patient to an unreasonable risk of harm. A legal claim for medical malpractice necessitates that the patient prove the health care professional owed the patient a duty to provide medical care within the accepted standards of medical practice, that the duty was breached, and that the breach caused injury to the patient; the injury claimed by the patient must be recognized by law as being possible to compensate.

malpresentation (mal-prez-en-ta'shun) A situation in which the presenting part of the fetus is one other than the vertex in an occiput position (e.g., brow, sinciput, face, acromion [transverse lie], breech).

mamil-, mamilli- Combining forms meaning nipple.

mamilla (mă-mil'ă), pl. mamillae **1.** A nipple. **2.** Any nipple-like protrusion.

mamillary (mam'ĭ-ler-e) Relating to a nipple.

mamilliplasty (mă-mil'ĭ-plas-te) Reparative or esthetic surgery of the nipple. Also called theleplasty.

mamillitis (mam-ĭ-li'tis) Inflammation of a nipple.

mamma (mam'ă), pl. mammae A mammary gland; a breast, male or female.

mammaplasty (mam'ă-plas-te) See mammoplasty.

mammary (mam'er-e) Relating to the breasts.

mammectomy (mă-mek'to-me) See mastectomy.

mammitis (mam-i'tis) See mastitis.

mammo- Combining form meaning breast.

mammogram (mam'ŏ-gram) An x-ray picture of a breast produced by mammography.

mammography (mă-mog'ră-fe) A diagnostic imaging technique for detecting breast neoplasia.

   baseline m. A surveillance mammogram taken to establish the condition of breast tissue at a point in time.

   screening m. A surveillance mammogram in which a basic number of views are taken to assess the integrity of breast tissue.

mammoplasty (mam'o-plas-te) Plastic surgery of the breast. Also called mammaplasty; mastoplasty.

   augmentation m. Enlargement of breast size by implanting a silicone bag filled with silicone gel, saline, or air, or a combination of the three; the implant may be placed beneath the breast tissue or beneath the pectoralis major muscle.

   reconstructive m. Insertion of an implant to replace a breast that has been removed partly or completely; may be performed at the time the breast is removed or at a later date.

   reduction m. Any of various techniques for decreasing breast size, generally by removing a portion of breast tissue from the center and lower areas of the breast; the nipple and areola are retained in a skin pedicle and repositioned.

mammotroph (mam'o-trōf) A cell of the anterior portion of the pituitary (hypophysis) that produces the hormone prolactin; a prolactin cell.

mammotrophic (mam-o-trof'ik) Stimulating the development, growth, and function of the mammary glands.

maneuver (mă-noo'ver) A procedure requiring skill and dexterity.

   Bracht's m. A maneuver used in breech delivery in which the breech is allowed to deliver spontaneously up to the navel, then the body of the fetus is held (without pressure) against the mother's pubic symphysis and moderate suprapubic pressure is applied by an assistant.

   Brandt-Andrews m. A method of delivering the placenta during the last (third) stage of labor; pressure is applied with the fingers of one hand just above the symphysis to elevate the uterus into the abdomen and at the same time express the placenta into the vagina; gentle cord traction with the other hand is used to guide the placenta into the birth canal.

   corkscrew m., Woods corkscrew m. See Woods maneuver.

   Credé's m. (1) A method of expressing the placenta, after the infant has been delivered, by squeezing or kneading the body of the uterus to produce placental separation; it usually traumatizes the placental site, therefore it is not generally recommended. Also called Credé's method. (2) The application of one drop of a 2% solution of silver nitrate onto each eye of the newborn infant to prevent gonococcal conjunctivitis; may cause inflammation and eye discharge within the first 24 hours of life. (3) The use of manual pressure on the bladder, especially a paralyzed bladder, to express urine.

   Leopold's m.'s Four maneuvers to

determine the fetal position in the uterus: (1) palpation of the uterine fundus over the abdomen to determine what fetal part occupies the fundus (i.e., head or breech); (2) deep, gentle pressure on the sides of the abdomen to determine the position of the fetal back and extremities; (3) grasping of the lower portion of the abdomen with the thumb and finger of one hand, just above the pubic symphysis, to ascertain whether the presenting part has engaged; (4) deep palpation into the pelvic brim on either side with the first three fingers of each hand to assess the direction of the head and to determine the extent to which it has descended into the pelvis.

McDonald m. See McDonald technique, under technique.

McRobert's m. Maneuver used in the management of shoulder dystocia; the patient's legs are flexed acutely upon her abdomen, which causes the pubic symphysis to rotate toward the patient's head and the angle of the pelvic inclination to be reduced; the impacted fetal shoulder is thereby released.

Mauriceau m. A method of extracting the aftercoming head in partial breech presentation when the chin is directed posteriorly (occiput anterior position) and the rest of the body has been delivered; the body of the fetus straddles the forearm of the operator, the middle and index fingers of one of the operator's hands are pressed over the maxilla to maintain flexion of the head, two fingers of the operator's other hand are placed forklike over the neck and shoulders to exert gentle downward traction until the suboccipital region appears under the maternal pubic symphysis, and then the body is elevated toward the mother's abdomen until

the mouth, nose, and brow are delivered over the perineum. Also called Mauriceau-Smellie-Veit maneuver.

Mauriceau-Smellie-Veit m. See Mauriceau maneuver.

modified Prague m. A method of delivering the fetal head in breech presentation when the back of the head remains directed posteriorly (occiput posterior position) and the rest of the body has been delivered; one hand of the operator supports the shoulders from below while the other hand gently draws the body upward toward the maternal abdomen, thus flexing the head within the birth canal, which permits delivery of the back of the head over the perineum.

modified Ritgen's m. Maneuver for conducting a controlled delivery of the head in vertex presentation to prevent injuries to the nervous system of the fetus and to the maternal perineal musculature; gentle forward pressure is applied on the chin with one hand placed on the maternal perineum (just in front of the coccyx) while the back of the head is held against the pubic symphysis with the other hand; the maneuver is performed between contractions, when the vaginal opening is distended to 5 cm or more.

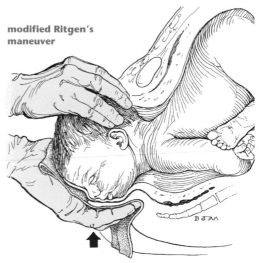

modified Ritgen's maneuver

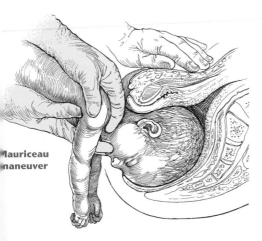

Mauriceau maneuver

Mueller-Hillis m. A procedure of uncertain reliability in predicting the possibility of cephalopelvic disproportion. In an occiput presentation, fundal pressure is applied to determine if the head can descend into the maternal pelvis. If no disproportion exists, the head readily enters the pelvis. However, inability to push the head into the pelvis does not necessarily indicate vaginal delivery is impossible.

Pinard's m. A method of extracting a fetal foot in frank breech presentation; two fingers are passed along the fetal thigh to the knee to push it away from the midline and flex the leg; the foot is then readily grasped and brought down and out.

Rubin's m.'s Maneuvers for the management of shoulder dystocia, (1) by rocking of the fetal shoulders from side to side with the hands on the mother's abdomen, (2) by reaching the most accessible of the fetal shoulders and pushing it toward the front of the chest of the fetus to reduce the shoulder-to-shoulder distance.

Scanzoni m. Forceps rotation of the head when it presents with its back directed posteriorly (occiput posterior position); the head is rotated slowly through a 180 degree arc; then the instrument is removed and reapplied for delivery of the head with its back directed anteriorly (occiput anterior position).

Sellick m. A technique used to facilitate endotracheal intubation in which pressure is applied to the cricoid cartilage to occlude the esophagus.

Stillman m. Modification of the Scanzoni maneuver; the head is repeatedly rotated through an arc of 15 to 30 degrees until the head is in the occiput anterior (OA) position.

Woods m. Maneuver for management of shoulder dystocia with impacted anterior shoulder; the operator's hand is placed behind the posterior shoulder of the fetus; the shoulder is then progressively rotated 180 degrees in a corkscrew manner, thus dislodging the impacted anterior shoulder. Also called corkscrew maneuver; Woods screw maneuver.

Zavanelli's m. Maneuver for managing shoulder dystocia, perfomed when vaginal delivery cannot be effected; consists of (1) returning the head to the occiput anterior (OA) position or the occiput posterior (OP) position if it has rotated from either, (2) slowly pushing the head back into the vagina, and (3) performing a cesarean delivery.

mark (mark) A skin blemish.

port-wine m. See nevus flammeus, under nevus.

stretch m.'s See striae atrophicae, under stria.

marker (mark'er) A characteristic by which a cell or molecule can be identified or a disease can be recognized.

cutaneous m. Any of various skin changes that serve as a sign of an internal (frequently malignant) disease.

genetic m. Any character that serves as a signpost of the presence or location of a gene in an individual in a given population.

tumor m. A substance secreted by a tumor and released into the blood and other body fluids; detection of its presence aids diagnosis of the tumor; examples include alpha-fetoprotein (AFP) for hepatoma and chorionic embryonic antigen (CEA) for colon cancer.

marrow (mar'o) A medulla, especially of bone.

bone m. The soft tissue occupying the cavities of bones; it produces most of the cells that circulate in the blood (erythrocytes, leukocytes, and megakaryocytes). Also called marrow; medulla of bone.

red m. The marrow found mainly within the spongy tissues of ribs, breastbone, and the ends of the long bones; it is the site of production of red blood cells and granular white blood cells.

yellow m. The material located mainly within the large cavities of large bones; consists mainly of fat cells and a few immature blood cells.

marsupialization (mar-soo-pe-al-ĭ-za'shun) Surgical procedure for eradication of a cyst, whereby the cystic sac is opened and emptied, its anterior wall removed, and its edges sutured to the margins of the surrounding tissue.

masculinization (mas-ku-lin-ĭ-za'shun) 1. The normal development of secondary male characteristics. 2. See virilization.

mask (mask) 1. A shield designed to cover the nose and mouth to preserve antiseptic conditions (i.e., in operating rooms), or to prevent the spread of an infectious disease when caring for patients. 2. A device for administration of inhalation anesthesia.

m. of pregnancy Popular term for melasma gravidarum; see under melasma.

masochism (mas'o-kizm) The derivation of pleasure from being subjected to physical or psychological pain or abuse either by oneself or by others; may be sought for sexual gratification or to relieve guilt.

masochist (mas'o-kist) One who derives pleasure (often sexual pleasure) from being subjected to physically or psychologically painful or humiliating experiences by others or by the self.

mass (mas) A body of coherent material.

inner cell m. See embryoblast.

massage (mă-sahzh') The therapeutic pressing,

rubbing, kneading, or tapping of selected areas of the body.

uterine m. Gentle massaging of the fundus of a lax uterus through the abdominal wall; performed during separation and expulsion of the placenta (third stage of labor), or immediately after its delivery.

mastalgia (mas-tal'je-ă) See mastodynia.

mastatrophy, mastatrophia (mas-tat'rŏ-fe, mas-tă-tro'fe-ă) Atrophy of the breasts.

mastectomy (mas-tek'tŏ-me) Removal of the breast. Also called mammectomy.

extended radical m. Mastectomy that includes removal of the underlying chest muscles, axillary lymph nodes, and the internal mammary nodes.

modified radical m. Removal of the breast, connective tissue covering the pectoralis major muscle (but not the muscle), and the axillary lymph nodes.

partial m. See segmental mastectomy.

radical m. Removal of the breast, underlying pectoral muscles, axillary lymph nodes, and associated skin and subcutaneous tissue. Also called Halsted's operation.

segmental m. Removal of part of the breast (e.g., quadrantectomy, lumpectomy) or of a growth in the breast, along with only enough breast tissue to ensure that the margins of the removed specimen are free of tumor. Also called breast conservation treatment; partial mastectomy.

simple m. Removal of the whole breast only. Also called total mastectomy.

total m. See simple mastectomy.

subcutaneous m. Removal of the breast with preservation of overlying skin, areola, and nipple, to facilitate reconstruction of the breast form.

mastitis (mas-ti'tis) Inflammation of breast tissue. Also called mammitis.

chronic cystic m. See fibrocystic change of the breast, under change.

infectious m. Acute condition in which one breast (often only one quadrant) becomes tender, reddened, swollen, and hot; the patient develops fever and appears ill; occurs as a complication of breast-feeding, usually (not exclusively) affecting first-time mothers; caused by a microorganism, especially *Staphylococcus aureus*, which gains entry through cracks in the nipple. Also called puerperal mastitis; postpartum mastitis; lactational mastitis.

interstitial m. Inflammation of connective tissue within the breast.

lactational m. See infectious mastitis.

phlegmonous m. Diffuse breast inflammation, sometimes accompanied by abscess formation.

plasma cell m. A chronic benign condition usually seen in perimenopausal women; characterized mainly by dilatation and obstruction of lactiferous ducts with masses containing dried secretions and plasma cells; may cause nipple retraction resembling breast cancer.

postpartum m. See infectious mastitis.

puerperal m. See infectious mastitis.

masto-, mast- Combining forms meaning breast.

mastodynia (mas-to-din'e-ă) Pain in the breast. Also called mastalgia.

mastopathy (mas-top'ă-the) Any disease of the breast.

mastopexy (mas'to-pek-se) Procedure for correction of sagging breasts; it involves repositioning of the areola and nipple in a higher location, above the level of the inferior fold of the breast (inframammary fold), and tightening of the skin for support.

mastoplasty (mas'to-plas-te) See mammoplasty.

mastoptosis (mas-to-to'sis) Sagging breasts.

mastotomy (mas-tot'ŏ-me) A surgical cut into a breast.

masturbation (mas-tur-ba'shun) Self-manipulation of the genitals for sexual excitement.

maternity (mă-ter'nĭ-te) **1.** The state of being a mother or pregnant. **2.** Relating to childbirth (e.g., an area of the hospital).

matrilineal (ma-trĭ-lin'e-al) In genetics, inherited through the maternal line.

maturate (mach'u-rāt) To bring to maturity; to cause to ripen.

maturation (mach-u-ra'shun) **1.** The process of attaining full development. **2.** The process by which a primitive cell reaches its final structure and functional capacity.

sexual m. See puberty.

mature (mă-chur') **1.** Fully developed. **2.** To attain full development.

maytansine (ma-tan'sēn) An antineoplastic alkaloid derived from the wood and bark of several varieties of the mandrake plant; used in chemotherapy. See also podophyllotoxin; vinca alkaloids, under alkaloid.

measles (me'zelz) A highly contagious disease marked by high fever, cough, inflammation of respiratory tract, eruption of white (Koplik's) spots in the mouth, and a reddish skin rash; caused by a paramyxovirus; incubation period is about 10 days; complications that may sometimes occur include pneumonia and encephalitis. Maternal infection during pregnancy causes a high risk of abortion and low-birthweight infants. Also called hard measles; rubeola.

German m. See rubella.

hard m. See measles.

neonatal m. Measles occurring in a newborn infant exposed to the virus through a near-term maternal infection.

slapped-cheek m. Popular term for erythema infectiosum (a manifestation of parvovirus infection). See erythema infectiosum, under erythema.

meatus (me-a'tus), pl. meatuses, meatus An anatomic passageway, or its opening.

external m. of female urethra See external orifice of female urethra, under orifice.

internal m. of urethra See internal orifice of urethra, under orifice.

mechanism (mek'a-nizm) **1.** The means by which some result is obtained. **2.** An aggregation of parts that interact to perform a common function.

Duncan m. Separation of the placenta from the uterine wall beginning at the placental periphery; blood from the implantation site exits immediately through the vagina followed by the placenta, which descends sideways into the vagina, presenting the maternal surface at the vulva.

Schultze m. Separation of the placenta from the uterine wall beginning at the center; blood from the implantation site accumulates behind the placenta and membranes; its weight then pushes the center of the placenta toward the uterine cavity and eventually into the vagina; the placenta presents the fetal surface at the vulva; the accumulated blood follows.

meconiorrhea (mĕ-ko-ne-o-re'ă) Passage of an abnormally large amount of meconium by the newborn infant.

meconium (mĕ-ko'ne-um) The dark green intestinal contents formed before birth and first present in the ileum at 75 to 80 days of gestation; composed of desquamated intestinal cells, skin cells, and fetal hair (lanugo) swallowed by the fetus with the amniotic fluid. See also meconium aspiration syndrome and meconium plug syndrome, under syndrome; meconium ileus, under ileus.

mediad (me'de-ad) Toward the midline.

medial (me'de-al) **1.** Relating to the middle. **2.** Situated near the median plane of the body or an organ. **3.** Relating to the middle layer of a blood vessel wall.

median (me'de-an) **1.** Situated in the middle or midline; central. **2.** In statistics, denoting the middle value (i.e., the point at which half of the plotted values are on one side and half on the other).

medicine (med'ĭ-sin) **1.** The science concerned with diagnosing and treating disease and the maintenance of health. **2.** Any substance used in the treatment of disease.

clinical m. The study and practice of medicine at the bedside, i.e., by direct examination and observation of patients as opposed to theoretical, classroom, or laboratory study.

critical care m. Medical subspecialty concerned with the care of medical and surgical patients whose conditions are life-threatening and require comprehensive care and constant monitoring; it involves relevant areas of anesthesiology, surgery, internal medicine, and pediatrics. Also called intensive care medicine.

emergency m. The branch of medicine concerned with the acutely (often suddenly) ill or injured person.

intensive care m. See critical care medicine.

neonatal m. See neonatology.

perinatal m. See perinatology.

medicolegal (med-ĭ-ko-le'gal) Relating to overlapping aspects of the health professions and the law, especially those medical matters called before a court of law; applied to matters concerning damages, which may include injuries due to medical negligence or malpractice, medical evidence of injury in a civil action, mental competence of people who have drawn legal documents, commitment of the mentally ill to mental institutions, and the use of tests for determining paternity; may also relate to such matters as a person's right to die, sterilization, artificial insemination, *in vitro* fertilization, surrogacy, and the right to confidentiality (particularly in the context of AIDS).

medionecrosis (me-de-o-nĕ-kro'sis) Tissue death in the middle layer of arterial walls.

m. of the aorta See cystic medial necrosis, under necrosis.

medium (me'de-um), pl. media, mediums **1.** A substance through which something is transmitted. **2.** An intervening substance. **3.** Culture medium.

contrast m. In radiology, a substance (e.g., barium) that blocks the passage of x rays or any other form of radiation; introduced into or around a structure to provide contrast with surrounding tissues and allow visualization of the structure in x-ray or fluoroscopic examinations; those materials used intravenously or intra-arterially (e.g., in intravenous pyelography, angiography) usually consist of iodinated compounds. Also called radiopaque medium; radiopaque substance.

radiopaque m. See contrast medium.

medroxyprogesterone acetate (med-rok-se-pro-jes'ter-ōn as'ĕ-tāt) A synthetic progestin used in the treatment of endometriosis, endometrial neoplasia, and hormone replacement therapy of the menopause, and as a long-acting injectable contraceptive.

medulla (mĕ-dul'ă), pl. medullae **1.** Any centrally located soft tissue. **2.** The marrow of bone or any similar structure. **3.** Any part of an organ situated more centrally than the cortex.

m. of bone See bone marrow, under marrow.

m. of lymph node The inner, darker portion of the lymph node, composed of a stroma of reticular fibers containing cordlike masses of lymphocytes, plasma cells, and macrophages, separated by lymph sinuses.

m. oblongata The oblong, caudal portion of the brainstem extending from the lower margin of the pons to the beginning of the spinal cord, at the level of the upper border of the first cervical vertebra; it contains the involuntary centers controlling the heart, blood vessels, and respiratory organs.

m. of ovary The inner portion of the ovary, composed of loose fibroelastic tissue containing smooth muscles, lymphatics, nerves, and a mass of large contorted blood vessels; it is surrounded by a thick cortex containing the ovarian follicles and corpora lutea.

mega- Combining form meaning large.

megacephalic (meg-ă-sĕ-fal'ik) See macrocephalic.

megacephalous (meg-ă-sef'ă-lus) See macrocephalous.

megacephaly (meg-ă-sef'ă-le) See macrocephaly.

megacolon (meg-ă-ko'lon) Abnormally large colon.

congenital m. Condition resulting from absence of ganglion (nerve) cells at the junction of the rectum and colon; the aganglionic area of the intestine is unable to relax during normal intestinal movements, producing constriction, constipation, and distention of the colon; eventually the entire colon (including the appendix) may become dilated; in the newborn infant, symptoms include a distended abdomen, failure to pass

meconium, and vomiting of a bilious material. Also called Hirschsprung's disease; congenital aganglionic megacolon.

congenital aganglionic m. See congenital megacolon.

megavoltage (meg-ă-vol'tij) Electromotive force in excess of one million volts; used in radiation therapy.

megestrol (mĕ-jest'trol) A synthetic antineoplastic and progestational drug. It is potentially hazardous to the fetus, especially when taken between 5 and 10 weeks of gestation.

meiosis (mi-o'sis) A special type of cell division that occurs only in the ovaries and testes during maturation of the germ cells (oocyte and spermatocyte, forerunners of the ovum and spermatozoon). It consists of two consecutive cell divisions occurring in rapid succession, designated: *meiosis I*, the first of the two divisions; homologous chromosomes pair off (at which time DNA is replicated), then the chromosomes split longitudinally and the cell divides into two new cells, each with half the number of chromosomes (haploid number). Also called reduction division; first meiotic division. *Meiosis II*, the second division, follows the first in rapid succession but without additional DNA replication; the end result is four daughter cells (gametes), each containing half the number of chromosomes found in the general body cells. Also called second meiotic division. Compare with mitosis.

meiotic (mi-ot'ik) Relating to meiosis.

melanoma (mel-ă-no'mă) A malignant tumor derived from pigment-producing cells (melanocytes), occurring usually in the skin and

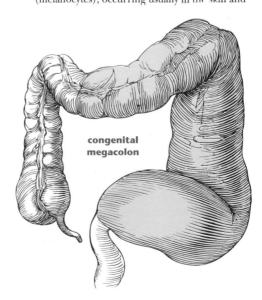

congenital megacolon

(less commonly) the eye, oral cavity, genitalia, and other sites that contain melanocytes. Melanomas vary in appearance and rate of growth and metastasis, but generally they grow and spread rapidly and have four distinguishing characteristics known as the ABCD of melanoma: *asymmetry*, one half of the tumor is unlike the other half; *border* is irregular, scalloped, and poorly circumscribed; *color* varies from one area of the tumor to another; *diameter* is, as a rule, larger than 6 mm. The tumor pigment ranges from light brown and white to red and bluish black. Also called malignant melanoma.

malignant m. Term used interchangeably with melanoma.

malignant m. of vagina A rare melanoma occurring singly or in groups as polypoid or pedunculated growths, usually on the anterior wall and lower half of the vagina, and causing vaginal bleeding and discharge; seen primarily in postmenopausal women.

malignant m. of vulva An uncommon but aggressive malignancy, usually arising in the labia minora and clitoris as a pigmented, raised lesion, sometimes causing itching and bleeding.

melanosis (mel-ă-no'sis) Abnormal deposits of dark pigments in various organs or tissues.

m. coli Pigmentation of gastrointestinal mucosa associated with cathartic abuse.

vulvovaginal m. A noncancerous, flat, darkly pigmented lesion on the vulvar skin or the vagina.

melasma (mě-laz'mă) Areas of brown patches on the skin, most commonly of the face and neck; caused by hormonal action (i.e., in the use of oral contraceptives). Also called chloasma.

m. gravidarum Increased pigmentation on the forehead and across the cheeks and nose occurring sometimes during pregnancy. Also called chloasma of pregnancy; mask of pregnancy.

melphalan (mel'fă-lan) An antineoplastic alkylating agent whose action prevents cell division primarily by cross-linking strands of DNA. It is potentially hazardous to the fetus, especially when taken between 5 and 10 weeks of gestation.

membrane (mem'brān) 1. A thin, pliable layer of tissue that covers a surface, lines a cavity, connects two structures, or divides a space or organ. 2. A limiting protoplasmic surface.

anal m. In the embryo, the posterior portion of the bilayered cloacal membrane after it is subdivided by the urorectal septum. See also urogenital membrane.

decidual m. See decidua.

exocelomic m. A layer of flat cells forming the external lining of the blastocyst. Also called Heuser's membrane.

fetal m.'s The extraembryonic structures that protect the developing embryo or fetus and provide for its nourishment, respiration, excretion, and hormonal secretions; they include the amnion, chorion, allantois, yolk sac, decidua, and all structures of the placenta.

Heuser's m. See exocelomic membrane.

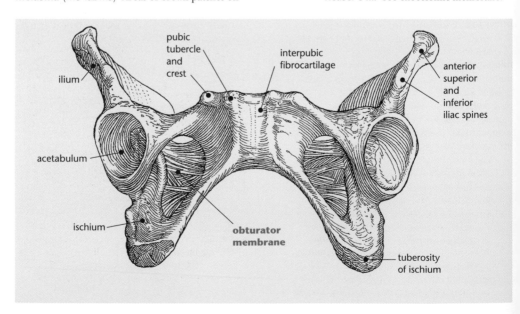

mucous m. A membrane whose surface is moistened by mucous glands; it lines tubular structures as well as the alimentary, respiratory, and urogenital tracts.

obturator m. The thin membrane of interlacing white fibers that almost completely closes the obturator foramen of the hipbone; it leaves a small canal for the passage of the obturator nerve and vessels.

perineal m. See inferior fascia of urogenital diaphragm, under diaphragm.

serous m. A membrane whose surface is covered with a film of thin serous-like fluid; it lines the pleural, peritoneal, and pericardial cavities of the body, and exposed surfaces of protruding organs.

urogenital m. In the embryo, the anterior portion of the cloacal membrane after it is subdivided by the urorectal septum. See also anal membrane.

virginal m. See hymen.

membranous (mem'bră-nus) Relating to membrane.

menacme (mĕ-nak'me) The time in a woman's life between onset of menstruation (menarche) and the natural cessation of menstruation and ovarian function (physiologic menopause).

menarche (mĕ-nar'ke) The first menstrual period, usually occurring at about the age of 12 to 13 years.

premature m. Menarche occurring before the age of 10 years and in the absence of other secondary sexual development.

menarcheal, menarchial (mĕ-nar'ke-al) Relating to the menarche.

meninges (mĕ-nin'jēz) Specifically, the membranes covering the brain and spinal cord (pia mater, arachnoid, dura mater).

meningitis (men-in-ji'tis) Inflammation of the membranes covering the brain and spinal cord. Routes of infection include cerebrospinal fluid and bloodstream pathways (e.g., lumbar punctures, skull fractures and penetrating wounds, and brain surgery).

acute bacterial m. Meningitis generally characterized by headache, irritability, fever, lethargy, neck stiffness, and presence of large numbers of polymorphonuclear leukocytes in a cloudy (normally clear) cerebrospinal fluid; caused by a variety of bacteria, especially *Escherichia coli* (affecting chiefly newborn infants), *Haemophilus influenzae, Neisseria meningitidis* (the cause of epidemics), and *Streptococcus pneumoniae* (affecting most frequently infants and old people and those with head injuries). If untreated, the disease

may be fatal. Also called acute pyogenic meningitis.

acute chemical m. Meningitis caused by irritating substances introduced or released into the cerebrospinal fluid (e.g., certain spinal anesthetics, contents of intradural cysts).

acute lymphocytic m. See aseptic meningitis.

acute nonpyogenic m. See aseptic meningitis.

acute pyogenic m. See acute bacterial meningitis.

aseptic m. Meningitis characterized by intense headache, nausea, vomiting, neck stiffness, an increase of lymphocytes in the cerebrospinal fluid, normal glucose levels, and an absence of bacteria; usually caused by viruses, most frequently by coxsackieviruses, echoviruses, and the genital herpes (herpes simplex II) virus. Also called acute lymphocytic meningitis; acute nonpyogenic meningitis.

meningomyelocele (mĕ-ning-o-mi'ĕ-lo-sēl) Outpouching of the membranes covering the spinal cord through an abnormal gap (spina bifida) in the vertebral column; the protrusion is devoid of a skin covering and contains spinal cord tissue and/or nerve roots. Also called myelomeningocele.

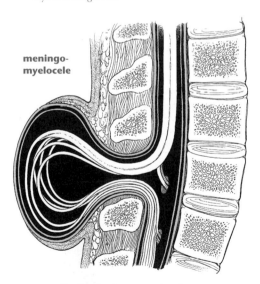

meningo-myelocele

meno- Combining form meaning the menses.

menometrorrhagia (men-o-met-ro-ra'je-ă) Uterine bleeding occurring at irregular intervals and in varying amounts and duration of flow.

menopausal (men-o-paw'zal) Relating to the menopause.

menopause (men'o-pawz) The permanent cessation of menstruation. The term is commonly used interchangeably with climacteric. Popularly called change of life. See also climacteric.

>**artificial m.** See iatrogenic menopause.

>**iatrogenic m.** Permanent cessation of menstruation resulting from surgical procedures (removal of the ovaries or the uterus, or both) or from radiation therapy or chemotherapy. Also called artificial menopause; surgical menopause.

>>**natural m.** See physiologic menopause.

>>**physiologic m.** Permanent cessation of menstruation resulting from the normal cessation of ovarian function, usually between the ages of 45 and 55 years. Also called natural menopause.

>>>**premature m.** Cessation of ovarian function at an abnormally early age.

>>>**surgical m.** See iatrogenic menopause.

menorrhagia (men-o-ra'je-ă) Excessive or prolonged menstrual flow. Also called hypermenorrhea.

menoschesis (mĕ-nos'kĕ-sis) Suppression of the menses.

menses (men'sēz) See menstruation.

menstrual (men'stroo-al) Relating to menstruation.

menstruation (men-stroo-a'shun) Bleeding that occurs with the cyclic breakdown and shedding of the uterine mucosa in the absence of pregnancy; it is normally preceded by discharge of an ovum from the ovary and usually occurs at intervals of approximately 28 days (from the start of one menstrual period to the start of the next) and lasts 3 to 5 days. Also called menses. See also menstrual cycle, under cycle; menstrual period, under period.

>**anovular m., anovulatory m.** Menstruation without ovulation; occurs normally from the first through the following 12 to 18 menstruations and just before the menopause.

>**painful m.** See dysmenorrhea.

>**vicarious m.** Bleeding from sites other than the uterus (e.g., the nose), occurring at the time when normal menstruation takes place.

menton (men'ton) A craniometric point on the lower jaw, at the lowermost point of its median plane.

mentum (men'tum) The chin; the point of reference in a face presentation (e.g., mentum anterior).

meperidine (mĕ-per'ĭ-dēn) A narcotic analgesic with multiple actions similar to those of morphine.

meprobamate (mĕ-pro'bă-māt) A minor tranquilizer used to treat anxiety. It may be associated with fetal malformations when taken in the first trimester of pregnancy.

mercaptopurine (mer-kap-to-pū'rēn) An anticancer drug. Adverse effects include nausea, vomiting, mouth ulcers, and appetite loss; may cause fetal malformations and low birth weight when taken during pregnancy.

mesentery (mez'en-ter-e) The double layer of peritoneum attaching various organs to the body wall and conveying to them their blood vessels and nerves. The term is commonly used in reference to the peritoneal fold attaching the small intestine to the posterior abdominal wall.

meso-, mes- Prefixes meaning intermediate, connecting.

mesoblast (mez'o-blast) In embryology, a cell of the early mesoderm.

mesoderm (mez'o-derm) In embryology, the middle layer of embryonic cells (between the ectoderm and endoderm); it gives rise to the deep layer of the skin, connective tissues, vascular and genitourinary systems, and most skeletal and smooth muscles.

mesometrium (mez-o-me'tre-um) The portion of the broad ligament of the uterus, below the attachment of the ovary, and extending to the lateral wall of the pelvis.

mesonephros (mes-o-nef'ros) An intermediate excretory organ of the embryo, eventually replaced by the kidney; in the male, its duct system is retained as the epididymis and the vas deferens (deferent duct). Also called wolffian body.

mesosalpinx (mez-o-sal'pinks) The upper free portion of the broad ligament of the uterus, above the attachment of the ovary and investing the fallopian (uterine) tube.

mesovarium (mez-o-va're-um) The short fold of peritoneum attaching the ovary to the posterior layer of the broad ligament.

mestranol (mes'tră-nol) The 3-methyl ether of the estrogen ethynyl estradiol; used in oral contraceptives.

metabolism (mĕ-tab'o-lizm) The sum of the chemical changes occurring in the living body by which energy is provided for vital processes and by which new substances are produced and assimilated for growth and maintenance.

>**basal m.** The minimum amount of energy required to maintain vital functions in an individual at complete physical and mental rest. Also called basal metabolic rate (BMR).

metacyesis (met-ă-si-e'sis) See ectopic pregnancy, under pregnancy.

metamorphosis (met-ă-mor'fŏ-sis) A change in

form and/or function.

acute fatty m. See acute fatty liver of pregnancy, under liver.

metaphase (met'ă-fāz) The stage of cell division in which the contracted chromosomes, each consisting of two chromatids, are aligned along the equatorial plane of the cell prior to separation of the chromatids.

metaplasia (met-ă-pla'ze-ă) An abnormality of cell differentiation in which one type of adult cell is replaced by a different type of mature cell that is not normal for the tissue involved.

squamous m. Transformation of columnar or cuboidal epithelium into a normal-looking stratified squamous epithelium; occurs commonly in the endocervix.

metastasis (mĕ-tas'tă-sis), pl. metastases **1.** The process by which cancerous cells form secondary tumors that are discontinuous with the primary tumor, in parts of the body distant from the original site; it is the most important feature distinguishing malignant from benign tumors. **2.** The secondary cancerous tumor thus formed.

metastasize (mĕ-tas'tă-sīz) To spread by metastasis.

methamphetamine hydrochloride (meth-am-fet'ă-mēn hi-dro-klo'rīd) A sympathomimetic drug that stimulates the central nervous system and depresses intestinal motility, thus allaying hunger. Drug abusers take it orally or intravenously; it produces psychological dependence. Abuse during pregnancy results in increased incidence of preterm labor, placental abruption, fetal distress, intrauterine growth retardation, low birth weight, and postpartum hemorrhage. Also known by the slang terms meth and speed.

method (meth'ud) A manner of performing an act, especially a systematic way of performing an examination, operation, or test. See also maneuver; procedure; technique.

barrier m. Method of contraception that relies on the employment of any device for preventing the entrance of sperm into the cervical canal and uterine cavity (e.g., male and female condoms, diaphragm, cervical cap, and spermicidal agents).

Billings m. See cervical mucus rhythm method.

calendar rhythm m. A periodic abstinence method of contraception that depends on recording the menstrual pattern for several months to determine the time of ovulation.

cervical mucus rhythm m. A periodic abstinence method of contraception in which the time of ovulation is determined by

observing changes in the amount, consistency, and elasticity of cervical mucus secretions during the interval between two menstrual periods. Also called Billings method.

Crede's m.'s See Crede's maneuver, under maneuver.

hormonal m. Any method of contraception based on the use of hormones or their synthetic analogs; included are oral contraceptives and the injectable or implantable long-acting progestins.

immunofluorescence m. A method of determining the presence or location of an antigen by using a corresponding antibody labeled with a fluorescent substance.

Lamaze m. A method of psychophysiologic preparation for the birth process; it involves educating the pregnant woman about her body functions and the physiology of labor, emphasizing exercise, breathing techniques, and relaxation; usually requires the assistance of a partner or 'coach.'

rhythm m., periodic abstinence m. Any birth control method predicated on abstinence from sexual intercourse for a few days before, during, and after the expected day of ovulation. Also called natural family planning.

symptothermal m. A combination of the cervical mucus and temperature methods of contraception.

temperature rhythm m. A periodic abstinence method of contraception in which the time of ovulation is determined by observing and recording the slight changes in basal body temperature that take place during the ovarian cycle; rectal or vaginal temperature is taken every morning upon awakening.

Uchida m. See Uchida procedure, under procedure.

withdrawal m. See coitus interruptus, under coitus.

methotrexate (meth-o-trek'sāt) A drug with antineoplastic properties. Adverse effects include nausea, vomiting, mouth sores, and, if taken during pregnancy, fetal defects and low birth weight.

metolazone (mĕ-tol'ă-zōn) Diuretic drug used in the treatment of high blood pressure (hypertension) and the reduction of fluid retention in such conditions as kidney disorders, heart failure, and premenstrual syndrome. Possible side-effects include weakness and lethargy; taken during the first trimester of pregnancy causes increased risk of congenital defects.

metopion (mĕ-to'pe-on) Craniometric point on

the sagittal plane between the two frontal eminences.

metra (me'tra) Greek for uterus.

metria (me'tre-ă) Inflammatory condition of the uterus after childbirth.

metritis (mĕ-tri'tis) Inflammation of the uterus.

metrodynamometer (me-tro-di-nă-mom'ĕ-ter) Instrument for measuring the force of uterine contractions.

metromalacia (me-tro-mă-la'she-ă) Abnormal softening of the uterus.

metronidazole (met-ro-ni'dă-zōl) Antibiotic drug effective against anaerobic bacteria (e.g., in tooth abscesses and peritonitis) and protozoan infections (e.g., amebiasis, giardiasis, and trichomoniasis). Adverse effects include loss of appetite, abdominal pain, dark colored urine, and taste disturbance. Because laboratory studies have found that it causes mutations in bacteria and cancer in rodents, usage in the first trimester is generally not recommended, although short-term studies have not substantiated adverse findings in humans.

metropathia hemorrhagica (me-tro-path'e-ă hem-o-raj'ik-ă) Abnormal, profuse, and prolonged uterine bleeding associated with cyst formation in the endometrium.

metropathic (me-tro-path'ik) Relating to disease of the uterus.

metropathy (mĕ-trop'ă-the) Any disease of the uterus.

metrophlebitis (mĕ-tro-flĕ-bi'tis) Inflammation of the uterine veins occurring only during pregnancy and immediately after childbirth.

metroptosis (mĕ-tro-to'sis) See prolapse of the uterus, under prolapse.

metrorrhagia (mĕ-tro-ra'je-ă) Bleeding from the uterus occurring any time between menstrual periods; causes include acute inflammation of the cervix, a benign tumor, endometrial or cervical cancer and, at midcycle, may be due to ovulation. Also called intermenstrual bleeding.

metrorrhea (me-tro-re'ă) Discharge of mucus or pus from the uterus.

metrorrhexis (me-tro-rek'sis) See hysterorrhexis.

metrosalpingitis (me-tro-sal-pin-ji'tis) Inflammation of the uterus and one or both fallopian (uterine) tubes.

metroscope (me'tro-skōp) See hysteroscope.

metrostaxis (me-tro-stak'-sis) A slight continuous bleeding from the uterus.

metrostenosis (me-tro-stĕ-no'sis) Constriction of the uterine cavity.

metrotomy (me-trot'ŏ-me) See hysterotomy.

miconazole (mi-kon'ă-zōl) An antifungal drug specifically useful in the treatment of candidiasis.

microadenoma (mi-kro-ad-ĕ-no'ma) A noncancerous glandular tumor, smaller than 10 mm in diameter.

microaneurysm (mi-kro-an'u-rizm) Areas of small vessel distention seen in conditions such as chronic hypertension; visible in the retina of diabetes mellitus patients.

microangiopathic (mi-kro-an-je-o-path'ik) Relating to any disease of small blood vessels.

microangiopathy (mi-kro-an-je-op'ă-the) Disease

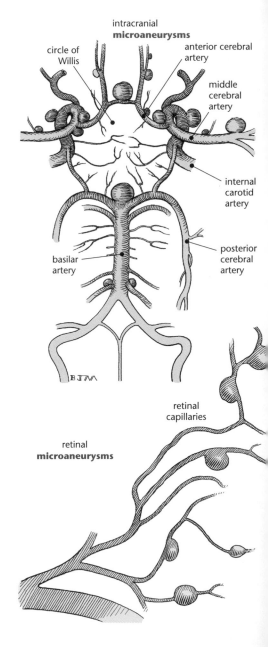

intracranial **microaneurysms**

circle of Willis

anterior cerebral artery

middle cerebral artery

internal carotid artery

posterior cerebral artery

basilar artery

retinal capillaries

retinal **microaneurysms**

of the small blood vessels, especially of the capillaries.

diabetic m. Diffuse thickening of vascular basement membranes, especially of capillaries of the skin and medulla of the kidney.

thrombotic m. A combination of arteriolar and capillary wall thickening resulting in a narrow lumen with deposition of minute plugs of platelet aggregates and fibrin.

microcarcinoma (mi-kro-kar-sĭ-no′mă) An early stage in the spread of carcinoma in which stromal infiltration is limited but there are multiple and confluent malignant projections, with a high risk of lymphatic involvement; the size of the tumor is no greater than 10 mm in length and 5 mm in width.

microgenitalism (mi-kro-jen′ĭ-tal-izm) Abnormal smallness of the external genital organs.

microinvasion (mi-kro-in-va′zhun) The earliest, limited stage in the spread of a cancerous tumor to adjacent tissues to a depth no greater than 3 mm, with no confluent extensions, and no lymphatic or blood vessel invasion.

micropenis (mi-kro-pe′nis) An abnormally small penis; in the newborn, one less than 2 cm in length from the pubic bone to the tip.

micturition (mik-tu-rish′un) The act of urinating. Also called urination.

mid- Combining form meaning middle.

midforceps (mid-for′seps) See midforceps delivery, under delivery.

midmenstrual (mid-men′stroo-al) Midway between two menstrual periods.

midpain (mid′pān) See intermenstrual pain, under pain.

midpelvis (mid-pel′vis) The portion of the pelvis extending anteriorly from the inferior margin of the pubic symphysis, laterally to the ischial spines, and posteriorly to the sacrum at the junction of the third and fourth sacral vertebrae; its average anteroposterior diameter is 11.5 cm; its interspinous diameter is 10.5 cm.

contracted m. A midpelvis in which the sum of the interspinous and posterior sagittal diameters is 13.5 cm or less.

midsection (mid-sek′shun) A surgical cut through the middle of an organ.

midwife (mid′wīf) A person who assists a woman in childbirth.

certified nurse m. A formally trained person with credentials in obstetrics, usually a registered nurse, who provides care to a woman during pregnancy and childbirth and cares for both mother and infant immediately following childbirth, usually with physician backup in case of emergencies or complications.

lay m. A person without formal training in obstetrics who attends a woman in childbirth and the puerperium.

midwifery (mid-wi′fer-e, mid-wif′ĕ-re) The care provided by a midwife in a hospital, birthing center, or home.

mifepristone (mif-pris′tōn) A progestational and glucocorticoid antagonist; may be used to induce menses before the missed period, as an abortifacient in early pregnancy, or to treat hypercortisolism in patients with nonpituitary Cushing's syndrome. Trade name: RU486.

milk (milk) **1.** The secretion of the mammary glands for nourishment of the young; contains protein, a sugar (lactose), and fats. **2.** An aqueous suspension.

uterine m. Secretion produced by uterine glands that nourishes the implanted fertilized ovum.

witch's m. Milk-like fluid sometimes secreted by the breasts of newborn infants of either sex.

minipill (min′ĭ-pil) See progestin-only pill, under pill.

minocycline (mĭ-no-si′klēn) An antibiotic of the tetracycline group used to treat a variety of infections. Intrauterine exposure may cause permanent discoloration of the developing teeth.

miniabortion (min-ĭ-ă-bor′shun) See menstrual aspiration, under aspiration.

miscarriage (mis-kar′ij) Popular term for spontaneous abortion. See under abortion.

miscarry (mis-kar′e) To deliver a nonviable fetus.

mitogen (mi′to-jen) A substance derived from plants or microorganisms that causes cells (particularly lymphocytes) to undergo cell division.

pokeweed m. (PWM) A mitogen for B lymphocytes, derived from the plant *Phytolacca americana.*

mitogenesis (mi-to-jen′ĕ-sis) The initiation of mitosis.

mitogenic (mi-to-jen′ik) Inducing cell mitosis.

mitosis (mi-to′sis) Process in which a cell divides and forms two daughter cells, each normally receiving the same chromosome and DNA content as that of the original cell. Compare with meiosis.

mitotic (mi-tot′ik) Relating to mitosis.

mitral (mi′tral) **1.** Relating to the mitral (left atrioventricular) valve of the heart. **2.** Shaped like a bishop's miter or a turban.

mittelschmerz (mit′el-shmarts) A dull, fleeting abdominal pain occurring between two menstrual periods, at the time of ovulation.

mixture (miks'tur) **1.** An aggregation of two or more substances that are not chemically combined. **2.** A pharmaceutical preparation containing an insoluble substance suspended in a liquid by means of a viscid material.

> **Brompton m.** See Brompton cocktail, under cocktail.

molding (mōld'ing) **1.** The process of shaping, as with a mold. **2.** The temporary change in shape of the fetal head as it passes through the birth canal.

mole (mōl) **1.** Popular term for a nevocellular nevus. See nevocellular nevus, under nevus. **2.** An intrauterine mass.

> **atypical m.** An acquired pigmented lesion of the skin that has clinical and histologic characteristics different from a typical common mole (nevocellular nevus); may have macular and/or papular components; has well-defined irregular borders, is typically larger than most acquired common moles (over 6 mm), has pigment variegation ranging from tan to dark brown, and occurs on both sun-exposed and nonexposed areas of the body, especially on the trunk. Also called dysplastic nevus.

> **carneous m., blood m.** An ovum or early embryo surrounded by clotted blood, which contains degenerated chorionic villi.

> **hydatid m.** See hydatidiform mole.

> **hydatidiform m.** An abnormal pregnancy in which a mass of clear vesicles resembling a bunch of grapes grows within the uterus from proliferation of placental tissues; initial symptoms are usually those of early pregnancy, including a positive pregnancy test and vomiting (often severe); characteristic symptoms include bleeding (usually during the first trimester), passage of vesicles, and a uterus too large for the estimated time of gestation; designated *complete hydatidiform m.* when there is no fetus present, and *incomplete hydatidiform m.* when a fetus is present in addition to the mole. Also called hydatid mole; molar pregnancy.

> **invasive m.** A hydatidiform mole that invades the uterine wall; it may completely penetrate the wall and be associated with uterine rupture. Also called chorioadenoma destruens; chorioadenocarcinoma.

> **partial m.** Focal molar changes in placental villi with variability in the degree of hydropic change (i.e., vesicle formation); a living fetus may be present at times.

molimina (mo-lim'ĭ-nă) An individually characteristic constellation of premenstrual symptoms such as bloating, cramping, and emotional lability secondary to the influence of ovarian steroids.

molluscum contagiosum (mo-lus'kum kon-tă-je-o'sum) Infectious skin eruption of small, white wartlike lesions containing a cheesy substance, typically seen on the trunk and the genital and anal areas; caused by a poxvirus, transmitted by direct contact.

monad (mon'ad) **1.** A one-cell organism. **2.** A single chromosome formed after the second division in meiosis.

monilial (mo-nil'e-al) Relating to the fruit molds; frequently used incorrectly with reference to *Candida.*

moniliasis (mon-ĭ-li'ă-sis) See candidiasis.

monitor (mon'ĭ-tor) **1.** To maintain a close, constant watch on a patient's condition. **2.** Any device used in monitoring.

monitoring (mon'ĭ-tor-ing) **1.** A close, sometimes continuous, watch, observation, or supervision (as of a patient considered at risk). **2.** Periodic or continuous surveillance or testing to provide early warning of adverse effects (e.g., exposure to toxic substances or radioactivity).

> **auscultatory fetal m.** Assessment of the fetal heart tones with a head stethoscope (fetoscope) during labor.

> **biologic m.** The measuring of a pollutant (either a chemical or its metabolite) in a biological specimen to assess the extent of exposure and the effect of that exposure on an individual (e.g., in the workplace); typically, specimens are blood, urine, or exhaled air. The measurement indicates the quantity of a chemical absorbed regardless of the route of absorption (ingestion, inhalation, skin contact). Since some chemicals are rapidly cleared from the body, correct timing of the specimen collection is necessary for accurate interpretation of the data.

> **electronic fetal heart rate m.** Monitoring of the fetal heart rate with any of various electronic devices; may be *external* (indirect), performed through the maternal abdominal wall, usually by pulsed ultrasonography (Doppler ultrasound); or it may be *internal* (direct), performed during labor with a spiral electrode attached directly on the scalp of the fetus.

mono-, mon- Combining forms meaning one.

monoamniotic (mon-o-am-ne-otik) Sharing one amniotic sac in the uterus; applied to twins.

monogametic (mon-o-gam-et'ik) See homogametic.

mononucleosis (mon-o-noo-kle-o'sis) Abnormal

increase of mononuclear white blood cells (monocytes) in circulating blood.

cytomegalovirus (CMV) m. Infectious disease resembling infectious mononucleosis but caused by CMV, a herpesvirus classified as human herpesvirus 5 (HHV-5); incubation period is 20 to 60 days; characterized by prolonged high fevers, headache, malaise, profound fatigue, muscle pains, and enlargement of the spleen; in contrast to infectious mononucleosis, involvement of throat and cervical nodes is uncommon; it is frequently seen in patients receiving transplanted organs from donors with prior CMV infections.

infectious m. Infectious disease caused by the Epstein-Barr virus (EBV), a herpesvirus classified as human herpesvirus 4 (HHV-4); symptoms occur after an incubation period of 1 to 2 months; they include fever, sore throat, and enlargement of the spleen and lymph nodes; blood contains a large number of atypical lymphocytes (i.e., infected lymphocytes that resemble monocytes). The virus can be carried in the throat and saliva of afflicted persons for several months after disappearance of clinical symptoms; occurs mostly in adolescents and young adults. Sometimes called glandular fever; popularly called mono, kissing disease.

monosome (mon'o-sōm) A chromosome without its homologous chromosome.

monosomic (mon-o-so'mik) Characterized by monosomy.

monosomy (mon'o-so-me) Condition in which one chromsome of a pair is missing so that there are 45 instead of the normal 46 chromosomes; seen in certain genetic disorders (e.g., Turner's

syndrome).

monozygotic (mon-o-zi-got'ik) Derived from a single fertilized ovum; applied to identical twins.

mons (monz), pl. montes A slight anatomic prominence.

m. pubis The pad of fatty tissue over the pubic symphysis in the female.

m. ureteris A slight prominence on the wall of the bladder at the entrance of each ureter.

morbidity (mor-bid'ĭ-te) **1.** A diseased (pathologic) condition. **2.** The proportion of patients with a particular disease during a given time period in a given unit of population.

mortality (mor-tal'ĭ-te) **1.** The condition of being mortal. **2.** The whole number of deaths in a given time or portion of a population. See also rate; ratio.

perinatal m. The sum of stillbirths and newborn deaths.

reproductive m. The sum of deaths related to pregnancy and deaths caused by techniques used to prevent pregnancy (i.e., intrauterine devices and oral contraceptives).

morula (mor'u-lă) A cluster of cells (blastomeres) resulting from the early division of the zygote; an early stage in the development of the embryo.

morulation (mor-u-la'shun) The formation of the morula.

mosaic (mo-za'ik) A person or tissue affected with mosaicism.

mosaicism (mo-sa'ĭ-sizm) The presence of two or more populations of cells within one person, some with a normal set of chromosomes, others with extra or missing chromosomes; caused by errors of cell division in the fertilized egg (zygote). Predominance of abnormal cells gives rise to chromosomal abnormality syndromes (e.g., Down's syndrome, Turner's syndrome).

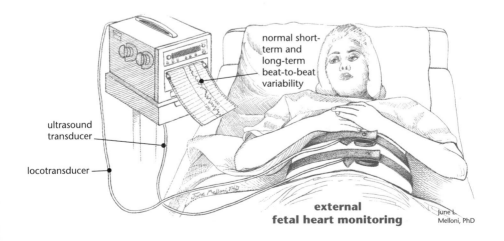

normal short-term and long-term beat-to-beat variability

ultrasound transducer

locotransducer

external fetal heart monitoring

June L. Melloni, PhD

movement (mōōv'ment) Motion; a change of place or position.

    fetal breathing m.'s Respiratory movements executed periodically by the fetus in the uterus which, by creating pressure changes, induce flowing of amniotic fluid in and out of the fetal lungs. Hypoxia or maternal cigarette smoking reduces fetal breathing movements, while high glucose levels (hyperglycemia) increase fetal breathing movements. The presence of fetal breathing movements is used as a measure of fetal well-being.

mucin (mu'sin) A viscous fluid composed of glycoproteins, secreted by mucous glands (e.g., salivary glands).

muco- Combining form meaning mucus.

mucocolpos (mu-ko-kol'pos) Abnormal accumulation of mucus within the vagina.

mucocutaneous (mu-ko-ku-ta'ne-us) Relating to both mucous membrane and skin (e.g., at the nasal, oral, vaginal, and anal orifices).

mucopurulent (mu-ko-pu'roo-lent) Containing mucus and pus; applied especially to discharges.

mucopus (mu'ko-pus) A purulent exudate; noted in the uterine cervical canal associated with chlamydial endocervicitis.

mucorrhea (mu-ko-re'ă) Excessive secretion of mucus.

    cervical m. Excessive discharge of clear, or slightly cloudy, mucus from endothelial cells of the uterine cervix.

mucosa (mu-ko'să) A mucous membrane; the inner lining of a cavity or tubular structure.

mucosanguineous (mu-ko-sang-gwin'e-us) Containing mucus and blood; applied to a discharge.

mucous (mu'kus) Relating to mucus.

mucus (mu'kus) The slippery suspension of mucin, desquamated cells, inorganic salts, and water, secreted by glands in a mucous membrane and serving to moisten and protect the membrane.

    cervical m. Mucus secreted by glands within the lining of the cervical canal; it undergoes periodic changes under hormonal influence: it is thin under the influence of estrogen, becoming thinnest and extremely elastic just before release of the ovum from the ovary (ovulation); under the influence of progesterone, it is thick, viscous and tenacious; during pregnancy, it becomes abundant and forms a thick plug (mucus plug) that completely fills and seals the canal.

muliebria (mu-le-eb're-ă) The female genital organs.

muliebris (mu-le-eb'ris) Relating to a female.

multi- Combining form meaning more than one; many.

multigravida (mul-tĭ-grav'ĭ-dă) A woman who has been pregnant more than once.

multipara (mul-tip'ă-ră) A woman who has completed two or more pregnancies in which each fetus reached the stage of viability, regardless of whether the infants were live or stillborn.

    grand m. A multipara who has completed six or more pregnancies.

multiparity (mul-tĭ-par'ĭ-te) The condition of being a multipara.

multiparous (mul-tip'ă-rus) Relating to a multipara.

multiple (mul'tĭ-pl) 1. Having more than one component. 2. Occurring in several sites at the same time.

mummification (mum-ĭ-fĭ-ka'shun) The drying and compression of a fetus that has died and remained in the uterus.

mural (mu'ral) Relating to the wall of a cavity or hollow organ.

muscle (mus'el) Tissue that serves to produce movement by its contraction; composed primarily of contractile cells.

    anal sphincter m., external Muscle of the anal canal. *Origin:* tip of coccyx, anococcygeal ligament. *Insertion:* perineal body. *Nerve supply:* inferior rectal and fourth sacral nerves. *Action:* closes anus.

    bulbocavernosus m., bulbospongiosus m. Muscle of the superficial urogenital region. In the female, *Origin:* perineal body. *Insertion:* fascia on dorsum of clitoris, corpus cavernosum of clitoris. *Nerve supply:* pudendal nerve. *Action:* constricts vaginal opening. In the male, *Origin:* median raphe of bulb, perineal body. *Insertion:* corpus cavernosum, root of penis. *Nerve supply:* pudendal nerve. *Action:* constricts urethra.

    coccygeus m. Muscle of the pelvic diaphragm. *Origin:* ischial spine, sacrospinous ligament. *Insertion:* coccyx, lower part of lateral border of sacrum. *Nerve supply:* third and fourth sacral nerves. *Action:* raises and supports pelvic floor. Also called ischiococcygeus muscle.

    gluteus maximus m. Muscle of the buttock. *Origin:* upper portion of ilium, sacrum and coccyx, sacrotuberous ligament, gluteal aponeurosis. *Insertion:* gluteal tuberosity of femur, iliotibial tract (band of fascia lata). Nerve supply: inferior gluteal nerve. *Action:* extends, abducts, and rotates thigh laterally.

    gluteus medius m. Muscle of the buttock. *Origin:* midportion of outer surface of ilium.

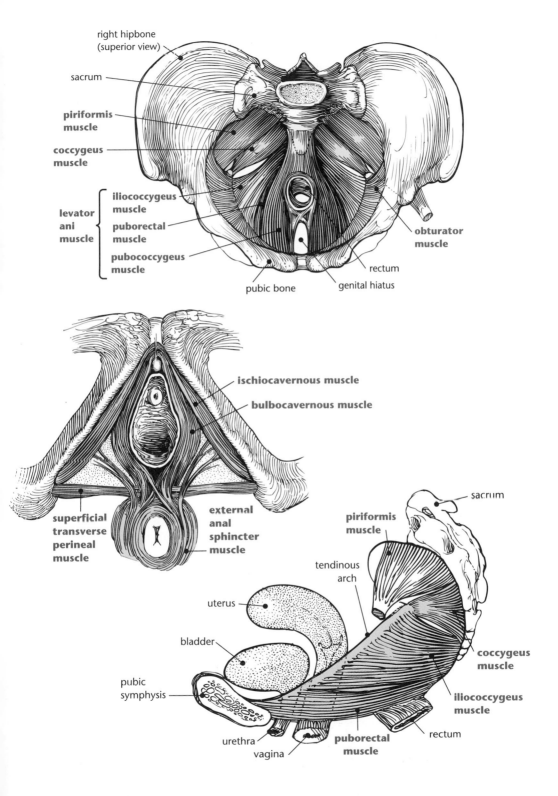

right hipbone
(superior view)

sacrum

piriformis muscle

coccygeus muscle

levator ani muscle {
iliococcygeus muscle
puborectal muscle
pubococcygeus muscle
}

obturator muscle

rectum

pubic bone

genital hiatus

ischiocavernous muscle

bulbocavernous muscle

superficial transverse perineal muscle

external anal sphincter muscle

piriformis muscle

sacrum

tendinous arch

uterus

bladder

pubic symphysis

urethra

vagina

puborectal muscle

coccygeus muscle

iliococcygeus muscle

rectum

Insertion: greater trochanter and oblique ridge of femur. *Nerve supply:* superior gluteal nerve. *Action:* abducts and rotates the thigh medially.

gluteus minimus m. Muscle of the buttock. *Origin:* lower portion of outer surface of ilium. *Insertion:* greater trochanter of femur. *Nerve supply:* superior gluteal nerve. *Action:* abducts and rotates the thigh medially.

iliococcygeus m. Muscle of the pelvic diaphragm. *Origin:* ischial spine, arching tendon over internal obturator muscle. *Insertion:* side of coccyx, perineal body between tip of coccyx and anal canal. *Nerve supply:* third and fourth sacral nerves. *Action:* constricts lower end of rectum and vagina, supports pelvic organs.

ischiocavernosus m. Muscle of the superficial urogenital region. *Origin:* ramus of ischium. *Insertion:* crus of clitoris (or penis). *Nerve supply:* perineal nerve. *Action:* maintains erection of clitoris (or penis).

ischiococcygeus m. See coccygeus muscle.

levator ani m. The main muscle of the pelvic diaphragm, composed of iliococcygeus, pubococcygeus, and puborectal muscles.

oblique m. of abdomen, external Muscle of the abdominal wall. *Origin:* inferior border of lower eight ribs. *Insertion:* anterior half of crest of ilium, linea alba through rectus sheath, inguinal ligament. *Nerve supply:* lower intercostal nerve. *Action:* flexes and rotates vertebral column, tenses abdominal wall, compresses abdominal organs.

oblique m. of abdomen, internal Muscle of the abdominal wall. *Origin:* iliac crest, thoracolumbar fascia, inguinal ligament. *Insertion:* lower three or four costal cartilages, linea alba by conjoint tendon to pubic bone. *Nerve supply:* lower intercostal nerve. *Action:* flexes and rotates vertebral column, tenses abdominal wall.

obturator m., internal Muscle of the pelvic diaphragm. *Origin:* pelvic surface of hipbone, internal margin of obturator foramen, obturator membrane. *Insertion:* greater trochanter of femur. *Nerve supply:* fifth lumbar nerve, first and second sacral nerves. *Action:* abducts and rotates thigh laterally.

pectoralis major m. Muscle of the chest. *Origin:* medial half of clavicle, sternum, and costal cartilages of fourth to sixth ribs; aponeurosis of external oblique muscle of abdomen; often at anterior extremity of sixth rib. *Insertion:* lateral lip of intertubercular groove of humerus. *Nerve supply:* lateral and medial pectoral nerves (C5, C6, C7, C8, T1).

Action: adduction and medial rotation of arm; draws arm forward.

pectoralis minor m. Muscle of the chest. *Origin:* anterior surface of ribs 3,4, and 5, near costal cartilages. *Insertion:* upper part of coracoid process. *Nerve supply:* lateral and medial pectoral nerves (C6, C7, C8). *Action:* draws shoulder forward and downward, raises rib cage.

piriformis m. Muscle of the pelvic diaphragm. *Origin:* front of sacrum, gluteal surface of ilium, sacroiliac joint. *Insertion:* greater trochanter of femur. *Nerve supply:* first and second sacral nerves. *Action:* rotates extended thigh laterally, abducts flexed thigh.

pubococcygeus m. Muscle of the pelvic diaphragm. *Origin:* back of pubic bone and obturator fascia. *Insertion:* front of coccyx, perineal body. *Nerve supply:* third and fourth sacral nerves. *Action:* supports pelvic organs.

puborectal m. Muscle of the pelvic diaphragm. *Origin:* back of pubic bone and pubic symphysis. *Insertion:* interdigitates to form a sling that passes behind the rectum. *Nerve supply:* third and fourth sacral nerves. *Action:* holds anal canal at 90° angle to rectum, supports pelvic organs.

pubovaginal m. Muscle of the pelvic diaphragm. In the female, the most medial fibers of the pubococcygeus muscle. *Origin:* pubic bone. *Insertion:* lateral wall of the vagina. *Nerve supply:* sacral and pudendal nerves. *Action:* aids in controlling micturition.

pyramidal m. Muscle of the abdominal wall. *Origin:* pubic bone, pubic symphysis. *Insertion:* linea alba. *Nerve supply:* last thoracic nerve. *Action:* tenses abdominal wall.

rectus m. of abdomen Muscle of the abdominal wall. *Origin:* pubic crest, pubic symphysis. *Insertion:* xiphoid process, fifth to seventh costal cartilages. *Nerve supply:* branches of the lower thoracic nerves. *Action:* tenses abdominal wall, draws thorax downward, flexes vertebral column.

sphincter m. of anus, external Striated (voluntary) muscle surrounding entire length of anal canal. *Origin:* tip of coccyx, anococcygeal ligament. *Insertion:* central tendon of perineum. *Nerve supply:* inferior rectal nerve, fourth sacral nerve. *Action:* closes anal canal and anus.

sphincter m. of anus, internal Smooth (involuntary) muscle forming a ring around the upper part of the anal canal. *Nerve supply:* branches from inferior hypogastric plexus. *Action:* closes anal canal and anus.

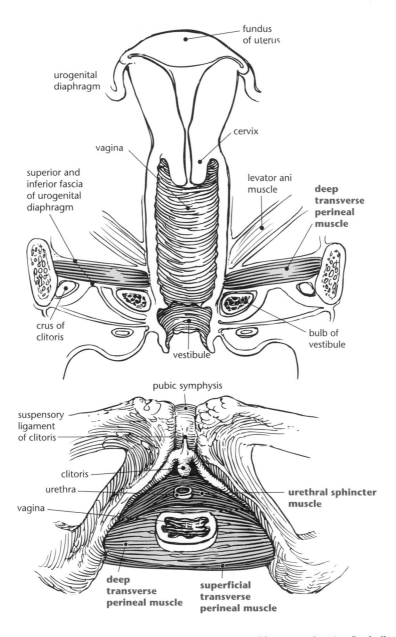

fundus of uterus

urogenital diaphragm

vagina

cervix

superior and inferior fascia of urogenital diaphragm

levator ani muscle

deep transverse perineal muscle

crus of clitoris

bulb of vestibule

vestibule

pubic symphysis

suspensory ligament of clitoris

clitoris

urethra

vagina

urethral sphincter muscle

deep transverse perineal muscle

superficial transverse perineal muscle

sphincter m. of urethra Muscle of the urogenital diaphragm. *Origin:* ramus of pubic bone. *Insertion:* fibers interdigitate around the urethra. *Nerve supply:* perineal nerve. *Action:* compresses the urethra.

sphincter m. of urinary bladder Thick muscular thickening around the internal urethral orifice. *Nerve supply:* vesical nerve. *Action:* acts as valve to close internal opening of urethra.

sphincter m. of vagina See bulbocavernosus muscle.

transverse m. of abdomen Muscle of the abdominal wall. *Origin:* seventh to twelfth costal cartilages, thoracolumbar fascia, iliac crest, inguinal ligament. *Insertion:* xiphoid process, linea alba, conjoint tendon to pubic bone. *Nerve supply:* lower intercostal nerve, iliohypogastric nerve, ilioinguinal nerve. *Action:* supports abdominal organs, tenses abdominal wall.

transverse m. of perineum, deep Muscle of the urogenital diaphragm. *Origin:* inferior ramus of ischium. *Insertion:* perineal body, external anal sphincter, vaginal wall. *Nerve supply:* perineal nerve. *Action:* supports pelvic organs.

transverse m. of perineum, superficial Muscle of the superficial urogenital region. *Origin:* ischium near tuberosity. *Insertion:* perineal body. *Nerve supply:* perineal nerve. *Action:* supports pelvic organs.

mutagen (mu'tă-jen) An agent (e.g., a radioactive substance, a chemical) that increases spontaneous genetic mutations by causing changes in DNA.

mutagenesis (mu-tă-jen'ĕ-sis) Production of a mutation.

insertional m. Mutation resulting from insertion of different material into a normal gene, especially the slow transformation induced by certain cancer-causing retroviruses.

mutagenic (mu-tă-jen'ik) Causing mutations.

mutagenicity (mu-tă-jĕ-nis'ĭ-te) The ability to induce basic and transmissible changes in the genetic material of a cell.

mutant (mu'tant) An organism or cell that differs from the parental strain as a result of carrying a gene that has undergone permanent and transmissible structural change.

mutation (mu-ta'shun) A permanent, heritable structural change in DNA.

point m. Mutation involving a minute section of a single gene (i.e., a change in a single base pair in the DNA molecule), as seen in sickle cell anemia.

myco- Combining form meaning fungus.

mycobacteria (mi-ko-bak-te're-ă) Microorganisms of the genus *Mycobacterium.*

Mycobacterium (mi-ko-bak-te're-um) Genus of Gram-positive aerobic bacteria (family Mycobacteriaceae); the principal habitat of some species is diseased or dead tissues.

M. avium complex (MAC) A bacterial complex that includes several strains of *Mycobacterium avium* and the immunologically related *Mycobacterium intracellulare,* most frequently found in respiratory secretions from persons with a tuberculous-like lung disease; it is the cause of a disseminated blood infection (MAC bacteremia) in AIDS patients. Distinguished from *Mycobacterium avium,* which causes disease primarily in birds. See also *Mycobacterium avium* complex bacteremia, under bacteremia.

M. avium-intracellulare (MAI) Species causing a nontuberculous lung disease in humans, similar to tuberculosis; occurs primarily in persons with underlying lung disease and as an opportunistic infection in AIDS patients.

M. bovis A species causing tuberculosis in cattle; an attenuated form is used to prepare the BCG vaccine.

M. fortuitum Species causing postoperative and posttraumatic wound infections.

M. tuberculosis The causative agent of tuberculosis in humans.

Mycoplasma (mi-ko-plaz'mă) A genus of bacteria that are the smallest free-living organisms presently known (about the same size as viruses); like viruses, they lack a rigid cell wall but, unlike viruses, they can reproduce outside living cells; some species cause disease (e.g., in the organs of reproduction of both females and males).

M. pneumonia Species causing pneumonia. Also called Eaton agent.

mycoplasma (mi-ko-plaz'mă) Any bacterium of the genus *Mycoplasma.*

T m.'s See *Ureaplasma urealyticus,* under *Ureaplasma.*

myelomeningocele (mi-ĕ-lo-mĕ-ning'go-sēl) See meningomyelocele.

myelosuppression (mi-ĕ-lo-soo'presh-un) Inhibition of the activity of bone marrow cells.

myo- Combining form meaning muscle.

myoblastoma (mi-o-blas-to'mă) Tumor composed of immature muscle cells.

granular cell m. See granular cell tumor, under tumor.

myocardiopathy (mi-o-kar-de-op'a-the) See cardiomyopathy.

myoma (mi-o'mă) See leiomyoma.

myometer (mi-om'ĕ-ter) Instrument for measuring the strength of a muscular contraction.

myometritis (mi-o-mĕ-tri'tis) Inflammation of the myometrium.

myometrium (mi-o-me'tre-um) The middle muscular layer of the uterine wall; composed of smooth (nonstriated) muscle fibers arranged in three layers: *external,* the layer continuing into the fallopian (uterine) tubes, round ligament of the uterus, and ligament of the ovary; *intermediate,* thickest layer containing the largest blood vessels; *internal,* layer in contact with the endometrium. Myometrium of the nonpregnant uterus is dense and firm; in pregnancy, it becomes greatly enlarged due to hypertrophy of the muscle cells.

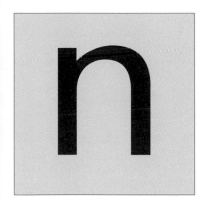

naloxone (nal-oks'ōn) A compound that blocks the action of narcotics, usually employed in treating respiratory depression (e.g., in patients who have received high narcotic doses during surgery and in newborn infants affected by maternal anesthetics administered during labor).

nano- **1.** (n) Prefix meaning one-billionth (10^{-9}). **2.** Combining form meaning dwarf.

nanosomia (nan-o-so'me-ă) See dwarfism.

nanus (nă'nus) See dwarf.

nape (nāp) The back of the neck. Also called nucha.

narco- Combining form meaning stupor.

narcosis (nar-ko'sis) A deep stuporous state produced by certain chemicals and physical agents.

narcotic (nar-kot'ik) **1.** Producing narcosis. **2.** A drug (natural or synthetic) intended for the relief of pain that also tends to produce insensibility, stupor, and sleep (i.e., it has both analgesic and sedative actions); narcotics have morphine-like pharmacologic action and, with prolonged use, may become addictive.

nasion (na'ze-on) A craniometric point in the middle of the nasofrontal suture.

natal (na'tal) **1.** Relating to birth. **2.** Relating to the buttocks.

natality (na-tal'ĭ-te) The birth rate.

nates (na'tēz) The buttocks.

natimortality (na-tĭ-mor-tal'ĭ-te) The proportion of stillbirths and newborn deaths to the birth rate.

nausea (naw'ze-ă) The imminent desire to vomit, often preceding or accompanying vomiting.

    n. gravidarum The nausea experienced by some women during pregnancy.

nauseant (naw'ze-ant) **1.** Inducing a desire to vomit. **2.** Any agent that induces nausea.

nauseate (naw'ze-āt) To cause a desire to vomit.

nauseous (naw'shus) Relating to nausea.

navel (na'vel) The umbilicus.

neck (nek) **1.** The part of the body between the head and trunk. **2.** Any relatively narrow area of a structure or organ (e.g., tooth, bladder, rib, femur).

    n. of womb See uterine cervix, under cervix.

necro-, necr- Combining forms meaning death; necrosis.

necrobiosis (nek-ro-bi-o'sis) The natural death of tissues with the concurrent replacement thereof.

    n. diabeticorum Condition characterized by patchy degeneration of the skin in which fat tissue is excessively involved in the concurrent degeneration and reparative process; usually associated with diabetes mellitus at the site of injection with animal-source insulins; seen less frequently since the availability of human insulin (i.e., of recombinant DNA origin).

necrose (nek'rōs) To undergo irreversible damage, decomposition, and death; applied to cells, tissues, and organs.

necrosis (nĕ-kro'sis) The total morphologic changes that follow irreversible injury and death of cells in a circumscribed area of living tissues and organs.

    acute tubular n. (ATN) A form of acute kidney failure usually occurring in association with a period of hypotension, especially from hemorrhage (e.g., in premature placental separation), shock, crush injury, or sepsis; characterized by absent or scanty urination for hours or several days followed by a gradually increasing flow of dilute urine, often reaching very large amounts. Also called lower nephron necrosis.

    colliquative n. See liquefactive necrosis.

    cystic medial n. (CMN) Focal accumulation of mucopolysaccharide in the middle layer of the aortic wall (especially of the ascending aorta) with fragmentation of the connective tissue, predisposing to dissecting aneurysms; seen sometimes in pregnant women. Also called medionecrosis of the aorta.

    fat n. Destruction of fatty tissue, seen in the female breast as a result of trauma; it is usually followed by inflammation and fibrosis, forming a benign hard mass that superficially resembles a cancerous growth. Also called adiponecrosis; steatonecrosis.

    fibrinoid n. A type of necrosis affecting particularly the middle layer of blood vessel walls; characterized by degeneration of normal structure and replacement by a material resembling fibrin; seen in autoimmune diseases (e.g., rheumatic fever, systemic lupus erythematosus).

liquefactive n. Complete and rapid dissolution of cells (including cell membranes) by enzymes, creating circumscribed areas of softened tissue with a semifluid exudate; characteristic of brain infarcts and localized bacterial infections (abscesses). Also called colliquative necrosis.

lower nephron n. See acute tubular necrosis.

postpartum n. of pituitary See Sheehan's syndrome, under syndrome.

renal papillary n. Necrosis of the papilla of the kidney resulting from deprivation of blood supply; usually occurs in patients with diabetes and pyelonephritis, in people who have habitually ingested large quantities of pain killers (analgesics), in sickle-cell disease, and in obstructive disease and infection of the urinary tract. Also called necrotizing papillitis.

subcutaneous fat n. of newborn A collection of sharply circumscribed reddish or purplish firm nodules on the cheeks, arms, thighs, and buttocks of newborn infants, appearing between days 1 and 7, and usually resolving within a few weeks; may also calcify; cause is unknown but a cold injury is thought to play a role.

necrospermia (nek-ro-sper'me-ă) Condition in which semen contains a high percentage of nonmotile spermatozoa.

necrotic (ně-krot'ik) Relating to dead cells or tissues.

needle (ne'dl) Any of various slender, sharp, solid or hollow implements for stitching, puncturing, injecting, or aspirating.

aneurysm n. A needle with a large blunt end for passing a ligature around a blood vessel.

aspirating n. A long, hollow needle for withdrawing fluid from a cavity.

atraumatic n. A surgical needle of small diameter that minimizes damage to tissue.

biopsy n. A hollow needle employed in obtaining tissue for microscopic examination.

disposable n. A needle intended to be discarded after a one-time use.

exploring n. A needle with a longitudinal groove for detecting the presence of fluid in a cavity or a tumor.

hypodermic n. A short, hollow needle for injecting fluids beneath the skin.

lumbar puncture n. A needle designed for entering the spinal canal to remove cerebrospinal fluid or to introduce medication.

surgical n. Any needle used in a surgical

procedure.

Vim-Silverman n. A biopsy needle for obtaining a small core of tissue (e.g., from the breast) for microscopic examination.

neglect (ně-glekt') **1.** To fail to care for or to give sufficient or proper attention to something (e.g., a responsibility). **2.** The act of neglecting something; a failure. **3.** The condition of being neglected.

negligence (neg'lĭ-jens) Failure to use care that a reasonably prudent person would exercise under similar circumstances, thereby exposing another to an unreasonable risk of harm. In order to have a legal claim against another for a negligent act, one must prove that a duty to exercise reasonable care was owed to the claimant, that the duty was breached and that the breach of duty caused an injury to the claimant which can legally be compensated. See also assumption of risk, under risk.

comparative n. The apportioning of the negligence of all parties, including the claimant, when determining responsibility for the claimant's losses. The award is reduced by the percent of negligence, if any, allocated to the claimant.

contributory n. An affirmative defense in a negligence claim wherein the claimant is proven to have contributed to his own loss by his own acts of negligence. In medical malpractice: failure of the patient to exercise reasonable care in following the physician's instructions concurrent with the physician's negligent conduct, and constituting a part of the proximate cause of the injury or loss for which compensation is being sought.

Neisseria (ni-se're-ă) Genus of bacteria (family Neisseriaceae) composed of Gram-negative microorganisms that occur in pairs and are parasitic in humans; some species cause disease.

N. gonorrhoeae A species causing gonorrhea and, in newborns, ophthalmia neonatorum.

N. meningitidis A species causing meningococcal meningitis.

neocystostomy (ne-o-sis-tos'tŏ-me) Surgical construction of a new connection between a ureter and the bladder to facilitate urine flow, either by inserting a ureter into a new site or by using a segment of defunctionalized ileum.

neodymium (ne-o-dim'e-um) Metallic element; symbol Nd, atomic number 60, atomic weight 144.24.

neonatal (ne-o-na'tal) Relating to the first 4 weeks of life.

neonate (ne'o-nāt) A newborn baby, from birth through the first 28 days of life. Also called newborn.

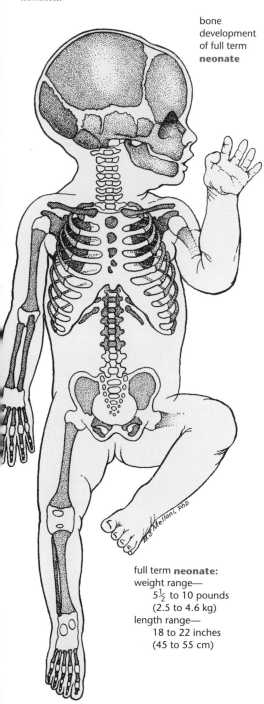

bone development of full term **neonate**

full term **neonate**:
weight range—
  $5\frac{1}{2}$ to 10 pounds
  (2.5 to 4.6 kg)
length range—
  18 to 22 inches
  (45 to 55 cm)

neonatologist (ne-o-na-tol'ŏ-jist) A specialist in neonatology.

neonatology (ne-o-na-tol'ŏ-je) The branch of medicine concerned with disorders of the newborn infant from birth through the first 28 days of life. Also called neonatal medicine.

neoplasia (nc-o-pla'ze-ă) The abnormal process that results in the formation and growth of a tumor (neoplasm). See also dysplasia.

  cervical intraepithelial n. (CIN) See cervical dysplasia, under dysplasia.

  gestational trophoblastic n. (GTN) See under disease.

  vaginal intraepithelial n. (VAIN) Abnormal cell growth occurring as single or multiple lesions within the epithelium of the vagina; it may progress and develop into carcinoma and occur with or without cervical or vulvar involvement. Depending on the thickness of epithelium involved, it is classified as VAIN I (mild), VAIN II (moderate), or VAIN III (severe); VAIN III is sometimes called carcinoma *in situ*.

  vulvar intraepithelial n. (VIN) See vulvar dysplasia, under dysplasia.

neoplasm (ne'o-plazm) An abnormal mass of tissue characterized by excessive growth that is uncoordinated with that of the surrounding normal tissues and persists in the same excessive manner after cessation of the stimuli that initiated the change. Also called tumor.

  borderline malignant n. Term used to describe tumors of low malignant potential.

neostomy (ne-os'tŏ-me) Surgical construction of a new artificial opening in a structure or organ.

neovagina (ne-o-vaj-i'nă) A surgically constructed vagina using a split-thickness skin graft, or a bowel segment, following total removal of the pelvic organs for the treatment of advanced cancer.

neovascularization (ne-o-vas-ku-lar-ĭ-za'shun) Abnormal formation of new blood vessels in any tissue.

nephro-, nephr- Combining forms meaning kidney.

nephrolith (nef'ro-lith) See kidney stone, under stone.

nephron (nef'ron) The functional unit of the kidney; it consists of the filtering unit (glomerulus), proximal and distal convoluted tubules, proximal and distal straight tubules, Henle's (nephronic) loop, and the connecting tubule. There are approximately one million nephrons in each kidney, the number declining with advancing age.

nephropathy (nĕ-frop'ă-the) Any disease of the kidney.

diabetic n. A complication of diabetes mellitus resulting from long-term high glucose levels in the blood; chief features include hypertension, damage to the filtration system of the kidney, and eventual kidney failure. Patients with either diabetes 1 or diabetes 2 may be affected; pregnancy tends to aggravate the condition.

nephrosis (nĕ-fro'sis), pl. nephroses **1.** General term denoting diseases of the kidneys that were thought to involve primarily the tubules; a non-inflammatory disease of the kidney. **2.** See nephrotic syndrome, under syndrome.

> **lower nephron n.** Obsolete term for acute tubular necrosis.

nephrostomy (nĕ-fros'tŏ-me) Surgical construction of an opening into the kidney pelvis for insertion of an external drainage tube.

> **percutaneous n.** Nephrostomy performed through the skin under the guidance of ultrasonography.

nephrotoxic (nef-ro-tok'sik) Destructive to the cells of the kidney.

nephrotoxicity (nef-ro-tok-sis'ĭ-te) The state of being nephrotoxic.

nerve (nerv) A cordlike structure composed of nerve fascicles that carries impulses between a part of the central nervous system (brain and spinal cord) and some other part of the body.

> **accelerator n.'s** Nerves serving to increase the rate of the heart contraction; they originate from the sympathetic trunk and innervate the heart muscle.

> **afferent n.** Any nerve that transmits impulses from the periphery of the body to the brain or spinal cord.

> **anococcygeal n.'s** Sensory nerves. *Origin:* coccygeal plexus. *Branches:* filaments. *Distribution:* skin over coccyx.

> **augmentor n.'s** Nerves of sympathetic origin that increase the force as well as the rate of the heart contraction.

> **auricular n.'s, anterior** Sensory nerves. *Origin:* auriculotemporal nerve. *Branches:* filaments. *Distribution:* skin of anterosuperior part of external ear, principally the helix and the tragus.

> **auricular n.'s, posterior** Motor and sensory nerves. *Origin:* facial nerve. *Branches:* auricular, occipital. *Distribution:* posterior auricular and occipital muscles, skin of external ear.

> **autonomic n.** Any nerve from either of the two divisions of the autonomic nervous system (i.e., the sympathetic or parasympathetic trunks).

> **axillary n.** Motor and sensory nerve. *Origin:* posterior cord of brachial plexus. *Branches:* posterior, anterior, cutaneous, articular. *Distribution:* deltoid and teres minor muscles, and neighboring skin.

> **n. of Bell** See thoracic nerve, long.

> **brachial plexus** See under plexus.

> **cavernous n.'s of clitoris** Parasympathetic, sympathetic, and afferent nerves. *Origin:* uterovaginal plexus through vaginal nerves. *Branches:* filaments. *Distribution:* corpus cavernosum of clitoris.

> **cervical n.'s** (C 1-8) Eight pairs of spinal nerves in the neck region, arising from the cervical segments of the spinal cord.

> **cervical plexus** See under plexus.

> **coccygeal n.** (C0) The lowest spinal nerve; it arises from the coccygeal segments of the spinal cord.

> **coccygeal plexus** See under plexus.

> **cranial n.'s** The twelve pairs of nerves connected directly with the brain, at its base: (I) olfactory, (II) optic, (III) oculomotor, (IV) trochlear, (V) trigeminal, (VI) abducent, (VII) facial, (VIII) vestibulocochlear, (IX) glossopharyngeal, (X) vagus, (XI) accessory, (XII) hypoglossal.

> **cutaneous n. of thigh, lateral** Sensory nerve. *Origin:* second and third lumbar nerves. *Branches:* anterior, posterior, filaments. *Distribution:* skin of lateral and anterior part of thigh.

> **cutaneous n. of thigh, posterior** Sensory nerve. *Origin:* first, second, and third sacral nerves. *Branches:* gluteal, perineal, femoral, sural. *Distribution:* skin of lower gluteal region, external genitalia, perineum, and posterior aspect of thigh and leg (calf).

> **dorsal n. of clitoris** Sensory and motor nerve. *Origin:* pudendal nerve. *Branches:* filaments. *Distribution:* urethra and clitoris.

> **efferent n.** Any nerve that transmits impulses from the brain or spinal cord to the periphery of the body.

> **genitofemoral n.** Sensory and motor nerve. *Origin:* first and second lumbar nerves. *Branches:* genital, femoral. *Distribution:* skin of labium majus, mons pubis, and adjacent surface of thigh, cremaster muscle, skin of scrotum.

> **gluteal n., inferior** Motor nerve. *Origin:* fifth lumbar nerve and first and second sacral nerves. *Branches:* filaments. *Distribution:* gluteus maximus muscle.

> **gluteal n., superior** Motor nerve. *Origin:* fourth and fifth lumbar nerves and first sacral nerve. *Branches:* superior, inferior, filaments.

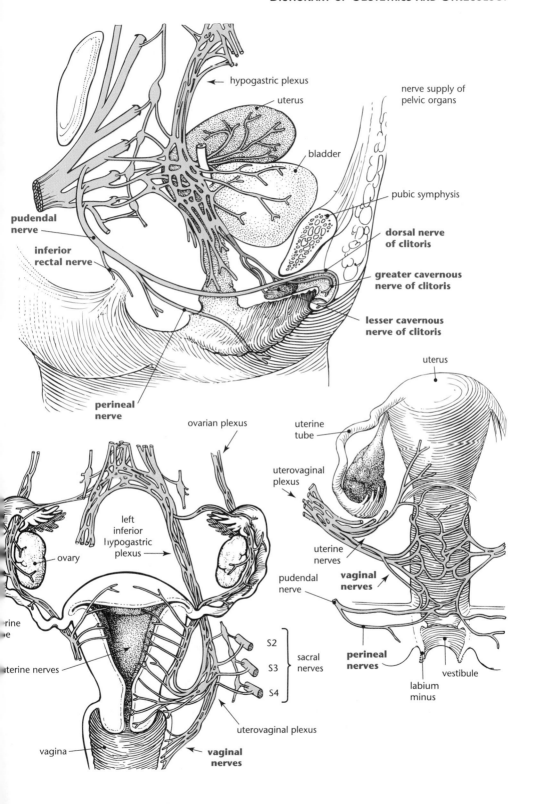

nerve supply of
pelvic organs

hypogastric plexus

uterus

bladder

pubic symphysis

**pudendal
nerve**

**dorsal nerve
of clitoris**

**inferior
rectal nerve**

**greater cavernous
nerve of clitoris**

**lesser cavernous
nerve of clitoris**

**perineal
nerve**

ovarian plexus

uterine
tube

uterus

uterovaginal
plexus

left
inferior
hypogastric
plexus

ovary

uterine
nerves

pudendal
nerve

**vaginal
nerves**

rine
e

uterine nerves

S2

S3

S4

sacral
nerves

**perineal
nerves**

vestibule

labium
minus

vagina

uterovaginal plexus

**vaginal
nerves**

Distribution: gluteus minimus and medius muscles, tensor muscle of fascia lata.

hemorrhoidal n. See rectal nerve, inferior.

iliohypogastric n. Motor and sensory nerve. *Origin:* first lumbar nerve. *Branches:* anterior cutaneous, muscular, lateral cutaneous. *Distribution:* skin of lower part of abdomen (above the mons pubis), lower abdominal muscles, skin of posterolateral gluteal region.

ilioinguinal n. Sensory nerve. *Origin:* first lumbar nerve. *Branches:* muscular, anterior labial, anterior scrotal, filaments. *Distribution:* muscles of lower abdominal wall, skin of mons pubis, superior and medial part of thigh, labium majus, root of penis, and upper part of scrotum.

intercostobrachial n. Sensory nerve. *Origin:* second and frequently third intercostal nerves. *Branches:* filaments. *Distribution:* skin of medial and posterior part of arm, axilla.

labial n.'s, anterior Sensory nerves. *Origin:* ilioinguinal nerve. *Branches:* filaments. *Distribution:* skin of anterior area of labia of female genitalia.

labial n.'s, posterior Sensory nerves. *Origin:* perineal nerve. *Branches:* filaments. *Distribution:* skin of posterior portion of labia and vestibule of vagina.

lumbar n.'s (L 1-5) Five pairs of spinal nerves, arising from the lumbar segments of the spinal cord.

mixed n. A nerve containing both afferent and efferent fibers.

motor n. An efferent nerve conveying impulses to skeletal muscles, inciting contraction.

obturator n., internal Sensory and motor nerve. *Origin:* fifth lumbar and first and second sacral nerves. *Branches:* muscular, filaments. *Distribution:* internal obturator and superior gemellus muscles.

occipital n., greater Sensory and motor nerve. *Origin:* median branch of dorsal division of second cervical nerve. *Branches:* muscular, filaments, medial, lateral, auricular. *Distribution:* scalp of top and back of head, semispinal muscle of head.

occipital n., lesser Sensory nerve. *Origin:* second cervical nerve. *Branches:* auricular, filaments. *Distribution:* skin of side of head and behind ear.

occipital n., third Sensory nerve. *Origin:* cutaneous part of third cervical nerve. *Branches:* medial, lateral. *Distribution:* skin of lower part of back of head.

parasympathetic n. Any nerve of the

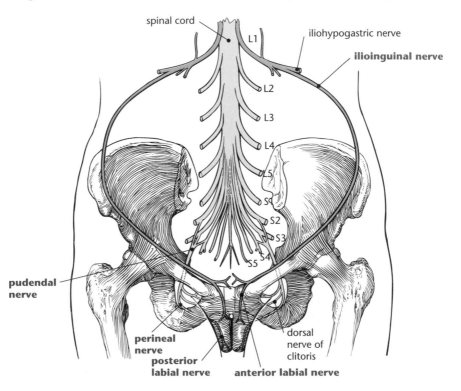

spinal cord

iliohypogastric nerve

ilioinguinal nerve

L1
L2
L3
L4
L5
S1
S2
S3
S4
S5

pudendal nerve

perineal nerve

posterior labial nerve

dorsal nerve of clitoris

anterior labial nerve

parasympathetic trunk (a division of the autonomic nervous system).

pectoral n., lateral Motor and sensory nerve. *Origin:* lateral cord of brachial plexus. *Branches:* filaments. *Distribution:* pectoralis major muscle.

pectoral n., medial Motor nerve. *Origin:* medial cord of brachial plexus. *Branches:* filaments. *Distribution:* pectoralis minor muscle and caudal part of pectoralis major muscle.

perineal n. Sensory and motor nerve. *Origin:* pudendal nerve. *Branches:* muscular, labial, posterior scrotal, nerve to urethral bulb. *Distribution:* urogenital diaphragm, skin of external genitalia, perineal muscles, mucous membrane of urethra.

pressor n. An afferent nerve that produces constriction of blood vessels, thereby increasing blood pressure.

pudendal n. Sensory, motor, and parasympathetic nerve. *Origin:* second, third, and fourth sacral nerves. *Branches:* inferior rectal nerve, perineal nerve, dorsal nerve of clitoris, dorsal nerve of penis. *Distribution:* external sphincter of anus, lining of lower anal canal, skin around anus, skin of posterior area of labia majora and scrotum, muscles of superficial urogenital region, urogenital diaphragm, muscles of perineum, lower vagina (about 2.5 cm), vestibule, prepuce and glans of clitoris and penis.

rectal n., inferior Sensory and motor. *Origin:* pudendal nerve. *Branches:* filaments. *Distribution:* external sphincter of anus, skin around anus, lining of anal canal.

sacral n.'s (S 1-5) Five pairs of spinal nerves, arising from the sacral segments of the spinal cord.

sacral plexus See under plexus.

sensory n. An afferent nerve that conducts impulses from a sense organ in the periphery of the body to the central nervous system.

spinal n.'s The 31 pairs of nerves arising from the spinal cord within the vertebral canal: eight cervical, 12 thoracic, five lumbar, five sacral, and one coccygeal.

sympathetic n. Any nerve of the sympathetic trunk (a division of the autonomic nervous system).

splanchnic n.'s, pelvic Preganglionic, parasympathetic, afferent nerves. *Origin:* second to fourth sacral nerves. *Branches:* filaments. *Distribution:* inferior hypogastric plexus, descending and sigmoid colon, pelvic viscera.

subcostal n. Sensory and motor nerve. *Origin:* 12th thoracic nerve. *Branches:* anterior cutaneous, lateral cutaneous. *Distribution:* skin of lower abdominal wall and side of gluteal region, some abdominal muscles.

supraclavicular n.'s, intermediate Sensory nerves. *Origin:* common trunk formed by third and fourth cervical nerves. *Branches:* filaments. *Distribution:* skin over pectoral and deltoid muscles.

supraclavicular n.'s, medial Sensory nerves. *Origin:* common trunk formed by third and fourth cervical nerves. *Branches:* filaments. *Distribution:* skin of medial infraclavicular region as far as the midline, sternoclavicular joint.

thoracic n.'s (T 1-12) Twelve pairs of spinal nerves, arising from the thoracic segments of the spinal cord.

thoracic n., long Motor nerve. *Origin:* fifth, sixth, and seventh cervical nerves. *Branches:* filaments. *Distribution:* all digitations of serratus anterior muscle.

thoracodorsal n. Motor nerve. *Origin:* sixth, seventh, and eighth cervical nerves. *Branches:* filaments. *Distribution:* latissimus dorsi muscle.

uterovaginal plexus See under plexus.

vaginal n.'s Sympathetic and parasympathetic nerves. *Origin:* uterovaginal plexus. *Branches:* filaments. *Distribution:* vagina, erectile tissue of vestibular bulbs.

vasomotor n. An efferent nerve of the autonomic nervous system conducting impulses to blood vessel walls, causing the vessels either to dilate or to constrict.

vomernasal n. Nerve present in the nasal septum of the fetus; it disappears before birth.

zygomatic n. Sensory nerve. *Origin:* maxillary nerve. *Branches:* zygomaticotemporal, zygomaticofacial. *Distribution:* skin of temple, skin over prominence of cheek (zygomatic arch).

nest (nest) A collection of similar entities (e.g., cells).

adrenal cortical n.'s Aggregations of small (3–4 mm), benign nodules found frequently in the broad ligament of the uterus.

neural (noor'al) **1.** Relating to the nervous system. **2.** Relating to the dorsal region of the embryo.

neurectomy (noo-rek'tŏ-me) Surgical removal of a nerve or nerve segment.

presacral n. Surgical excision of retroperitoneal nerves that overlie the terminal portion of the abdominal aorta and the surface of the sacrum and are the sensory innervation for the pelvic viscera. Used in the treatment of chronic pelvic pain most often secondary to endometriosis; its usage, however, is controversial because of inconsistent effectiveness.

neurocele (noor′o-sēl) The ventricles within the brain and the central canal within the spinal cord.

neurodermatitis (noor-o-der-mă-ti′tis) A localized itchy skin inflammation of nervous or psychological origin.

> **n. of vulva** See lichen simplex chronicus of vulva, under lichen.

neuroectoderm (noor-o-ek′to-derm) In embryology, the part of the ectoderm giving rise to the neural tube.

neurofibroma (noor-o-fi-bro′mă) A nonmalignant tumor originating in the connective tissue of nerves, forming a spindle-shaped enlargement of the affected nerve; it occurs most frequently in the skin.

neurofibromatosis (noor-o-fi-bro-mă-to′sis) Genetic disorder transmitted as a dominant inheritance, characterized by formation of multiple neurofibromas. Maternal neurofibromatosis may result in small-for-gestational-age infants.

> **n. I** A form involving cutaneous nerves and forming multiple soft tumors throughout the body that, during pregnancy, tend to increase in size and numbers. Also called von Recklinghausen's disease.

> **n. II** An acoustic form forming tumors in the eighth cranial nerves of both sides.

neurohypophyseal (noor-o-hi-po-fiz′e-al) Relating to the neurohypophysis. Also written neurohypophysial.

neurohypophysis (noor-o-hi-pof′ĭ-sis) The posterior lobe of the pituitary (hypophysis). Also called neural lobe of pituitary. See also adenohypophysis; hypophysis.

neuropeptide (noor-o-pep′tīd) Any of various substances (e.g., endorphin, vasopressin) present in neural tissue, especially the brain.

neurophysin (noor-o-fi′sin) Any of a group of soluble proteins produced in the hypothalamus (at the base of the brain); they transport the hormones vasopressin and oxytocin to the posterior part of the pituitary (neurohypophysis).

neurosis (noo-ro′sis), pl. neuroses Emotional maladjustment in which the individual regards his symptoms of this maladjustment as distressing and unacceptable but experiences anxiety when attempting to confront the symptoms; the individual's behavior does not violate societal norms.

> **posttraumatic n.** See posttraumatic stress disorder, under disorder.

neurotransmitter (noor-o-trans-mit′er) A substance (e.g., acetylcholine, catecholamines, monamines) that facilitates the transmission of impulses from one neuron to another, or between neurons and receptors of effector cells, at specialized regions (synaptic gaps) at the end of a presynaptic neuron.

neutron (noo′tron) (n) An uncharged subatomic particle, slightly heavier than a proton, present in the nuclei of atoms.

> **fast n.** A neutron with an energy level that exceeds 105 electron volts.

nevi (ne′vi) Plural of nevus.

nevoid (ne′void) Resembling a nevus.

nevus (ne′vus), pl. nevi A benign lesion of the skin present at birth; may be flat or elevated, smooth or warty, pigmented or nonpigmented.

> **n. anemicus** A congenital pale, flat, well-defined area on the skin; thought to be a functional defect of the blood vessels within the area, which, although otherwise normal, are hyperresponsive to vasoconstrictive stimuli; it often occurs in groups, but can also present as a single mark.

> **n. araneus** See spider telangiectasia, under telangiectasia.

> **blue n.** A uniform circumscribed deep blue coloration composed of heavily pigmented melanocytic cells in the deep layer (dermis) of the skin.

> **congenital nevocellular n.** A relatively large pigmented lesion, often covered with hairs; the melanocytic cells are located in the deepest layers of skin, involving also the subcutaneous fat, often associated with nerves; occasionally

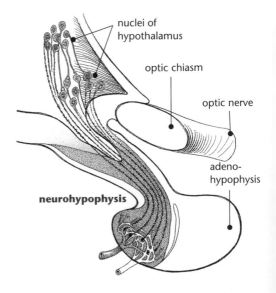

nuclei of hypothalamus

optic chiasm

optic nerve

adeno-hypophysis

neurohypophysis

may develop malignant potential.

dysplastic n. See atypical mole, under mole.

n. flammeus A purplish-red, vascular birthmark that is level with the skin surface and usually tends to be permanent. Also called port-wine stain; port-wine mark; port-wine hemangioma.

melanocytic n. See nevocellular nevus.

nevocellular n. Any of various circumscribed pigmented nevi composed of pigment-producing cells (melanocytes), present at birth or acquired in childhood, and varying from smooth to rough and from nonpalpable to nodular. Also called pigmented nevus; melanocytic nevus; commonly called mole.

pigmented n. See nevocellular nevus.

spider n. See spider telangiectasia, under telangiectasia.

n. vasculosus, n. vascularis See strawberry hemangioma, under hemangioma.

newborn (noo'born) A recently born baby; a neonate.

nicotine (nik'o-tēn) An alkaloid present in tobacco (*Nicotiana tabacum*); small doses stimulate and large doses depress autonomic ganglia; may have deleterious effects on pregnancy and the fetus; depending on the dose, they range from decreased placental blood flow to low birth weight, and increased risk of stillbirth or neonatal death.

nidation (ni-da'shun) Implantation of the early embryo (the fluid-filled blastocyst) into the inner lining of the uterus; occurs approximately 5 days after fertilization of the ovum.

nipple (nip'l) The pigmented protrusion at the apex of the breast, surrounded by the areola. Also called mammary papilla

accessory n. A nipple that develops anywhere on the sides of the thoracoabdominal wall along the mamillary lines.

nocturia (nok-tu're-ă) Waking to void more than once per night.

nocturnal (nok-tur'nal) Occurring at night; opposite of diurnal.

nodal (no'dal) Relating to a node.

node (nōd) **1.** A circumscribed mass of differentiated tissue. **2.** A swelling or protuberance, either normal or abnormal.

atrioventricular n. A small, roughly oval node made of interwoven modified cardiac muscle fibers and situated in the right atrial wall of the heart near the orifice of the coronary sinus, just dorsal to the basal attachment of the tricuspid (right atrioventricular) valve. From the atrium it transmits the cardiac impulse, through the Purkinje fibers, to the ventricular walls. Also called A-V node.

A-V n. See atrioventricular node.

axillary lymph n.'s Twenty to thirty large nodes of the axilla extending along the axillary veins: *anterior (pectoral)*, four or five nodes situated along the lower border of the pectoralis minor muscle; they receive lymph from the skin and muscles of the anterior and lateral walls of the upper body, and the central and lateral portions of the breast; *apical*, six to twelve nodes extending upward into the apex of the axilla, medial to the axillary vein; they

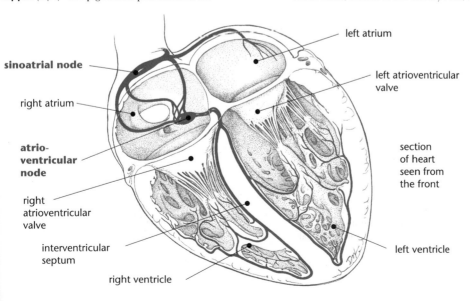

left atrium

sinoatrial node

left atrioventricular valve

right atrium

atrio-ventricular node

section of heart seen from the front

right atrioventricular valve

interventricular septum

left ventricle

right ventricle

receive lymph from the other axillary nodes; *central*, three or four nodes embedded in the axillary fat; they receive lymph from the other axillary nodes; *lateral*, four to six nodes situated medial to, and behind, the axillary vein; they receive lymph from the upper limb; *posterior (subscapular)*, six or seven nodes along the lower margin of the posterior wall of the axilla; they receive lymph from the lower back of the neck and the back of the trunk.

Cloquet's n. The highest of the deep inguinal lymph nodes, located on the lateral part of the femoral ring of the lower abdomen; when greatly enlarged, it could be mistaken for a femoral hernia. Also called Rosemüller's node; highest deep inguinal lymph node.

epigastric lymph n.'s, inferior Three or four nodes along the deep epigastric blood vessels; they receive lymph from the lower abdominal wall and empty into the external iliac nodes.

Hensen's n. See primitive knot, under knot.

iliac lymph n.'s, common Four to six nodes grouped around the common iliac artery, mostly lateral to the vessel and arranged chiefly in three chains: *medial, lateral*, and

intermediate; occasionally, there may be a *subaortic* node (in front of the fifth lumbar vertebra) and a *promontory* node (on the sacral promontory); they receive lymph from the external and internal iliac lymph nodes and drain into the lateral aortic nodes.

iliac lymph n.'s, external Eight to ten nodes along the external iliac vessels; designated *medial, intermediate*, and *lateral* depending on their location relative to the vessels; they receive lymph from the inguinal nodes, deep layers of the lower abdominal wall, inner thigh, glans of the clitoris (or penis), cervix, lower portion of the uterine body, upper part of the vagina, fundus of the bladder, membranous urethra, and prostate; they drain into the common iliac lymph nodes.

iliac lymph n.'s, internal The nodes surrounding the internal iliac blood vessels and the roots of their branches; they include the *sacral lymph nodes* (median and lateral) and the *obturator lymph node*; they receive lymph from all the pelvic organs, vagina, deep parts of the perineum, and muscles of the buttocks and back of the thigh; they drain into the

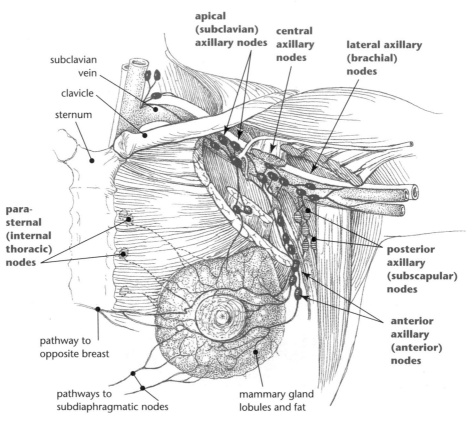

apical (subclavian) axillary nodes

central axillary nodes

lateral axillary (brachial) nodes

subclavian vein

clavicle

sternum

para-sternal (internal thoracic) nodes

posterior axillary (subscapular) nodes

anterior axillary (anterior) nodes

pathway to opposite breast

pathways to subdiaphragmatic nodes

mammary gland lobules and fat

common iliac lymph nodes.

inguinal lymph n.'s, deep One to three small nodes situated deep to the fascia lata and medial to the femoral vein, they receive lymph from the deep structures of the lower limb, glans of the clitoris (or penis), labia minora, and superficial inguinal lymph nodes; they empty into the external iliac lymph nodes.

inguinal lymph n., highest deep See Cloquet's node.

inguinal lymph n.'s, superficial Twelve to fifteen subcutaneous lymph nodes located below the inguinal ligament and extending along the proximal part of the great saphenous vein and its tributaries; designated *inferior*, lower nodes on the great saphenous vein, below the saphenous opening; *superolateral*, upper nodes along the circumflex iliac vein, lateral to the saphenous opening; *superomedial*, upper nodes along the superficial epigastric vein and superficial external pudendal vein, on the medial side of the opening; they receive lymph from the skin and subcutaneous tissues of the lower abdominal wall, external genitalia, buttocks, lower part of the anal canal, perianal area, and lower limb; they drain into the external iliac lymph nodes.

lymph n. A small, oval or kidney-shaped, encapsulated collection of lymphoid tissue, ranging in size from 2 to 20 mm in diameter; it is found interposed in the course of a lymphatic vessel, so that lymph passes through it on its way to the circulating blood; its functions are the production of lymphocytes

and the removal of foreign matter from the lymph. Lymph nodes are most numerous in the chest, posterior abdominal wall, pelvis, neck, and proximal ends of the limbs. A node may be enlarged because of a local infection, a systemic disorder, or a metastatic malignancy.

obturator lymph n. Node of the internal iliac group sometimes present in the obturator canal.

pelvic lymph n.'s The nodes receiving lymph from the pelvic organs and the wall of the pelvis; they include those of the external and internal iliac groups, which drain into the common iliac lymph nodes.

paravesical lymph n.'s Nodes located around the urinary bladder.

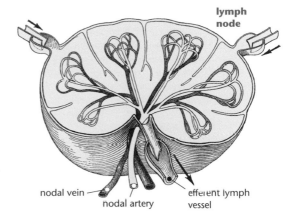

lymph node

nodal vein — nodal artery — efferent lymph vessel

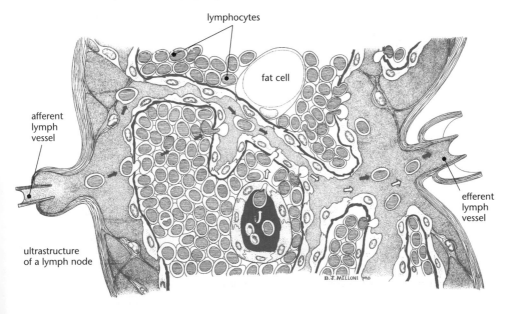

lymphocytes

fat cell

afferent lymph vessel

efferent lymph vessel

ultrastructure of a lymph node

pectoral lymph n.'s See axillary lymph nodes.

primitive n. See primitive knot, under knot.

Rosemüller's n. See Cloquet's node.

S-A n. See sinoatrial node.

sacral lymph n.'s Nodes of the internal iliac group: *median*, situated along the median sacral blood vessels and *lateral*, along the lateral sacral blood vessels; both groups receive lymph from the cervix, posterior pelvic wall, and rectum.

sentinel n. See signal node.

signal n. An enlarged, palpable, supraclavicular lymph node, especially on the left side, that is sometimes noted as the first presumptive sign of a malignant abdominal neoplasm. Also called sentinel node, Virchow's node.

sinoatrial n. An elongated node composed of interwoven modified cardiac muscle fibers, situated within the wall of the right atrium near the entrance of the superior vena cava; it receives fibers from both the sympathetic and parasympathetic nervous systems and is responsible for initiating each heart beat; it is often referred to as the pacemaker of the heart. Also called S-A node; sinus node.

sinus n. See sinoatrial node.

Virchow's n. See signal node.

nodose (no'dōs) Having nodes.

nodosity (no-dos'ĭ-te) 1. A knotlike projection or swelling. 2. The condition of having nodes.

nodular (nod'u-lar) 1. Having nodules. 2. Relating to a nodule.

nodulation (nod-u-la'shun) The condition of having nodules.

nodule (nod'ūl) A small node or closely packed aggregation of cells appearing distinct from surrounding tissue.

Sister Mary Joseph's n. A malignant nodule in the subcutaneous area of the navel, metastasized from intra-abdominal cancer.

nomogram, nomograph (nom'o-gram, nom'o-graf) A graph showing three graduated lines of different variables arranged in such a way that a straight line connecting two known values on two of the lines intersects the unknown value on the third line; used in estimating the surface area of the body, the two known values being the person's height and weight.

nondisjunction (non-dis-junk'shun) Failure of paired chromosomes to separate during cell division (meiosis or mitosis), so that both chromosomes are received by one daughter cell and none by the other, resulting in certain abnormal genetic conditions (e.g., Down's syndrome).

nonparous (non-par'us) See nulliparous.

nonviable (non-vi'ă-bl) Not capable of living independently; applied especially to a premature infant.

norethindrone (nor-eth'in-drōn) A progestin used in conjunction with an estrogen in oral contraceptives and in hormone replacement therapy; used alone in the treatment of endometriosis and amenorrhea.

norethynodrel (nor-ĕ-thi'no-drel) A progestin used in conjunction with an estrogen as an oral contraceptive and in the treatment of endometriosis.

normothermia (nor-mo-ther'me-ă) 1. A body temperature within the normal range. 2. Environmental temperature that does not affect the activity of body cells.

normotonic (nor-mo-ton'ik) Having normal muscular tone. Also called eutonic.

normotopia (nor-mo-to'pe-ă) The state of being in the normal or usual position.

normovolemia (nor-mo-vo-le'me-ă) The condition of having a normal blood volume.

noso- Combining form meaning disease.

nosocomial (nos-o-ko'me-al) 1. Relating to a hospital. 2. Originating in a hospital; applied to a newly acquired disease.

notch (noch) 1. An indentation or depression, usually on a bone, but occasionally applied to an organ. 2. A deflection on a graphic curve or wave.

sciatic n.'s Indentations on the posterior border of the hipbone. *Greater sciatic n.*, the deep indentation on the posterior border of the hipbone at the junction of the ilium and ischium, between the posterior inferior iliac spine and the ischial spine; it is converted into the greater sciatic foramen by the sacrospinous and sacrotuberous ligaments. *Lesser sciatic n.*, the notch on the posterior border of the ischium between the ischial spine and the tuberosity; it is converted into the lesser sciatic foramen by the sacrospinous and sacrotuberous ligaments.

vertebral n. One of two deep-pocketed indentations (superior and inferior) above and below the border of the pedicle of a vertebra on each side; the notches of two adjacent vertebrae form an intervertebral foramen, which transmits the spinal nerve and vessels.

notochord (no'to-kord) A supporting rod of cells in the embryo of all chordates; in vertebrates, it is replaced partly or wholly by the skull and vertebral column.

nucha (nu'kă) See nape.

pelvic lymph nodes

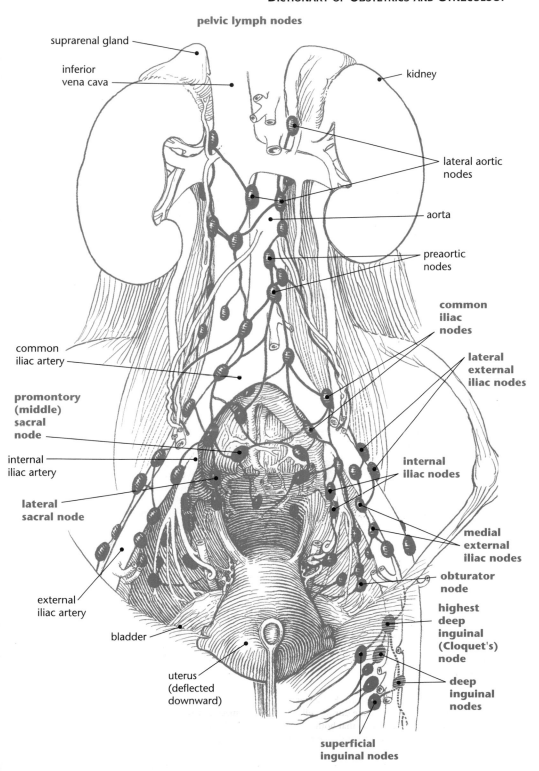

suprarenal gland

inferior
vena cava

kidney

lateral aortic
nodes

aorta

preaortic
nodes

**common
iliac
nodes**

common
iliac artery

**lateral
external
iliac nodes**

**promontory
(middle)
sacral
node**

internal
iliac artery

**internal
iliac nodes**

**lateral
sacral node**

**medial
external
iliac nodes**

**obturator
node**

external
iliac artery

**highest
deep
inguinal
(Cloquet's)
node**

bladder

**deep
inguinal
nodes**

uterus
(deflected
downward)

**superficial
inguinal nodes**

nuchal (nu'kal) Relating to the back of the neck.

nuclear (noo'kle-ar) Relating to a nucleus.

nucleated (noo'kle-āt-ed) Having a nucleus.

nuclei (noo'kle-i) Plural of nucleus.

nucleic acid (noo-kle'ik as'id) Any of a family of macromolecules, either DNA or various types of RNA, present in all living organisms and consisting mainly of a sugar moiety (pentose or deoxypentose), nitrogenous bases (purines and pyrimidines), and phosphoric acid.

nucleo-, nucl- Combining forms meaning nucleus.

nucleus (noo'kle-us), pl. nuclei **1.** The complex, usually spherical protoplasmic body near the center of the cell that is an essential organelle controlling the activities of the cell, including metabolism, growth, and reproduction; it contains the chromosomes and is surrounded by a pore-studded nuclear membrane, through which substances can pass to and from the surrounding cytoplasm. **2.** A localized mass of gray matter composed of cell bodies of excitable nerve cells (neurons) within the brain and spinal cord, where nerve fibers interconnect. **3.** The heavy, central, positively charged portion of the atom; it constitutes the mass of the atom, about which the electrons revolve in orbit.

  naked nuclei The characteristic vesicular nuclei, without cytoplasm, typically found in vaginal secretions during early pregnancy.

  paraventricular n. of hypothalamus A group of nerve cells in the anterior portion of the hypothalamus, near the third ventricle of the brain; some of the cells secrete the peptide oxytocin, which is carried to and stored in the posterior lobe of the pituitary (neurohypophysis). See also neurophysin; oxytocin.

  supraoptic n. of hypothalamus A group of nerve cells in the anterior portion of the hypothalamus, above the lateral border of the optic tract; some of the cells secrete the antidiuretic hormone vasopressin, which is carried to and stored in the posterior lobe of the pituitary (neurohypophysis). See also neurophysin; vasopressin.

nulligravida (nul-ĭ-grav'ĭ-da) A woman who has never been pregnant.

nullipara (nŭ-lip'ă-ră) A woman who has not delivered an offspring weighing 500 g or more, or of a gestation length of 20 weeks or longer.

nulliparity (nul-ĭ-par'ĭ-te) Condition of not having borne children.

nulliparous (nŭ-lip'ă-rus) Never having borne children. Also called nonparous.

nursing (ners'ing) **1.** Activities that constitute the duties of a nurse. **2.** Breast-feeding.

nutrient (noo'tre-ent) A nourishing constituent of food.

nutrition (noo-trish'un) **1.** The process through which a living organism takes in and assimilates food for growth and replacement of tissues. **2.** The study of foods in relation to the requirements of living organisms.

  enteral n. Introduction of nutrients via a tube inserted directly into the stomach or duodenum.

  total parenteral n. (TPN) Intravenous infusion of nutrients in place of oral intake. Also called total parenteral alimentation.

nympha (nim'fă), pl. nymphae See labia minora, under labium.

nympho-, nymph- Combining forms meaning the labia minora.

nympholabia (nim-fo-la'be-ă) Relating to the labia minora and labia majora.

nymphomania (nim-fo-ma'ne-ă) A female psychosexual disorder characterized by excessive and insatiable sexual desire.

nymphomaniac (nim-fo-ma'ne-ak) A woman affected with nymphomania.

nymphoncus (nim-fong'kus) Abnormal enlargement or swelling of the minor lips (labia minora) of the vulva.

nymphotomy (nim-fot'o-me) A surgical cut into a minor lip (labium minus) of the vulva.

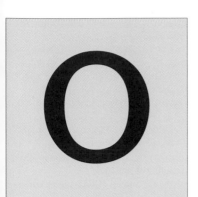

obesity (o-bēs'ĭ-te) Excessive accumulation of fat in the body.

    android o. Obesity characterized by excessive fat accumulation in the mid section of the body (i.e., in the abdominal wall and visceral-mesenteric structures); usually associated with increased risk of cardiovascular disease and diabetes mellitus. Also called central body obesity.

    central body o. See android obesity.

    gynoid o. Obesity in which excessive fat accumulates in the hips and buttocks.

    morbid o. Obesity that is so severe as to threaten health and limit activity.

oblique (o-blēk') Having a slanting direction; deviating from the vertical or horizontal.

obliquity (ob-lik'wĭ-te) See synclitism.

obstetric, obstetrical (ob-stet'rik, ob-stet're-kal) Relating to obstetrics.

obstetrician (ob-stĕ-trĭsh'un) A physician who is a specialist in obstetrics.

obstetrics (ob-stet'riks) (OB) The branch of medicine concerned principally with the management of pregnancy, labor, and the phenomena following childbirth to complete involution of the uterus.

    critical care o. The management of life-threatening emergencies during pregnancy and puerperium.

obstruction (obs-truk'shun) An impedance; a blockage or clogging.

    intestinal o. Bowel obstruction resulting from any of various conditions, especially from postoperative adhesions (e.g., from abdominal or pelvic surgery or from cesarean section); may become aggravated during pregnancy due to increasing compression of the bowel by the enlarging uterus; symptoms include abdominal pain, nausea, and vomiting.

OC-125 A murine monoclonal immunoglobulin developed to detect the serum marker CA-125 in the monitoring of a wide variety of tumors.

occipital (ok-sip'ĭ-tal) Relating to the back of the head.

occipitoatloid (ok-sip-ĭ-to-at'loid) Relating to the occipital bone and the first cervical vertebra, such as the articulation between the two bones.

occipitobregmatic (ok-sip-ĭ-to-breg-mat'ik) Relating to the back of the head and the bregma (a craniometric point); applied to a measurement of the skull. See also bregma.

occipitomental (ok-sip-ĭ-to-men'tal) Relating to the back of the head and the chin.

occipitoparietal (ok-sip-ĭ-to-pa-ri'ĕ-tal) Relating to the occipital and parietal bones of the skull.

occipitotemporal (ok-sip-ĭ-to-tem'po-ral) Relating to the occipital and temporal bones of the skull.

occiput (ok'sĭ-put) The back of the head.

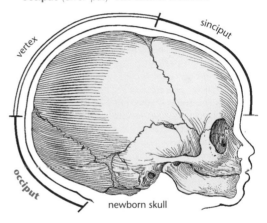

newborn skull

occlusion (o-kloo'zhun) **1.** The process of closing. **2.** An obstruction.

    cornual o. Closure of the lumen of a fallopian (uterine) tube at the site of its connection with the uterus; secondary to infection, endometriosis, leiomyomas, and, rarely, congenital malformation.

occult (ŏ-kult') Hidden (e.g., a concealed internal hemorrhage).

octa-, octi-, octo- Combining forms meaning eight.

octapeptide (ok-tă-pep'tĭd) A peptide composed of eight amino acid residues (e.g., the hormones oxytocin and vasopressin).

octoxynol 9 (ok-toks'ĭ-nol) A surface-acting agent, usually combined with spermicides for use in contraceptive devices.

oligemia (ol-ĭ-ge'me-ă) Deficient or reduced amount of blood in the body (e.g., resulting from hemorrhage).

oligo- olig- Combining forms meaning small; few.

oligoamnios (ol-ĭ-go-am'ne-os) See oligohydramnios.

oligohydramnios (ol-ĭ-go-hi-dram'ne-os) Severe deficiency of amniotic fluid, sometimes represented by only a few milliliters of a thick, viscid fluid; may be due to premature rupture of the membranes, obstruction of the fetal urinary tract, severe intrauterine growth retardation, or death of the fetus. Also called oligoamnios.

oligomenorrhea (ol-ĭ-go-men-o-re'ă) Reduction in the frequency of menstrual periods (i.e., occurring at intervals greater than 35 days).

oligospermia (ol-ĭ-go-sper'me-ă) Deficiency in the number of spermatozoa per unit volume of semen.

-oma Suffix meaning tumor; neoplasm (e.g., hemangioma).

omentum (o-men'tum) A fold of peritoneum in the abdominal cavity that connects various organs with each other or with the abdominal wall.

> **greater o.** A double fold of peritoneum resembling an apron and usually containing large deposits of fat; it descends a variable distance from the greater curvature of the stomach to the front of the small intestine, where it turns upon itself (thereby making four layers) and ascends to the top of the transverse colon.

> **lesser o.** The fold of peritoneum extending from the liver to the lesser curvature of the stomach and the beginning of the duodenum.

omo- Combining form meaning shoulder.

omoclavicular (o-mo-klă-vik'u-lar) Relating to the shoulder and collarbone (clavicle).

omphalic (om-fal'ik) Umbilical.

omphalo-, omphal- Combining forms meaning the umbilicus.

omphalocele (om'fă-lo-sēl) Congenital hernia of the umbilicus in which a small portion of the abdominal contents covered by a membranous sac protrudes into the base of the umbilical cord; the cord structures pass individually over the sac, coming together at its apex to form a normal-looking umbilical cord. It is often associated with chromosomal abnormalities (e.g., trisomy 13). Also called exomphalos. Compare with gastroschisis.

omphalopagus (om-fă-lop'ă-gus) Conjoined twins united at the abdominal wall, in the area of the navel.

omphalophlebitis (om-fă-lo-flĕ-bi'tis) Inflammation of the umbilical veins.

omphalorrhagia (om-fă-lo-ra'je-ă) Bleeding from the umbilicus.

omphalorrhea (om-fă-lo-re'ă) A discharge from the umbilicus.

omphalotomy (om-fă-lot'ŏ-me) The cutting of the umbilical cord at birth.

onanism (o'nă-nizm) See coitus interruptus, under coitus.

oncho-, onco- Combining forms meaning tumor; bulk; mass; hook.

oncocyte (on'ko-sīt) A granular, acidophilic tumor cell.

oncofetal (ong-ko-fe'tal) Relating to cancer and the fetus; used specifically in reference to substances occurring naturally in the fetus and in malignant tumors of the adult. See also carcinoembryonic antigen (CEA), under antigen.

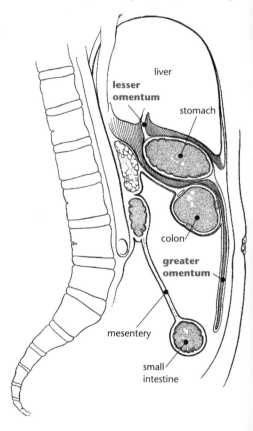

oncogene (ong'ko-jen) Any gene, viral or cellular (v-onc or c-onc), that is implicated in tumor formation.

> **retroviral o.** A fully tumorigenic version of a cellular proto-oncogene.

oncogenesis (ong-ko-jen'ĕ-sis) The origin of a tumor.

oncogenic, oncogenous (ong-ko-jen'ik, ong-koj'ĕ-nus) Causing tumor formation; may be a chemical, genetic, hormonal, viral, or radiation influence.

oncologist (ong-kol'ŏ-jist) A specialist in oncology.

oncology (ong-kol'ŏ-je) The study of the causes, characteristics, diagnosis, and treatment of cancer.

oncolysis (ong-kol'ĭ-sis) Destruction or reduction of any abnormal mass or tumor.

oncosis (ong-ko'sis) Condition characterized by the presence of tumors.

Oncovirinae (ong-ko-vir'ĭ-ne) A subfamily of tumor viruses (family Retroviridae) which, on the basis of morphology and antigenicity, are grouped into types A, B, C, and D; associated with malignant diseases.

oncovirus (ong-ko-vi'rus) Any virus of the subfamily Oncovirinae. See also oncogenic virus, under virus.

oo- Combining form meaning egg, ovum.

oocyte (o'o-sīt) A developing ovum in the ovary.

    primary o. Oocyte derived from an oogonium.

      secondary o. An oocyte resulting from the division of a primary oocyte.

oogenesis (o-o-jen'ĕ-sis) Formation of an ovum.

oogenetic (o-o-je-net'ik) Relating to oogenesis.

oogenic, oogenous (o-o-jen'ik, o-o-jen'us) Producing ova.

oogonium (o-o-go'ne-um), pl. oogonia One of the cells derived from a primordial germ cell by mitosis; oogonia form most of the ovarian tissue and serve as a source of oocytes.

ookinesia (o-o-kĭ-ne'ze-ă) The natural movements of the ovum during maturation and fertilization.

oolemma (o-o-lem'ă) The cell membrane of the ovum.

oophorectomy (o-of-ŏ-rek'tŏ-me) Removal of one or both ovaries. Also called ovariectomy.

oophoritis (o-of-ŏ-ri'tis) Inflammation of one or both ovaries; may occur secondary to an infection elsewhere in the body (e.g., mumps).

oophoro-, oophor- Combining forms meaning ovary.

oophorocystectomy (o-of-ŏ-ro-sis-tek'tŏ-me) Surgical removal of an ovarian cyst.

oophoron (o-of'ŏ-ron) Greek for ovum; egg.

oophorosalpingectomy (o-of'ŏ-ro-sal-pin-jek'tŏ-me) Surgical removal of an ovary and its corresponding fallopian (uterine) tube. Also called ovariosalpingectomy.

oophorosalpingitis (o-of'ŏ-ro-sal-pin-ji'tis) Inflammation of an ovary or ovaries and corresponding fallopian (uterine) tube. Also called ovariosalpingitis.

oophorotomy (o-of-ŏ-rot'ŏ-me) A surgical cut into an ovary. Also called ovariotomy.

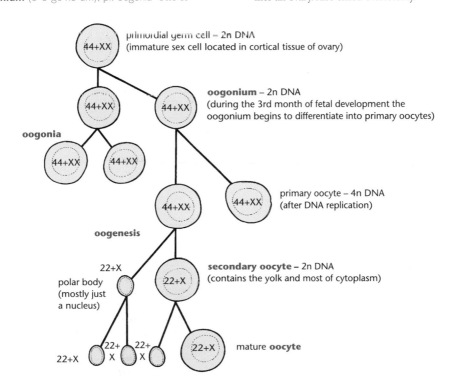

primordial germ cell – 2n DNA
(immature sex cell located in cortical tissue of ovary)

44+XX

oogonium – 2n DNA
(during the 3rd month of fetal development the oogonium begins to differentiate into primary oocytes)

44+XX   44+XX

oogonia

44+XX   44+XX

primary oocyte – 4n DNA
(after DNA replication)

44+XX   44+XX

oogenesis

22+X

polar body
(mostly just
a nucleus)

22+X   secondary oocyte – 2n DNA
(contains the yolk and most of cytoplasm)

22+X   22+X   22+X

22+X   mature oocyte

ooplasm (o'o-plazm) The cytoplasm of an ovum.

operation (op-er-a'shun) Any surgical procedure for remedying an injury, deformity, ailment, or dysfunction.

debulking o. The practice of reducing the bulk of carcinomatous tissue and removing, if possible, all gross disease in order to enhance the effectiveness of adjuvant treatment. Also called cytoreductive surgery.

Halsted's o. (1) See radical mastectomy, under mastectomy. (2) Operation for the repair of a direct inguinal hernia.

Irving's o. A method of female sterilization consisting of a double ligation of the fallopian (uterine) tubes with nonabsorbable sutures, division of the tubes between the sutures, freeing of the stumps from their peritoneal attachments, and either burying both distal and proximal stumps between the two layers of the broad ligament, or burying only the distal stumps and suturing the proximal stumps under the serous covering of the uterus, just anterior to each round ligament. Also called Irving's procedure; Irving's technique.

LeFort's o. A vaginal obliterative procedure in which the anterior and posterior vaginal walls are sutured together; a treatment for symptomatic pelvic relaxation when the medical condition of the patient precludes utilization of more extensive procedures.

McDonald's o. See McDonald's cerclage, under cerclage.

Madlener's o. Procedure for female sterilization consisting of lifting the middle third of each of the fallopian (uterine) tubes to create a loop, grasping and crushing the base of the loop with a clamp, ligating the crushed region of the loop with a nonabsorbable suture, and covering the ligature site with the round ligament to prevent adhesion formation. Also called Madlener's procedure; Madlener's technique.

Manchester o. High amputation of the uterine cervix and suturing together of the broad ligament bases in front of the shortened cervix; devised to relieve first and second degree prolapse of the uterus.

Marshall-Marchetti-Krantz o. An operation for correction of stress urinary incontinence. In the retropubic space sutures are placed in the periurethral, vaginal, or paravaginal tissue to elevate the urethrovesical junction; the elevated tissue is then sewn to the periosteum of the pubic symphysis.

modified Pomeroy's o. A version of the original Pomeroy's operation in which the tubal segment is ligated with two separate absorbable sutures instead of one.

Pomeroy's o. A method of female sterilization by partial resection of the fallopian (uterine) tubes; consists of lifting the middle third of each tube to create a loop, ligating the loop at its base with a single absorbable suture, resecting the ligated loop, and covering the wound surface with the round ligament to prevent adhesion formation. Also called Pomeroy's procedure; Pomeroy's technique.

radical o. A thorough procedure aimed at complete elimination of a disease or correction of a defect.

Sçanger o. See classic cesarean section, under section.

Shirodkar's o. See Shirodkar's cerclage, under cerclage.

Uchida o. See Uchida procedure, under procedure.

vaginal cuff o. Stage in a hysterectomy after the uterus has been separated from the vagina. The edges of the anterior and posterior vagina (the proximal portion of the vagina that had been attached to the uterine cervix) may then be sutured to achieve hemostasis in one of two ways: either approximating the anteroposterior edges thus closing the vagina, or edges may be sutured circumferentially to leave the proximal vagina open.

Wertheim's o. See modified radical hysterectomy, under hysterectomy.

operculum (o-per'ku-lum), pl. opercula **1.** Any anatomic structure resembling a lid or cover. **2.** The mucus plug sealing the opening of the cervix during pregnancy.

ophthalmia (of-thal'me-ă) Inflammation of the eye.

gonorrheal o. Acute purulent conjunctivitis caused by a gonorrheal infection.

o. neonatorum Acute purulent conjunctivitis of the newborn infant; may be due to infection acquired from its mother during passage through the birth canal (e.g., gonorrheal or chlamydial infection) or may be caused by a staphylococcal or a pseudomonal microorganism usually acquired as a nosocomial infection in the hospital nursery. Also called neonatal conjunctivitis.

ophthalmo-, ophthalm- Combining forms meaning eye.

opiate (o'pe-āt) Any preparation derived from opium, which has analgesic and sedative activity.

opioid (o'pe-oid) Any natural or synthetic compound that has morphine-like pharmacologic activity. Opioids are not derived

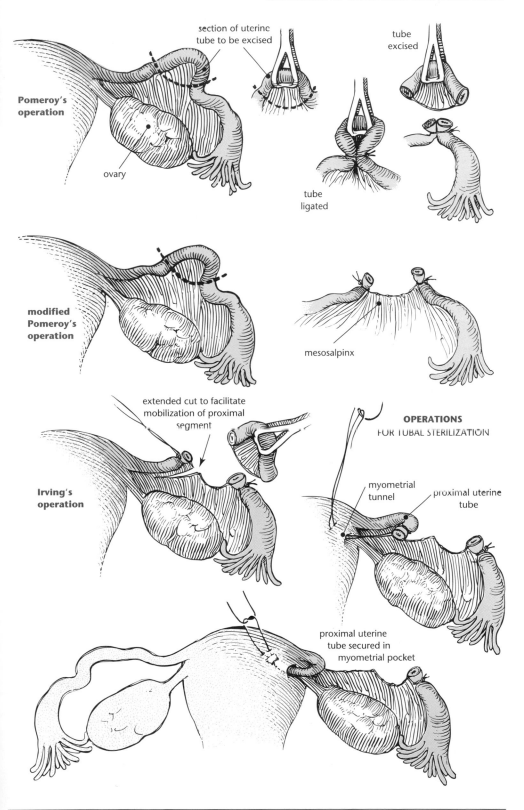

Pomeroy's operation

section of uterine tube to be excised

tube excised

ovary

tube ligated

modified Pomeroy's operation

mesosalpinx

Irving's operation

extended cut to facilitate mobilization of proximal segment

OPERATIONS FOR TUBAL STERILIZATION

myometrial tunnel

proximal uterine tube

proximal uterine tube secured in myometrial pocket

from opium.

endogenous o.'s Natural peptides that bind to opiate receptors in cell membranes; they are produced primarily in the central nervous system and include dynorphins, endorphins, and enkephalins.

opportunistic (op-or-too-nis'tik) **1.** Denoting a disease that occurs in people whose immune system is impaired by other infections or by ongoing drug therapy (e.g., chemotherapy). **2.** Denoting the organisms causing such a disease, and which do not cause disease (or cause only mild infections) in healthy people.

order (or'der) **1.** In biologic classification, the category just below the class and above the family. **2.** A directive, advisory instruction, or prescription for a specific course of action (e.g., preoperative or postoperative orders).

organ (or'gan) A distinct structural unit of the body that performs specific functions.

genital o.'s of the female See reproductive organs of the female.

genital o.'s of the male See reproductive organs of the male.

reproductive o.'s of the female The various organs in the female concerned with reproduction, namely the ovaries, fallopian (uterine) tubes, uterus, vagina, clitoris, labia majora and minora, bulb of the vestibule, greater vestibular glands, vestibule, and the mons pubis. Also called genital organs of the female.

reproductive o.'s of the male The various organs of the male concerned with reproduction, namely the penis, scrotum, testes, epididymides, deferent ducts, ejaculatory ducts, seminal vesicles, urethra, prostate, and the bulbourethral glands. Also called genital organs of the male.

o. of Rosenmüller See epoophoron.

target o. An organ that is influenced or stimulated by a hormone (e.g., the adrenal gland, which is stimulated by corticotropin, a pituitary hormone).

urinary o.'s The organs involved with the production and excretion of urine; composed of the kidneys, ureters, urinary bladder, and the urethra.

organism (or'ga-nizm) Any plant or animal.

TWAR (Taiwan acute respiratory) o. See *Chlamydia pneumoniae*, under *Chlamydia*.

organogenesis (or-ga-no-jen'ĕ-sis) In embryology, the formation of organs.

orgasm (or'gazm) The culmination of sexual intercourse or stimulation of the sex organs, accompanied in the male by ejaculation of semen

and in the female by involuntary contractions of the vagina.

orifice (or'ĭ-fis) An opening into a body cavity or tubular structure.

abdominal o. of uterine tube The opening at the lateral, fimbriated end of each fallopian (uterine) tube; through it, the ovum expelled by the ovary enters the tube on its way to the cavity of the uterus.

anal o. See anus.

external o. of female urethra The slitlike orifice with prominent margins directly in front of the opening of the vagina and behind the clitoris. Also called external meatus of female urethra.

external o. of uterus See external os of uterus, under os.

internal o. of urethra The crescentic opening at the apex of the bladder, leading to the urethra. Also called internal meatus of urethra.

internal o. of uterus See internal os of uterus, under os.

o. of ureter The slitlike termination of a ureter through the bladder wall at the posterolateral angle of the trigone.

o. of uterine tube The minute opening of a fallopian (uterine) tube into the superior angle of the cavity of the uterus on either side.

o. of vagina The external opening of the vagina, located just behind the external urethral orifice.

os (os), pl. ora Latin for mouth; orifice.

external o. of uterus The opening between the cervical canal and the cavity of the vagina; it is small and round or oval in young girls and women who have not borne children; in those who have given birth, it becomes a transverse slit bounded by the anterior and posterior lips of the cervix. Also called external orifice of the uterus; popularly called mouth of the uterus. See also labium anterius and labium posterius, under labium.

internal o. of uterus The opening between the cavity of the body of the uterus and the canal of the cervix. Also called internal orifice of the uterus.

os (os), pl. ossa Latin for bone.

osseocartilagenous (os-e-o-kar-tĭ-laj'ĭ-nus) Composed of both bone and cartilage.

ossification (os-ĭ-fĭ-kashun) **1.** Replacement of cartilage by bone. **2.** Formation of bone.

ossify (os'ĭ-fi) To change into bone.

osteo- Combining form meaning bone.

osteoblast (os'te-o-blast) A bone-forming cell, responsible for the formation of bone matrix.

osteocalcin (os-te-o-kal'sin) A calcium-binding protein present in the noncollagenous portion of bone matrix. The degree of serum concentration of osteocalcin has been used in assessments of bone formation.

osteochondrodysplasia (os-te-o-kon-dro-dis-pla'ze-ă) Abnormal development of both cartilage and bone.

osteoclast (os'te-o-klast) A large multinucleated cell found in the lacunae of bone; it plays an important role in the modeling of bone through selective absorption of bone tissue.

osteocranium (os-te-o-kra'ne-um) The skull of the fetus after ossification has begun.

osteocyte (os'te-o-sīt) A bone cell arising from an osteoblast; it is surrounded by a calcified matrix and plays a role in maintaining constituents of the matrix at normal levels.

osteogenesis (os-te-o-jen'ĕ-sis) The formation of bone.

    o. imperfecta (OI) A group of closely related genetic disorders caused by defective bone formation, all of which result in small-for-gestational-age fetuses; a common characteristic is bone fragility and susceptibility to fractures; depending on the degree of genetic defect, features may also include deformity of long bones, laxness of ligaments, blueness of scleras, and hearing impairment due to otosclerosis. A rare autosomal recessive variant causes multiple fractures beginning at birth; death occurs in the first year of life. Also called brittle bones; brittle bones disease.

osteogenic, osteogenetic (os-te-o-jen'ik, os-te-o-je-net'ik) Relating to bone formation; derived from bone.

osteomyelitis (os-te-o-mi-ĕ-li'tis) Inflammation of the bone marrow caused most commonly by pus-forming bacteria; the organisms usually gain entry to the bone via the bloodstream through a wound, penetrating injury, or surgical procedure; or it may spread from a neighboring focus of infection.

    postpartum o. Maternal osteomyelitis occurring shortly after giving birth; usually caused by a group B streptococcus.

osteoporosis (os-te-o-pŏ-ro'sis) Disease that appears to be the result of increased resorption of bone and slowing of bone formation; seen most frequently in the elderly of both sexes, especially postmenopausal women; occurs also in women who have had their ovaries removed; symptoms include bone pain, reduced height, bone deformity, and susceptibility to fractures; may be associated with other disorders (e.g., osteomalacia, multiple myeloma, hypopituitarism) or may be caused by certain drug therapies.

osteosclerosis (os-te-o-sklĕ-ro'sis) Abnormally increased density of bone.

osteoporosis

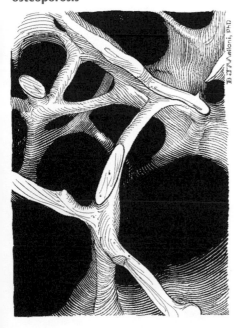

normal bone density

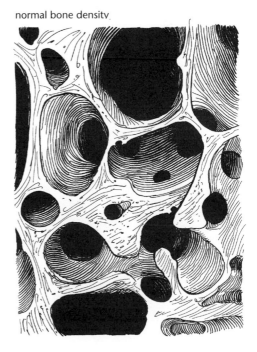

o. congenita See achondroplasia.

ostomy (os'tŏ-me) An artificial opening created surgically.

otoscope (o'to-skōp) Instrument containing magnifying lenses, a light, and a funnel-shaped tip; designed for inspection of the external ear canal and the eardrum; used also for vaginal inspection of a young child.

-ous Suffix meaning having (e.g., cancerous).

outlet (out'let) In anatomy, an opening or passageway that permits an outward movement.

   pelvic o. The lower aperture of the pelvis, bounded by the pubic arch, the ischial tuberosities, the sacrotuberous ligaments, and the tip of the coccyx.

ova (o'va) Plural of ovum.

ovarian (o-va're-an) Relating to the ovaries.

ovariectomy (o-va-re-ek'tŏ-me) See oophorectomy.

ovario-, ovari- Combining forms meaning ovary.

ovariocentesis (o-va-re-o-sen-te'sis) Therapeutic puncture of an ovarian cyst.

ovariocyesis (o-va-re-o-si-e'sis) Ovarian pregnancy.

ovariohysterectomy (o-va-re-o-his-ter-ek'tŏ-me) Removal of the ovaries and uterus.

ovariolysis (o-va-re-ol'ĭ-sis) The cutting away of adhesions that prevent the normal mobility of the ovary; a procedure used in the treatment of certain cases of female infertility.

ovariopexy (o-va-re-o-pek'se) The suturing of an ovary to the abdominal wall.

ovariorrhexis (o-va-re-o-rek'sis) Rupture of an ovary.

ovariosalpingectomy (o-va-re-o-sal-pin-jek'tŏ-me) See oophorosalpingectomy.

ovariosalpingitis (o-va-re-o-sal-pin-ji'tis) See oophorosalpingitis.

ovariotomy (o-va-re-ot'ŏ-me) See oophorotomy.

ovarium (o-va're-um) Latin for ovary.

ovary (o'vă-re) One of the paired sexual glands in which ova are formed; situated on either side of the uterus, near the free end of each fallopian (uterine) tube; it produces the female hormones estrogen and progesterone; the female gonad.

   large white o. See polycystic ovary.

   oyster o. See polycystic ovary.

   palpable postmenopausal o. An ovary measuring more than $1.5 \times 1 \times 0.5$ cm (the average size of a normally atrophied postmenopausal ovary) and which is felt on pelvic examination.

   polycystic o. A diseased, usually enlarged ovary containing multiple cysts filled with thin serous fluid and covered with a thick, pearly white capsule; seen in such conditions as Stein-Leventhal syndrome, abnormal bleeding, and virilism; it is associated with infertility. Also called oyster ovary; popularly called large white ovary.

   third o. An accessory ovary.

ovi- Combining form meaning egg.

ovicidal (o-vĭ-si'dal) Causing destruction of the ovum.

oviduct (o'vĭ-dukt) See uterine tube, under tube.

ovo- Combining form meaning egg.

ovotestis (o-vo-tes'tis) An abnormal gonad in which both testicular and ovarian tissues are present.

ovulation (o-vu-la'shun) The discharge of an ovum from the mature (vesicular) follicle of an ovary.

ovule (o'vūl) 1. The ovum in the ovarian follicle. 2. Any small egg-shaped structure.

ovulocyclic (o-vu-lo-sī'klik) Associated with, or occurring within, the ovulatory cycle.

ovum (o'vum), pl. **ova** The female reproductive cell which, when fused with the male cell (spermatozoon), forms the zygote. Also called egg. See also oocyte.

   blighted o. A fertilized ovum (zygote) that has ceased to develop and has degenerated; a common finding in early spontaneous abortions.

oximeter (ok-sim'ĕ-ter) Instrument used to photoelectrically measure the degree of oxygen saturation in the circulating blood.

   pulse o. A monitor used to measure oxygen saturation in arterial blood by passing a beam of red and infrared light through a pulsating capillary bed without pricking the skin; used especially in anesthetized patients. The monitor provides a continuous record of the oxygen level in the blood and sounds an alarm if the level falls too low.

oximetry (ok-sim'ĕ-tre) The use of an oximeter to determine oxygen saturation in the blood (i.e., the percent of red blood cells that have oxygen attached to them).

oxy- Combining form meaning oxygen; pointed; sharp.

oxycephalic (ok-se-sĕ-fal'ik) Relating to oxycephaly. Also called acrocephalic.

oxycephaly (ok-se-sef'ă-le) A skull enlarged in a vertical direction, with a peaked or cone shape; caused by early closure of the lambdoid and coronal sutures of the skull. Also called acrocephaly; popularly called tower skull.

oxygenate (ok sĭ-jen-āt) To supply oxygen.

oxygenation (ok-sĭ-jĕ-na shun) 1. The combination of oxygen with the blood pigment hemoglobin. 2. The supplying of oxygen (e.g., to

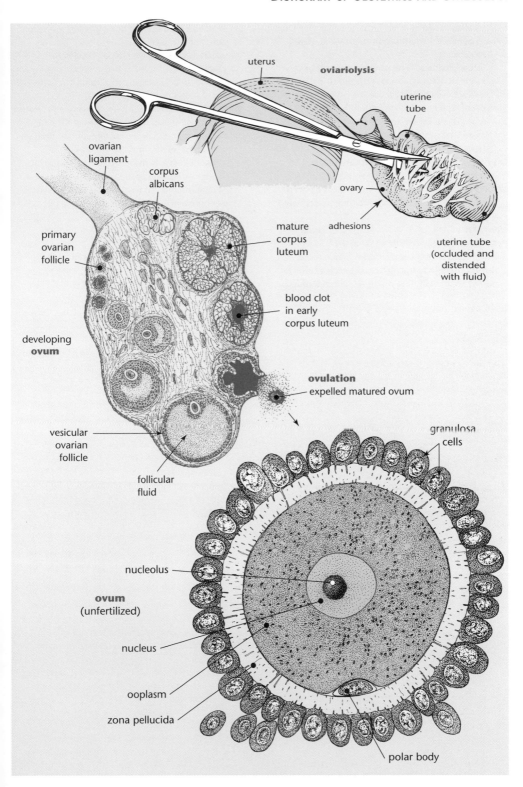

uterus

oviariolysis

uterine tube

ovarian ligament

corpus albicans

mature corpus luteum

ovary

adhesions

uterine tube (occluded and distended with fluid)

primary ovarian follicle

blood clot in early corpus luteum

developing **ovum**

ovulation
expelled matured ovum

vesicular ovarian follicle

granulosa cells

follicular fluid

nucleolus

ovum (unfertilized)

nucleus

ooplasm

zona pellucida

polar body

a tissue or to a person).

apneic o. See diffusion respiration, under respiration.

hyperbaric o. The administration of oxygen at greater than sea-level atmospheric pressure in a special chamber to increase the sensitivity of malignant cells to radiation therapy, and as a treatment for air and gas embolism, clostricial gangrene, acute carbon monoxide poisoning, and other conditions.

oxygenator (ok-sĭ-jĕ-na tor) Device for the mechanical oxygenation of venous blood.

oxyhemoglobin (ok-se-he-mo-glo'bin) The bright red hemoglobin combined with oxygen, present in arterial blood.

oxytetracycline (ok-sĭ-tet-ră-si'klēn) A broad spectrum antibiotic isolated from the actinomycete *Streptomyces rimosus*. When taken during pregnancy it may have deleterious effects on the fetus, including yellowing of developing teeth and inhibition of bone growth; may also cause maternal liver toxicity.

oxytocia (ok-se-to'se-ă) Rapid childbirth.

oxytocic (ok-se-to'sik) **1.** Relating to a rapid childbirth. **2.** Hastening the childbirth process by stimulating uterine contractions.

oxytocin (ok-se-to'sin) (OXT) Hormone produced in the hypothalamus (at the base of the brain) and stored in the posterior lobe of the pituitary prior to its release into the circulation; it stimulates smooth muscle contractions; causes strong contraction of the pregnant uterus and ejection of milk from the breast (distinguished from prolactin, a hormone that stimulates milk production).

oxyuriasis (ok-se-u-ri'ă-sis) Infestation with pinworms.

oxyuricide (ok-se-u'rĭ-sīd) An agent that kills pinworms.

oxyurid (ok-se-u'rid) Pinworm.

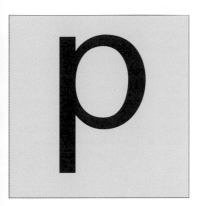

pachy- Prefix meaning thick.

pachytene (pak'e-tēn) In meiosis, the stage in the prophase of the first meiotic division in which paired homologous chromosomes shorten, thicken, and intertwine; then they split longitudinally (remaining attached by a centromere), forming two chromatids; thus each homologous chromosome pair becomes a set of four chromatids (a tetrad). See also diplotene; leptotene; zygotene.

pack (pak) **1.** To fill a cavity or orifice (e.g., to control bleeding). **2.** Any material so used. **3.** To wrap the body or a part with sheets, blankets, or other material for therapeutic purposes.

packer (pak'er) An instrument for introducing an absorbent material into a body cavity or orifice.

packing (pak'ing) **1.** The application of a pack. **2.** The material used to fill a wound or cavity.

paclitaxel (pak-lĭ-taks'el) An anticancer drug for treating refractory ovarian cancer (i.e., ovarian cancer that has progressed in spite of standard treatment); its mechanism of action appears to be cytotoxicity through inhibition of cell division. Trade name: Taxol.

pad (pad) **1.** A soft, cushion-like material used to protect a vulnerable part or as a filling in a depressed area to hold a dressing in place. **2.** A collection of soft tissue serving as a cushion between structures or to fill a space.

　abdominal p. A pad made of several layers of gauze used in surgical procedures of the abdomen (e.g., to absorb secretions or to protect the viscera).

　ischiorectal fat p. A pad of fat extending upward from the anal region in the ischiorectal fossa.

　retropubic fat p. A large quantity of fat located in the U-shaped space between the pubic symphysis and the bladder and extending posteriorly on each side of the bladder.

　sucking p., suctorial p. The pad of encapsulated fat in the cheek, between the buccinator and masseter muscles; it is especially prominent in infants, believed to help prevent the cheek from being sucked in while the baby nurses. Also called adipose body of the cheek.

-pagus Combining form meaning a union (e.g., craniopagus).

pain (pān) A physical or mental sensation of distress or suffering.

　bearing-down p. Pain due to uterine contraction during the second stage of labor, usually accompanied by spontaneous expulsive forces.

　calf p. Pain in the calf muscles; when occurring after parturition, it may be due to a superficial injury to the muscles resulting from inappropriate placement of the patient's leg on the leg holder of the delivery table.

　intermenstrual p. Pelvic pain occurring midway between two menstruations. Also called midpain.

　intractable p. Pain that is not relieved by analgesic medications.

　labor p. Pain caused by the rhythmic contraction of the pregnant uterus at the onset of parturition; characteristically it increases in frequency, duration, and severity as the moment of birth approaches.

pair (pār) Two similar entities regarded together as a functional or structural unit.

　base p. Either of the two pairs of purine–pyrimidine bases that make up the DNA molecule; they are joined by hydrogen bonds.

palpable (pal'pă-bl) Perceptible through touch.

palsy (pawl'ze) Paralysis.

　Bell's p. See facial nerve palsy.

　Erb-Duchenne p. See under paralysis.

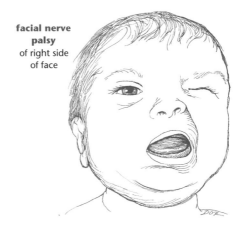

facial nerve palsy of right side of face

facial nerve p. Temporary paralysis or weakness of the muscles on one side of the face; thought to be caused, in the adult, by a viral infection. In the neonate, it usually results from pressure on the facial nerve by forceps during delivery; when occurring in spontaneous delivery, it may be caused by undue pressure on the nerve from the maternal sacrum; recovery usually occurs within a few weeks. Also called Bell's palsy.

pan- Prefix meaning all.

panendoscope (pan-en'dŏ-skōp) A tubular instrument equipped with an optic system designed for wide-angle visualization of the interior of the bladder and urethra.

panhypopituitarism (pan-hi-po-pĭ-tu'ĭ-tar-izm) Condition characterized by absence or deficiency of all the hormones produced by the anterior portion of the pituitary. Also called Simmonds' disease.

panhysterosalpingectomy (pan-his-ter-o-sal-pin-jek'tŏ-me) Surgical removal of the uterus (including the cervix) and the fallopian (uterine) tubes.

panhysterosalpingo-oophorectomy (pan-his-ter-o-sal-pin'go o-of-ŏ-rek'tŏ-me) Surgical removal of the uterus (including the cervix), fallopian (uterine) tubes, and ovaries.

Pap See Papanicolaou.

Papanicolaou (pă-pă-nik'o-lōō) (George N. Papanicolaou, 1883–1962) A Greek-U.S. physician, anatomist, and cytologist; the name is usually shortened to Pap. See Pap smear, under smear; Pap test, under test.

papilla (pă-pil'ă), pl. papillae A small projection from the surface of any tissue.

    mammary p. See nipple.

papillitis (pap-ĭ-li'tis) 1. Inflammation of the optic disk. Also called neuropapillitis. 2. Inflammation of a papilla of the kidney (renal papilla).

    necrotizing p. See renal papillary necrosis, under necrosis.

papilloma (pap-ĭ-lo'mă) A noncancerous tumor that arises from the outermost layer (epithelium) of skin and mucous membranes and develops fingerlike projections from the surface. Also called papillary tumor; villoma.

    choroid plexus p. Papilloma arising in the ventricles of the brain; most commonly seen in children in association with hydrocephalus.

    ductal p. of breast See intraductal papilloma of breast.

    intraductal p. of breast Papilloma arising from the inner lining of a lactiferous duct near the nipple and usually causing a clear, often bloody, discharge from the nipple. Also called

ductal papilloma of breast.

    p. venereum See condyloma acuminatum, under condyloma.

papillomatosis (pap-ĭ-lo-mă-to'sis) The presence of numerous papillomas.

    laryngeal p. Papillomatosis of the larynx, seen in children born of women infected with genital warts; the infant aspirates the human papillomavirus (hPV) while passing through the infected birth canal; types 6 and 11 of the virus are the strains implicated.

papillomatous (pap-ĭ-lo'mă-tus) Relating to a papilloma.

Papillomavirus (pap-ĭ-lo-mă-vi'rus) A genus of DNA viruses (family Papovaviridae); some species have been associated with malignancy with a predilection for squamous epithelium.

papillomavirus (pap-ĭ-lo-mă-vi'rus) Any member of the genus *Papillomavirus*.

    human p. (hPV) A species with several serotypes; types 1 and 2 cause common and plantar warts; types 6, 11, 16, 18, and 31 cause genital warts.

Papovaviridae (pap-o-vă-vir'ĭ-de) A family of double-stranded DNA viruses that may be transmitted to vertebrates by direct contact, indirectly (by arthropods carrying the virus), or by airborne particles; includes viruses causing warts and papillomas.

papovavirus (pap-o-vă-vi'rus) Any virus of the family Papovaviridae.

papular (pap'u-lar) Relating to papules.

papulation (pap-u-la'shun) Development or formation of papules.

papule (pap'ul) A superficial, solid elevation on the skin less than 1 cm in diameter; can arise from the superficial or deep layers of the skin (epidermis or dermis), or from a combination of the two.

    moist p. See condyloma latum, under condyloma.

papulosis (pap-u-lo'sis) The presence of numerous papules.

    bowenoid p. Multiple reddish brown, warty papules occurring on the external genitalia and perianal region of both sexes; grossly, they resemble genital warts (condylomata acuminata); histologically, they have features of squamous cell carcinoma *in situ* indistinguishable from Bowen's disease; DNA sequences of herpesvirus (HPV) type 16 are frequently found in the lesions.

para- Prefix meaning beside; beyond; resembling; secondary; diverging from the normal.

para (par'ă) Denoting a woman's past pregnancies that have reached the period of viability, regardless of whether the infant is dead or alive at the time of delivery; used in conjunction with numerals to designate the number of pregnancies (e.g., para I, para II). The term refers to pregnancies, not fetuses; thus a woman who has given birth to twins at the end of her first pregnancy is still para I.

parabiosis (par-ă-bi-o'sis) **1.** Union of two organisms; may occur naturally (e.g., conjoined twins) or may be produced artificially in experimental animals. **2.** Temporary loss of conductivity of a nerve.

paracentesis (par-ă-sen-te'sis) Aspiration of fluid from a body cavity through a fine needle or any other hollow instrument; tapping. When not further modified, the term usually refers to removal of fluid from the abdominal cavity.

paracentral (par-ă-sen'tral) Off center or situated near a central structure.

paracervix (par-ă-ser'viks) The inferior portion of the parametrium; specifically, the connective tissue extending on both sides of the cervix, between the two layers of the broad ligament, and supporting the uterine vessels.

parachordal (par-ă-kor'dal) Situated near the notochord of the embryo.

paracolpium (par-ă-kol'pe-um) Tissues near the vagina.

paracystic (par-ă-sis'tik) Situated near the bladder. Also called paravesical.

paralysis (pă-ral'ĭ-sis), pl. paralyses Loss of muscular function resulting from disease or injury in the motor pathways of the nervous system or from lesions in the muscles themselves.

    bilateral p. See diplegia.

    Erb-Duchenne p. Paralysis of the upper musculature of an infant's arm (deltoid, biceps, anterior brachial, and long supinator muscles); caused by trauma to the brachial plexus or to the roots of the fifth and sixth cervical nerves during birth. Also called Erb-Duchenne palsy.

    immunologic p., immune p. See immunologic tolerance, under tolerance.

    Klumpke's p. Paralysis of the small muscles of the hand resulting from a traction injury to the lower portion of the brachial plexus; most commonly seen in newborns, usually caused by traction during delivery.

    obstetric p. Paralysis of the dorsiflexor and evertor muscles of the foot, causing dropfoot, as a result of injury to the common peroneal nerve during childbirth by improper placement of the patient in leg holders or stirrups.

paramenia (par-ă-me'ne-ă) Abnormal menstruation.

paramethadione (par-ă-meth-ă-di'on) Anticonvulsant drug administered orally. First trimester intrauterine exposure has deleterious effects on the fetus, such as increased risk of spontaneous abortion and multiple anomalies, including tetralogy of Fallot.

parametria (par-ă-me'tre-ă) Plural of parametrium.

parametric (par-ă-met'rik) Situated near the uterus.

parametritis (par-ă-mĕ-tri'tis) Inflammation of the parametrium. Also called pelvic cellulitis.

parametrium (par-ă-me'tre-um), pl. parametria Extraperitoneal tissue (connective tissue and smooth muscle) contained within the broad ligaments of the uterus; clinically important as an area of potential spread of malignancies of the uterine cervix.

paraplegia (par-ă-ple'jă) Paralysis of both legs and the lower part of the body. During the second stage of labor, the paraplegic woman experiences no pain, even during vigorous uterine contractions; the expulsive reflexes characteristic of this stage are also absent, therefore she needs to be instructed to bear down when contractions occur.

parasalpingitis (par-ă-sal-pin-ji'tis) Inflammation of tissues surrounding the fallopian (uterine) tubes.

parasympathomimetic (par-ă-sim-pă-tho-mĭ-met'ik) Denoting drugs that produce effects similar to those of parasympathetic nerves.

paraumbilical (par-ă-um-bil'ĭ-kal) Adjacent to the navel.

paravaginal (par-ă-vaj'ĭ-nal) Adjacent to the vagina.

paravesical (par-ă-ves'ĭ-kal) See paracystic.

parenteral (pă-ren'ter-al) Taken into the body through a route other than the gastrointestinal tract (e.g., by subcutaneous, intramuscular, or intravenous injection).

parieto-occipital (pă-ri'ĕ-to ok-sip'ĭ-tal) Relating to the parietal and occipital bones of the skull or to the corresponding lobes of the cerebrum.

parity (par'ĭ-te) The state of having borne children.

paroophoron (par-o-of'ŏ-ron) A group of coiled, vestigial tubules in the broad ligament between the epoophoron and the uterus; they are the remnants of the excretory part of the mesonephros and are best seen in very young children.

parous (par'us) Having borne one or more children.

parovarian (par-o-va're-an) Situated next to or

near an ovary.

part (part) A portion.

abdominal p. of ureter The portion of the ureter extending from the kidney to the brim of the pelvis; situated behind the peritoneum; it is approximately the same length as the pelvic part of the ureter.

pelvic p. of ureter The part of the ureter that extends from the brim of the pelvis to the urinary bladder; it is approximately the same length as the abdominal part of the ureter.

presenting p. In obstetrics, the portion of the fetus closest to the birth canal and which is felt through the cervix on vaginal examination; the presenting part indicates the position of the fetus in the uterus during labor.

particle (par'tĭ-kl) A minute portion of matter.

alpha p. A positively charged particle ejected from the nucleus of a radioactive atom; an ionized atom of helium, it consists of two neutrons and two protons.

beta p. An electron, either positively charged (positron) or negatively charged (negatron), emitted from an atomic nucleus during beta decay of a radionuclide.

Dane p. The complete virion of the hepatitis B virus; composed of a DNA central core and an outer layer containing surface antigen.

partogram (par'to-gram) A graphic representation for the purpose of managing labor which compares the progress of a labor with established parameters of a normal labor.

parturient (par-tu're-ent) Relating to childbirth.

parturifacient (par-tu-re-fa'shent) Inducing labor.

parturition (par-tu-rish'un) The process of giving birth; childbirth.

Parvovirus (par-vo-vi'rus) A genus of infectious viruses (family Parvoviridae).

P. B19 Small DNA virus that causes erythema infectiosum.

patch (pach) **1.** A flat, nonpalpable, circumscribed area more than 1 cm in diameter, differing in color from the surrounding surface. **2.** A small piece of material containing a pharmaceutical compound, placed on the skin for transdermal administration of the medication.

blood p. A treatment for post-spinal headache in which blood from the patient is placed in the epidural space at a previous dural puncture site in an effort to plug a 'leak' of spinal fluid.

estradiol p. Any patch affixed to intact skin to continuously provide exogenous estrogen through a rate-limiting membrane; used in systemic hormone replacement therapy to alleviate symptoms of estradiol deficiency in menopausal women (e.g., symptoms of postmenopausal osteoporosis).

mucous p. The superficial grayish patch in the oral mucosa occurring in secondary syphilis.

patent (pa'tent) **1.** Open, unobstructed. **2.** Apparent.

patho-, -pathy, path- Combining forms meaning disease.

pathogen (path'ŏ-jen) A disease-causing microorganism.

pathogenesis (path-o-jen'ĕ-sis) The abnormal biochemical and pathophysiologic mechanisms that lead to disease.

pathogenic (path-o-jen'ik) Causing disease.

pathogenicity (path-o-jĕ-nis'ĭ-te) The capacity to produce disease.

pathway (path'wa) **1.** The linked nerve fibers providing a structural course for nerve impulses. **2.** A sequence of chemical reactions by which one substance is converted into another.

pattern (pat'ern) **1.** A characteristic arrangement or configuration. **2.** A characteristic set of actions.

pulsative p. A rhythmic pattern (e.g., the release of a hormone by the cells that produce it).

sinusoidal fetal heart rate p. A fetal heart rate tracing characterized by: 120 to 160 beats/minute with regular oscillations, 5 to 15 beats/minute, 2 to 5 cycles/minute long-term variability, fixed or flat short-term variability, oscillation of the sinusoidal waveform above or below a baseline, and absent accelerations.

peau d'orange (po'dŏ-rahnj') An abnormal dimpled condition of the skin resembling the skin of an orange; seen in some forms of breast cancer.

pectineal (pek-tin'e-al) Relating to the pubic bone or to any comb-like structure.

pectoral (pek'tŏ-ral) Relating to the chest.

pedi-, ped- Combining forms meaning child; feet.

pederasty (ped'ĕr-as-te) Anal intercourse, especially between man and boy.

pedophilia (pe-do-fil'e-ă) Engaging in sexual fantasies and activities with children as a repeatedly preferred or exclusive method by an adult. It includes any form of heterosexual or homosexual activity.

pedophilic (pe-do-fil'ik) Relating to pedophilia.

pelvi-, pelvo- Combining forms meaning pelvis.

pelvic (pel'vik) Relating to the pelvis.

pelvicephalometry (pel-vĭ-sef-ă-lom'ĕ-tre) Comparative measurement of the maternal pelvis and fetal head.

pelvimeter (pel-vim´ĕ-ter) A caliper-type instrument for measuring the diameters of the pelvis.

    Breisky's p. Pelvimeter used to measure the anteroposterior diameter of the pelvic outlet.

    Thom's p. Pelvimeter used to measure the transverse diameter of the pelvic outlet.

pelvimetry (pel-vim´ĕ-tre) Measurement of diameters of the female pelvis in pregnancy to determine whether the woman is likely to develop difficult labor due to disproportion between the fetal head and maternal pelvis.

    clinical p. See manual pelvimetry.

    combined p. Pelvimetry made both within the body with the examiner's hand and outside the body with a pelvimeter.

    instrumental p. Pelvic measurement conducted with a pelvimeter.

    manual p. Estimation of the pelvic size by measuring the diagonal conjugate with a physical examination; the examiner introduces the index and middle fingers into the vagina and carries them over and up the anterior surface of the sacrum until the sacral promontory is felt with the tip of the middle finger; with the finger held in place, the hand is elevated against the pubic arch and the point of contact is marked on the hand; the hand is then withdrawn and the distance between the tip of the middle finger and the mark on the hand is measured with a rigid scale; this measurement is the diagonal

conjugate and, if greater than 12.5 cm, it may be assumed that it is adequate for a vaginal delivery. Also called clinical pelvimetry.

    radiologic p. See x-ray pelvimetry.

    x-ray p. A precise method, using ionizing radiation, of determining the capacity and morphology of the maternal bony pelvis, and the attitude and position of the fetal presenting part. Measurements of the critical diameters of the maternal pelvis (e.g., the transverse diameter of the midpelvis and transverse diameter of the pelvic inlet) are used as a guide for predicting the possibility of a vaginal delivery. X-ray pelvimetry is indicated when the potential benefit exceeds the risk of radiation exposure to the fetus (e.g., in anticipated vaginal delivery of a breech presentation) and is usually obtained during active labor. Also called radiologic pelvimetry. See also magnetic resonance imaging, under imaging; computed tomography, under tomography; fetopelvic index, under index.

pelviotomy (pel-ve-ot´ŏ-me) **1.** Surgical division of the pubic joint. **2.** Incision into the pelvis of the kidney.

pelvis (pel´vis), pl. pelvises, pelves **1.** The basin-shaped skeletal structure at the lower end of the trunk, composed of the two hipbones and the sacrum and coccyx; it supports the spinal column and rests on the lower limbs. Also called bony pelvis. **2.** A funnel-like dilatation.

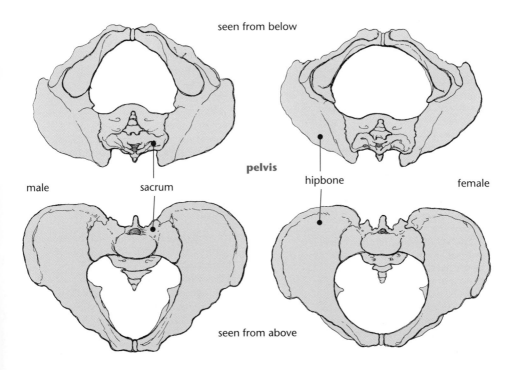

seen from below

pelvis

male   sacrum   hipbone   female

seen from above

achondroplastic p. A broad, flattened pelvis, as seen in achondroplastic dwarfs.

android p. An elliptical or heart-shaped pelvis in which the posterior sagittal diameter of the inlet is shorter than the anterior sagittal. Also called funnel-shaped pelvis; brachypellic pelvis.

anthropoid p. A pelvis with a long, narrow, oval inlet; its anteroposterior diameter exceeds its transverse diameter. Also called pithecoid pelvis; dolichopellic pelvis.

bony p. See pelvis (1).

brachypellic p. See android pelvis.

contracted p. A pelvis characterized by diminished diameters of the inlet, outlet, or midpelvis, or a combination of the three.

cordate p. A pelvis with an inlet that is somewhat heart-shaped; caused by thrusting forward of the sacrum.

dolichopellic p. See anthropoid pelvis.

double Naegele p. See Robert pelvis.

false p. See major pelvis.

funnel-shaped p. See android pelvis.

greater p. See major pelvis.

gynecoid p. A pelvis with an inlet that has a well-rounded oval shape; it represents the average or normal female pelvis. Also called mesatipellic pelvis.

p. of kidney See renal pelvis.

kyphotic p. A pelvis that, due to kyphoscoliosis, has a shortened transverse diameter at the outlet and appears funnel-shaped with a marked inclination.

lesser p. See minor pelvis.

lordotic p. A pelvis that is deformed by an anterior curvature in the lumbar region of the vertebral column.

major p. The false pelvis; the portion of the pelvis above the oblique plane of the pelvic brim; its cavity is part of the abdomen. Also called false pelvis; greater pelvis.

mesatipellic p. See gynecoid pelvis.

minor p. The true pelvis; a narrowed continuation of the major pelvis, below and behind the pelvic brim; in the female, it is typically short, wide, and curved. Also called true pelvis; lesser pelvis.

Naegele p. An obliquely contracted pelvis in which there is complete ankylosis of one sacroiliac synchondrosis or complete fusion of the sacrum with one hipbone.

p. obtecta A pelvis associated with severe kyphosis, in which the vertebral column extends horizontally across the pelvic inlet.

pithecoid p. See anthropoid pelvis.

platypellic p. See platypelloid pelvis.

platypelloid p. An exceedingly flat pelvis in which the transverse diameter of the pelvic inlet is far greater than the anteroposterior diameter. Also called platypellic pelvis.

rachitic p. A grossly distorted pelvis secondary to the ravages of rickets, which can involve virtually every bone of the pelvis and lower spine.

renal p. The funnel-shaped dilatation formed by the junction of the calices of the kidney through which urine passes into the ureter. Also called pelvis of kidney.

Robert p. A transversely contracted pelvis in which the lateral parts of the sacrum (sacral alae) are lacking bilaterally, resulting in extreme narrowing of the pelvis. Sometimes called double Naegele pelvis.

scoliotic p. An obliquely deformed pelvis, seen in association with scoliosis.

spondylolisthetic p. A pelvis tilted posteriorly to the degree that the body of the fifth lumbar vertebra is situated on a plane in front of the body of the sacrum.

stove-in p. One in which, as a result of a severe compression injury, part of the pelvis is driven into the pelvic cavity.

true p. See minor pelvis.

pelvisacral (pel-vĭ-sa'kral) Relating to the pelvis and sacrum.

pelviscope (pel'vĭ-skōp) Instrument provided with a light source for inspecting the interior of the pelvis.

penetrance (pen'ĕ-trans) The frequency with which a heritable trait is manifested by individuals carrying a gene coding for it, irrespective of variation in the degree of expression (e.g., retinoblastoma). Compare with expressivity.

penicillamine (pen-ĭ-sil-a'mēn) A chelating agent used in treating lead poisoning and hepatolenticular degeneration (Wilson's disease). Intrauterine exposure may cause connective tissue abnormalities such as cutis laxa.

penicillin (pen-ĭ-sil'in) Any of a family of antibiotic compounds; derived from the fungus *Penicillum notatum* (natural penicillin) or produced synthetically. Penicillin suppresses synthesis of bacterial cell walls, which results in eventual death of the cell when the penicillin-poisoned bacteria outgrows its cell wall.

pentazocine (pen-taz'o-sēn) A narcotic analgesic with addiction potential. Abuse of the drug during pregnancy produces fetal growth retardation and withdrawal symptoms in the newborn infant.

pentobarbital (pen-to-bar'bĭ-tal) A drug with sedative properties sometimes used to treat insomnia. Intrauterine exposure may cause withdrawal symptoms and hemorrhage in the newborn infant.

penumbra (pĕ-num'bră) In radiation therapy, peripheral radiation surrounding the full x-ray beam.

peptide (pep'tīd) One of various compounds consisting of two or more amino acid residues.

    vasoactive intestinal p. (VIP) See under polypeptide.

Peptostreptococcus (pep-to-strep-to-kok'us) A genus of Gram-positive bacteria found normally in the respiratory, intestinal, and female genital tracts; also found in certain pus-forming infections.

per- Prefix meaning through; largest amount.

percutaneous (per-ku-ta'ne-us) Effected or performed through the skin.

perforation (per-fŏ-ra'shun) 1. A hole made in a tissue or organ by disease or injury (e.g., of the tympanic membrane by sharp objects or by middle ear infection and of the stomach by a peptic ulcer). 2. The act of piercing.

    cervical p. Perforation of the uterine cervix; may be caused by the downward displacement or partial expulsion of an intrauterine device (IUD), by wires or knitting needles while performing an illegal abortion, or during therapeutic procedures such as cervical dilatation, sounding of the uterus, cervical conization, or insertion of an intracavitary radium applicator (e.g., a colpostat or tandem).

    uterine p. Perforation of the wall of the uterus; may occur accidentally while sounding the uterus, performing a dilatation and curettage, or during insertion of an intrauterine contraceptive device.

perfusion (per-fu'zhun) The passage of fluid through the blood vessels of an organ or tissue.

peri- Prefix meaning around; about.

perianal (per-e-a'nal) Situated around the anus. Also called circumanal.

pericolpitis (per-ĭ-kol-pi'tis) See perivaginitis.

pericystic (per-ĭ-sis'tik) Surrounding the bladder, the gallbladder, or a cyst.

perimetric (per-ĭ-met'rik) Surrounding the uterus.

perimetritis (per-ĭ-mĕ-tri'tis) Inflammation of the perimetrium.

perimetrium (per-ĭ-me'tre-um) The outer, serous layer of the uterine wall.

perinatal (per-ĭ-na'tal) Relating to the period of time preceding and following birth, from completion of 20 weeks of gestation through the first 28 days after birth.

perinate (per'ĭ-nāt) An infant 1 week before birth to 1 week after birth.

perinatology (per-ĭ-na-tol'ŏ-je) The branch of obstetrics and pediatrics concerned with the study and treatment of mother and infant in the last stages of pregnancy and early days after birth. Also called perinatal medicine.

perineal (per-ĭ-ne'al) Relating to the perineum.

perineo- Combining form meaning perineum.

perineoplasty (per-ĭ-ne'o-plas-te) Reparative surgery of the perineum (e.g., to correct a relaxed condition of the musculature).

perineorrhaphy (per-ĭ-ne-or'ă-fe) Suturing of the perineum to repair lacerations or other injuries.

perineotomy (per-ĭ-ne-ot'ŏ-me) See episiotomy.

perineum (per-ĭ-ne'um) The diamond-shaped area between the thighs extending from the coccyx to the pubic bone, just below the pelvic floor; superficially, it is the area between the vulva and the anus in the female and the scrotum and the anus in the male.

    obstetric p. The area between the posterior commissure of the labia majora and the anterior margin of the anus.

period (pe're-od) 1. A portion of time. 2. Popular name for an occurrence of menstruation.

    embryonic p. The first 4 to 8 weeks of gestation.

    fertile p. The time in the midportion of the menstrual cycle when ovulation takes place and conception is most likely to occur; usually 10 to 18 days after the first day of the last menstruation.

    fetal p. The gestation period from the eighth week to term.

    gestation p. The time between conception and parturition; period of pregnancy.

    incubation p. The time between infection with a disease-causing microorganism and the appearance of the first symptoms of the disease. Also called incubative stage, latent period.

    instant p. See menstrual aspiration, under aspiration.

    intrapartum p. See labor; delivery.

    latent p. (1) An apparently inactive period (e.g., the time elapsed between exposure to an injurious agent, such as radiation or poisons, and manifestation of effects, or between the application of a stimulus and a response to the stimulus). Also called latent stage. (2) See incubation period.

    menstrual p. The 3 to 5 days of the menstrual cycle during which menstruation occurs. See also menstruation.

missed p. Failure of menstruation to occur in any given month.

neonatal p. The span of life from birth to 28 days. May be divided into: *neonatal p. I*, from birth through 23 hours, 59 minutes; *neonatal p. II*, from 24 hours of life through 6 days, 23 hours, 59 minutes; and *neonatal p. III*, from the 7th day of life through 27 days, 23 hours, 59 minutes. Also called neonatal interval.

perinatal p. The span of fetal and neonatal periods (i.e., from the 20th week of completed gestation through the 28th day after birth). May be divided into: *perinatal p. I*, from 28 weeks of completed gestation through the 7th day of life; *perinatal p. II*, from 20 weeks of gestation through 27 days after birth. Also called perinatal interval.

puerperal p. The period beginning just after childbirth and the return of the uterus to its original state; usually lasts about 6 weeks.

safe p. Time in the menstrual cycle when conception is least likely to occur; usually lasting from about 10 days before to 10 days after the first day of menstruation. Variability in ovulation time from month to month makes this an unreliable contraceptive method.

transitional p. The first 6 hours after birth during which the newborn infant is observed to detect signs of distress or abnormality.

peritoneocentesis (per-ĭ-to-ne-o-sen-te'sis) Aspiration of fluid from the abdominal cavity with a fine needle or any other hollow instrument. Also called abdominocentesis; paracentesis.

peritoneoscopy (per-ĭ-to-ne-os'kŏ-pe) See laparoscopy.

peritoneum (per-ĭ-to-ne'um) The serous membrane lining the abdominal and pelvic cavities and covering most of the organs contained within.

parietal p. The peritoneum lining the wall of the abdominal and pelvic cavities.

visceral p. The peritoneum adhering to the surface of abdominal and pelvic organs.

periumbilical (per-ĭ-um-bil'ĭ-kal) Surrounding the navel.

periureteritis (per-ĭ-u-re-ter-i'tis) Inflammation of tissues that surround the ureters.

periurethritis (per-ĭ-u-re-thri'tis) Inflammation of tissues about the urethra.

perivaginal (per-ĭ-vaj'i-nal) Adjacent to or near the vagina.

perivaginitis (per-ĭ-vaj-i-ni'tis) Inflammation of tissues adjacent to the vagina. Also called pericolpitis.

pessary (pes'ă-re) A device generally made of Lucite, rubber, or plastic, individually fitted and thus available in various sizes; it is placed in the vagina to support the uterus or cervical stump after hysterectomy (e.g., Hodge and Risser pessaries), or to reduce vaginal herniations, such as cystocele and rectocele, or prolapse of the vagina after hysterectomy (e.g., ring, inflatable ball, cube, Gellhorn, and donut pessaries).

ball p. A hollow plastic ball that, by pressing against the vaginal wall, reduces a cystocele or a rectocele; used when the perineum is relatively adequate for retention of the device.

bee cell p. A hexagonal pessary made of sponge rubber for elevating the cervix and to reduce a cystocele or a rectocele; used when the perineum is adequate for holding it in place. Also called cube pessary.

cube p. See bee cell pessary.

diaphragm p. See contraceptive diaphragm, under diaphragm.

donut p., doughnut p. An inflatable pessary shaped like a doughnut; formerly made of red rubber, currently made of silicone; its use is much like that of the ring pessary .

Gehrung p. A rigid pessary resembling two U letters, inverted and attached; designed to help reduce a cystocele by pressing against, and arching, the anterior vaginal wall.

Hodge p. An elongated, curved, ovoid pessary; one end is placed behind the symphysis, the other in the posterior-superior end (fornix) of the vagina; used to hold a retroverted uterus in place after it has been manually brought into its normal forward position. Also called Smith-Hodge pessary.

inflatable p. A ring-shaped pessary made of soft rubber that, once in place, is inflated with air. Also called Millex pessary.

Gellhorn p. A pessary shaped like a collar button that provides a ringlike platform for the cervix; it is stabilized by a stem that rests upon the perineum; used to correct a markedly prolapsed uterus when the perineal body is reasonably adequate for retention of the pessary.

Milex p. See inflatable pessary.

ring p. A ring placed around the cervix; when in place, it elevates the cervix and distends the vaginal wall, thus reducing a cystocele or a rectocele.

Risser p. A modification of the Hodge pessary; it has a wider bar and deeper notch giving it a larger weight bearing area with less likelihood of causing soft tissue necrosis.

Smith-Hodge p. See Hodge pessary.

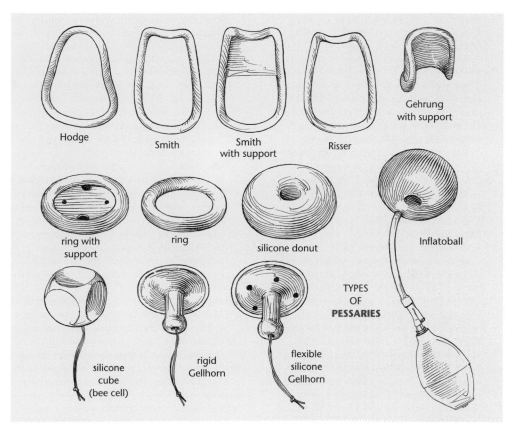

Hodge

Smith

Smith with support

Risser

Gehrung with support

ring with support

ring

silicone donut

Inflatoball

silicone cube (bee cell)

rigid Gellhorn

flexible silicone Gellhorn

TYPES OF PESSARIES

petit mal (pĕ-te' mahl) See absence epilepsy, under epilepsy.

P-fimbriae (pe-fim'bre-ă) Tiny hairlike appendages on the surface of certain *Escherichia coli* strains by means of which they attach to receptors of epithelial cell membranes (e.g., those of the urogenital tract), thereby initiating infection.

pharyngitis (far-in-ji'tis) Inflammation of tissues lining the pharynx.

    acute streptococcal p. Abrupt sore throat, headache, fever, malaise, and enlarged lymph nodes of the neck; children may additionally experience nausea, vomiting, and abdominal pain; caused by species of *Streptococcus*, especially group A, and occasionally groups C or G; may lead to scarlet fever. Infection of the pharynx with other species of *Streptococcus* may lead to rheumatic fever. Commonly called strep throat.

    gonococcal p. Sexually transmitted infection of the pharynx; may cause sore throat, discomfort in swallowing, and, rarely, a mucopurulent discharge with swelling of the uvula; caused by *Neisseria gonorrhoeae* acquired through orogenital contact with a gonorrhea-infected individual. Also called pharyngeal gonorrhea.

pharyngo-, pharyng- Combining forms meaning pharynx.

pharynx (far'inks) The musculomembranous tubular cavity, lined with mucous membrane, extending from the back of the nasal and oral cavities to the beginning of the trachea and esophagus.

phase (fāz) **1.** A relatively distinct part of a process or cycle. **2.** A portion of matter present in a nonhomogeneous system (e.g., an ingredient of an emulsion) that is physically and mechanically separable.

    acceleration p. See under active phase of labor.

    active p. of labor A phase of cervical dilatation during labor, said to begin at 3 cm; it can be further subdivided into an *acceleration phase, phase of maximum slope*, and *deceleration phase*. The minimum normal rate of dilatation during the active phase of labor for a nullipara is 1.2 cm/h, and 1.5 cm/h for a multipara. Failure to achieve these rates of dilatation results in disordered labor. See also arrest disorders and protraction disorders, under disorder; disordered labor, under labor.

deceleration p. See under active phase of labor.

excitement p. In the sexual response cycle, early sexual arousal in both male and female in response to stimulation. In the female, it is characterized by vaginal lubrication, enlargement of the shaft and glans of the clitoris, engorgement of the labia, distention of the upper two-thirds of the vagina, darkening of the vaginal walls, erection of the breasts and nipples with flushing of the skin (sex flush), increased muscle tension, and elevation of blood pressure. See also plateau phase; resolution phase.

follicular p. See secretory phase.

latent p. See latent period, under period.

latent p. of labor A phase of parturition that begins when the mother perceives the onset of regular uterine contractions, and ends when the active phase begins. This interval is considered to be normal at less than 20 hours in a nullipara and less than 14 hours in a multipara. A latent phase of a duration beyond these limits is considered abnormal and identified as a prolonged latent phase. See also arrest disorders and protraction disorders, under disorder; disordered labor, under labor.

luteal p. See secretory phase.

p. of maximum slope See under active phase of labor.

plateau p. In the sexual response cycle, the preorgasmic stage in both male and female. In the female, the expansion or ballooning of the upper two thirds of the vagina increases while the lower vagina tightens, the clitoris retracts, and the labia coloring deepens due to continued engorgement. See also excitement phase, orgasm, resolution phase.

preovulatory p. See secretory phase.

proliferative p. See secretory phase.

prolonged latent p. of labor An abnormal pattern of labor in which the latent phase of labor lasts longer than 20 hours in nulliparas or 14 hours in multiparas. See also prolonged labor, under labor.

resolution p. The stage of the sexual response cycle immediately following orgasm, characterized in the female by gradual return of the genital and related organs to their unstimulated state; may last as long as 30 minutes. See also excitement phase; plateau phase.

secretory p. In the menstrual cycle, the time following ovulation when, under the influence of estrogen and progesterone from the corpus luteum, the endometrium becomes highly vascularized and edematous. As glands become coiled and tortuous, and begin to secrete a clear fluid, their function is reflected in specific histologic changes that can then be used to date their stage of development. Also called luteal phase; preovulatory phase; proliferative phase. See also luteal phase deficiency, under deficiency.

phencyclidine (fen-si'klĭ-dēn) Hallucinogenic drug that can produce profound psychological disturbances; toxicity includes necrosis of muscle and liver and severe hypertension. Intrauterine exposure may have deleterious effects on the fetus, including abnormal features, nystagmus, hypertonicity, and respiratory distress, and withdrawal symptoms in the newborn infant. Commonly called angel dust; PCP (phencyclidine pill).

phenindione (fen-in-di'ōn) Anticoagulant drug administered orally. Intrauterine exposure has a significant risk of causing fetal malformations.

phenmetrazine (fen-met'rǎ-zēn) An appetite depressant drug. Intrauterine exposure during the first trimester of pregnancy has an increased risk of causing skeletal and visceral defects in the fetus.

phenomenon (fĕ-nom'ĕ-non) Any occurrence or manifestation.

Arias-Stella p. The hypersecretory appearance of secretory glands which can be confused with neoplasia. At one time thought to be associated with ectopic pregnancy; however, it can also occur with normal pregnancy and after clomiphene therapy.

dawn p. The abrupt increase of blood sugar (glucose) levels between 5:00 and 9:00 a.m., occurring in diabetic persons receiving insulin therapy.

Lyon p. Phenomenon of X chromosome inactivation first proposed by the geneticist Mary Lyon: One of the two X chromosomes in female somatic cells is inactivated early in embryonic life, while the second X remains condensed; either the paternal or the maternal X chromosome is randomly inactivated in any one cell; however, the same chromosome is involved in clonal descendants of that cell.

phenotype (fe'no-tī p) The entire observable characteristics of an individual, resulting from interactions of the environment and the individual's genetic make-up (genotype).

phenytoin (fen'ĭ-to-in) Anticonvulsant and

antiarrhythmic drug administered orally. Maternal ingestion during pregnancy has been implicated in causing neonatal deficiency of blood clotting factors II, VII, IX, and X (with increased risk of fetal hemorrhage at delivery), multiple anomalies, and mental retardation.

pheochromocytoma (fe-o-kro-mo-si-to'mă) A tumor arising within the medulla of an adrenal (suprarenal) gland or sympathetic paraganglia characterized by production of catecholamines (norepinephrine and epinephrine); manifested by hypertension that may be episodic and severe, rapid heartbeat, palpitations, flushing or pallor, and weight loss.

phimosis (fi-mo'sis) A narrowing or constriction, especially an abnormally small opening of the prepuce, which prevents full retraction of the prepuce behind the glans of the penis; it may be a developmental defect or the consequence of inflammation.

> **prefimbrial p.** Constriction of a fallopian (uterine) tube at the level of its abdominal opening.

phlebitis (flē-bi'tis) Inflammation of a vein.

> **deep p.** See deep thrombophlebitis, under thrombophlebitis.

> **superficial p.** Inflammation of one of the veins near the skin, producing a red, tender, and swollen area along the path of the vein, which may feel like a rope beneath the skin.

phlebo-, phleb- Combining forms meaning vein.

phlebothrombosis (fleb-o-throm-bo'sis) Blood clotting within a vein without apparent antecedent inflammation, frequently occurring in varicose veins of the legs. Predisposing factors (in the absence of varicosities) include congestive heart failure, postoperative periods, prolonged immobilization, pregnancy, and local infection.

phlegmasia (fleg-ma'ze-ă) Obsolete term for inflammation.

> **p. alba dolens** See puerperal thrombophlebitis, under thrombophlebitis.

phlegmon (fleg'mon) Acute inflammatory reaction to infection of subcutaneous tissues.

> **parametrial p.** A complication of cesarean delivery caused by a bacterial infection; characterized by formation of a unilateral solid mass within the leaves of the broad ligament, most frequently limited to the base of the ligament, and accompanied by persistent fever.

phosphatidate phosphohydrolase (fos-fă-ti'dāt fos-fo-hi'dro-lās) (PAPase) An enzyme that promotes the breakdown of phosphatidic acid to form phosphatidylcholine, a major phospholipid of surfactant.

phosphatidic acid (fos-fă-tid'ic aš'id) An acid

that results from the partial hydrolysis of a phospholipid and that on hydrolysis yields two fatty acid molecules and one molecule each of glycerol and phosphoric acid.

phosphatidylcholine (fos-fă-ti-dil-ko'lēn) (PC) A phospholipid compound resulting from condensation of phosphatidic acid and choline; it is a major component of cell membranes and accounts for almost 50% of the phospholipids of surfactant. Also called lecithin.

phosphatidylglycerol (fos-fă-ti-dil-glis'er-ol) (PG) A phosphatidic acid constituent of amniotic fluid, appearing at about 35 weeks of gestation and increasing in amount thereafter; its concentration in the amniotic fluid is an important indicator of fetal lung maturation.

phosphatidylinositol (fos-fă-ti-dil-ĭ-no'sĭ-tol) A phospholipid that is a component of cell membranes.

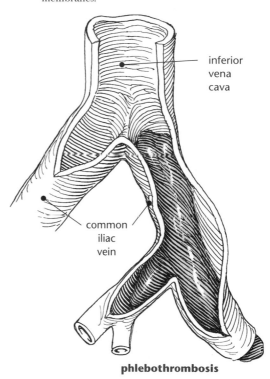

inferior
vena
cava

common
iliac
vein

phlebothrombosis

phosphodiesterase (fos-fo-di-es'ter-ās) One of a group of enzymes that promotes the splitting of phosphodiester bonds, such as those between nucleotides.

phospholipase (fos-fo-lip'ās) An enzyme that catalyzes the breakdown of a phospholipid.

phospholipid (fos-fo-lip'id) Any of several waxy compounds containing phosphoric acid and comprising a major component of cell membranes.

phosphor-, phospho-, phos- Combining forms meaning phosphorus.

phosphoric acid (fos-for'ik as'id) A strong mineral acid that is an important metabolite.

phosphorylation (fos-for-ĭ-la'shun) Introduction of a phosphate group into an organic molecule; a metabolic process.

phosphorus (fos'fo-rus) A nonmetallic element, symbol P, atomic number 15, atomic weight 30.974. It occurs in nature always in combined form, as inorganic phosphates in minerals and water, and as organic phosphates in all living cells. It is an essential element for energy in many biologic processes; recommended dietary allowances for pregnant women: 1200 mg.

photon (fo'ton) A unit or quantum of electromagnetic energy.

phototherapy (fo-to-ther'ă-pe) The use of light (visible, ultraviolet, or laser) for the treatment of neonatal hyperbilirubinemia, psoriasis, or certain neoplasms.

Phthirus pubis (thir'us pu'bis) A sucking louse, parasitic of coarse hair of humans, particularly in the pubic region, but also the hair of the chest, axillae, eyebrows, and eyelashes. Also called crab; crab louse; pubic louse.

phyto-, phyt- Combining forms meaning plants.

phytoestrogen (fi-to-es'tro-gen) Estrogen found in herbs (e.g., dong quai, black cohosh, damiana, and licorice) or other plant sources (e.g., soybeans and yams).

phytohemagglutinin (fi-to-hem-ă-gloo'tĭ-nin) (PHA) A protein of plant origin that clumps (i.e., agglutinates) red blood cells; also acts as a mitogen, stimulating lymphoid cells to divide, replicate their DNA, and transcribe RNA.

pica (pi'kă) The ingestion of unwholesome substances during pregnancy (e.g., dry laundry starch, flour, and clay). The practice may be unrelated to physiologic craving.

pile (pīl) A hemorrhoid.

    sentinel p. A thickening or tag of mucous membrane, resembling a hemorrhoid, located at the end of an anal fissure.

pileus (pi'le-us) A caul.

pill (pil) A small mass of solid medication intended to be swallowed whole. Reference to 'the pill' denotes an oral contraceptive.

    birth-control p. See oral contraceptive, under contraceptive.

    bread p. A placebo made of bread.

    morning-after p. See postcoital contraceptive, under contraceptive.

    pep p. Popular name for a pill containing

an amphetamine or any other stimulant of the central nervous system.

    postcoital p. See postcoital contraceptive, under contraceptive.

    progestin-only p. A pill containing a microdose of progestin only (rather than in combination with estrogen); administered daily as a contraceptive.

pilo- Combining form meaning hair.

pilocystic (pi-lo-sis'tik) Cystlike and containing hair, such as certain tumors.

pilonidal (pi-lo-ni'dal) Having hair as a main characteristic (e.g., certain cysts).

pilosis (pi-lo'sis) See hirsutism.

pinworm (pin'werm) A nematode worm *Enterobius vermicularis* (family Oxyuridae) occurring worldwide as an intestinal parasite of animals and humans, especially children; may infest the vagina through fecal soiling of the vaginal opening, causing intense itching and inflammation of the affected area. Also called seatworm; threadworm.

pit (pit) Any normal or abnormal surface indentation.

    anal p. See proctodeum.

pituitary (pĭ-tu'ĭ-tar-e) **1.** Relating to the hypophysis. Also called hypophyseal. **2.** See hypophysis.

placenta (plă-sen'tă) The disk-shaped organ through which the fetus derives its nourishment (via the umbilical cord); it is an organ for fetomaternal physiologic exchange, attached on one side to the interior wall of the uterus and on the other it is connected to the fetus by means of the umbilical cord; at term it weighs 400 to 600 g and measures 15 to 20 cm in diameter and 2 to 4 cm in thickness; the maternal surface is velvety and spongy; the fetal surface is smooth, covered by amniotic membrane; the fetal membranes arise from its margin. See also amnion; chorion; cotyledon; chorionic villi, under villus.

    accessory p. See succenturiate placenta.

    p. acreta An abnormally adherent placenta; may be implanted directly on the muscular layer of the uterine wall due to partial or total absence of the normally intervening layer of modified endometrium (decidua basalis); based on the degree of wall penetration by placental tissue, it is classified as: *p. acreta vera* (superficial but exceptional adherence), *p. increta* (invasion of uterine muscular wall), or *p. percreta* (full thickness penetration of uterine wall). It is associated with postpartum hemorrhage which, when massive, may lead to hypotension. Predisposing factors include previous cesarean section, placenta previa,

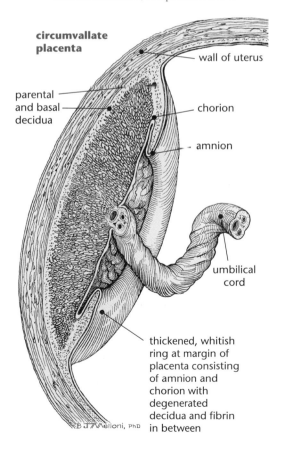

fetal
side of
placenta

placenta

chorion

umbilical
cord

maternal
side of
placenta

cotyledon

amnion

umbilical
arteries

umbilical
vein

umbilical cord

umbilical cord attached to its margin.

p. biloba See bilobate placenta.

bilobate p., bilobed p. A placental anomaly occurring with a single fetus; the placenta is partially divided into two lobes, which are connected by major fetal blood vessels before they unite to enter the umbilical cord. Also called placenta biloba; placenta bipartita.

p. bipartita See bilobate placenta.

circummarginate p. A placenta with its margin raised in a ringlike fashion due to an undercutting of the margin by a groove, which is filled with decidua and fibrin. Also called marginate placenta.

circumvallate p. A variety of extrachorial placenta characterized by the presence of a central depression on its fetal surface, surrounded by a dense, grayish-white ring composed of a double fold of membranes with degenerated decidua and fibrin between the folds; it is associated with increased rates of slight to moderate second-trimester bleeding, premature marginal separation, early delivery, fetal malformations, and perinatal death.

**circumvallate
placenta**

wall of uterus

parental
and basal
decidua

chorion

amnion

umbilical
cord

thickened, whitish
ring at margin of
placenta consisting
of amnion and
chorion with
degenerated
decidua and fibrin
in between

previous uterine curettage, more than six deliveries (grand multiparity), and treatment for Asherman's syndrome.

p. acreta vera See under placenta acreta.

battledore p. A placenta that has the

RB J7Melloni, PhD

271

p. diffusa See placenta membranacea.

p. duplex A single-fetus placenta with two entirely separate lobes, each with its own blood vessels. Compare with bilobate placenta.

extrachorial p. A placental anomaly characterized by an abnormal disproportion of the chorionic plate and basal plate dimensions; may result in a circumvallate or a circummarginate placenta.

fenestrated p. A rare anomaly characterized by absence of portions of the placenta, most frequently involving only chorionic villi.

fundal p. A placenta implanted in the fundus of the uterus, the usual site.

p. increta See under placenta acreta.

low-lying p. A placenta implanted in the lower segment of the uterus where the edge of the placenta is near, but does not reach, the internal opening of the cervix.

marginal p. previa See under placenta previa.

marginate p. See circummarginate placenta.

p. membranacea Placenta in which functioning villous stems and their branches persist over the entire chorion, and which is covered with a thin membrane; it occasionally causes severe hemorrhage during the third stage of labor since it does not readily separate from the uterine wall. Also called placenta diffusa.

partial p. previa See under placenta previa.

p. percreta See under placenta acreta.

p. previa A placenta implanted over or at the edge of the internal opening of the cervix, causing sudden, painless, and profuse bleeding usually in the third trimester or close to the end of the second trimester. Classified as *total p. previa*, when it completely covers the internal cervical opening; *partial p. previa*, when it only partially covers the opening; and *marginal p. previa*, when the edge of the placenta is at the edge of, but does not cover, the opening. Incidence increases with advancing age, multiparity, and scarring from previous cesarean section. Also called placental presentation.

retained p. Placental tissue that remains attached to the uterine wall after delivery, usually causing postpartum hemorrhage; frequently occurs in placenta acreta, in manual removal of the placenta, and in unrecognized succenturiate placenta.

ring-shaped p. A rare anomaly in which the entire placenta is annular or horseshoe-shaped; it is associated with increased rates of antepartum and postpartum hemorrhage and fetal growth retardation.

succenturiate p. One or more accessory lobes that often have vascular connections of fetal origin and are developed in the membranes distant from the primary placenta; may be retained in the uterus after expulsion of the primary placenta, causing postpartum hemorrhage. Also called accessory placenta.

total p. previa See under placenta previa.

triplex p. A single-fetus placenta with three entirely separate lobes, each with its own blood vessels.

placental (plă-sen'tal) Relating to the placenta.

placentation (plas-en-ta'shun) The development of the placenta and its structural relationship to maternal and fetal tissues.

hemochorioendothelial p. Term used to describe placental development with reference to its blood supply (i.e., maternal blood, which bathes the chorionic villi, and fetal blood within the fetal capillaries traversing the intravillous spaces).

placentitis (plas-en-ti'tis) Inflammation of the placenta, usually caused by a bacterial infection ascending from the birth canal.

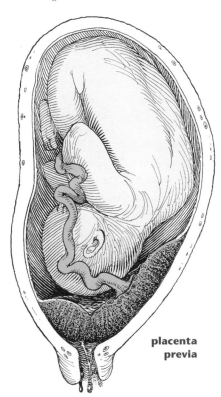

placenta previa

placentography (plas-en-tog'ră-fe) X-ray visualization of the placenta after injection of a radiopaque substance.

placentotherapy (plas-en-to-ther'ă-pe) The therapeutic use of extracts prepared from placental tissue.

plagio- Combining form meaning oblique.

plagiocephaly (pla-je-o-sef'ă-le) A deformity of the skull in which one side is more developed anteriorly and the other side posteriorly. Usually the skull becomes gradually symmetrical after 9 months to 2 years of age.

plane (plān) **1.** A flat or level surface. **2.** An imaginary surface formed by extension through two points or an axis. **3.** A particular level; a stage in surgical anesthesia.

　　interspinous p. A horizontal plane transecting the body at the level of the anterior superior iliac spine of the hipbone.

　　intertubercular p. See transtubercular plane.

　　midinguinal p. The vertical plane passing through the middle of the inguinal ligament.

　　pelvic p. of greatest dimension The roomiest portion of the pelvic cavity extending from the middle of the posterior surface of the pubic symphysis anteriorly to the junction of the second and third sacral vertebrae posteriorly; in the average pregnant woman,

the anteroposterior diameter is approximately 12.75 cm and its transverse diameter is around 12.5 cm.

　　pelvic p. of inlet The rounded or oval opening of the true (minor) pelvis, bounded anteriorly by the upper border of the pubis, laterally by the iliopectineal line, and posteriorly by the sacral promontory. Also called superior aperture of minor pelvis; superior pelvic strait.

　　pelvic p. of least dimension The midpelvis plane, extending from the lower margin of the pubic symphysis through the ischial spines to the apex of the sacrum; in the average pregnant woman, the anteroposterior diameter measures approximately 11.5 cm and its transverse diameter is around 10 cm. Also called pelvic plane of midpelvis.

　　pelvic p. of midpelvis See pelvic plane of least dimension.

　　pelvic p. of outlet The plane across the lower opening of the true (minor) pelvis, bounded anteriorly by the pubic symphysis and the sides of the pubic arch, laterally by the ischial tuberosities, and posteriorly by the tip of the coccyx. Also called inferior aperture of minor pelvis; inferior pelvic strait.

　　principal p. The plane containing the central ray of a radiation beam, used for

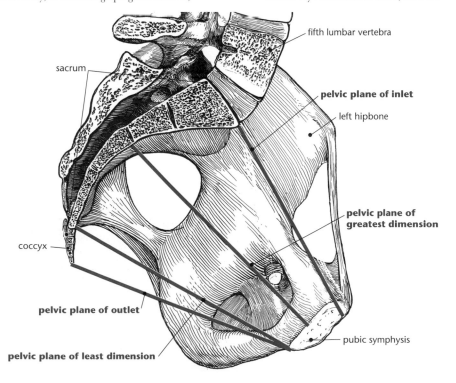

fifth lumbar vertebra

sacrum

pelvic plane of inlet

left hipbone

pelvic plane of greatest dimension

coccyx

pelvic plane of outlet

pelvic plane of least dimension

pubic symphysis

diagnosis and treatment.

transtubercular p. The horizontal plane at the level of the tubercles of the iliac crest of the hipbone; usually the same level as the lower part of the fifth lumbar vertebra. Also called intertubercular plane.

umbilical p. The horizontal plane passing through the navel.

planigraphy (plă-nig'ră-fe) See tomography.

plaque (plak) An elevated flat-topped lesion, primarily originating in the epidermis.

-plasia Suffix meaning formation (e.g., hyperplasia).

plasma (plaz'mă) **1.** The fluid component of blood in which its formed elements are suspended; distinguished from serum. **2.** The fluid component of lymph.

antihemophilic human p. Normal human plasma that has had its original antihemolytic properties preserved; used in temporary arrest of bleeding in hemophilic patients.

fresh frozen p. (FFP) Plasma that has been frozen within 6 hours of withdrawal from donor.

plasmapheresis (plaz-mă-fĕ-re'sis) Removal of plasma from withdrawn blood and reinfusion of the blood's formed elements suspended in a sterile plasma substitute (e.g., saline).

plasmid (plaz'mid) An extrachromosomal, self-replicating genetic element in bacteria that is not essential for bacterial growth but has a role in such activities as drug resistance and toxin production; plasmids are valuable in molecular biology as vectors for cloned segments of DNA.

-plasty Suffix meaning molding or shaping (e.g., rhinoplasty).

plate (plāt) **1.** In anatomy, any flattened, relatively thin structure. **2.** In microbiology, a glass culture receptacle, such as the Petri dish. **3.** A smooth, flat metal device of uniform thickness, used for approximating fractured bones. **4.** A thin perforated structure for covering defects sustained during injury or surgery.

basal p. Placental tissues on the maternal side of the placenta; composed of syncytium (lining the outer aspect of the intervillous space), a layer of fibrinoid deposits, and decidua (adjoining the myometrium).

chorionic p. Placental tissues on the fetal side of the placenta, giving rise to the chorionic villi; composed of amniotic epithelium (lining the fetal aspect), connective tissue (conveying the main branches of the umbilical vessels), and a layer of cellular and syncytial trophoblasts (lining the inner aspect of the intervillous space).

medullary p. See neural plate.

neural p. The middle ectodermal thickening in the embryo from which the neural tube develops; the anlage of the brain and spinal cord (central nervous system). Also called medullary plate.

obstetrical measuring p. A calibrated plate for calculating the digital measurements of the true conjugate (anteroposterior diameter of the pelvic inlet) without a pelvimeter.

platyhieric (plat-e-hi-er'ik) Having an abnormally flat sacrum.

platypellic, platypelloid (plat-e-pel'ik, plat-e-pel'oid) Having a wide and flattened pelvis.

pleo- Combining form meaning more.

pleomastia (ple-o-mas'te-ă) See polymastia.

plethysmography (pleth-iz-mog'ră-fe) The process of measuring and recording variations in the size of a part produced by changes in the circulation of blood within it.

impedance p. (IPG) Technique for diagnosing deep venous thrombosis (DVT) by recording the blood volume changes within the leg by means of skin electrodes around the leg and a pneumatic cuff around the thigh; venous obstruction will diminish the normal changes occurring with inflation and rapid deflation of the thigh cuff. The technique is less sensitive for DVT of the calf than of the proximal veins; also pressure exerted by the pregnant uterus on the inferior vena cava or the common iliac veins can produce a false-positive result.

plethysmometer (pleth-iz-mom'ĕ-ter) Instrument for measuring the degree of fullness of a hollow structure, usually a blood vessel.

pleura (ploor'ă) The double-layered serous membrane enveloping the lungs and lining the interior walls of the chest cavity.

pleuro-, pleur- Combining forms meaning the pleura; a side; rib.

plexus (plek'sus), pl. plexuses An interwoven network of nerves, veins, arteries or lymphatic vessels.

abdominal aortic p. A network of autonomic nerves in front of and alongside the abdominal aorta between the origins of the superior and inferior mesenteric arteries; the plexus is formed by branches from the celiac plexus and the first and second lumbar splanchnic nerves; it sends an extension below the level of the bifurcation of the aorta, where it is known as the superior hypogastric plexus.

anococcygeal p. See coccygeal plexus.

anterior coronary p. of heart See right coronary plexus of heart.

autonomic p.'s Plexuses composed of sympathetic and parasympathetic nerves and ganglia in combination with visceral afferent fibers; located in the thorax (cardiac plexus), abdomen (celiac plexus), and pelvis (hypogastric plexus); from the plexuses, branches are distributed to the viscera.

axillary lymphatic p. A plexus of lymphatic channels in the axilla that drain into axillary nodes.

brachial p. A plexus composed of the ventral primary divisions of the fifth to eighth cervical nerves and first thoracic nerve, with possible contributions from the fourth cervical and second thoracic nerves. The various nerves unite to form three trunks: upper trunk of the plexus (formed by the fifth and sixth cervical nerves), lower trunk of the plexus (formed by the eighth cervical and first thoracic nerves), and middle trunk of the plexus (formed by the seventh cervical nerve alone). Each trunk splits into anterior and posterior divisions: the anterior divisions of the upper and middle trunks unite to form a lateral cord; the anterior division of the lower trunk, after receiving some nerve fibers from the seventh cervical nerve, forms the medial cord; the posterior divisions of all three trunks unite to form the posterior cord. Most of the branches of the brachial plexus originate from the cords in the axilla and supply the muscles and skin of the entire upper limb.

cavernous p. of clitoris An autonomic nerve plexus of the clitoris, derived from the vesical plexus and located in the cavernous tissue at the root of the clitoris.

choroid p. A network of fringelike folds of the pia mater fused with the epithelial lining (ependyma) of the third and fourth and lateral ventricles of the brain and containing numerous blood vessels and nerves; branches of the internal carotid and posterior cerebral arteries supply the plexuses of the third and lateral ventricles, the posterior cerebellar arteries supply the plexus in the fourth ventricle. The choroid plexus regulates the intraventricular pressure by secretion and absorption of cerebrospinal fluid.

coccygeal p. A small plexus formed by the anterior branches of the fifth sacral and coccygeal nerves, supplemented by some fibers from the anterior branch of the fourth sacral nerve; it forms a small trunk that pierces the coccygeal muscle to enter the pelvis; anococcygeal nerves arise from the plexus to innervate the skin around the coccyx. Also

called anococcygeal plexus.

dangling choroid p. Term employed in describing an early sign of hydrocephalus; the fetal choroid plexus in the dependent lateral ventricle of the brain separates from its normal position adjacent to the medial ventricular wall and drifts toward the lateral wall, where it remains in contact with the wall. The defect is observed sonographically.

Frankenhauser's p. A group of myelinated and nonmyelinated nerve fibers located in the uterosacral ligaments and innervating primarily the uterus, including the cervix.

hypogastric p.'s Plexuses of autonomic nerve fibers located in the pelvis just below the bifurcation of the aorta: *Inferior hypogastric p.'s*, two networks of nerves located in front of the lower sacrum, composed of the right and left hypogastric nerves, pelvic splanchnic nerves, and pelvic parasympathetic nerves; branches of the right and left inferior hypogastric plexuses innervate pelvic organs and blood vessels. *Superior hypogastric p.*, a network of nerves located between the bifurcation of the aorta and the promontory of the sacrum (usually to the left side of the median plane), where it receives contributions from the third and fourth lumbar splanchnic nerves before dividing into the right and left hypogastric nerves which descend to the inferior hypogastric plexuses, as well as contribute to the testicular or ovarian plexus; branches innervate the pelvic organs and blood vessels.

inguinal lymphatic p. A plexus of lymphatic channels in the iliopectineal fossa, distributed along the femoral artery and vein.

lumbar p. A plexus of nerves located in front of the transverse processes of the lumbar vertebrae; it is composed of the anterior primary divisions of the first three lumbar nerves, the larger portion of the fourth lumbar nerve, and a branch from the last thoracic nerve.

lumbosacral p. The combined lumbar and sacral plexuses.

lymphatic p. Any plexus of interconnecting lymph channels that absorb colloidal material and transport it to larger vessels for drainage into lymph nodes.

mammary arterial p. An extensive network of anastomosing branches of the lateral and internal thoracic arteries, and intercostal arteries; they form a circular plexus around the areola, and a deeper plexus in the region of the acinar structures of the female breast.

mammary lymphatic p. A rich network of

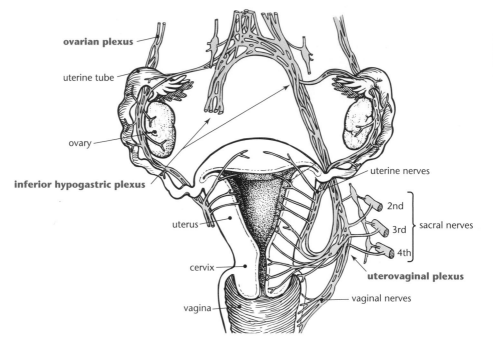

ovarian plexus
uterine tube
ovary
inferior hypogastric plexus
uterine nerves
uterus
2nd
3rd } sacral nerves
4th
cervix
uterovaginal plexus
vaginal nerves
vagina

lymph vessels divided into two planes, a superficial (subareolar) plexus and a deep (fascial) plexus; both originate in the interlobular spaces and in the wall of the lactiferous ducts, collecting lymph from the central parts of the gland, the skin, areola, and nipple; most of the superficial plexus drains laterally to the axillary lymph nodes; most of the deep fascial plexus drains medially to the internal mammary and mediastinal lymph nodes.

mammary venous p. A circular venous plexus around the base of the nipple and areola that radiates throughout the female breast, draining mostly toward the axilla to the axillary vein by way of the lateral thoracic vein; also drained by the internal thoracic vein, which empties into the brachiocephalic vein.

ovarian p. A network of autonomic nerve fibers distributed to the ovary and fallopian (uterine) tube; formed by branches from the renal and aortic plexuses and reinforced below by branches from the superior and inferior hypogastric plexuses.

pampiniform p. In the female, a venous plexus in the broad ligament that drains the ovary and fallopian (uterine) tube and empties into the ovarian vein; it communicates with the uterine plexus; during pregnancy both the pampiniform and uterine plexuses enlarge. In the male, a venous plexus that is the chief

constituent of the spermatic cord; it drains the testis and epididymis and empties into the testicular vein.

pudendal p. Plexus located in the posterior pelvis and formed by the anterior primary divisions of the second and third sacral nerves and the entire fourth sacral nerve; it supplies the pelvic viscera and the external genitalia. Considered by some to be part of the sacral plexus.

rectal venous p. A network of veins surrounding the rectum; in the female it communicates with the vaginal and uterine plexuses, and in the male with the vesical plexus. It consists of two divisions: *Internal rectal venous p.*, situated beneath the epithelium of the rectum and anal canal; it drains chiefly into the superior rectal vein. *External rectal venous p.*, situated outside the muscular coats of the rectum; it drains into the superior, middle, and inferior rectal veins.

right coronary p. of heart Autonomic nerve fibers derived from the superficial part of the cardiac plexus and partly from the deep part of the cardiac plexus (right side); it accompanies the right coronary artery, and distributes branches to the right atrium and right ventricle. Also called anterior coronary plexus of heart.

sacral p. A plexus of nerve fibers located in the posterior wall of the pelvis, formed by the anterior primary divisions of the fourth lumbar to the third sacral nerves; it supplies the buttocks, perineum, lower extremities, and pelvic viscera; it gives rise to the sciatic nerve.

uterine venous p. A venous plexus on both sides of the uterus within the broad ligament, closely associated with the vaginal and ovarian plexuses; drained by the uterine veins into the internal iliac vein.

uterovaginal p. Plexus located in the base of the broad ligament and derived from the inferior hypogastric plexus; it sends fibers to the vagina, cervix, and the body of the uterus.

vaginal venous p. A venous plexus around the vagina that is closely associated with the uterine, vesical, and rectal venous plexuses; drained by vaginal veins into the internal iliac vein.

vertebral venous p.'s Four venous plexuses along the vertebral column: *External vertebral venous p.*, situated outside the length of the vertebral column and divided into anterior and posterior plexuses; they drain the muscles around the vertebral column. *Internal vertebral venous p.*, situated inside the vertebral canal and divided into anterior and posterior plexuses; they drain the structures within the vertebral canal.

vesical p. An autonomic nerve plexus along the side of the bladder; an extension of the inferior hypogastric plexus.

vesical venous p. A network of veins surrounding the base of the bladder, linked below with the vaginal plexus in the female and with the prostatic plexus in the male; it is drained by vesical veins into the internal iliac vein.

plica (pli'kă) pl. plicae **1.** A fold (e.g., of skin or membrane). **2.** A matted condition of the hair resulting from filth and parasites.

p. triangularis of tonsil In fetal life, a free fold of mucous membrane covering the anteroinferior part of the palatine tonsil. After birth, the fold houses lymphoid tissue and becomes part of the tonsil. It is rarely present in adults. Also called triangular fold of tonsil.

plication (pli-ka'shun) The folding and suturing of muscles or connective tissues (e.g., for the treatment of stress incontinence), or of the wall of a hollow organ to reduce its size.

Kelly p. See anterior colporrhaphy, under colporrhaphy (2).

Kennedy p. See anterior colporrhaphy, under colporrhaphy (2).

plug (plug) Anything that stops up an orifice or passage.

cervical p. See mucous plug.

epithelial p. A group of epithelial cells temporarily blocking the nostrils of the fetus.

meconium p. syndrome See under syndrome.

mucus p. A thick, viscous plug of accumulated mucous secretions filling the cervical canal during pregnancy. Also called cervical plug.

pneumatosis (nu-mă-to'sis) The abnormal presence of air or gas in any body tissue.

p. intestinalis Gas within the bowel wall, appearing in the x-ray image as a string of submucosal bubbles; caused by bacterial invasion of the bowel wall; most commonly seen in newborn infants with necrotizing enterocolitis.

pneumaturia (nu-mă-tu're-ă) Passage of gas in the stream of urine due to entrance of air into the bladder through an abnormal opening or channel (e.g., a fistula).

Pneumocystis carinii (nu-mo-sis'tis kar-in'e) A parasitic protozoan, commonly occurring in nature, which causes pneumocystis carinii pneumonia in debilitated humans, especially infants and those individuals whose immune system is compromised (e.g., by disease or chemotherapy). It has little or no virulence for people with normal immune function. See also pneumocystis carinii pneumonia, under pneumonia.

pneumocystosis (noo-mo-sis-to'sis) See pneumocystis carinii pneumonia, under pneumonia.

pneumonia (noo-mo'ne-ă) Inflammation of lung tissue, usually involving the air sacs (alveoli) and development of areas of tissue consolidation; caused by a variety of microorganisms (e.g., bacteria, viruses, fungi, parasites) or by chemical or physical agents. In pregnancy, pneumonia may not be tolerated as well as in the nonpregnant state due to the usual pregnancy-induced changes in the respiratory physiology.

aspiration p. Pneumonia caused by inhalation of foreign material (e.g., food particles, vomited debris, throat secretions).

atypical p. See mycoplasmal pneumonia.

bacterial p. Any pneumonia caused by bacteria (e.g., *Streptococcus pneumoniae, Haemophilus influenzae, Staphylococcus aureus*).

chemical p. Pneumonia caused by aspiration of any chemical substance that is toxic to the lungs (e.g., aspiration of meconium by a fetus or by an infant at the time of birth).

chlamydial p. Pneumonia caused by the

bacterium *Chlamydia trachomatis*, seen in infants during the first 3 to 11 weeks after birth; usually acquired from an infected maternal cervix during vaginal delivery.

Eaton agent p. See mycoplasmal pneumonia.

mycoplasmal p. The most common form of pneumonia affecting school-age children and young adults; it is generally a mild illness caused by the bacterium *Mycoplasma pneumoniae*, beginning insidiously after a 3-week incubation period; it does not result in consolidation of lung tissue, which is typical of bacterial pneumonias (hence the synonym 'atypical' pneumonia). Distinguished from viral pneumonia by the presence of cold agglutinin. Also called primary atypical pneumonia; Eaton agent pneumonia.

pneumocystis carinii p. An opportunistic pneumonia occurring predominantly in individuals with impaired immunity, such as premature or malnourished infants, children with primary immunodeficiency diseases, patients undergoing chemotherapy for cancer or organ transplantation, and patients in the last stage of an HIV infection (AIDS); caused by the protozoan *Pneumocystis carinii*, through airborne transmission. The organism multiplies in the pulmonary air sacs (alveoli), which become filled with a pink frothy mass. Also called pneumocystosis.

primary atypical p. See mycoplasmal pneumonia.

viral p. Pneumonia caused by any of a variety of viruses; may be complicated by a secondary bacterial infection.

pneumonitis (noo-mo-ni'tis) Inflammation of the lungs.

lymphocytic interstitial p., lymphoid interstitial p. (LIP) Extensive infiltration of lung tissue with lymphocytes and plasma cells frequently associated with increased incidence of malignant lymphoma; may be diffuse or involve a circumscribed area of the lung; it has been described in association with AIDS.

pneumothorax (noo-mo-tho'raks) Accumulation of air between the two layers of the pleura (pleural space); may be due to trauma (e.g., air leakage from an accidental puncture of a lung), or may result from spontaneous rupture of a bulla on the lung surface. In newborn infants it occurs chiefly after meconium aspiration, positive pressure resuscitation, or as a complication of artificial ventilation.

catamenial p. Recurrent right pneumothorax occurring concurrently with menstruation; a rare condition associated with endometriosis due to implantation of endometrial tissue on the pleura.

tension p. A life-threatening condition occurring when lungs and heart are compressed by the accumulated air in the pleural space, compromising ventilation.

Pneumovirus (noo-mo-vi'rus) A genus of viruses that includes the respiratory syncytial virus.

podophyllin (pod-o-fil'in) Caustic resin extracted from the roots of the May apple *(Podophyllum peltatum)*; it has been used as a paint to treat genital warts, skin tumors, and senile keratoses, and as a laxative taken internally; it may cause central nervous system damage; first-trimester fetal exposure causes multiple anomalies.

podophyllotoxin (pod-o-fil-o-tok'sin) A highly toxic compound with antineoplastic and laxative properties. Two semisynthetic derivatives (etoposide and teniposide) are less toxic and used in chemotherapy. See also maytansine; vinca alkaloids, under alkaloid.

pogonion (po-go'ne-on) The most anterior midpoint of the lower jaw; a craniometric point. Also called mental point.

point (point) 1. A minute spot or area. 2. The sharp or tapered end of an instrument. 3. A specific position, condition, or degree. 4. A minute orifice.

craniometric p.'s Fixed points on the skull used as standard landmarks from which skull measurements are taken.

cutoff p. In test interpretation, the value used to separate positive from negative results; a designated limit.

McBurney's p. The spot on the lateral third of a line between the right anterior superior iliac spine and the umbilicus; used to estimate the location of the appendix; the spot is especially tender in acute appendicitis. The appendix is gradually displaced upward, above the McBurney's point, after the first trimester of pregnancy.

mental p. See pogonion.

midinguinal p. The point on the inguinal ligament halfway between the pubic symphysis and the anterior superior iliac spine.

occipital p. The most posterior point of the occipital bone, situated in the median plane at the tip of the external occipital protuberance; the distance between the occipital point and the glabella (between the eyebrows) represents the maximum anteroposterior dimension of the skull.

pole (pōl) 1. Either end of an axis. 2. Either of two points with opposite physical properties.

animal p. The site of an early ovum, near its nucleus, where the polar bodies are formed in succession and where segmentation begins. Also called germinal pole.

germinal p. See animal pole.

polio- Combining form meaning the gray matter of the brain and spinal cord.

polio (po'le-o) Commonly used abbreviated version of poliomyelitis.

poliomyelitis (po-le-o-mi-e-li'tis) An infectious disease caused by the poliovirus, serotypes 1, 2, and 3; most infections are subclinical; some are mild febrile diseases without involving the nervous system and lasting only a few days with complete recovery; a third, *paralytic p.*, is the form most commonly affecting children; initial symptoms are fever, muscle pain, sore throat, and headache, lasting from 2 to 6 days; after several symptom-free days, headache recurs accompanied by fever, nausea, stiff neck, and spinal rigidity; involvement of the medulla oblongata causes impairment of swallowing and cardiopulmonary functions, usually with a fatal outcome. Maternal poliovirus infection during pregnancy may have deleterious effects on the fetus (e.g., cardiovascular abnormalities). Commonly called polio.

poliovirus (po-le-o-vi'rus) The virus (genus *Enterovirus*) that causes poliomyelitis, with an average incubation period of 7 to 14 days; it has a predilection for the central nervous system, especially the anterior columns of the brainstem and spinal cord; serologic types 1, 2, and 3 have been recognized.

poly- Combining form meaning many, much.

polyamine (pol-e-am'ēn) Any of a group of substances that are synthesized within cells and are widely distributed among living forms; some (e.g., spermine and spermidine) are found in increased amounts in the decidua of the pregnant uterus and play an important role in tissue growth and cell hypertrophy.

polyarteritis (pol-e-ar-tĕ-ri'tis) Inflammation of several arteries.

p. nodosa (PAN) A systemic disease marked by degenerating (necrotizing) inflammation of small to medium-sized arteries anywhere throughout the body except in the lungs; characteristically, arteries of the kidneys and viscera are involved; it affects mostly young adults, especially males, and is frequently associated with hepatitis B antigens; symptoms depend on the organs involved; generally, they include fever, malaise, and weight loss. When occurring during pregnancy, the condition is often associated with an unfavorable maternal outcome. Also called periarteritis nodosa.

polychemotherapy (pol-e-ke-mo-ther'ă-pe) See combination chemotherapy, under chemotherapy.

polycystic (pol-e-sis'tik) Containing several cysts. See also polycystic ovary disease, under disease.

polyembryoma (pol-e-em-bre-o'mă) A rare highly malignant germ cell tumor composed of several embryoid bodies that, morphologically, resemble normal early embryos; formed in the ovary, and most commonly in the testis, usually as a component of other germ cell tumors.

polyhydramnios (pol-e-hi-dram'nĭ-os) Excessive accumulation of amniotic fluid, usually greater than 2000 ml; occurs frequently in diabetic women.

polygalactia (pol-e-gă-lak'shea) Excessive secretion of milk.

polymastia (pol-e-mas'ti-ă) The presence of accessory breasts or breast tissue along the embryonic milk line. Also called accessory breasts; secondary breasts; supernumerary breasts; pleomastia.

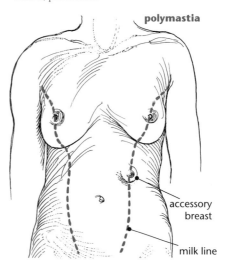

polymastia

accessory breast

milk line

polymenorrhea (pol-e-men-o-re'ă) Menstruation occurring at intervals shorter than 21 days.

polymer (pol'ĭ-mer) A complex substance formed by the joining of small, simple molecules (monomers).

polymerization (pol-ĭ-mer-ĭ-za'shun) The chemical joining of several monomers to form a polymer.

polymerase (pol-im'er-ās) An enzyme that promotes polymerization.

polymorphism (pol-e-mor'fizm) 1. Occurring in various forms either during the development of individuals or as adults within a single species. 2.

The presence of two or more recognizable characteristics (phenotypes) within a species.

restriction fragment length p. (RFLP) Variation in the length of DNA fragments generated by the enzymatic action of a specific endonuclease.

polymyositis (pol-e-mi-o-si'tis) An inflammatory disorder characterized primarily by skeletal muscle pain and tenderness; it may also affect the skin and connective tissue; the muscles most often affected are those of the pelvic and shoulder girdles and pharynx; often associated with occult malignant tumors (e.g., of the breast, ovary, lung, stomach); when skin changes are prominent, the disorder is called dermatomyositis.

polyneuropathy (pol-e-noo-rop'ă-the) A disorder affecting several peripheral nerves, usually associated with systemic disorders such as diabetes mellitus, especially in women of childbearing age; or may be due to the effects of drugs or exposure to environmental toxins.

polyovular (pol-e-ov'u-lar) Relating to more than one ovum.

polyovulation (pol-e-ov-u-la'shun) The maturation and release of several eggs in one ovarian cycle.

polyp (pol'ip) A space-occupying tumor arising from the mucous membrane of a hollow structure (e.g., uterus, bladder, colon, nose).

adenomatous p. A benign polyp composed of glandular tissue; may be pedunculated or broad-based (sessile).

cervical p. A relatively common, usually benign polyp, most frequently seen in women over 20 years of age; some may cause intermenstrual or postintercourse bleeding; a few may undergo malignant change; usually designated *endocervical p.*, a soft, fragile, pedunculated or broad-based growth that originates within the cervical canal and ranges

in size from a few millimeters to several centimeters, frequently protruding through the cervical opening into the vagina; or *ectocervical p.*, to describe a pale, flesh-colored, smooth, and rounded (sometimes elongated) growth arising from the surface of the vaginal portion of the cervix (i.e., the portion that protrudes into the vagina); can undergo size and shape change during pregnancy.

ectocervical p. See under cervical polyp.

endocervical p. See under cervical polyp.

endometrial p. A pedunculated or sessile polyp arising singly or in groups from the epithelium of the uterine cavity, usually from the fundus, and ranging in size from 2 mm in diameter to a large mass filling the uterine cavity, sometimes projecting through the cervical opening into the vagina; occurs most commonly during the perimenopausal period, frequently causing postmenopausal bleeding. Very rarely, endometrial polyps undergo cancerous transformation.

hyperplastic p. A benign, sessile polyp, usually no larger than 5 mm in diameter, lying on top of a mucosal fold (e.g., of the large intestine) and producing no symptoms.

inflammatory p. See pseudopolyp.

neoplastic p. A polyp composed of cells that develop the capacity for uncontrolled proliferation, which results in a cancerous process.

pedunculated p. Polyp attached to the tissue of origin by a slender stalk.

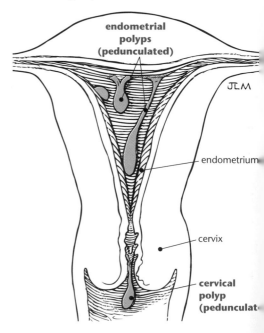

endometrial
polyps
(pedunculated)

JLM

endometrium

cervix

cervical
polyp
(pedunculat...

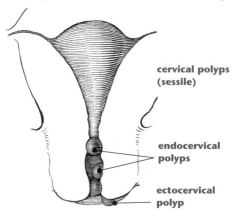

cervical polyps
(sessile)

endocervical
polyps

ectocervical
polyp

placental p. Polyp composed of degenerating chorionic villi, developed from placental tissue that has remained attached to the uterine wall after delivery; it prevents complete involution of the uterus and causes late postpartum hemorrhage.

sessile p. Polyp attached to the tissue of origin by a broad base.

urethral p. A benign, elongated growth developed within the urethra (usually the distal portion); it sometimes protrudes through the urethral orifice.

polypectomy (pol-ĭ-pek'tŏ-me) Removal of a polyp.

polypeptide (pol-e-pep'tīd) Compound composed of two or more amino acids joined by peptide linkage.

vasoactive intestinal p. (VIP) A peptide hormone synthesized in the pituitary and present throughout the body with high concentrations in the nervous system and the gut; it causes relaxation of smooth muscles in the blood vessels, intestines, and genitourinary tract; stimulates conversion of glycogen to glucose; enhances the breakdown of lipids and secretion of insulin; stimulates pancreatic and intestinal secretion; inhibits gastric acid production; and increases secretion of the hormone prolactin. Also called vasoactive intestinal peptide.

polyploidy (pol'e-ploĭ-de) An abnormal increase in the number of chromosomes by exact multiples of the number of chromosomes present in normal diploid cells. Also called tetraploidy.

polypold (pol'e-poid) Resembling a polyp.

polyposis (pol-e-po'sis) The occurrence of several polyps. See also familial adenomatous polyposis syndrome, under syndrome.

polypotome (po-lip'ŏ-tōm) A cutting surgical instrument for removing polyps.

polypous (pol'e-pus) Resembling or characterized by the presence of polyps.

polyspermia (pol-e-sper'me-ă) Excessive secretion of semen.

polyspermy (pol-e-sper'me) The entry of more than one spermatozoon into the ovum during fertilization.

polythelia (pol-e-the'le-ă) The presence of more than two nipples. Also called hyperthelia.

polyunsaturated (pol-e-un-sach'ĕ-ra-ted) Containing two or more double bonds between carbon molecules; applied especially to essential fatty acids.

polyuria (pol-e-u're-ă) The excessive and frequent passage of urine. See also urinary frequency, under frequency.

porphyria (por-fe'rc-ă) Any of a group of disorders characterized by disturbance of the metabolism of blood pigment (heme) due to deficiency of various enzymes in the body; each causes a distinct pattern of overproduction, accumulation, and excretion of intermediates (porphyrins) of heme production. Some forms (e.g., the acute intermittent form) become apparent first during pregnancy.

portio (por'she-o), pl. portiones Latin for part.

p. vaginalis cervicis The portion of the uterine cervix that protrudes into the vagina.

p. supravaginalis cervicis The upper portion of the uterine cervix; anteriorly, it is separated from the bladder by connective tissue; posteriorly, it is located in front of the rectouterine pouch.

position (pŏ-zish'un) **1.** The place or location of an object, structure, body, or body part in relation to others. **2.** The place occupied. **3.** The placement of the body in a particular way to facilitate specific diagnostic or therapeutic procedures.

dorsosacral p. See lithotomy position.

fetal p. The relationship of a designated point on the presenting part of the fetus to a designated point in the right or left side of the maternal pelvis. See also fetal attitude, under attitude; lie; presentation.

frontoanterior p., FA p. Cephalic fetal presentation with the brow directed anteriorly and toward the right (RFA) or the left (LFA) side of the maternal pelvis.

frontoposterior p., FP p. Cephalic fetal presentation with the brow directed posteriorly and to the right (RFP) or the left (LFP) side of the maternal pelvis.

frontotransverse p., FT p. Cephalic fetal presentation with the brow directed transversely toward the right (RFT) or the left (LFT) iliac fossa of the maternal pelvis.

genupectoral p. See knee–chest position.

high pelvic p. See Trendelenburg's position.

knee–chest p. A prone position in which the patient rests on the knees and chest with arms crossed and forearms supporting the head; assumed for rectal examination.

lateral recumbent p. See Sims' position.

lithotomy p. A supine position with the patient's buttocks at the end of the examining or operating table, the hips and knees fully flexed, the thighs abducted and externally rotated. Also called dorsosacral position.

mentoanterior p., MA p. A face presentation with the chin directed anteriorly toward the right (RMA) or the left (LMA) side of the maternal pelvis.

mentoposterior p., MP p. A face presentation with the chin directed posteriorly toward the right (RMP) or the left (LMP) side of the maternal pelvis.

mentotransverse p., MT p. A fetal presentation with the chin directed transversely toward the right (RMT) or the left (LMT) iliac fossa of the maternal pelvis.

obstetrical p. See Sims' position.

occipitoanterior p., OA p. Cephalic fetal presentation with the occiput directed anteriorly and to the right (ROA) or the left (LOA) side of the maternal pelvis.

occipitoposterior p., OP p. Cephalic fetal presentation with the occiput directed posteriorly toward the right (ROP) or the left (LOP) side of the maternal pelvis.

occipitotransverse p., OT p. Cephalic fetal presentation with the occiput transversely directed toward the right (ROT) or the left (LOT) iliac fossa of the maternal pelvis.

sacroanterior p., SA p. A breech fetal presentation with the sacrum directed anteriorly toward the right (RSA) or the left (LSA) side of the maternal pelvis.

sacroposterior p., SP p. A breech fetal presentation with the sacrum directed posteriorly toward the right (RSP) or the left (LSP) side of the maternal pelvis.

sacrotransverse p., ST p. A breech fetal presentation with the sacrum directed transversely toward the right (RST) or the left (LST) iliac fossa of the maternal pelvis.

semiprone p. See Sims' position.

Sims' p. Position in which the patient lies on the left side with the right thigh acutely flexed and the left thigh slightly flexed; the left arm is behind the body; it is used to facilitate certain procedures (e.g., vaginal and rectal examinations, curettement of the uterus, intrauterine irrigation after labor, tamponade of vagina). Also called semiprone position; lateral recumbent position; obstetrical position.

Trendelenburg's p. Position in which the patient is supine on an operating table, inclined at various angles (usually from 30 to 45 degrees); the head is lower and the knees are higher than the rest of the body; the table is angulated at the knees, permitting the legs and feet to hang over it. Also called high pelvic position.

positive (poz'ĭ-tiv) **1.** Having a value opposite another (negative) value. **2.** Indicating the presence of a condition (especially one being tested) or the occurrence of a response.

false-p. See false-positive.

post- Prefix meaning situated behind; subsequent to.

postabortal (pōst-ă-bor'tal) Relating to the period following an abortion.

postbrachial (pōst-bra'ke-al) Relating to the posterior part of the upper arm.

postcoital (pōst-ko'ĭ-tal) Relating to postcoitus.

postcoitus (pōst-ko'ĭ-tus) The period immediately following sexual intercourse (coitus).

postdatism (pōst'dāt-izm) See prolonged pregnancy, under pregnancy.

posteroanterior (po-ster-o-an-tēr'e-or) From the back to the front.

posterolateral (po-ster-o-lat'er-al) Behind and to one side.

posteromedial (po-ster-o-me'de-al) Behind and toward the middle.

posteromedian (po-ster-o-me'de-an) A central position of the back of the body or a part.

postmature (pōst-mă-tur') See postterm.

postmenopausal (pōst-men-o-paw'zal) Occurring after the menopause.

postnatal (pōst-na'tal) Occurring after birth.

postnatal blues See postpartum depression, under depression.

postoperative (pōst-op'er-ă-tiv) Occurring after a surgical operation.

postpartum (pōst-par'tum) Relating to the period after childbirth.

postpubertal (pōst-pu'ber-tal) Relating to the period immediately after puberty.

postterm (pōst'term) Denoting a fetus that remains in the uterus beyond 42 weeks of gestation.

posture (pos'chur) The physical disposition of the body as a whole.

fetal p. See fetal attitude, under attitude.

potency (po'ten-se) **1.** The quality of having strength or great control. **2.** A capacity for growth. **3.** A comparative expression of drug activity; determined by the dose required to produce a particular effect of given intensity, relative to a standard of reference; it varies inversely with the magnitude of the dose required to produce the effect.

sexual p. The ability of a male to perform sexually; often used to mean the ability to have and maintain adequate erection of the penis during sexual intercourse.

pouch (pouch) **1.** A small sac or pocket-like space, especially occurring as an outgrowth of a larger structure; an anatomic receptacle that resembles a bag. **2.** A surgically constructed bag.

abdominovesical p. The peritoneal pouch between the distended bladder and anterior abdominal wall.

continent p. A large-volume abdominal reservoir created from a segment of bowel; it is designed with an abdominal outlet for intermittent introduction of a catheter to remove the pouch contents; constructed after resection of pelvic organs in the surgical treatment of advanced cancer of the pelvic viscera.

craniobuccal p. See Rathke's pouch.

Douglas' p. See rectouterine pouch.

Indiana p. A continent pouch designed as a urinary reservoir; it is constructed with a segment of colon into which the ureters are transplanted for diversion of the urine flow; the urinary conduit to the abdominal wall is usually made with a segment of the terminal ileum but sometimes a section of the sigmoid colon or the transverse colon is preferred. See also continent pouch.

p. of Luschka In embryology, an angled recess of the endoderm at the roof of the primitive pharynx, which forms the pharyngeal bursa.

neurobuccal p. See Rathke's pouch.

Rathke's p. In embryology, the outpocketing of the embryonic mouth (stomodeum) formed when the embryo is about 3 weeks old and subsequently forming the anterior lobe of the pituitary (hypophysis). Also called craniobuccal pouch, neurobuccal pouch.

rectouterine p. The pouchlike space between the posterior wall of the uterus and the anterior wall of the rectum. Also called Douglas' pouch; Douglas' space; rectouterine space.

uterovesical p. The peritoneal pouch between the uterus and the bladder, bounded laterally by the round ligaments of the uterus. Also called vesicouterine pouch.

vaginal p. See female condom, under condom.

vesicouterine p. See uterovesical pouch.

Poxviridae (poks-vir'ĭ-de) A family of large, double-stranded DNA viruses.

poxvirus (poks-vi'rus) Any virus of the family Poxviridae.

pre- Prefix meaning before in time or space.

preanal (pre-a'nal) In front of the anus.

preanesthetic (pre-an-es-thet'ik) Prior to induction of anesthesia.

preaortic (pre-a-or'tik) In front of the aorta.

precancer (pre-kan'ser) A lesion that is known to

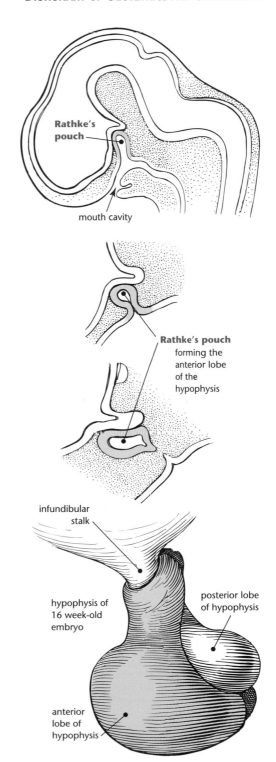

Rathke's pouch

mouth cavity

Rathke's pouch forming the anterior lobe of the hypophysis

infundibular stalk

hypophysis of 16 week-old embryo

posterior lobe of hypophysis

anterior lobe of hypophysis

have the potential to become a cancer.

precancerous (pre-kan'ser-us) Denoting a lesion that precedes, develops into, or has a high risk of becoming a cancer. Also called premalignant; sometimes used synonymously with carcinoma *in situ.*

precipitin (pre-sip'ĭ-tin) An antibody that reacts with its specific soluble antigen, causing the antigen to separate from solution and form solid clumps (i.e., to agglutinate).

precocious (pre-ko'shus) Exhibiting the characteristics of precocity.

precocity (pre-kos'ĭ-te) An exceedingly early development of physical, mental, or sexual characteristics.

> **sexual p.** See precocious puberty, under puberty.

preeclampsia (pre-e-klam'se-ă) A form of pregnancy-induced hypertension characterized by proteinuria and edema. Although it occurs most often after 20 weeks of gestation, it may develop earlier in gestations complicated by trophoblastic disease or in multifetal pregnancies. Formerly called toxemia of pregnancy.

preemie (pre'me) See premature infant, under infant.

pregnancy (preg'nan-se) Condition of the female from the time of conception to delivery of the embryo or fetus. A full-term pregnancy usually spans 40 weeks. Also called gestation.

> **abdominal p.** Implantation of a fertilized ovum on a surface within the abdominal cavity, usually resulting from the expulsion of a tubal pregnancy.

> **adolescent p.** Pregnancy in girls under 19 years of age.

> **ampullar tubal p.** Implantation of the fertilized ovum within the wide, lateral end (ampulla) of the uterine tube; it is the most common of tubal ectopic pregnancies.

> **biochemical p.** In *in vitro* fertilization, the state in which the onset of menstruation is a few days late and human chorionic gonadotropin (hCG) can be detected in the woman's blood.

> **cervical p.** Implantation of a fertilized ovum in the lining of the cervical canal; a rare form of ectopic pregnancy.

> **combined intrauterine and ectopic p.'s** Implantations of fertilized ova occurring simultaneously within and outside the uterine cavity.

> **compound intrauterine and ectopic p.'s** Implantation within the uterus (usually a normal pregnancy) superimposed on an ectopic implantation, usually after the embryo

of the ectopic pregnancy has died.

> **cornual p.** Pregnancy occurring in women with a double uterus; the fertilized ovum implants within a (usually rudimentary) horn of the uterus.

> **ectopic p.** Implantation of the fertilized ovum outside of the uterine cavity; may occur in the uterine tubes, abdominal cavity, cervix, and ovaries. On rare occasions, implantations within the liver, spleen, and vaginal wall have been reported. Also called eccyesis; extrauterine pregnancy; metacyesis. Popularly, simply called ectopic.

> **extrauterine p.** See ectopic pregnancy.

> **fallopian p.** See tubal pregnancy.

> **false p.** See pseudocyesis.

> **heterotypic p.** Ectopic pregnancy occurring with a coexisting intrauterine pregnancy; the ectopic implantation may occur anywhere, but it is most common in a uterine tube and in the cervix.

> **high-risk p.** Pregnancy in which the mother, fetus, or newborn is or will be at increased risk of having a disease or of dying before or after delivery; contributing factors include poor nutrition, absence of prenatal care, genetic disorders and unwanted pregnancy; appearance of abruptio placentae or pre-eclampsia-eclampsia also places the pregnancy at high risk.

> **interstitial tubal p.** An uncommon type of ectopic pregnancy in which the fertilized ovum implants in the portion of uterine tube that is located within the uterine wall.

> **intraligamentous p.** Implantation within the broad ligament of the uterus.

> **intramural p.** Pregnancy that occurs within the uterine wall.

> **isthmic tubal p.** Ectopic pregnancy in which the fertilized ovum implants within the narrowest portion (isthmus) of the uterine tube; it is the second most common of tubal ectopic pregnancies.

> **molar p.** See hydatidiform mole, under mole.

> **multiple p.** Pregnancy with two or more fetuses.

> **multiple tubal p.** Simultaneous implantation of two or more fertilized ova within a single uterine tube, or in both tubes.

> **ovarian p.** A rare form of ectopic pregnancy implanting on the ovary. See also Spielberg's criteria, under criterion.

> **phantom p.** See pseudocyesis.

> **postterm p.** See prolonged pregnancy.

> **prolonged p.** Pregnancy that has reached 42

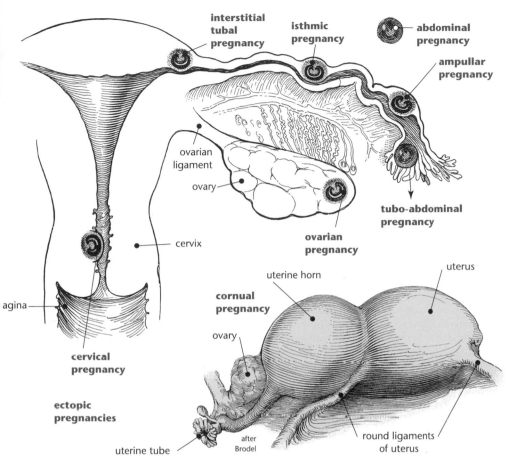

interstitial tubal pregnancy

isthmic pregnancy

abdominal pregnancy

ampullar pregnancy

ovarian ligament

ovary

tubo-abdominal pregnancy

cervix

ovarian pregnancy

uterus

uterine horn

cornual pregnancy

ovary

agina

cervical pregnancy

ectopic pregnancies

uterine tube

after Brodel

round ligaments of uterus

weeks of gestation from the first day of the last menstrual period. Also called postterm pregnancy.

spurious p. See pseudocyesis.

tubal p. Ectopic pregnancy occurring within a fallopian (uterine) tube, termed ampullary, isthmic, or interstitial, depending on the site of implantation. Also called fallopian pregnancy salpingocyesis.

tubo-abdominal p. An uncommon type of ectopic pregnancy in which the fertilized ovum implants in the fimbriated, lateral end of the uterine tube and then gradually extends out of the tube and into the peritoneal cavity.

tubo-ovarian p. Ectopic pregnancy in which the amniotic sac is adhered to both the fimbriated, lateral end of the uterine tube and its neighboring ovary.

tubo-uterine p. An uncommon type of ectopic pregnancy in which implantation of the fertilized ovum occurs in the interstitial portion of the uterine tube (i.e., the portion located within the uterine wall).

pregnane (preg'nān) A saturated steroid hydrocarbon, precursor of the female hormone progesterone and of several hormones of the adrenal cortex.

pregnanediol (preg-nān-di'ol) The chief metabolic end product of the female hormone progesterone; its concentration in the urine is an indicator of the status of the corpus luteum function.

pregnanetriol (preg-nān-tri'ol) A precursor in the biosynthesis of the hormone hydrocortisone.

pregnant (preg'nant) The state of having a developing offspring within the body. Also called gravid.

pregnene (preg'nēn) An unsaturated steroid derivative of pregnane.

prelacteal (pre-lak'te-al) Before establishment of full milk flow.

premalignant (pre-mă-lig'nant) See precancerous.

premature (pre-mă-chōōr') Occurring before the

expected, usual, or normal time.

prematurity (pre-mă-chōōr'ĭ-te) The state of being premature.

premedication (pre-med-ĭ-ka'shun) A drug or drugs administered prior to induction of anesthesia to allay apprehension and produce sedation, or to prevent or minimize anticipated or possible adverse reactions (e.g., a corticosteroid may be administered prior to the administration of an organic iodine contrast material when there is increased likelihood of an allergic reaction to the contrast substance).

premenarche (pre-mě-nar'ke) The period before menstruation is established (i.e., before the menarche).

premenopause (pre-men'o-pawz) The transitional period of marked menstrual irregularity occurring prior to the permanent cessation of ovarian function and menstruation; it represents the irregular maturation of ovarian follicles, with or without ovulation.

premenstrual (pre-men'stroo-al) Relating to the time of month prior to the onset of the menstrual flow.

prenatal (pre-na'tal) Before birth. Also called antenatal.

preoperative (pre-op'er-ă-tiv) Relating to the period before a surgical operation.

preparation (prep-ă-ra'shun) **1.** Readiness. **2.** Something that has been made ready for use (e.g., a pharmaceutical agent).

    spermicidal p. Any of various vaginal creams, gels, suppositories, and foams that kill sperm; it also acts as a mechanical barrier to the entry of sperm into the cervical canal.

prepuce (pre'pūs) A fold of thin skin overlapping the glans clitoridis (or the glans penis); it is the tissue removed at a circumcision. Also called foreskin.

presentation (pre-zen-ta'shun) The position of the fetus in the uterus in relation to the birth canal at the time of labor. Also called fetal presentation. See also fetal attitude, under attitude; lie; position.

    breech p. Presentation of the fetal pelvis, named according to three basic forms: *frank breech p.*, when the legs of the fetus are fully extended over the anterior surface of its body; *complete breech p.*, when both thighs are flexed on the abdomen and both legs are flexed at the knee; *footling breech p.*, when one leg (single footling breech) or both legs (double footling breech) are extended below the level of the fetal buttocks.

    bregma p. A transient cephalic presentation in which the large fontanel (at the top of the head) is the presenting part and the head is partly extended. Also called sinciput presentation; military attitude.

    brow p. A transient cephalic presentation in which the brow is the presenting part and the head is partly flexed.

    cephalic p. Presentation in which the fetal head is the presenting part; may be called bregma, brow, face, or vertex presentation, depending on the region of the head that is the presenting part. Also called head presentation.

    complete breech p. See under breech presentation.

    compound p. Presentation in which there is a prolapse of an extremity alongside the presenting part into the birth canal.

    p. of the cord See funic presentation.

    face p. A cephalic presentation in which the whole face is foremost in the birth canal; the head is sharply extended at the neck and the occipital region of the head is in contact with the back.

    fetal p. See presentation.

    footling breech p. See under breech presentation.

    frank breech p. See under breech presentation.

    funic p. Presentation in which the umbilical cord has prolapsed below the level of the presenting part before rupture of the membranes occurs; loops of the cord are palpated through the membranes on pelvic examination. The condition is associated with high fetal mortality and maternal complications. Also called presentation of the cord. See also prolapse of umbilical cord, under prolapse.

    head p. See cephalic presentation.

    occiput p. See vertex presentation.

    placental p. See placenta previa, under placenta.

    shoulder p. Presentation occurring when the fetus is in transverse lie (i.e., the long axis of the fetus is at right angle to the maternal long axis); hence, one shoulder is the presenting part.

    sinciput p. See bregma presentation.

    transverse p. See transverse lie, under lie.

    vertex p. A cephalic presentation in which the occipital region of the head (the vertex) is the presenting part; the head is sharply flexed, with the chin in contact with the chest. Also called occiput presentation.

pressoreceptor (pres-o-re-sep'tor) See baroreceptor.

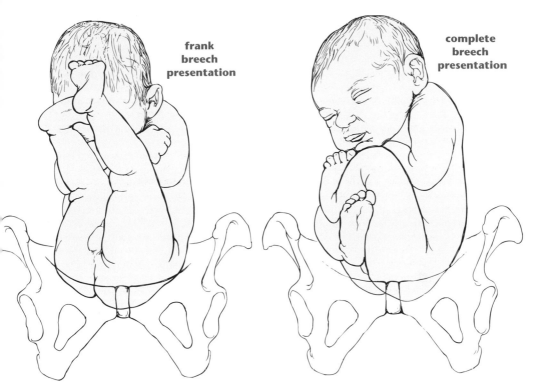

frank breech presentation

complete breech presentation

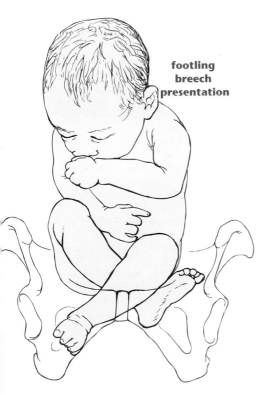

footling breech presentation

pressure (presh′ur) A force exerted against resistance.

> **alveolar p.** The pressure within the terminal air sacs (alveoli) of the lungs.
>
> **amniotic p.** The pressure within the membranes enveloping the fetus (amniotic sac) secondary to a uterine contraction.
>
> **arterial p.** Blood pressure within the systemic arteries.
>
> **blood p.** (BP) Pressure exerted by circulating blood on the arterial walls; maintained by the contraction of the left ventricle, the resistance of the small arteries (arterioles) and capillaries, the elasticity of the arterial walls, and the volume and viscosity of the blood; it is expressed in relation to the ambient atmospheric pressure.
>
> **central venous p.** (CVP) Pressure of blood in the superior or inferior vena cava.
>
> **continuous positive airway p.** (CPAP) Technique used in respiratory therapy in which pressure within the lung airways is mechanically maintained above ambient pressure throughout the respiratory cycle, preventing collapse of the airway.
>
> **diastolic p.** The force exerted on the blood vessels when the heart relaxes; specifically the lowest pressure during any given ventricular

cycle.

expiratory p. The pressure of gas in a patient's airway during exhalation (e.g., when receiving artificial ventilation).

maximum safety p. In anesthesiology, the upper limit of positive pressure permitted in an anesthesia-breathing apparatus or other related devices; exceeding the limit is considered hazardous to the patient.

mean arterial p. (MAP) The average arterial pressure throughout a complete cardiac cycle. It is calculated (in mmHg) by dividing by three the sum of the systolic pressure and twice the diastolic pressure.

minimum safety p. In anesthesiology, the lower limit of positive pressure permitted in an anesthesia-breathing apparatus or other related devices; pressure below the limit is considered ineffective.

negative p. Pressure that is less than that of the ambient atmosphere.

negative end-expiratory p. (NEEP) The negative pressure in the lung airways at the end of expiration, as in artificial ventilation.

oncotic p. Osmotic pressure exerted by colloids in solution.

osmotic p. The pressure that must be exerted to overcome the pressure that substances in solution exert against a barrier (e.g., a semipermeable membrane) to pull solvent into the solution through the barrier.

positive end-expiratory p. (PEEP) Technique used in respiratory therapy in which the amount of gases remaining in the lung airways at the end of exhalation is mechanically maintained above ambient pressure.

pulmonary capillary wedge p. (PCWP) Pressure obtained by wedging the tip of a catheter in a small pulmonary artery; blocking the blood flow provides an indirect measurement of the pressure within the left atrium of the heart.

pulse p. The difference between the systolic (maximal) and diastolic (minimal) blood pressures.

systolic p. The pressure exerted on the blood vessels when the heart contracts; specifically, the highest pressure reached during any given ventricular cycle.

transmural p. The pressure within a hollow organ relative to the pressure outside its walls.

zero end-expiratory p. (ZEEP) Airway pressure that equals ambient pressure at the end of expiration.

presystolic (pre-sis-tol'ik) Relating to the interval before a systole.

prevesical (pre-ves'ĭ-kal) In front of the bladder.

primigravida (pri-mĭ-grav'ĭ-dă) A woman who has been pregnant only once. Also called gravida I.

primipara (pri-mip'ă-ră) A woman who has completed one pregnancy to the stage of fetal viability, regardless of whether it was a single or multiple birth, or whether the fetus was live or stillborn. Also called para I.

primiparous (pri-mip'ă-rus) Denoting a primipara.

primitive (prim'ĭ-tiv) Embryonic; primary.

primordium (pri-mor'de-um) A group of cells in an early embryo indicating the first trace of a developing organ or structure of the body; usually denoting a theoretical stage later than anlage.

pro- Prefix meaning before; precursor of.

probe (prōb) **1.** A slender flexible rod with a blunt tip for exploring a body cavity or channel, or a wound. **2.** In genetics, a reagent capable of recognizing the clone of concern in a complex mixture of many DNA or RNA sequences. **3.** To explore.

procarbazine hydrochloride (pro-kar'bă-zēn hi-dro-klo'rīd) An anticancer drug. Intrauterine exposure may cause fetal malformations and low birth weight.

procedure (pro-se'jur) A series of steps undertaken to accomplish something; may be for diagnostic, therapeutic, or surgical purposes.

Irving's p. See Irving's operation, under operation.

loop electrosurgical excision p. (LEEP) A method of removing tissue for biopsy (e.g., from the uterine cervix) using an electrosurgical unit that supplies low levels of electrical current for cutting with a thin (0.2 mm) stainless steel wire.

Lord's p. Procedure for the management of hemorrhoids by relieving spasm of the anal sphincter; the sphincter is gently dilated with a finger after injecting an anesthetic into it and the perianal area; the relaxed sphincter allows the hemorrhoids to recede.

Madlener's p. See Madlener's operation, under operation.

McDonald's p. See McDonald's cerclage, under cerclage.

McIndoe's p. Surgical procedure for the construction of an artificial functioning vagina; a channel is created by dissecting the tissues between the urethra and bladder anteriorly and the perineal body and rectum posteriorly; the channel is then covered with a split-thickness skin graft.

Pomeroy's p. See Pomeroy's operation,

under operation.

sling p. Surgical procedure employed in the management of stress urinary incontinence; a strip of fascia or synthetic material is passed under the urethra, at the level of the urethrovesical junction, for support and partial obstruction of the urethra.

swim-up p. In *in vitro* fertilization (IVF), a method of preparing semen specimens that contain high quality spermatozoa; the specimen is centrifuged several times to concentrate the spermatozoa in pellets of solid material at the bottom of the centrifuge tubes; a fluid is poured on top, followed by incubation at body temperature for 30 to 60 minutes. The most motile spermatozoa swim out of the solid mass into the fluid, leaving the less active ones at the bottom of the tube.

Uchida p. Procedure for sterilization; saline–epinephrine solution is injected under the mucosa of the uterine tube, at its midportion, to separate the mucosa from the tube muscle; the mucosa is then cut open; a segment of the denuded tube is pulled out, ligated, and excised under traction; the proximal end retracts when released. Also called Uchida method.

process (pros'es) **1.** In anatomy, a marked prominence; a projection; an extension from a part. **2.** A series of actions that achieve a specific result.

acromial p. See acromion.

articular p. of sacrum One of two rounded processes projecting upwardly from the base of the sacrum; it bears a hyaline-coated, concave surface for articulation with the inferior articular facet of the fifth lumbar vertebra.

articular p. of vertebra One of the small projections on the upper and lower surfaces of a vertebra, on either side. *Inferior articular p. of vertebra*, one of a pair of downward projections from the lamina of a vertebra, bearing a hyaline-coated facet for articulation with the vertebra below. *Superior articular p. of vertebra*, one of a pair of upward projections from the junction of the pedicle and lamina, bearing a hyaline-coated facet for articulation with the vertebra above.

coracoid p. A thick, strong, curved bony process arising from the superior border of the shoulder blade (scapula), partly overhanging the glenoid fossa; it provides attachment for the short head of the biceps muscle, and the coracobrachial and pectoralis minor muscles; it also provides attachment for the conoid and

coracoacromial ligaments. The process can be felt below the lateral third of the collarbone (clavicle).

mamillary p. of vertebra A small, rough elevation on the superior articular process of a lumbar vertebra for muscle attachment.

odontoid p. of axis A toothlike process of the second cervical vertebra that protrudes sharply upward from the vertebral body to articulate with the first cervical vertebra. Also called dens.

spinous p. of vertebra The elongated process that projects backward from the junction of the laminae of the vertebral arch; it provides attachment for ligaments and muscles of the back and neck. See also vertebral spine, under spine.

vaginal p. of peritoneum See processus vaginalis peritonei.

processus (pro-ses'us) Latin for process.

p. vaginalis peritonei In embryology, a sacculation of the lower anterior peritoneum protruding into the inguinal canal; normally, it obliterates completely before birth or shortly thereafter; in the female, it accompanies the round ligament; in the male, it precedes the descent of the testis into the scrotum and eventually separates from the abdominal cavity, forming the tunica vaginalis. Also called vaginal process of peritoneum.

persistent p. vaginalis peritonei A congenital defect in which the vaginalis peritonei fails to obliterate at birth, sometimes giving rise to an oblique inguinal hernia. Also called canal of Nuck, Nuck's diverticulum.

procidentia (pro-sĭ-den'she-ă) Complete prolapse of an organ.

proctatresia (prok-tă-tre'ze-ă) See imperforate anus, under anus.

proctitis (prok-ti'tis) Inflammation of the mucous membrane of the rectum, usually caused by rectal gonorrhea, chlamydia infection, candidiasis, or syphilis. Symptoms include passage of blood, mucus, or pus with the stools, painful ineffectual straining to defecate (tenesmus), and pain in the anus and rectum.

radiation p. Proctitis resulting from radiation therapy of the genital organs and causing mucosal changes usually localized to the anterior wall of the rectum, near the site of maximal dosage; changes range from thickening to atrophy and ulceration of the mucosa; principal symptoms include diarrhea and abdominal cramps, which may begin months or even years after the radiation treatment.

procto-, proct- Combining forms meaning anus; rectum.

proctocele (prok'to-sēl) See rectocele.

proctocolpoplasty (prok-to-kol'po-plas-te) Surgical closure of an abnormal channel (fistula) between the rectum and vagina.

proctodeum (prok-to-de'um) An ectodermal depression of the embryo at the point where the anal orifice will eventually develop. Also called anal pit.

proctoperineoplasty (prok-to-per-ĭ-ne'o-plas-te) Plastic surgery of the anus and surrounding tissues (perineum). Also called rectoperineorrhaphy.

proctosigmoidoscopy (prok-to-sig-moi-dos'ko-pe) Examination of the sigmoid colon, rectum, and anal canal with a sigmoidoscope; if a flexible instrument is used, the descending colon may also be examined; usually indicated when there have been changes in bowel habits, lower abdominal and perineal pain, prolapse of the rectum on defecation, itchiness (pruritis), or the passage of blood, mucus, or pus in the stool; also performed routinely as a screening technique to detect cancer.

product (prod'ukt) Any substance resulting from a natural process, or that is manufactured synthetically.

> **cleavage p.** A substance produced by the splitting of large, complex molecules into simpler ones.

> **fibrin/fibrinogen p.** Any of several small peptides formed in the breakdown of the proteins fibrin and fibrinogen. Also called fibrin-split product; split product.

> **fibrin-split p.** See fibrin/fibrinogen product.

> **split p.** See fibrin/fibrinogen product.

profile (pro'fīl) **1.** A simple outline. **2.** A summary. **3.** A collection of data (e.g., medical data) subject to tests.

> **biophysical p.** (BPP) In obstetrics, assessment of fetal well-being taking into consideration fetal body movements and their relationship to fetal heart rate (FHR), position of arms and legs (normally flexed), and amount of fluid in the amniotic sac; data are obtained with ultrasound scanning and external monitoring.

> **urethral pressure p.** A record of the resistance exerted by the urethral muscles to fluid flow, used for detecting weakness of the urethral sphincter mechanism; a liquid or gas is infused into the bladder with a catheter; the catheter is slowly withdrawn and the pressure at several points within the urethra is recorded.

progestational (pro-jes-ta'shun-al) **1.** Conducive to conception. **2.** Having effects similar to those of progesterone; applied to certain pharmaceutical preparations.

progesterone (pro-jes'tĕ-rōn) Steroid hormone, produced in the ovary by the corpus luteum, necessary for establishment and maintenance of pregnancy; it stimulates changes in the uterine wall in preparation for implantation of the fertilized ovum. Deficiency of progesterone during the secretory phase of the menstrual cycle is implicated in some cases of infertility. See also luteal phase deficiency, under deficiency.

progestin (pro-jes'tin) General term for a synthetic or natural drug that acts on the uterine lining. Also called progestational agent.

progestogen (pro-jes'to-jen) An agent that produces biologic effects similar to those of progesterone.

progression (prŏ-gresh'un) **1.** An advancement (e.g., of a disease). **2.** The forward movement of spermatozoa.

prohormone (pro-hor'mōn) A precursor of a hormone.

prolactin (pro-lak'tin) (PRL) A hormone that stimulates milk secretion; produced in the anterior lobe of the pituitary (adenohypophysis).

prolactinoma (pro-lak-tĭ-no-mă) The most common pituitary tumor arising from chromophobe cells that secrete prolactin. Sometimes associated with nonpuerperal galactorrhea and menstrual disturbances.

prolan (pro'lan) Obsolete term. See human chorionic gonadotropin (hCG), under gonadotropin.

prolapse (pro-laps') The downward displacement of a body part or organ.

> **cord p.** See prolapse of umbilical cord.

> **mitral valve p.** Posterior displacement of the posterior (occasionally the anterior) leaflet of the mitral valve, occurring in mid- or late systole, and often producing a click that may be followed by a late systolic murmur; may cause back flow (regurgitation) of blood through the valve; found with increased incidence in Marfan's syndrome and atrial septal defect; it is associated with an increased frequency of arrhythmias.

> **occult cord p.** See under prolapse of umbilical cord.

> **overt cord p.** See under prolapse of umbilical cord.

> **p. of rectum** Protrusion of the inner lining of the rectum through the anus; may involve (rarely) the full thickness of the rectum.

p. of umbilical cord Descent of the umbilical cord toward the cervix during childbirth; it may lie next to the presenting part (occult cord prolapse) or below the presenting part (overt cord prolapse). See also funic presentation, under presentation.

p. of uterus Descent of the uterus into the vagina due to stretching and laxity of its supporting structures. Also called descensus uteri; metroptosis; and (popularly) falling of the womb.

vaginal vault p. A herniation of the upper vagina occurring subsequent to a hysterectomy, at the site of the incision.

promontory (prom'on-tor-e) A projecting part.

pelvic p. See promontory of sacrum.

p. of sacrum The most prominent anterior border of the sacrum, facing the pelvic cavity, at its junction with the fifth lumbar vertebra. Also called pelvic promontory.

promoter (pro-mo'ter) **1.** In neoplasia, a chemical substance that has no cancer-causing activity but is capable of enhancing development of a cancerous tumor in a tissue previously exposed to a carcinogen. **2.** In genetics, the area on DNA in which RNA polymerase binds and initiates synthesis of messenger RNA (mRNA), thereby the transcription of genetic code information.

promotion (pro-mo'shun) In chemical carcinogenesis, the stage in the process of cancerous tumor development in which one or more chemicals known as promoters (e.g., drugs, hormones, phorbol compounds) act upon previously initiated cells (i.e., cells that have been exposed to, and permanently changed by

another chemical); the promoters by themselves cannot cause tumor formation and their effect is reversible. See also initiation.

pronephros (pro-nef'ros) In embryology, the earliest kidney tissue, consisting of a series of rudimentary tubules.

pronucleus (pro-noo'kle-us) One of two nuclei (haploid nuclei) undergoing fusion, as of an egg and sperm at the time of fertilization.

pro-opiomelanocortin (pro-o'pe-o-mel-ă-no-kor'tin) (POMC) A large peptide molecule synthesized by the action of a single messenger RNA (mRNA) at a variety of sites in the body; it is the precursor of adrenocorticotropic hormone (ACTH), melanocyte-stimulating hormone (MSH), lipoprotein, and endorphin.

prophase (pro'fāz) The first stage of cell division (mitosis or meiosis) in which the chromosomes become visible, the nucleus begins to lose its identity, and the centrioles migrate to opposite poles of the cell.

prophylactic (pro-fĭ-lak'tik) **1.** Tending to prevent disease; applied to procedures, drugs, or equipment. **2.** Popular name for a condom.

prophylaxis (pro-fĭ-lak'sis) Measures taken to prevent disease.

propylthiouracil (pro-pil-thi-o-u'ră-sil) (PTU) A drug that inhibits production of thyroid hormones; used in the treatment of hyperthyroidism. Intrauterine exposure may cause hypothyroidism and goiter in the infant.

prorenin (pro-re'nin) The inactive precursor of the enzyme renin.

prostacyclin (pros-tă-si'klin) A prostaglandin produced by endothelial cells of the

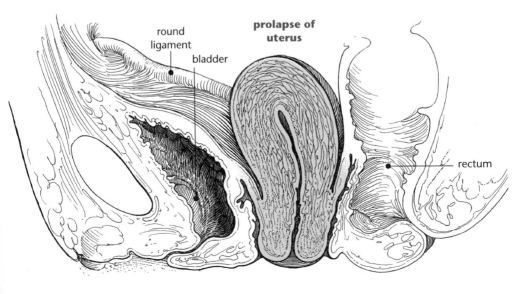

round ligament
bladder
prolapse of uterus
rectum

cardiovascular system; it inhibits platelet aggregation and helps maintain the integrity of the endothelial cells. Also called prostaglandin I_2 (PGI$_2$).

prostaglandin (pros-tă-glan'din) (PG) Any of a group of hormone-like, lipid-soluble compounds derived from long-chain polyunsaturated fatty acids and occurring in nearly all body tissues and fluids (including amniotic fluid); prostaglandins have a multitude of physiologic actions (e.g., stimulation of smooth muscle contraction, dilatation of peripheral blood vessels, suppression of stomach secretion, increase of blood flow in kidney, dilatation of bronchial tubes); their production is inhibited by nonsteroidal anti-inflammatory drugs (e.g., aspirin). Concentration of vasodilating prostaglandins is elevated during normal pregnancy.

 p. E$_2$ (PGE$_2$) An agent that stimulates contraction of the myometrium, marketed as a vaginal suppository indicated for the termination of pregnancy between 12 and 20 weeks of gestation. Formulations include an endocervical or vaginal gel used for ripening the cervix when labor is to be induced.

 p. F$_2$α (PGF$_2$α) A synthetic preparation that stimulates contraction of smooth muscle (e.g., of the uterus and bronchi); used to induce abortion, usually as an instillation into the amniotic fluid; it also has vasoconstrictive properties and has been used to control postpartum hemorrhage due to uterine atony.

 p. I$_2$ (PGI$_2$) See prostacyclin.

prosthesis (pros-the'sis), pl. prostheses An artificial replacement for a missing or dysfunctional body part, fabricated and fitted to meet the individual requirement of the intended user.

 penile p. A device surgically implanted within the penis to permit adequate rigidity for coitus in the treatment of erectile dysfunction; currently available models include a semirigid rod, and a two-cylinder inflatable device. Also called penile implant.

prosthion (pros'the-on) (PR) A craniometric point at the midpoint of the alveolar rim of the maxilla; it is the most anterior projection, between the two central incisors.

protein (pro'tēn) Any of a group of complex nitrogenous substances that contain amino acids as their fundamental structural units, are present in cells of all plants and animals, and function in all aspects of chemical and physical activity of the cells.

 androgen-binding p. (ABP) A protein formed in the Sertoli cells of mature males; it binds the hormones testosterone and dihydrotestosterone in the lumen of the seminiferous tubules of the testes, concentrating them in the tubule epithelium for sperm formation and in the epididymis for sperm maturation.

 p. C A protein constituent of blood plasma that prevents coagulation of blood. Deficiency of protein C causes recurrent thrombophlebitis.

 p. G Any of several proteins that act as mediators between activated cell receptors and their enzymes; the resulting chain of events alters the concentration of intracellular messengers (e.g., cyclic adenosine monophosphate [cyclic AMP]), which in turn alter the behavior of other target proteins within the cell.

 glucose transport (GLUT) p. A member of a transmembrane segment transporter superfamily.

 heat shock p. Any protein that is synthesized within cells in response to abnormally high body temperature and other environmental stresses.

 parathyroid hormone-related p. (PTH-rP) A protein expressed in myometrium during the latent phase of parturition; believed to play a role in that phase of the parturition process.

 pregnancy p.'s Proteins usually produced by the body of a pregnant woman or by the placenta; may be present only during pregnancy (pregnancy specific) or may be found also in persons undergoing estrogen therapy or taking oral contraceptive, or in those with certain malignancies.

 proto-oncogene p. A product of an oncogene that normally has no cancer-causing or transforming properties, but is involved in the regulation or differentiation of cell growth. See also oncogene.

 zinc finger p. An important part of the conformation pattern of DNA binding domains in which multiple amino acid repeat units are each held in a finger-like shape by a zinc ion.

proteinuria (pro-te-nu're-ă) Excretion of protein in the urine in amounts greater than the normal daily levels; an average-size healthy person normally excretes up to 150 mg of protein per day.

 gestational p. Proteinuria occurring during pregnancy in the absence of disease.

proteo-, prot- Combining forms meaning protein.

proto-, prot- Combining forms meaning earliest; primitive.

protocol (pro'to-kol) A detailed description or plan of action.

    Bagshawe p. A multidrug regimen for the treatment of gestational trophoblastic disease.

    clinical p. A detailed plan for the study of a medical problem and/or performance of a treatment.

    rape p. The organized, structured steps followed during a medical examination of a rape victim for the dual purpose of obtaining evidence for a criminal investigation and treating the patient. It includes a detailed history of the assault; a gynecological history of the victim to assess risks of impregnation and transmission of disease; a history of the victim's activities in the interval between the assault and the examination (e.g., eating, drinking, bathing, douching, urinating, defecating) which may affect findings of the examination; an inspection of the whole body, especially the perineum and vulva, to document location and extent of external injuries, photographing the injuries or noting them in a diagram; a vaginal and cervical examination with a speculum; collection of specimens from both outside and within the body for laboratory examination; and a detailed description of the findings.

proto-oncogene (pro-to ong'ko-jēn) A normal DNA component of vertebrate cells thought to be a homolog of viral oncogenes, important in normal cellular differentiation.

protuberance (pro-too'ber-ans) A prominence or bulge, usually rounded or blunt.

    p. of chin See mental protuberance.

    external occipital p. A prominence on the back of the skull, at the middle of the outer surface of the occipital bone, midway between the foramen magnum and the summit of the bone; it is the attachment site for the nuchal ligament.

    internal occipital p. A prominence at the midpoint of the inner surface of the occipital bone next to the confluence of the sinuses.

    mental p. The anterior prominence of the chin at the midline of the lower border of the mandible. Also called protuberance of chin.

    parietal p. See parietal eminence, under eminence.

Providencia (pro-vĭ-den'se-ă) Genus of Gram-negative bacteria that have been found in human feces and urine. Some species are associated with diarrhea and urinary tract infections.

provirus (pro-vi'rus) The DNA sequences of a virus that are integrated into the DNA of the host cell and transmitted from one cell generation to the next without destroying the host cell. Proviruses are often associated with cell transformation into cancerous cells and are a key feature of retrovirus biology.

proximal (prok sĭ-mal) Nearest the midline or point of origin; opposite of distal.

proximate (prok'sĭ-māt) Nearest; in immediate relation to something else. In medical malpractice, the term is applied to the negligent act that caused the injury of concern.

pruritic (proo-rit'ik) Relating to pruritus.

pruritic urticarial papules and plaques of pregnancy (PUPPP) A self-limited cutaneous eruption developed sometimes in pregnant women; consists of intensely itchy red patches, appearing first on the skin around the navel and spreading throughout the abdomen, thighs, and limbs; occurs almost exclusively in first pregnancies, usually during the third trimester, and disappears within 2 weeks after delivery.

pruritus (proo-ri'tus) Persistent and severe itching of clinically normal skin; may be due to a systemic disease (e.g., chronic kidney failure, thyroid dysfunction, Hodgkin's disease, drug abuse).

    p. gravidarum Generalized pruritus occurring during pregnancy, usually the third trimester; thought to be a sign of reduced liver function resulting from impedance of bile flow within the liver.

    p. vulvae Intense itching of the vulvar skin and mucous membranes.

pseudo- Combining form meaning false.

pseudocyesis (soo-do-si-e'sis) Development of pregnancy symptoms in a nonpregnant woman (e.g., menstrual abnormalities, abdominal enlargement, and breast changes). Also called false pregnancy; phantom pregnancy; spurious pregnancy.

pseudofolliculitis (soo-do-fo-lik-u-li'tis) Condition characterized by papules and pustules surrounding ingrown hairs, typically affecting shaved areas of the skin; may occur in women who shave their pubic hair to conform to a bikini swimsuit.

pseudohermaphrodite (soo-do-her-maf'ro-dīt) An individual possessing the characteristics of pseudohermaphroditism. See also hermaphrodite.

    female p. An individual who has ovaries and the genetic make-up of a female but whose external genitalia are morphologically those of a male.

    male p. An individual who has testes and

the genetic make-up of a male but whose external genitalia are morphologically those of a female.

pseudohermaphroditism (soo-do-her-maf'ro-dit-izm) Condition in which the individual has internal sex organs that are distinctly of one sex but has superficial sex characteristics that are either ambiguous or of the opposite sex. Erroneously called hermaphroditism.

pseudomenopause (soo-do-men'o-pawz) Temporary arrest of the menses, artificially induced by reducing the production of endogenous estrogen and progesterone to low levels; used in the medical treatment of endometriosis.

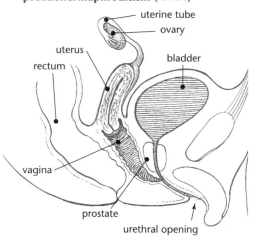

pseudohermaphroditism (female)

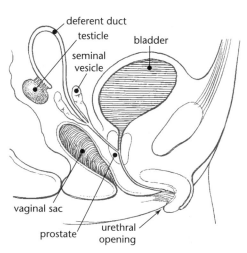

pseudohermaphroditism (male)

Pseudomonas (soo-do-mo'nas) A genus of widely distributed Gram-negative motile bacteria; some species cause disease in humans.

P. aeruginosa A species found in human feces and skin; it is a frequent cause of infections of the lungs and urinary tract.

pseudomyxoma (soo-do-mik-so'ma) A gelatinous, epithelial tumor resembling a myxoma.

p. peritonei Extensive accumulation of tenacious, semisolid mucin in the abdominal cavity; secreted by multiple peritoneal implants originating from a mucin-secreting, cancerous tumor (cystadenocarcinoma) of the ovary or appendix.

pseudoneoplasm (soo-do-ne'o-plazm) See pseudotumor.

pseudopolyp (soo-do-pol'ip) A mass composed of inflammatory tissue and protruding from a mucous membrane; it has no malignant potential. Also called inflammatory polyp.

pseudopregnancy (soo-do-preg'nan-se) **1.** A hormonal treatment for endometriosis using oral contraceptives on a daily basis in an effort to create high levels of progestins as seen in pregnancy and thus effect involution of endometrial implants. **2.** See pseudocyesis.

pseudopuberty (soo-do-pu'ber-te) Development of secondary sexual characteristics without gametogenesis (i.e., without ovulation in girls and spermatogenesis in boys).

precocious p. Pseudopuberty occurring at an abnormally early age, before 8 years in girls and 10 years in boys.

pseudotumor (soo-do-too'mor) The appearance of symptoms and signs that indicate the presence of a tumor in the absence of one, followed by spontaneous recovery. Also called pseudoneoplasm.

p. cerebri A frequently self-limited condition characterized by increased intracranial pressure thought to be caused by overproduction or underabsorption of cerebrospinal fluid; symptoms and signs include headache, stiff neck, swelling of the optic nerve head (papilledema), and blurred vision; most commonly seen in overweight young women; in pregnancy, it is usually detected at midpregnancy, resolving after childbirth. Also called benign intracranial hypertension.

psoriasis (so-ri'ă-sis) A chronic, recurrent skin disorder marked by well-defined reddish plaques covered with silvery scales, occurring mostly on the knees, elbows, trunk, and sometimes scalp. May be associated with nail changes (onycholysis) and sometimes with severe arthritis.

pustular p. A rare variety of psoriasis characterized by a generalized rash of sterile pustules on reddish, inflamed skin, accompanied by high fever, malaise, pain in the joints, elevated white blood cell count, and other systemic symptoms; when occurring during pregnancy, it is thought to be an acute exacerbation of an existing mild psoriasis precipitated by the pregnant state. Also called von Zumbush's psoriasis.

von Zumbush's p. See pustular psoriasis.

psycho-, psych- Combining forms meaning the mind.

psychoprophylaxis (si-ko-pro-fĭ-lak'sis) See Lamaze method, under method.

psychosexual (si-ko-seks'u-al) Relating to the emotional factors of sex.

psychosis (si-ko'sis), pl. psychoses A severe mental disorder in which the ability to think, communicate, respond emotionally, and interpret reality is impaired to such a degree that all aspects of a person's life are affected, rendering that individual unable to meet the ordinary demands of life; frequently, the person also has regressive behavior, hallucinations, and delusions; caused by organic and/or emotional factors.

postpartum p. Any psychosis occurring 4 to 6 weeks after delivery, frequently requiring hospitalization; considered by some to be a manifestation of a latent or underlying psychotic condition.

Pthirus pubis (thir'us pu'bis) A parasite infecting the pubic hair and causing intense itching; transmitted by sexual contact or by contact with infested bedding or towels. Commonly called crab louse; pubic louse.

pubarche (pu-bar'ke) The growth of pubic hair at the beginning of puberty.

pubertal, puberal (pu'ber-tal, pu'ber-al) Relating to puberty.

pubertas (pu-ber'tas) Latin for puberty.

p. praecox See precocious puberty, under puberty.

puberty (pu'ber-te) The span of time during which, under the influence of hormonal activity, sexual maturation occurs; generally the period extends between the ages of 8 and 16 years in girls, and between 10 and 17 years in boys; age of onset varies with genetic, health, and socioeconomic factors; in the female, it begins with development of breast buds (thelarche) and culminates with establishment of cyclic menstruation (menarche) and reproductive function.

complete isosexual precocious p. See constitutional precocious puberty.

constitutional precocious p. Precocious puberty occurring in an otherwise normal child; characterized by an abnormally early sexual maturation but developing in a normal sequence; in the female, it includes increased secretion of hormones with cyclic menstruation, accompanied by ovulation and sexual reproduction capability; the cause is unknown. Also called complete isosexual precocious puberty; idiopathic precocious puberty; true precocious puberty. Compare with precocious pseudopuberty, under pseudopuberty.

delayed p. Puberty that has failed to occur by the usual age (i.e., 16 years in girls, 17 years in boys).

heterosexual precocious p. Abnormal condition in which sexual maturation occurs prematurely and does not correspond to the genetic sex of the child (i.e., virilization in girls, feminization in boys). Compare with isosexual precocious puberty.

idiopathic precocious p. See constitutional precocious puberty.

incomplete isosexual precocious p. Abnormally early development of a single secondary sex characteristic, usually breasts in girls or pubic and axillary hair.

isosexual precocious p. Sexual maturation that occurs prematurely but corresponds to the normal genetic sex of the child (i.e., feminization in girls, virilization in boys). Compare with heterosexual precocious puberty.

precocious p. Sexual maturation occurring at an abnormally early age, usually before the age of 8 years in girls and 9 years in boys; may be caused by a variety of disease processes, including brain lesions and disorders involving the adrenal (suprarenal) glands, testes, and ovaries. Also called pubertas praecox. See also constitutional precocious puberty.

true precocious p. See constitutional precocious puberty.

pubescence (pu-bes'ens) The beginning of sexual maturity.

pubescent (pu-bes'ent) One who is reaching the age of sexual maturity.

pubic (pu'bik) Relating to the pubic bone or area.

pubis (pu'bis) **1.** See pubic bone, under bone. **2.** The region over the pubic bone. **3.** The hair of the pubic region.

pubomadesis (pu-bo-mă-de'sis) Loss or absence of pubic hair.

pubovesical (pu-bo-ves'ĭ-kal) Relating to the

pubic bone and the bladder.

pubovesicocervical (pu-bo-ves-ĭ-ko-ser'vĭ-kal)
Relating to the pubic bone, bladder, and uterine
cervix. See also pubovesicocervical fascia, under
fascia.

pudendal (pu-den'dal) Relating to the genitals.

pudendum (pu-den'dum), pl. pudenda The
external genitals, especially the female genitals;
the vulva.

puerpera (pu-er'per-ă) A woman who has just
given birth.

puerperal (pu-er'per-al) Relating to the
puerperium.

puerperalism (pu-er'per-al-izm) Any disease
associated with the puerperium.

puerperium (pu-er-pe're-um) The postpartum
period, from the end of labor to the return of the
uterus to normal size, usually from 3 to 6 weeks.

pump (pump) An apparatus for drawing a liquid or
gas to or from any part.

    breast p. A suction pump (manual or
electric) for removing milk from a lactating
breast.

    insulin p. A battery-powered pump
equipped with a syringe and needle, designed
for the continuous subcutaneous infusion of
insulin in specifically programmed doses; used
in the management of diabetes mellitus.

    terbutaline p. A portable pump designed
for the long-term subcutaneous administration
of low doses of the beta-adrenergic agonist
terbutaline; used for the tocolysis (i.e.,
inhibition of uterine contractions) of preterm
labor. Its purpose is to reduce the incidence of
tachyphylaxis by using a lower dose of
terbutaline to achieve tocolytic effectiveness.

punctate (pungk'tāt) Having multiple tiny dots.

punctation (pungk-ta'shun) **1.** A minute spot. **2.**
The condition of being punctate.

puncture (pungk'chur) **1.** To pierce with a pointed
instrument. **2.** A minute hole made with a
needle.

    lumbar p. Procedure in which a hollow
needle is inserted into the subarachnoid space
of the lower spinal canal (between two lumbar
vertebrae) to withdraw cerebrospinal fluid for
diagnostic purposes, or to inject an anesthetic.
Also called spinal puncture; spinal tap;
rachicentesis; rachiocentesis.

    spinal p. See lumbar puncture.

purpura (pur'pu-ră) The occurrence of
spontaneous bleeding into the skin, resulting in
multiple pigmented patches of varying sizes; may
also occur in mucous membranes and the serous
lining of the intestines.

    p. fulminans A neonatal condition

secondary to severe protein C deficiency.

    idiopathic thrombocytopenic p. (ITP)
Purpura associated with immune destruction
of blood platelets. It occurs in two forms: *acute
idiopathic thrombocytopenic p.*, a self-limited
disorder seen mainly in children after a viral
infection (e.g., rubella, infectious
mononucleosis); and *chronic idiopathic
thrombocytopenic p.*, a disorder of long standing,
with multiple remissions and relapses seen in
adults, mostly women of childbearing age.
Incidence of relapses seems to increase during
pregnancy. Also called immune
thrombocytopenic purpura.

    immune thrombocytopenic p. See idiopathic
thrombocytopenic purpura.

purpuric (pur-pu'rik) Relating to purpura.

purulent (pu'roo-lent) Producing, consisting of, or
containing pus.

pus (pus) A yellowish liquid or semisolid

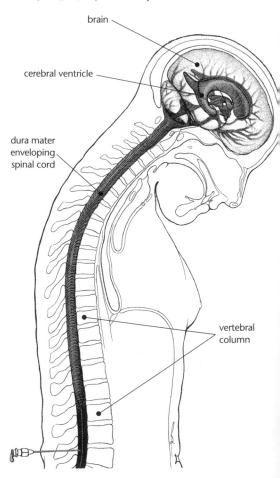

brain

cerebral ventricle

dura mater
enveloping
spinal cord

vertebral
column

lumbar puncture

substance, which is a product of inflammation and is composed of dead white blood cells (leukocytes) and other cellular debris in a thin liquid (liquor puris); it often contains the microbiologic agent responsible for the inflammation.

pustule (pus'tūl) A small localized accumulation of pus in the skin.

pyelo-, pyel- Combining forms meaning the pelvis of the kidney.

pyelocystitis (pi-ĕ-lo-sis-ti'tis) Inflammation of the bladder and kidney pelvis.

pyelogram (pi'e-lo-gram) An x-ray image of the kidney pelvis and ureter.

pyelography (pi-ĕ-log'ră-fe) The making of x-ray images of the kidney pelvis and ureter after introduction of a contrast medium into the structures.

> **antegrade p.** Pyelography in which the contrast medium is injected directly into the kidney pelvis through a percutaneous needle puncture; usually performed to detect an obstruction (e.g., by tumor, stone, or stricture), or to evaluate the result of recent surgery (e.g., transplantation of a ureter for urinary diversion).

> **intravenous p.** Pyelography in which the contrast medium is injected through a vein; usually performed to assess the structure and excretory function of the kidney (parenchyma, calices, and pelvis), and of the ureters and bladder. Normally, the contrast medium is rapidly excreted in the urine. Also called excretory urography.

> **retrograde p.** Pyelography in which the contrast medium is injected through a catheter

introduced via the bladder and ureter; usually performed to assess the structure and integrity of the collecting system of the kidney (i.e., of the ureter, pelvis, and calices). Also called ureteropyelography.

pyo- Combining form meaning pus.

pyocele (pi'o-sēl) Distention of a body cavity due to accumulation of pus.

pyocolpos (pi-o-kol'pos) Accumulation of pus in the vagina.

pyocyst (pi'o-sist) A pus-containing cyst.

pyometra (pi-o-me'tră) Accumulation of pus in the uterus.

pyometritis (pi-o-me-tri'tis) Inflammation of the wall of the uterus with accumulation of pus in the uterine cavity.

pyo-ovarium (pi'o o-va're-um) An ovarian abscess.

pyopagus (pi-op'ă-gus) Conjoined twins united at the lower back, in the area of the sacrum.

pyophysometra (pi-o-fi-so-me'tră) The presence of pus and gas in the uterine cavity.

pyosalpingitis (pi-o-sal-pin-ji'tis) Suppurative inflammation of a fallopian (uterine) tube.

pyosalpingo-oophoritis (pi-o-sal-ping'go o-of-ŏ-ri'tis) Suppurative inflammation of a fallopian (uterine) tube and the corresponding ovary.

pyosalpinx (pi o-sal'pinks) Accumulation of pus in a fallopian (uterine) tube.

pyrexia (pi-rek'se-ă) Fever.

pyrimidine (pǐ-rim'ǐ-dēn) The essential substance of several organic bases, some of which are components of nucleic acid (i.e., of DNA and RNA).

pyro- Combining form meaning heat, produced by heat.

pyrosis (pi-ro'sis) See heartburn.

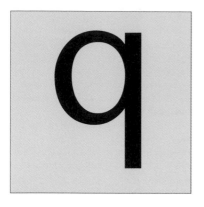

quadrant (kwod'rant) (Q) **1.** One quarter of a circle. **2.** In anatomy, one of the four areas into which certain roughly circular parts of the body are divided for descriptive purposes (e.g., the breast, abdomen, eardrum).

quadrantectomy (kwod-ran-tek'to-me) Removal of one quarter of an organ, especially a breast in the surgical treatment of a tumor.

quadri- Combining form meaning four.

quadruplet (kwod'rup-let) One of four offspring born at one birth.

quasidominance (kwa-zi-dom'ĭ-nans) Direct transmission, from generation to generation, of a recessive trait occurring in inbreeding populations; it results from the mating of a homozygous affected person with a heterozygous carrier of the same recessive gene; the pedigree pattern superficially resembles that of a dominant trait, hence the name.

quickening (kwik'en-ing) A slight abdominal sensation first felt by a pregnant woman about the fourth or fifth month of pregnancy, caused by the movement of the fetus within the uterus.

quinacrine (kwin'ă-krin) A bright yellow compound originally used to treat malaria; now used against infections with the protozoon *Giardia lamblia* (giardiasis). Possible adverse effects include nausea, vomiting, and yellow discoloration of the skin; prolonged use may cause blood disorders (e.g., aplastic anemia). First-trimester intrauterine exposure may cause fetal malformations.

quinidine (kwin'ĭ-din) An alkaloid from cinchona bark, used in the management of irregular heartbeats (cardiac arrhythmia). Intrauterine exposure may cause blood platelet reduction (thrombocytopenia) in the newborn infant.

quinine (kwi'nīn) A bitter alkaloid from cinchona bark used in the treatment of malaria. Intrauterine exposure has caused malformations of the central nervous system, heart, gastrointestinal tract, and the limbs of the infant.

quintuplet (kwin-tup'let) One of five offspring born at one birth.

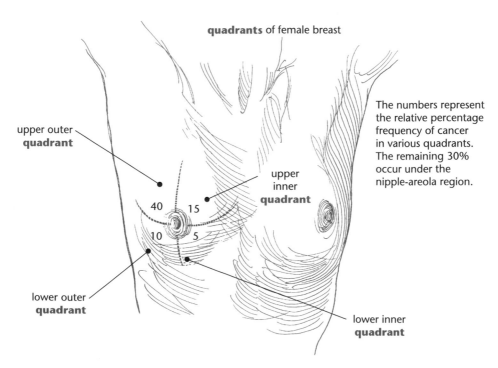

quadrants of female breast

upper outer **quadrant**

upper inner **quadrant**

lower outer **quadrant**

lower inner **quadrant**

40 15
10 5

The numbers represent the relative percentage frequency of cancer in various quadrants. The remaining 30% occur under the nipple-areola region.

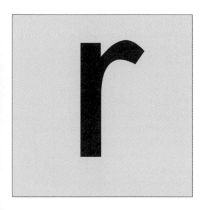

rachial (ra′ke-al) Spinal.

rachicentesis, rachiocentesis (ra-ke-sen-te′sis, ra-ke-o-sen-te′sis) See lumbar puncture, under puncture.

rachio-, rachi- Combining forms meaning spine.

rad (rad) A unit of radiation exposure representing the absorbed dose; 1 rad represents absorption of 100 ergs of energy per gram of tissue. The term is an acronym for radiation absorbed dose. In the International System of Units (SI), the unit of deposition of energy by radiation exposure is the gray (Gy); 1 gray = 100 rad = 1 joule (J) of energy.

radiant (ra′de-ant) **1.** Emitting heat or light rays. **2.** A central point from which rays diverge. **3.** Emitted as radiation.

radiation (ra-de-a′shun) **1.** The high-speed emission and projection of energy (waves or particles). **2.** A bundle of diverging white fibers interconnecting different parts of the brain.

  corpuscular r. Radiation consisting of a stream of subatomic particles that have a specific mass (e.g., protons, electrons, neutrons, and alpha or beta particles). Compare with electromagnetic radiation.

  electromagnetic r. Forms of energy that have no mass and travel in waves at the speed of light; they differ in wavelength, frequency, and photon energy (e.g., x rays, gamma rays, radio and infrared waves, visible light, and ultraviolet and cosmic radiation). Compare with corpuscular radiation.

  external r. Radiation therapy in which the radiation source (e.g., a standard orthovoltage x-ray machine) is located at a distance from the body.

  hyperfractionated r. Radiation treatment in which the total dose of radiation is divided into smaller doses and given more than once a day.

  interstitial r. Local radiation in which the radiation source is placed within the tissue under treatment, usually in the form of pellets or needles.

  intracavitary r. Local radiation in which the radiation source is placed in a body cavity.

  intraoperative r. A type of external radiation in which a large dose of radiation is applied to the tumor bed and surrounding tissues at the time of surgery.

  intraperitoneal r. Instillation of a radioactive colloid, such as radiophosphorus (^{32}P), into the peritoneal cavity.

  ionizing r. Electromagnetic radiation (e.g., x rays, gamma rays) or corpuscular radiation (e.g., protons, electrons) capable of producing electrically charged atoms (ions) in its passage through matter.

  local r. Therapeutic radiation from a source in direct proximity to the tissues under treatment. See also brachytherapy.

  postoperative r. Radiation applied after surgery to destroy cancerous cells that may remain in the area.

  preoperative r. Radiation of a cancerous growth before surgery (e.g., to shrink a large tumor to facilitate its removal).

  scattered r. Radiation that is dispersed in a random manner as a result of collision of the particles, photons, or waves with encountering matter. Also called secondary radiation.

  secondary r. See scattered radiation.

radical (rad′ĭ-kal) Descriptive term applied to a form of treatment characterized by extreme, extensive, or innovative measures. Opposite of conservative.

radiogram (ra′de-o-gram) See roentgenogram.

radiograph (ra′de-o-graf) The processed photographic film produced in radiography.

radiography (ra-de-og′ră-fe) The making of an image of an internal body part by transmitting x rays through the body onto a sensitized film. Also called roentgenography.

radioimmunoassay (ra-de-o-im-u-no-as′a) (RIA) Any of a variety of sensitive laboratory techniques using radioactive reagents for detection of antigen–antibody reactions either directly or indirectly; used to measure the concentration of an antibody or of substances against which a specific antibody can be produced.

radioisotope (ra-de-o-i′so-tōp) Any isotope of an element that is naturally radioactive or artificially made radioactive.

radionecrosis (ra-de-o-nĕ-kro′sis) Destruction of tissues by radiation.

radiopelvimetry (ra-de-o-pel-vim′ĕ-tre) An x-ray technique for determining the size and shape of the pelvis.

radiopotentiation (ra-de-o-po-ten-she-a'shun) The action of certain chemical compounds in enhancing the effect of radiation on cells.

radiopotentiator (ra-de-o-po-ten-she-a'tor) Any drug that has radiopotentiation properties.

radioreaction (ra-de-o-re-ak'shun) Any reaction to radiation, especially a skin reaction.

radioresistance (ra-de-o-re-zis'tans) The relative resistance of cells or tissues to the destructive effects of a usual dose of radiation.

radiosensitivity (ra-de-o-sen-sĭ-tiv'ĭ-te) The relative susceptibility of biologic tissues or substances to the action of radiation.

radiotherapist (ra-de-o-ther'ă-pist) A physician who specializes in radiation therapy.

radiotherapy (ra-de-o-ther'ă-pe) See radiation therapy, under therapy.

rape (rāp) An illegal, nonconsensual act of sexual penetration of any body orifice, usually carried out by force or other forms of duress, including intimidation, deceit, impairment of the victim's senses (by any means), or any other method used to overcome the physical and psychological resistance of the victim. Physical damage inflicted upon the female victim may include bruising of the vaginal walls or cervix, swelling of the labia, and tearing of the anus and the area between the anus and genitals (perineum). Psychological damage (posttraumatic stress disorder) usually has an acute phase lasting from a few days to a few weeks, characterized by fear and anger manifested in various ways, depending on the person's usual coping reactions. Symptoms range from talkativeness, crying, trembling, and shock, to apparent indifference and acquiescence or even inappropriate smiling. The long-term psychological effects of rape may include flashbacks, nightmares, depression, anxiety, and aversion to sex. The medical examination of a rape victim should follow an established rape protocol. Also called aggravated sexual assault; criminal sexual conduct; sexual assault; sexual battery. See also rape protocol, under protocol.

   anger r. Sexual assault that is not premeditated but seems to be triggered by a stressful situation (e.g., if the rapist feels he has been wronged by the victim and his anger prompts him to get revenge).

   date r. Sexual assualt occurring during a social engagement.

   power r. Premeditated sexual assault (frequently accompanied by precrime rape fantasies), usually perpetrated by an immature male intent on demonstrating power; injury to the victim usually results from the coercive nature of the act rather than from the need to injure.

   sadistic r. Premeditated sexual assault, often involving ritualistic torture of the victim, causing violent injury or even death.

   statutory r. The act of sexual penetration usually by an adult with a minor. May also include two minors if the age difference between the two is significant.

rate (rāt) Strictly, a measured quantity, or a counted value, per unit time in which there is a distinct relationship between the two (i.e., between the quantity or value and the unit of time). The term is often used less strictly in epidemiologic and demographic studies to express values or quantities that are dimensionless in time.

   basal metabolic r. (BMR) See basal metabolism, under metabolism.

   birth r. The number of births in a given population per year or any other unit of time.

   death r. See mortality rate.

   erythrocyte sediment ation r. (ESR) The rate (in millimeters per hour) of settling of red blood cells when anticoagulated blood is allowed to stand under standard conditions in a vertical glass column. Used mainly as an index of inflammation. Also called sedimentation rate.

   fertility r. The actual production of live births, expressed as the number of live births per 1000 women aged 15 through 44 years during a given period, usually 1 year.

   fetal death r. The number of stillbirths occurring in 1 year per 1000 infants born (including live births and stillbirths) in that same year. Also called stillbirth rate.

   fetal heart r. (FHR) The number of fetal heartbeats per minute, normally ranging from 120 to 160.

   growth r. The growth increase (absolute or relative) expressed in units of time.

   infant mortality r. The relation of the number of deaths in the first year of life to the total number of live births in the same population during the same period of time.

   maternal mortality r. The number of maternal deaths resulting from the reproductive process in a given geographic area in 1 year per 100,000 live births that occurred in the same area during the same year.

   morbidity r. The number of persons with a particular disease in a specified time per given unit of the total population.

   mortality r. The relation between the number of registered deaths in a specified area and the total population during a given period, usually 1 year. Also called death rate.

neonatal mortality r. The number of deaths of newborn infants under 28 days of age in a given year per 1000 live births of that same year.

perinatal mortality r. The number of deaths of newborn infants less than 7 days of age plus the number of fetal deaths after 28 weeks of gestation in a given year per 1000 live births of that same year.

prevalence r. The total number of individuals in a population who have a disease at a specified point in time divided by the total population at risk at that particular time.

pulse r. The number of beats per minute of a peripheral arterial pulse.

respiratory r., r. of respiration The rate of breathing; the number of inspirations per minute.

sedimentation r. See erythrocyte sedimentation rate.

stillbirth r. See fetal death rate.

survival r. The proportion of individuals, studied over a period of time, of those who are alive at the beginning of the study, who are alive at the end of the study (e.g., the proportion of surviving patients studied over 5 years).

ratio (ra'she-o) A proportion.

A̅/B̅ r. See systolic/diastolic ratio.

lecithin–sphingomyelin (L/S) r. The ratio of lecithin to sphingomyelin in amniotic fluid; employed in determining the maturity of the fetal lungs and predicting respiratory problems.

maternal mortality r. The number of maternal deaths resulting from the process of reproduction per 100,000 live births.

systolic/diastolic r. A quantitative assessment of velocities of umbilical artery flow; often used to assess the fetal condition. Also called A/B ratio.

ray (ra) **1.** A straight beam of electromagnetic radiation (e.g., heat, light). **2.** A linear anatomic structure.

alpha r., α r. A ray composed of a stream of high-velocity, positively charged particles (alpha particles) ejected from radioactive substances.

beta r., β r. A ray composed of negatively charged particles (beta particles), especially electrons, ejected from radioactive substances, with a velocity greater than that of the alpha particles; beta rays have a greater penetrating power than alpha rays.

gamma r., γ r. A stream of photons emitted

spontaneously by the nucleus of an atom during the radioactive decay process; analogous to the x ray but of shorter wavelength.

roentgen r. See x ray.

x r., roentgen r. An electromagnetic ray with a very short wavelength, generated at the point of impact of a stream of high-speed cathode electrons on a target of an x-ray tube.

re- Prefix meaning backward; again.

reaction (re-ak'shun) **1.** Any response to a stimulus. **2.** The observable color change in, or produced by, indicators or reagents in chemical analysis.

adverse r. An undesirable and sometimes life-threatening reaction to a therapeutic drug.

allergic r. A reaction stimulated by exposure to a substance (allergen) to which the individual has become sensitized.

decidual r. The physiologic changes occurring within the endometrium in response to progesterone stimulation; it begins after ovulation, starting the process of decidua development in preparation for implantation of the blastocyst.

Herxheimer's r. See Jarisch-Herxheimer reaction.

immune r. See immune response, under response.

Jarisch-Herxheimer r. An inflammatory condition sometimes occurring 2 to 8 hours after instituting antibiotic therapy for syphilis; characterized by chills, fever, headache, muscle pain, and mild low blood pressure; believed to be an allergic reaction to the rapid release of treponemal antigen. Also called Herxheimer's reaction.

polymerase chain r. (PCR) Technique for a rapid *in vitro* amplification of a short stretch of DNA; applications include genetic testing, detection of pathogens which are difficult to isolate, mutation analysis, DNA sequencing, diagnosis of disease, and analysis of evolutionary relationships.

zona r. A change in the zona pellucida occurring after a sperm has entered the ovum by penetrating the zona and plasma membrane of the ovum; the ovum becomes impenetrable to other sperm, thus preventing polyploidy; the reaction is stimulated by enzymes released by the acrosome of the fertilizing sperm.

receptor (re-sep'tor) **1.** A large protein molecule on the surface of a cell membrane, or sometimes in the cytoplasm or the nucleus; it selectively binds to a specific substance (e.g., a hormone or neurotransmitter), producing a biologic effect that is specific to that binding. **2.** The small structure in which a sensory nerve fiber terminates; a sensory end-organ.

estrogen r. A receptor that binds estrogens, found particularly in cells of the breast and uterus. The presence of high levels of estrogen receptors in the cytoplasm of excised tumor cells is an indicator of a likely response to hormonal therapy.

progesterone r. Hormonal receptor that has a high affinity for progesterone. High levels occurring in the cytoplasm of excised tumor cells are a sensitive indicator of a likely response to hormonal therapy.

recombinant (re-kom'bĭ-nant) Term applied to an organism, chromosome, or DNA with a new combination of genes resulting from the introduction of genetic material from an outside source.

record (rek'ord) A collection of related data.

medical r. A confidential record documenting a patient's medical history and history of medical care, including illness, diagnoses, treatment, and results of treatment. It serves as a basis for the planning and continuity of the patient's care; it provides a means of communication among physicians and other professionals involved in the therapy; it serves as a basis for review, study, and evaluation of the patient's condition; it furnishes documentary evidence of the patient's care; it serves to protect the legal interests of the patient, hospital, and responsible health practitioner; it also provides data for use in research and education.

uniform perinatal r. A record that provides the same data for every pregnant patient to assist the physician in evaluating risk factors in pregnancy.

recto- Combining form meaning the rectum.

rectoabdominal (rek-to-ab-dom'ĭ-nal) Relating to the rectum and the abdomen.

rectocele (rek'to-sēl) A hernial protrusion of the rectum into the posterior vaginal wall; caused by disruption of the connective tissue (rectovaginal fascia) between the rectum and vagina, which weakens the wall; usually occurs during childbirth. Also called proctocele.

rectoperineorrhaphy (rek-to-per-ĭ-ne-or'ă-fe) See proctoperineoplasty.

rectosigmoid (rek-to-sig'moid) The rectum and the sigmoid colon considered together, especially the section of the bowel where these two portions meet.

rectourethral (rek-to-u-re'thral) Relating to the rectum and urethra.

rectouterine (rek-to-u'ter-ĭn) Relating to the rectum and uterus.

rectovaginal (rek-to-vaj'ĭ-nal) Relating to the rectum and vagina.

rectovesical (rek-to-ves'ĭ-kal) Relating to the rectum and bladder.

rectum (rek'tum) The portion of the intestinal tract extending from the sigmoid colon (at the level of the sacrum) to the anal canal.

recurrence (re-kur'ens) A return of a morbid process after a period of abatement.

reflex (re'fleks) **1.** An involuntary and immediate response to a stimulus. **2.** Turned backward.

abdominal r. Contraction of the abdominal wall musculature elicited by light stroking of the overlying skin.

bladder r. See micturition reflex.

Ferguson r. During pregnancy, uterine contraction is induced by mechanical stretching of the cervix.

grasp r. A normal neonatal reflex characterized by the immediate grasping of a finger placed in the palm of the infant's hand.

let-down r. The sudden and rapid ejection of milk from the alveoli into the ducts of the lactating breasts; it causes a typical prickly sensation and may or may not be followed by spontaneous expression of milk. The reflex is initiated by liberation of the hormone oxytocin from the posterior portion of the

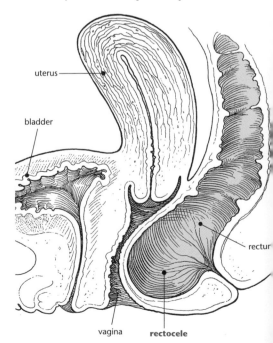

uterus

bladder

rectum

vagina   **rectocele**

pituitary (neurohypophysis), which in turn causes contraction of the alveoli and milk ducts in the breast. It may be triggered by stimulation of the mother's nipples (particularly by suckling) or by her emotional response to her baby (e.g., hearing the baby's cry). Also called milk ejection reflex; milk let-down reflex.

micturition r. Any of the reflexes controlling effortless urination and the subconscious ability to retain urine within the bladder. Also called bladder reflex; urinary reflex; vesical reflex.

milk-ejection r., milk let-down r. See let-down reflex.

Moro's r., Moro's embrace r. A normal neonatal reflex occurring in response to loud noises or sudden changes in position; characterized by tensing of muscles, a wide embracing motion of the arms, and extension of the thighs, legs, and fingers, except the thumb and index finger, which remain in a 'C' position. Also called startle reflex.

neck-righting r. A normal neonatal reflex elicited by turning the infant's head to the right or the left, which causes the shoulder of the opposite side to rotate.

oral r. Normal reflex elicited when the corner of the mouth of a newborn infant is touched; the bottom lip lowers on the same side and the tongue moves forward and toward the examiner's finger.

rooting r. A normal neonatal reflex characterized by turning of the head in the direction of a light touch on the cheek, and pursing of the lips in preparation for sucking.

primitive r. Any of the reflexes occurring naturally in the newborn; an indication of normal neuromuscular development; it occurs in the adult only in certain degenerative disorders.

startle r. See Moro's reflex.

sucking r. The sucking movement elicited by touching the roof of the infant's mouth (e.g., with a nipple or the tip of a finger); a normal neonatal reflex.

trunk-incurvation r. A normal neonatal reflex elicited by firmly running a finger down the side of the vertebral column; the infant's spine curves laterally in the direction of the stimulus.

urinary r. See micturition reflex.

vesical r. See micturition reflex.

reflux (re'fluks) A backward flow.

gastroesophageal r. (GER) Reflux of the stomach and duodenal contents into the esophagus.

vesicoureteral r. Abnormal flow of urine from the bladder back into a ureter during urination.

refusal (re-fu'zal) The act of withholding permission, acceptance, or compliance.

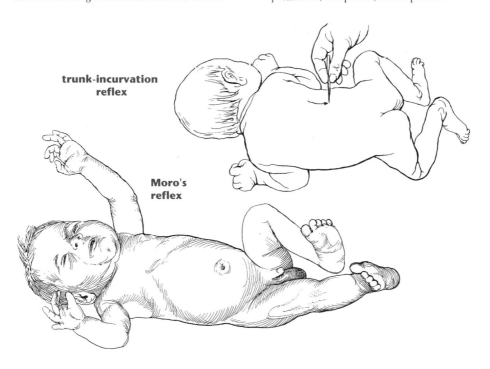

trunk-incurvation reflex

Moro's reflex

r. to treat Refusal of a health professional to initiate or continue treatment of a person or a group of people.

treatment r. Refusal of a person to accept treatment (medical or psychiatric), or unwillingness to comply with the physician's instructions or prescribed regimens. If the person is legally incompetent, or a minor, the concept may include a third party authorized to make decisions on the patient's behalf.

regimen (rej'ĭ-men) A regulated activity or procedure (e.g., exercise, diet, chemotherapy) designed to achieve hygienic or therapeutic ends.

CMF r. An adjunctive treatment for carcinoma of the breast consisting of cyclophosphamide, methotrexate, and fluorouracil.

MAC r. A chemotherapeutic regimen consisting of methotrexate, dactinomycin (actinomycin D), and chlorambucil for treating malignant gestational trophoblastic disease.

region (re'jun) 1. An arbitrary division, or continuous area on the surface of the body, with more or less definite boundaries. 2. A body part with a special nervous or vascular supply. 3. A portion of an organ that has a special function.

abdominal r.'s The nine regions into which the abdomen is divided by imaginary planes, namely the right and left hypochondriac, epigastric, right and left lumbar, umbilical, right and left inguinal, and pubic.

epigastric r. The upper middle area of the abdomen, just below the breastbone (sternum).

hinge r. A short sequence of amino acids present in the three-lobed, Y-shaped immunoglobulin molecule; it is situated between the two short arms of the 'Y', which allows movement when necessary (e.g., when binding to an antigen, the Y-shape changes to a taut T-shape).

hypochondriac r.'s The two upper and lateral areas of the abdomen, about the cartilages of the ribs.

hypogastric r. See pubic region.

iliac r.'s See inguinal regions.

infraclavicular r. The region of the chest just below the collarbone (clavicle).

inguinal r.'s The two regions of the abdomen lateral to the pubic region and about the inguinal canals. Also called iliac regions.

nuchal r. The region of the back of the neck.

perineal r. The region overlying the pelvic outlet; for descriptive purposes, it is usually divided into two triangles by a transverse line connecting the ischial tuberosities: a triangle of the anal region posteriorly and a triangle of the urogenital region (perineum) anteriorly.

promoter r. See promoter.

pseudoautosomal r. The region at the tip of the short arm of the Y chromosome; so named because, during meiosis, the X- and Y-linked copies of this region are homologous to each other, like pairs of autosomes (i.e., of any chromosome other than the sex chromosomes).

pubic r. The lowest midabdominal region, between the inguinal regions. Also called hypogastric region.

sacral r. The region of the lower back overlying the sacrum.

sex-determining r. (SRY) A region on the short arm of the Y chromosome, believed to control development of the male sex.

supraclavicular r.'s The hollow areas above the collarbones (clavicles).

umbilical r. The central part of the abdomen surrounding the navel.

relationship (re-la'shun-ship) An association; a kinship; a connection.

physician/patient r. The rights and responsibilities assumed by both a physician and the patient who has sought the physician's medical assistance; usually they include confidentiality and trust and it may be collaborative in nature.

sadomasochistic r. A complementary relationship, usually sexual, in which one partner enjoys suffering while the other enjoys inflicting pain or humiliation.

rem (rem) Acronym for roentgen-equivalent-man. A unit of radiation dose equivalent to the amount of absorbed ionizing radiation that is required to produce a biologic effect equivalent to the absorption of 1 rad of x or gamma rays. See also equivalent dose, under dose.

renin (re'nin) An enzyme formed in the kidneys and released into the bloodstream; it has an important role in the formation of angiotensin (a potent pressor substance) and thereby in the regulation of blood pressure, and possibly in cardiovascular disorders.

reoxygenation (re-ok-sĭ-gen-a'shun) Exposure of tumor cells to oxygen by close proximity to capillary flow, which renders the cells radiosensitive (i.e., subject to destruction by radiation therapy). Those cells located away from capillaries (farther than 100 mm) are hypoxic and are not killed by radiation.

replication (rep-lĭ-ka'shun) The process of

duplicating something.

DNA r. The unwinding of the two strands of a DNA molecule and subsequent formation of identical strands; a process initiated by enzymatic action.

report (re-port') A detailed account of the results of a study or investigation.

pathology r. The end product of a pathologic procedure indicating the result of the procedure; it may be a number (as in chemical tests), the name of a disease-causing microorganism, or a diagnosis (such as cancer) based on the microscopic characteristics of a tissue section.

repositor (re-poz'ĭ-tor) Instrument for repositioning a prolapsed or dislocated organ, especially the uterus.

reproduction (re-pro-duk'shun) The process of producing offspring.

assisted r. Reproduction achieved with the aid of any of several technologies involved in direct retrieval of oocytes from the ovary (e.g., *in vitro* fertilization [IVF], gamete intrafallopian transfer [GIFT], tubal embryo transfer [TET]).

resect (re-sekt') To remove surgically.

resectable (re-sek'tă-bl) Capable of being surgically removed.

resection (re-sek'shun) Surgical removal of tissue or body parts.

cornual r. A sterilization procedure consisting of removal of a wedge of tissue that includes the portion of fallopian (uterine) tube located within the wall of the uterine horn (cornu), along with adjacent cornual tissue.

resistance (re-zis'tans) **1.** Any passive force that retards the action of another, active, force. **2.** The ability of an organism to remain relatively unchanged when exposed to the action of an antagonistic agent.

drug r. In reference to cells or microorganisms, a state of diminished or total lack of response to drugs that ordinarily inhibit growth or cause death of target cells or organisms. Formerly called drug-fast. Compare with drug resistance, under tolerance.

peripheral r. See total peripheral resistance.

total peripheral r. (TPR) The sum of resistance to the flow of blood through the blood vessels. Also called peripheral resistance.

respiration (res-pĭ-ra'shun) (R) **1.** The processes through which an organism acquires oxygen and releases carbon dioxide. **2.** The act of breathing.

artificial r. See artificial ventilation, under ventilation.

assisted r. See assisted ventilation, under ventilation.

controlled r. See controlled ventilation, under ventilation.

diffusion r. Introduction of air into the lungs by means of an intratracheal catheter. Also called apneic oxygenation.

external r. The interchange of gases in the lungs.

mouth-to-mouth r. See mouth-to-mouth resuscitation, under resuscitation.

positive pressure r. See continuous positive pressure ventilation (CPPV) and intermittent positive pressure ventilation (IPPV), under ventilation.

respirator (res'pĭ-ra-tor) An apparatus for administering artificial ventilation.

pressure-controlled r. A respirator that supplies a predetermined pressure of gases during inhalation.

volume-controlled r. A respirator that supplies a predetermined volume of gases during inhalation.

response (re-spons') A reaction to a specific stimulus.

immune r. A specific response resulting in immunity; it includes an initial (afferent) phase during which responsive cells are primed by antigen, a central response during which antibodies (immunoglobulins) are formed, and an efferent response in which immunity is carried out by antibodies. Also called immune reaction, immunoreaction.

supine pressor r. See rollover test, under test.

restitution (res-tĭ-tu'shun) See external rotation, under rotation.

resuscitation (re-sus-ĭ-ta'shun) An act of resuscitating, or the state of being resuscitated.

cardiopulmonary r. (CPR) Administration of external cardiac compression and mouth-to-mouth resuscitation to restore breathing and heart muscle contraction.

mouth-to-mouth r. Restoration of breathing by placing one's mouth over the patient's mouth (and nose if the patient is a small child) and blowing rhythmically at a rate of about 20 cycles per minute. Also called mouth-to-mouth respiration.

neonatal r. The series of steps employed to initiate, or restore, spontaneous breathing in a newborn infant immediately after birth and applied progressively as needed; they generally include: prevention of heat loss, oropharyngeal suctioning, oxygen administration, chest compression,

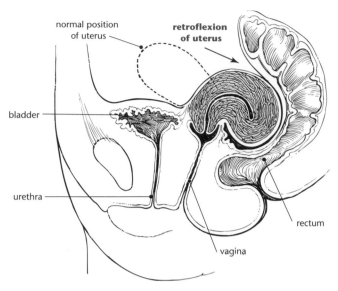

normal position of uterus

retroflexion of uterus

bladder

urethra

rectum

vagina

endotracheal suctioning, and administration of medications.

retardation (re-tar-da'shun) Delayed or diminished development.

fetal growth r. See intrauterine growth retardation.

intrauterine growth r. (IUGR) Birth weight that is below average, usually below the 10th percentile for the infant's gestational age. Also called fetal growth retardation.

retention (re-ten'shun) **1.** The holding back of body wastes that are normally discharged. **2.** The ability to remember.

13-*cis*-retinoid acid See isotretinoin.

retinopathy (ret-ĭ-nop'ă-the) Any degenerative noninflammatory disease of the retina.

r. of prematurity (ROP) Eye condition sometimes occurring in premature infants, characterized by constriction and obliteration of the capillary bed of the retina followed by formation of new blood vessels extending into the vitreous, retinal hemorrhages, fibrosis, and eventual retinal detachment; associated with exposure to elevated concentrations of oxygen; in most cases the process is reversed before fibrosis occurs. Formerly called retrolental fibroplasia.

retraction (re-trak'shun) Shrinking or drawing back.

retro- Combining form meaning backward.

retrocecal (ret-ro-se'kal) Behind the first portion of the large intestine (cecum), in the lower right side of the abdomen.

retrocervical (ret-ro-ser've-kal) Behind the uterine cervix.

retrocession (ret-ro-sesh'on) A backward slumping of the cervix and vaginal apex.

retrodisplacement (ret-ro-dis-plās'ment) Any backward displacement.

retroflexion (ret-ro-flek'shun) Backward bending of an organ.

r. of uterus Extreme backward bending or angulation of the body of the uterus while the cervix remains in its normal position. Compare with retroversion of uterus.

retrograde (ret'ro-grād) Moving or flowing in a backward direction.

retromammary (ret-ro-mam'er-e) Behind the mammary glands.

retroposition (ret-ro-pŏ-zish'un) Any type of backward displacement of an organ.

adherent r. of uterus A fixed retroposition of the uterus caused by adhesions; seen in a variety of pelvic inflammatory conditions (e.g., sexually transmitted infections, endometriosis, pyosalpinx, hydrosalpinx).

retrosternal (ret-ro-ster'nal) Behind the breastbone (sternum).

retrouterine (ret-ro-u'ter-in) Behind the uterus.

retroversion (ret-ro-ver'zhun) Backward tilting of an organ in its entirety.

r. of uterus Backward inclination of the entire uterus (including the cervix) toward the hollow of the sacrum. Compare with retroflexion of uterus.

retroverted (ret-ro-vert'ed) Inclined backward.

Retroviridae (ret-ro-vir'ĭ-de) A family of viruses, 100 nm in diameter, that have RNA-dependent polymerases; it includes the tumor viruses.

retrovirus (ret-ro-vi'rus) Any virus of the family

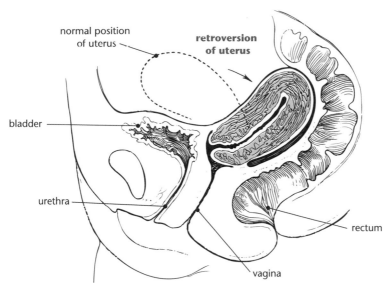

normal position of uterus

retroversion of uterus

bladder

urethra

rectum

vagina

Retroviridae. Retroviruses are named for their ability to convert RNA into DNA and thus use genetic material of the cells they infect to make the proteins they need to survive, causing several diseases in the process. Retroviruses include the cancer-causing virus HTLV (human T-cell leukemia/lymphoma virus), and HIV (human immunodeficiency virus) which causes AIDS (acquired immune deficiency syndrome); these viruses have an affinity for T4 (helper) lymphocytes.

rhabdomyosarcoma (rab-do-mi-o-sar-ko'ma) A malignant soft-tissue tumor.

    embryonal r. A malignant tumor composed of loose spindle-celled tissue and areas of cross-striations; arises in many parts of the body of young children, especially the head, neck, and lower genitourinary tract.

    embryonal r. of vagina An uncommon highly malignant vaginal tumor of infants and young children; it develops in the submucosal vaginal tissue (usually the anterior wall), spreading rapidly under the intact epithelium and causing the mucosa to bulge and form enlarging grapelike clusters, which may protrude through the vaginal orifice. Also called botryoid sarcoma; sarcoma botryoides.

rhombocele (rom'bo-sēl) The natural terminal expansion of the spinal canal, located within the lumbar portion of the spinal cord.

rhythm (rith'm) The pattern of recurrence of a biologic cycle (e.g., the heartbeat).

    circadian r. A regular recurrence in cycles of approximately 24-hour intervals.

    diurnal r. A regular occurrence during daylight hours.

    infradian r. A regular recurrence in cycles of more than 24-hour intervals.

    r. method See under method.

    ultradian r. A regular recurrence in cycles of less than 24-hour intervals.

rickets (rik'ets) Disease of infants and young children caused by vitamin D deficiency, resulting in defective bone growth.

ridge (rij) A linear elevation (e.g., on a bone).

rima (ri'ma), pl. rimae A cleft, fissure, slit, or elongated opening.

    r. pudendi See vulval cleft, under cleft.

ring (ring) **1.** In anatomy, a circular band of tissue surrounding an opening. **2.** In chemistry, an arrangement of atoms graphically representable as a circle. **3.** Any circular device.

    abdominal r. See deep inguinal ring.

    Bandl's r. See pathologic retraction ring.

    deep inguinal r. The oval orifice in the transverse fascia of the external oblique muscle marking the deep opening of the inguinal canal. Also called abdominal ring; internal inguinal ring.

    external inguinal r. See superficial inguinal ring.

    Falope r. A nonreactive rubber band used for occluding each fallopian (uterine) tube as a procedure for sterilization; the ring is placed around a 2.5-cm loop of the tube, at the junction of its proximal and middle thirds. Also called silastic band; silastic ring; Yoon ring.

    femoral r. The abdominal or superior oval opening of the conical femoral canal underlying the inguinal ligament at the groin; it is bounded posteriorly by the pectineus muscle, medially by the lacunar ligament and laterally by the femoral vein. It is normally filled with extraperitoneal fatty and lymphoid tissues and is a potential site of hernia.

internal inguinal r. See deep inguinal ring.

pathologic retraction r. A markedly pronounced and persistent ring usually associated with protracted labors; the lower uterine portion becomes abnormally stretched and thin-walled, a sign of impending rupture. Also called Bandl's ring.

physiologic retraction r. A retraction ring formed during normal labor; it marks the boundary between the thickened, actively contracting upper portion of the uterus and the passively expanding lower portion.

retraction r. A transverse, ringlike ridge on the inner surface of the uterus formed during labor at the junction of the isthmus and body of the uterus.

silastic r. See Falope ring.

subcutaneous inguinal r. See superficial inguinal ring.

superficial inguinal r. The orifice in the aponeurosis of the external oblique muscle forming the external opening of the inguinal canal. Also called external inguinal ring;

subcutaneous inguinal ring.

umbilical r. The opening in the abdominal connective tissue (linea alba) of the fetus through which pass the umbilical arteries and vein.

Yoon r. See Falope ring.

ringworm (ring'wurm) See tinea.

risk (risk) **1.** The probability of suffering harm or a loss. **2.** In toxicology, the probability that a substance will inflict injury under specified conditions of use.

assumption of r. In negligence law, especially in reference to medical malpractice, the doctrine that a person who consents to a treatment, procedure, or omission of either, with the knowledge that injury may reasonably result, relinquishes the future complaint that injury was caused by negligence on the part of the practitioner. In medical professional liability, assumption of risk provides a valid defense from suit only when medical treatment was administered with proper care. See also negligence.

roentgen (rent'gen) (R, r) A unit of radiation exposure equal to 2.58×10^{-4} coulomb per kilogram.

roentgeno- Combining form meaning x rays.

roentgenogram (rent-gen'o-gram) A processed photographic film on which an image is produced by x rays striking a sensitized film after their passage through a portion of the body. Also called radiogram; x-ray picture; commonly called x-ray.

roentgenography (rent-gen-og'rǎ-fe) See radiography.

body-section r. See tomography.

sectional r. See tomography.

roentgenometry (rent-gě-nom'e-tre) **1.** Measurement of the therapeutic dosage of x rays. **2.** Measurement of the penetrating power of x-rays.

room (room) A limited area enclosed by walls in a building.

birthing r. A hospital room in which women undergo both labor and delivery; it is provided with infant warmers and resuscitation equipment. See also birth center, under center.

delivery r. A hospital room into which women in labor are taken for delivery.

labor r. (LBR) A hospital room in which women in labor are monitored prior to delivery. Also called predelivery room.

predelivery r. See labor room.

recovery r. (RR) (1) A hospital room (usually adjoining an operating or delivery room) that

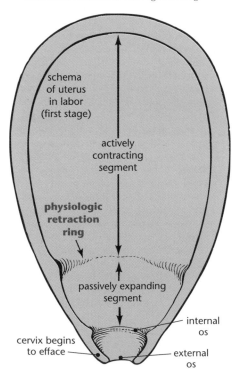

schema of uterus in labor (first stage)

actively contracting segment

physiologic retraction ring

passively expanding segment

internal os

cervix begins to efface

external os

is provided with equipment and personnel for continuous monitoring of postoperative patients immediately following anesthesia, and where special attention is focused on airway management and control of pain, nausea, and vomiting. (2) A hospital room where postoperative patients are briefly placed after release from the postanesthesia room, prior to discharge from the hospital.

rooming-in (room'ing in) The practice of allowing a newborn baby to stay in the mother's hospital room, in a bassinet, rather than in the nursery during the hospital stay.

root (root) The origin, attaching part, or proximal end of a structure.

r.'s of brachial plexus The five roots forming the brachial plexus of the arm, consisting of the anterior (ventral) rami of the fifth, sixth, seventh, and eighth cervical nerves and the greater part of the first thoracic nerve; they fuse with one another to form three trunks.

r. of clitoris The proximal part of the clitoris, consisting of two diverging corpora cavernosa that lie deeply in close apposition with the periosteum of the ischiopubic rami.

rotation (ro-ta'shun) **1.** Movement around an internal axis. **2.** In obstetrics, the turning of the fetal head or presenting part during birth, whereby the head becomes accommodated to the birth canal.

external r. The spontaneous turning of the fetal head when it reaches the level of the ischial spines during labor; the back of the head (occiput) may turn either anteriorly toward the pubic symphysis or posteriorly toward the sacrum. Also called restitution.

internal r. The return of the rotated infant's head to its natural alignment with the shoulders, after the head's complete emergence from the maternal vulva.

manual r. Maneuver used when the back of the fetal head (occiput) is persistently directed posteriorly, either toward the right or the left sacroiliac joint and engagement of the head has occurred (i.e., the head has entered the level of the ischial spines); a hand with the palm upward is introduced into the vagina and the head is grasped, with the fingers on the side of the head that is to be turned toward the anterior position and the thumb on the opposite side; the head is then slowly rotated anteriorly.

-rrhage Combining form meaning excessive discharge (e.g., hemorrhage).

-rrhaphy Combining form meaning suture (e.g.,

herniorrhaphy).

-rrhea Combining form meaning a flow (e.g., diarrhea).

RU 486 Trade name for mifepristone.

rubella (roo-bel'ă) Contagious viral disease, usually mild and of short duration, but capable of causing fetal abnormalities from maternal infection during the first 3 months of pregnancy; characterized by malaise, headache, fever, enlarged lymph nodes (especially behind the ears), and a maculopapular rash. Caused by the rubella virus (genus *Rubivirus*); incubation period is 2 to 3 weeks. Also called German measles.

rubeola (roo-be'ŏ-lă, roo-be-o'lă) See measles.

Rubivirus (roo-bĭ-vi'rus) A genus of viruses (family Togaviridae) that, unlike other members of the Togaviridae family, are not transmitted by arthropods; humans are the only vertebrate hosts; includes the rubella (German measles) virus.

ruga (roo'gă), pl. rugae A fold or wrinkle.

vaginal rugae The transverse folds in the lining of the vagina. Also called vaginal folds.

rugal (roo'gal) Creased, corrugated.

rule (rool) A guide.

delivery date r. See Naegele's rule.

Naegele's r. Estimation of the day of childbirth by counting back 3 months from the first day of the last menstrual period and adding 7 days. Also called delivery date rule.

rupture (rup'chur) **1.** A tearing or bursting of an organ or body part. Distinguished from dehiscence. **2.** Popular term for a hernia.

premature r. of membranes Rupture of the membranes occurring at any time before the onset of labor, regardless of the length of gestation.

preterm r. of membranes Rupture of the membranes before 38 weeks of gestation.

prolonged premature r. of membranes Rupture of the membranes occurring 24 hours before the onset of labor.

r. of uterus Rupture of the uterine wall; classified as *complete*, when the tear traverses the whole thickness of the wall and the uterine cavity opens into the peritoneal cavity; *incomplete*, when the peritoneal covering of the uterus remains intact and there is therefore no communication between the uterine and peritoneal cavities. Rupture of the uterus may occur during childbirth under certain predisposing conditions (e.g., the presence of fibroids, an abnormally adherent placenta, scarring from a previous cesarean section, uterine anomalies, prolonged labor due to malposition of the fetus), or by misuse of forceps, application of strong pressure on the uterine fundus, and extensive use of uterine stimulants (e.g., oxytocin, prostaglandins, ergot infusions). Predisposing factors not associated with labor include choriocarcinoma, uterine cancer, and invasive hydatidiform mole.

rutherford (ruth'er-ford) Unit of radioactivity, equal to the amount of radioactive material undergoing 1 million disintegrations per second.

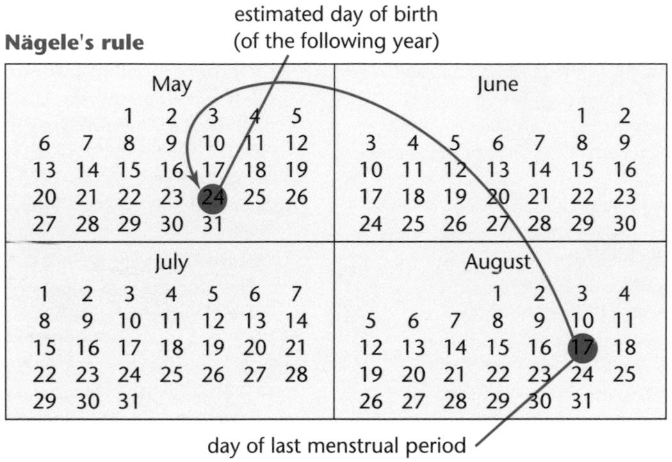

Nägele's rule

estimated day of birth
(of the following year)

May						June					
		1	2	3	4	5				1	2
6	7	8	9	10	11	12	3	4	5	6	7	8	9
13	14	15	16	17	18	19	10	11	12	13	14	15	16
20	21	22	23	**24**	25	26	17	18	19	20	21	22	23
27	28	29	30	31			24	25	26	27	28	29	30

July						August					
1	2	3	4	5	6	7			1	2	3	4
8	9	10	11	12	13	14	5	6	7	8	9	10	11
15	16	17	18	19	20	21	12	13	14	15	16	**17**	18
22	23	24	25	26	27	28	19	20	21	22	23	24	25
29	30	31					26	27	28	29	30	31

day of last menstrual period

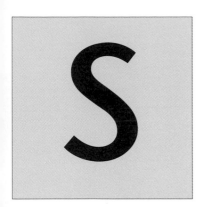

sac (sak) A pouchlike anatomic structure.

abdominal s. The part of the embryonic sac that develops into the peritoneal cavity of the abdomen.

air s. See pulmonary alveolus, under alveolus.

dural s. The continuation of the loose sheath of the spinal dura mater below the terminal part of the spinal cord; it surrounds the cauda equina and filum terminale and ends at the lower border of the second sacral vertebra.

gestation s. The membranes enveloping the fetus or embryo, composed of the fused chorion and amnion.

greater s. of peritoneum The main part of the peritoneal cavity, between the parietal and visceral layers of the peritoneum; it extends across the whole breadth of the abdomen, and from the diaphragm to the pelvis. Also called greater peritoneal cavity.

hernial s. The lining of a hernia (e.g., the pouch of peritoneum that lines an umbilical hernia).

lesser s. of peritoneum The smaller part of the peritoneal cavity; a diverticulum of the greater sac of peritoneum, situated behind the lesser omentum; it extends upward as far as the diaphragm, and downward between the layers of the greater omentum, to its opening through the epiploic foramen where it communicates with the greater sac of peritoneum. Also called omental bursa; omental sac; lesser peritoneal cavity.

omental s. See lesser sac of peritoneum.

vitelline s. See yolk sac.

yolk s. The highly vascular umbilical vesicle enveloping the nutritive yolk of an embryo; it is attached to the embryo's midgut. Also called vitelline sac.

sacculation (sak-u-la'shun) **1.** The process of sac

formation. **2.** The presence of sacs.

s. of uterus The presence of an abnormal pouchlike enlargement in the uterine wall most commonly developed in the anterior part of the wall.

sacrad (sak'rad) Toward the sacrum.

sacral (sa'kral) Relating to the sacrum.

sacro-, sacr- Combining forms meaning sacrum.

sacrococcygeal (sa-kro-kok-sij'e-al) Relating to the sacrum and the coccyx.

sacroiliac (sa-kro-il'e-ak) Relating to the sacrum and ilium.

sacrum (sa'krum) A slightly curved, triangular bone composed of five fused vertebrae, forming the back of the pelvis; it articulates with the corresponding ilium on each side, and with the last lumbar vertebra above and the coccyx below.

tilted s. A forward displacement of the sacrum resulting from separation of the sacroiliac joints.

sadism (sa'dizm) The derivation of pleasure from inflicting physical or psychological pain or abuse on others.

sexual s. A psychosexual disorder in which the infliction of physical or psychological pain on another person is the only or the preferred means of attaining sexual excitement.

sadist (sād'ist) A person who practices sadism.

sadomasochism (sa-do-mas'ŏ-kizm) A condition in which submissive (masochistic) and aggressive (sadistic) attitudes coexist in an individual's social and/or sexual relationships.

sagittal (saj'ĭ-tal) In an anteroposterior direction (i.e., occurring or situated in the median plane of the body or in a plane parallel to it).

salpingectomy (sal-pin-jek'tŏ me) Removal of a fallopian (uterine) tube. Also called tubectomy.

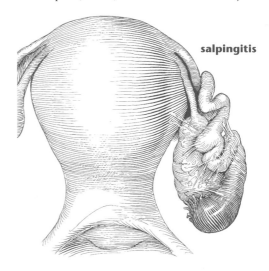

salpingitis

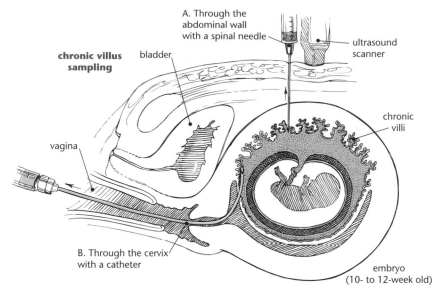

A. Through the abdominal wall with a spinal needle

ultrasound scanner

chronic villus sampling **bladder**

chronic villi

vagina

B. Through the cervix with a catheter

embryo (10- to 12-week old)

salpingemphraxis (sal-pin-jem-frak'sis) Obstruction of a fallopian (uterine) tube or a eustachian (auditory) tube.

salpinges (sal-pin'jez) Plural of salpinx.

salpingian (sal-pin'je-an) Relating to a fallopian (uterine) tube or to a eustachian (auditory) tube.

salpingitis (sal-pin-ji'tis) Inflammation of one or both fallopian (uterine) tubes; may be caused by infection with a single organism or occur as a polymicrobial infection; most frequently implicated are *Neisseria gonorrhoeae, Chlamydia trachomatis,* and *Ureaplasma urealyticus.*

salpingitis ithmica nodosa (sal-pin-ji'tis ith'mĭ-că no-do'să) (SIN) A noninflammatory condition of the narrowest portion of a uterine tube in which the epithelial lining of the tubal lumen extends deeper into the tube's muscular layer, forming a tiny pouch (diverticulum); may be associated with (not necessarily the cause of) tubal ectopic pregnancy.

salpingo-, salping- Combining forms meaning tube.

salpingocele (sal-ping'go-sēl) Herniation of a fallopian (uterine) tube.

salpingocyesis (sal-ping-go-si-e'sis) See tubal pregnancy, under pregnancy.

salpingography (sal-ping-gog'ră-fe) X-ray examination of a fallopian (uterine) tube after infusion of a radiopaque substance through the cervix; usually performed to diagnose tubal occlusion.

salpingolysis (sal-ping-gol'ĭ-sis) The release of adhesions from a fallopian (uterine) tube.

salpingoneostomy (sal-ping-go-ne-os'tŏ-me) See salpingostomy.

salpingo-oophorectomy (sal-ping'go o-of-ŏ-rek'tŏ-me) Surgical removal of a fallopian (uterine) tube and its corresponding ovary. Also called tubo-ovariectomy; salpingo-ovariectomy.

salpingo-oophoritis (sal-ping'go o-of-ŏ-ri'tis) Inflammation of a fallopian (uterine) tube and its ovary. Also called tubo-ovaritis.

salpingo-ovariectomy (sal-ping'go o-var-e-ek'tŏ-me) See salpingo-oophorectomy.

salpingoperitonitis (sal-ping'go-per-i-tŏ-ni'tis) Inflammation of a fallopian (uterine) tube and its adjacent peritoneum.

salpingoplasty (sal-ping'go-plas-te) Reparative surgical operation on a fallopian (uterine) tube. Also called tuboplasty.

salpingorrhaphy (sal-ping-gor'ă-fe) Suturing of a fallopian (uterine) tube.

salpingostomy (sal-ping-gos'tŏ-me) The surgical creation of a new opening in an occluded fallopian (uterine) tube; performed to restore its patency, especially when the occlusion is at the wide (ampullary) end of the tube. Also called salpingoneostomy.

salpingotomy (sal-ping-got'ŏ-me) An incision made into a fallopian (uterine) tube.

    linear s. A longitudinal incision made on the wide (ampullary) segment of a fallopian (uterine) tube to remove an ectopic pregnancy.

salpinx (sal'pinks), pl. salpinges Latin for tube.

sampling (sam'pling) The acquisition and examination of a sample.

    chorionic villus s. (CVS) Sampling of placental tissue (chorionic villi) for genetic analysis to detect chromosomal defects in the developing fetus; cells of the villi are considered most often to reflect the total genetic composition (karyotype) of the fetus, except in cases of placental mosaicism (i.e., when the placenta has two cell populations differing in chromosomal constitution), which occurs about 1% of the time. Tissue may be obtained through the cervix or through an abdominal puncture with a needle and syringe under the guidance of ultrasound visualization. The sampling is performed at approximately 10 to 12 weeks of gestation. Also called chorionic villus sampling test.

fetal scalp blood s. Sampling of capillary blood from the fetal scalp (sometimes the buttocks), obtained during the course of labor to determine the acid–base status (pH) of the blood for identifying a fetus in distress. An illuminated endoscope is introduced through the dilated cervix, a narrow incision, no more than 2 mm deep, is made on the scalp and blood is aspirated into a capillary tube treated with heparin, and the blood pH is then promptly measured. The sampling is performed only after the membranes have ruptured.

percutaneous umbilical blood s. (PUBS) Sampling of fetal blood from the umbilical cord by transabdominal aspiration under ultrasound guidance. The specimen thus obtained can be used for various biochemical and hematologic tests. Also called cordocentesis.

sangui-, sanguino- Combining forms meaning blood.

sanguineous (sang-gwin'e-us) Relating to blood.

sanguinolent (sang-gwin'ō-lent) Blood-tinged.

sanguinopurulent (sang-gwĭ-no-pu'roo-lent) Containing blood and pus.

saniopurulent (sa-ne-o-pu'roo-lent) Denoting a blood-tinged discharge mixed with pus.

sanioserous (sa-ne-o-se'rus) Denoting blood-tinged serum.

sarco- Combining form meaning flesh.

sarcoid (sar'koid) Resembling flesh.

sarcoma (sar-ko'mă) Cancerous tumor composed of connective tissue.

botryoid s., s. botryoides See embryonal rhabdomyosarcoma of vagina, under rhabdomyosarcoma.

endometrial stromal s. (ESS) A bulky, infiltrating, malignant tumor of the uterine lining, capable of spreading early and extensively; usual symptoms include uterine enlargement, pelvic pain, and irregular bleeding; seen most commonly in older women.

Ewing's s. An uncommon, rapidly growing, malignant tumor of a single bone, affecting predominantly long tubular and pelvic bones; occurs in children and young adults. Also called Ewing's tumor.

Kaposi's s. (KS) Malignant skin tumor occurring in multiple sites, especially the lower legs, and spreading to mucous membranes, lymph nodes, and internal organs; initial lesions are small red papules that enlarge and fuse to form purple to brown plaques and nodules; usually a slowly progressive disease, its course is much more aggressive when occurring as an opportunistic disease in AIDS patients.

sarcomatoid (sar-ko'mă-toid) Resembling a sarcoma.

sarcomatous (sar-ko'mă-tus) Relating to sarcoma.

satellite (sat'e-līt) Any structure, lesion, mass, or radiologic density associated with another, usually larger, entity.

satyriasis (sat-ĭ-ri'a-sĭs) Insatiable sexual desire or behavior in the male; the counterpart of nymphomania in the female.

scale (skāl) 1. A thin, flaky piece of epithelium that is partly adherent to the skin. 2. To shed such material. 3. A set of graduated marks (as on an instrument or device) serving as a standard of measurement.

scan (skan) 1. To survey by a continuous sweep of a sensing device. 2. A graphic record of an area or volume so obtained (e.g., of the distribution of a radioactive element within an organ). The term is an abbreviated form of the word scintiscan and is often used preceded by the structure examined (e.g., brain scan, bone scan), the device or technology used (e.g., CAT scan, radionuclide scan, ultrasound scan), or the technique used (e.g., perfusion scan, ventilation scan). See also tomography.

scanner (skan'er) A sensing device that scans a region point by point in a continuous systematic manner.

scanning (skan'ning) The act of surveying an area or region by a continuous sweep of a sensing device. The term is usually preceded by the technology or sensing device used (e.g., PET scanning). See also tomography.

scintiscanner (sin-tĭ-skan'er) A device that automatically scans a region of the body to produce an image of a radiation-emitting isotope in tissues.

scinticisternography (sin-tĭ-cis-tern-og'ră-fe) The process of injecting a radioactive substance into the subarachnoid space, then recording its concentration with a scintiscanner; used for diagnosing hydrocephalus and for studying the flow of cerebrospinal fluid. Also called test for hydrocephalus.

scintigraphy (sin-tig'ră-fe) Injection of a radioactive substance and determination of its distribution in the tissues with the aid of a scintiscanner.

sclero-, scler- Combining forms meaning hard.

sclerosis (sklĕ-ro'sis) Hardening of tissues due to proliferation of connective tissue, frequently originating in sites of chronic inflammation.

> **amyotrophic lateral s.** (ALS) Disease of motor neurons characterized by degeneration of the lateral motor tracts of the spinal cord, causing progressive atrophy of muscles and exaggerated reflexes. Commonly called Lou Gehrig's disease.

> **tuberous s.** Rare disorder inherited as an autosomal dominant trait; major features include mental retardation, convulsions, and small skin nodules composed of fibroelastic and blood vessel proliferation; the brain contains hard benign tumors, which sometimes obstruct circulation of cerebrospinal fluid. Also called epiloia; Bourneville's disease.

sclerotic (sklĕ-rot'ik) Relating to sclerosis.

sclerous (sklĕ'rus) Hardened.

-scope Combining form meaning instrument for viewing (e.g., endoscope).

-scopy Combining form meaning observation, especially with a specially designed instrument (e.g., proctoscopy).

score (skor) An evaluative record, usually expressed numerically.

> **Apgar s.** A numerical expression of the condition of a newborn infant on a scale of 0 to 10, usually recorded at 1 and 5 minutes after delivery. Numerical values are assigned to the status of skin color, heart rate, respiratory effort, muscle tone, and reflex irritability. The findings become a permanent part of the child's health record.

> **Bishop s.** A numerical expression reflecting the status of the uterine cervix and fetal presenting part; used for determining the likelihood of the successful induction of labor.

> **Brewer s.** A numerical expression, ranging from 0 to 3, for predicting the likelihood of developing gestational trophoblastic tumors in subsequent pregnancies after the first occurrence of a molar pregnancy.

screen (skrēn) 1. A structure with a flat surface, such as one against which images are projected, or one used in fluoroscopy. 2. A substance used

as protection against a deleterious influence (e.g., ultraviolet rays). 3. To conduct a screening.

screening (skrēn'ing) The process of examining large groups of people for a given disease or trait.

> **genetic s.** Any method of identifying individuals in a given population at high risk of having, or transmitting to their children, a specific genetic disorder.

> **gestational diabetes s.** The administration of tests to identify pregnant women with diabetes mellitus. See glucose tolerance test, under test.

seatworm (sēt'werm) See pinworm.

secobarbitol (seh-ko-bar'bĭ-tal) A short-acting, fast-onset sedative and hypnotic. May cause hemorrhagic disease of the newborn. Trade name: Seconal.

secretion (se-kre'shun) 1. The process by which a cell or gland produces and releases a specific substance. 2. The substance produced.

> **fetoplacental s.'s** Proteins and steroid hormones secreted into the maternal circulation; the proteins are synthesized by the placenta (e.g., human chorionic gonadotropin [hCG] and human placental lactogen [hPL]); the steroid hormones (e.g., progesterone and estrogens) are produced by the placenta but derived from maternal or fetal precursor steroids.

section (sek'shun) 1. The act of cutting. 2. One of several component segments of a structure. 3. A thin slice of tissue suitable for examination under the microscope. 4. A cut surface.

> **C s.** See cesarean section.

> **cervical cesarean s.** See lower segment cesarean section.

> **cesarean s.** (CS) An incision through the abdominal and uterine walls for extraction of the fetus; it may be vertical or, more commonly, horizontal. Also called abdominal delivery; commonly called C section.

> **classic cesarean s.** A cesarean section in which the upper segment (fundus) of the uterus is vertically incised. Also called corporeal cesarean section; Sçanger operation.

> **corporeal cesarean s.** See classic cesarean section.

> **extraperitoneal cesarean s.** A horizontal cesarean section made in the lower segment of the uterus, after displacing the peritoneum upward and the bladder downward.

> **low cesarean s.** See lower segment cesarean section.

> **lower segment cesarean s.** A cesarean section in which the uterus is entered by a transverse incision through the lower uterine

segment, either transperitoneally or extraperitoneally. Also called cervical cesarean section; low cesarean section.

   postmortem cesarean s. Cesarean section performed on a woman just after her death, or when her death is imminent.

   transperitoneal cesarean s. Cesarean section performed with an incision through the uterovesical fold of peritoneum.

   vaginal cesarean s. A very rarely performed cesarean section done through the vagina and lower uterine segment. This approach is discouraged by most authorities.

secundigravida (sĕ-kun-dĭ-grav'ĭ-dă) A woman who has been pregnant twice.

secundines (se-kun'dinz) See afterbirth.

secundipara (se-kun-dip'ă-ră) A woman who has given birth twice. Formerly called bipara. See also para.

seizure (se'zhur) **1.** An attack; a sudden onset of a disease or symptom. **2.** An abrupt and temporary change in the electrical activity of the superficial layer of the brain (the cerebral cortex); manifested clinically by a change in consciousness or by a sensory, motor, or behavioral symptom.

   absence s. A sudden, transient (10 to 30 second) break of consciousness of thought or activity, sometimes accompanied by rapid eyelid flutterings; seen in absence epilepsy.

Also called petit mal seizure.

   catamenial s. Epileptic seizure activity that is exacerbated during menstruation.

sella turcica (se'lă tur'sĭ-kă) A depression with two prominences (anterior and posterior) on the upper surface of the sphenoid bone at the base of the skull, resembling a Turkish saddle; it houses the pituitary (hypophysis). Frequently called sella.

semen (se'men) The thick whitish ejaculation of the male reproductive organs, composed chiefly of spermatozoa, a fructose-rich fluid from the seminal vesicles, and secretions from the prostate. Also called seminal fluid.

seminal (sem'ĭ-nal) Relating to the semen.

semination (sem-ĭ-na'shun) See insemination.

seminiferous (se-mĭ-nif'er-us) Conveying semen.

sensitive (sen'sĭ-tiv) **1.** Responsive to external stimulation. **2.** Susceptible (e.g., to the action of a drug). **3.** In immunology, the increased capacity to respond specifically to an antigen.

sensitivity (sen-sĭ-tĭ-vĭ-te) The state of being sensitive.

   diagnostic s. Applied to a screening test: the proportion of individuals who truly have a disease in a screened population, and who are identified as such by the screening test (i.e., it is a measure of the probability that a person with a disease will be correctly identified by the screening test).

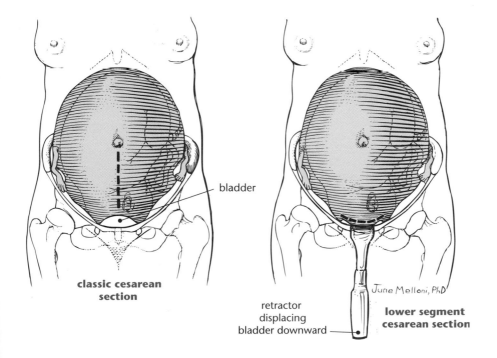

bladder

classic cesarean section

retractor displacing bladder downward —

June Melloni, PhD

lower segment cesarean section

sensor (sen'sor) Any device designed to respond to a physical stimulus (e.g., temperature, light, motion), generating electrical signals for measurement or control.

separation (sep-ă-ra'shun) The act of dividing, detaching, or keeping apart.

    premature s. of placenta See abruptio placentae.

    symphyseal s. Destabilization of the anterior articulation of the pubic bones beyond the physiologic relaxation induced by pregnancy, which may result in painful ambulation. It is manifest typically in the last trimester of pregnancy but may also occur postpartum.

sepsis (sep'sis) The systemic response to infection, characterized by (but not limited to) two or more of the following features: elevation of body temperature, heart rate, respiratory rate, and white blood cell count.

septa (sep'tă) Plural of septum.

septal (sep'tal) Relating to a septum or partition.

septate (sep'tāt) Divided into compartments by a septum.

septectomy (sep-tek'tŏ-me) Surgical removal of a septum.

septic (sep'tik) Relating to sepsis.

septo-, sept- Combining forms meaning septum.

septum (sep'tum), pl. **septa** A thin wall or partition between two cavities or masses of soft tissue.

    atrial s. See interatrial septum.

    interatrial s. The partition between the right and left atria of the heart. Also called atrial septum.

    interventricular s. The musculomembranous partition dividing the right and left ventricles of the heart. Also called ventricular septum.

    longitudinal vaginal s. A developmental anomaly consisting of a fibrous partition within the vagina, which divides the structure lengthwise into two; caused by failure of the mullerian ducts to fuse during embryonic life.

    placental septa Incomplete partitions that divide the maternal surface of the placenta into 15 to 20 compartments (cotyledons).

    rectovaginal s. The thin layer of fascia separating the vagina from the anterior wall of the rectum. The equivalent in the male is the rectovesical septum.

    transverse vaginal s. An abnormal partition across the width of the vagina, usually at mid-level; caused by faulty canalization of the vagina during embryonic development.

    urorectal s. In the embryo, a partition within the cloaca, dividing it into a posterior rectal portion and an anterior urogenital channel.

    ventricular s. See interventricular septum.

sequence (se'kwens) A series of items or events, one following another.

    twin-reversed arterial perfusion s. A rare but serious complication of monozygotic twinning thought to be secondary to serious placental vascular anastomoses. Inadequate perfusion of one twin results in lethal anomalies, such as absence of the heart (acardia) and the head (acephaly); the remaining twin is at risk for *in utero* heart failure.

serocystic (sēr-o-sis'tik) Composed of serum-filled cysts.

seropurulent (sēr-o-pu'roo-lent) Containing serum and pus; applied to a discharge.

serosanguinous (sēr-o-sang-gwin'us) Containing serum and blood; applied to a discharge.

serum (se'rum), pl. **serums**, **sera** 1. The clear fluid moistening serous membranes. 2. A loosely used term denoting serum that contains antitoxins, used for therapeutic and diagnostic purposes. 3. See blood serum.

    blood s. The clear, fluid portion of blood that is left after fibrinogen (a protein) and the cellular elements of blood are removed by coagulation; distinguished from plasma, the

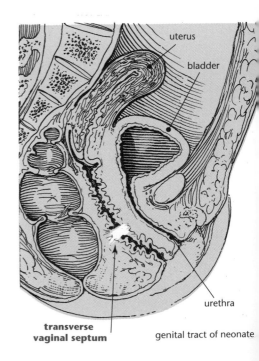

uterus

bladder

urethra

transverse vaginal septum

genital tract of neonate

cell-free liquid portion of uncoagulated blood.

sessile (ses'il) Attached by a broad base rather than a pedicle; applied to certain polyps and tumors.

sex (seks) The classification of organisms as male or female according to their reproductive characteristics.

> **chromosomal s.** An individual's sex determined by the presence or absence of the Y chromosome in the spermatozoon at the time of its union with the ovum. Also called genetic sex.

> **genetic s.** See chromosomal sex.

> **gonadal s.** Sex determined by the presence of either testes or ovaries.

> **morphologic s.** Sex determined by the structure and form of the external genitalia. Also called phenotypic sex.

> **phenotypic s.** See morphologic sex.

sex-linked (seks' linkt) Carried in a sex (X or Y) chromosome; applied to a gene.

sheath (shēth) An enveloping structure.

> **contraceptive s.** See condom.

> **crural s.** See femoral sheath.

> **femoral s.** A funnel-shaped sheath located behind, and just below, the inguinal ligament; divided into three compartments by two vertical partitions: the lateral compartment contains the femoral artery, the middle one contains the femoral vein, the medial one (femoral canal) contains lymphatic vessels and a lymph node. Also called crural sheath.

shield (shēld) 1. Any protective device or substance that serves as a barrier or screen. 2. To afford protection (e.g., from radiation).

> **breast s.** A rubber cap or dome for protecting inflamed or irritated nipples from contact with clothing.

> **Dalkon s.** An intrauterine device made of a plastic polymer with a polyfilamentous string (tail) which may have served as a wick for introducing pathogenic organisms into the uterine cavity, resulting in subsequent infectious morbidity. The subject of intensive litigation in the 1970s and 1980s.

> **embryonic s.** The disk in the blastoderm from which the embryo proper develops.

> **lead s.** In radiology, a lead screen for protecting patients or personnel from radiation.

> **nipple s.** A round plate with a short central projecting tube fitted with a rubber nipple; used to protect the irritated nipples of a nursing woman; the pressure from the infant's mouth is attenuated by the resistance of the rubber nipple.

shock (shok) A condition characterized by inadequate blood circulation through vital organs; clinical manifestations include pale clammy skin, weak rapid pulse, lowered blood pressure, and sometimes unconsciousness.

> **anaphylactic s.** See anaphylaxis.

> **cardiogenic s.** Shock resulting from inability of the heart to adequately pump blood through the vital organs due to a disease of the heart.

> **hypovolemic s.** Shock resulting from loss of circulating blood volume (e.g., due to hemorrhage).

> **neurogenic s.** Shock resulting from inadequate vasomotor tone; often seen in spinal cord injury.

> **septic s.** Shock resulting from a severe infection, most commonly a bacterial infection often associated with heavy invasion of the circulation with bacteria, or the release of bacterial toxins into the blood; the infective agents can also be viruses or protozoa.

show (sho) See bloody show.

shunt (shunt) 1. An abnormal communication between two natural channels; it may be congenital (e.g., between heart chambers, between chambers and blood vessels, or between blood vessels), or it may be an anastomosis surgically created to bypass an obstruction (e.g., to divert blood, cerebrospinal fluid, urine, or intestinal contents from one site to another). 2. To bypass or divert; to provide with a shunt surgically.

> **left-to-right s.** A diversion of blood either from the left to the right side of the heart through an abnormal opening (septal defect) between the atria or ventricles, or from the systemic to the pulmonary circulations through an abnormal channel (patent ductus arteriosus) between the aorta and the pulmonary trunk.

> **portacaval s.** A surgical communication made between the portal vein and the vena cava.

> **portasystemic s., portal-systemic s.** Any surgical communication established between the portal vein or its tributaries and those of the inferior vena cava.

> **ventriculoperitoneal s.** The establishment of a channel between a cerebral ventricle and the peritoneum by means of plastic tubing to allow circulation of the cerebrospinal fluid; performed for the treatment of hydrocephalus.

shunting (shun'ting) The surgical establishment of a shunt.

sievert (se'vert) (Sv) In the International System of Units (SI), the unit of ionizing radiation effective dose; 1 Sv equals 100 rem. See also effective dose and equivalent dose, under dose.

sigmoid (sig'moid) Having the shape of the letter S; applied to the distal portion of the descending colon (adjoining the rectum).

sigmoidectomy (sig-moi-dek'tŏ-me) Removal of part of the sigmoid colon; removal of the sigmoid flexure.

sigmoidoscope (sig-moi'do-skōp) Instrument for inspecting the interior of the sigmoid colon. Sometimes called sigmoscope.

sigmoidoscopy (sig-moi-dos'kŏ-pe) Visual examination of the interior of the sigmoid colon with a sigmoidoscope.

>**fiberoptic s.** Sigmoidoscopy performed with a flexible optical instrument that transmits images through a bundle of parallel fibers made of glass or plastic.

sign (sīn) Any objective evidence indicative of disease that is perceptible to the examiner. Some signs are deliberately elicited by means of tests for diagnostic purposes.

>**Baart de la Faille's s.** A finding associated with an interstitial pregnancy marked by a softening of the uterus compatible with an early pregnancy modified by a broad, soft-based extension outward.

>**banana s.** An abnormal curvature of the fetal cerebellum, as observed in ultrasonography; it is a sign of spina bifida.

>**Calkin's s.** The change in shape of the uterus at the time of delivery, from discoid to ovoid, indicating separation of the placenta.

>**Chadwick's s.** Bluish coloration of the vagina and cervix due to congestion of blood vessels; considered a probable sign of early pregnancy.

>**Cullen's s.** Bluish coloration of the skin around the navel, seen in intraperitoneal hemorrhage. Also called periumbilical ecchymosis.

>**double-bubble s.** The x-ray appearance of two distended sites in the gastrointestinal tract, one in the stomach and the other in the duodenum, due to the presence of gas. In the fetus, the distentions are filled with fluid and are observed by ultrasonography.

>**Goodell's s.** Bluish coloration and softening of the uterine cervix, suggestive but not conclusive of an early pregnancy.

>**halo s.** A radiologic sign of a dead or dying fetus; the subcutaneous layer of fat over the fetal head appears elevated.

>**Hegar's s.** Increased softening of the lower portion of the uterus (isthmus), occurring about 6 to 8 weeks after the onset of the last menstrual period; it is detected through bimanual palpation and is a reasonably reliable sign of early pregnancy.

>**Ladin's s.** A small soft area on the anterior aspect of the uterocervical junction, at the midline; a probable sign of pregnancy.

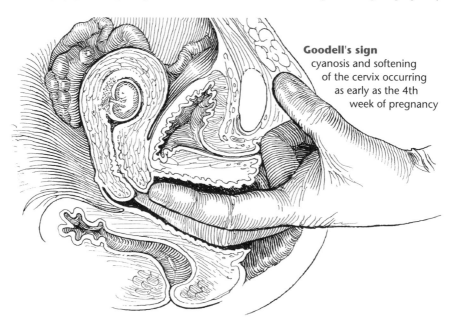

Goodell's sign
cyanosis and softening
of the cervix occurring
as early as the 4th
week of pregnancy

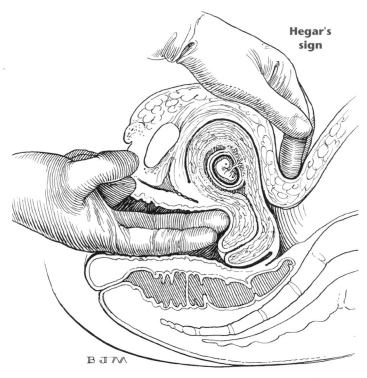

Hegar's sign

B JM

Latzko's s. See intermittent hydrosalpinx, under hydrosalpinx.

lemon s. A concave or flattened frontal contour of the fetal cranium, detected by ultrasonography; it results from scalloping of the frontal bones and may indicate the presence of spina bifida.

McDonald's s. Flexibility of the uterus at the uterocervical junction, detected at 7 to 8 weeks of gestation.

placental s. See implantation bleeding, under bleeding.

Robert's s. The presence of gas in the fetal great vessels observed in x-ray pictures, indicating intrauterine death of the fetus.

Spalding's s. Overlapping of the fetal skull bones observed in x-ray pictures, indicating intrauterine death of the fetus.

vital s.'s (VS) Breathing, heartbeat, sustained blood pressure, and temperature; the signs of life.

signaling (sig'nal-ing) The act of communicating something to incite an action.

preimplantation s. The phenomenon whereby the embryo induces the production of early pregnancy factor (EPF) by the maternal ovary to facilitate implantation.

sincipital (sin-sip'ĭ-tal) Relating to the forehead and upper part of the head.

sinciput (sin'sĭ-put) The upper frontal surface of the head.

sinus (si'nus) **1.** Any cavity within a bone normally filled with air. **2.** A wide channel normally conveying body fluids (i.e., blood, lymph, or aqueous humor). **3.** Abnormal channel or tract (e.g., one leading from an abscess, permitting escape of pus).

anal s. One of several small recesses, between folds of mucous membrane, in the posterior upper end of the anal canal. Also

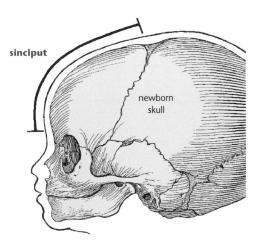

sinciput

newborn skull

called anal crypt.

lactiferous s. The normal enlargement of a milk (lactiferous) duct within the breast, just before it enters the nipple. It serves as a reservoir of milk.

pilonidal s. An abnormal pit or tract containing hairs, usually occurring in the upper part of the cleft between the buttocks. Also called pilonidal fistula.

skull (skul) The bony framework of the head; includes the bones encasing the brain and the bones of the face.

tower s. See oxycephaly.

smear (smēr) A specimen spread thinly on a glass slide for examination under the microscope; it may or may not be fixed and stained prior to examination.

cervical s. General term for specimens obtained from the uterine cervix or cervical canal (e.g., for the detection of infection, cancer, or infertility, or for hormonal evaluation).

cytologic s. A thin layer of cells spread on a glass slide, then fixed and stained for examination under a microscope. Also called cytosmear.

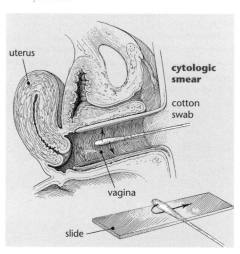

FGT cytologic s. Female genital tract cytologic smear; any cytologic smear obtained from the female genital tract.

Pap s., Papanicolaou s. A smear containing cells from the vaginal wall and the uterine cervix. See also Pap test, under test; Bethesda System of Classification, under classification.

vaginal s. A smear of secretions collected from the vaginal walls with a cotton-tipped applicator or a wooden spatula.

VCE s. A cytologic smear obtained from the vagina, cervix, and cervical canal (endocervix), spread separately on one slide in that order, and fixed; used for identification of the sites of disease.

wet Pap s. A Pap smear that is spread on a slide and immediately examined under the microscope.

snare (snār) An instrument with a wire loop for removing a polyp or tumor by tightening the loop around its base.

sodomy (sod'o-me) Sexual practice in which the penis is introduced into the anus or mouth of another person, male or female.

solution (sŏ-loo'shun) **1.** A mixture of a gaseous, liquid, or solid substance (solute) with a liquid or noncrystalline solid (solvent), and from which the dissolved substance can be recovered. **2.** The process of making such a mixture.

hypertonic s. A solution that has higher osmotic pressure than a standard of reference (e.g., a solution of sodium chloride having a higher osmotic pressure than blood plasma); often denotes a solution that, when surrounding a cell, causes water to leave the cell through the semipermeable cell membrane.

intra-amniotic hyperosmotic s.'s Solutions (e.g., hypertonic saline and hyperosmotic urea) injected into the amniotic sac during the second trimester of pregnancy to induce abortion. Because of complications (sometimes fatal), this method of inducing abortion has been largely replaced by dilatation and evacuation (D & E).

Lugol's s. A solution of 5% iodine and 10% potassium iodide containing 126 ng/ml of iodine, used in screening for cervical neoplasia. See also Schiller's test, under test.

saline s. A solution of any salt, especially of table salt (sodium chloride) in purified water. Commonly called saline.

Schiller's s. A solution of 1 g of pure iodine and 2 g of potassium iodide dissolved in 300 cm³ of water, used in screening for cervical neoplasia. See also Schiller's test, under test.

somato- Combining form meaning body.

somatotropin (so-mă-to-tro'pin) See growth hormone, under hormone.

somatosexual (so-mă-to-sek'shoo-al) Relating to the physical sexual (as opposed to psychosexual) characteristics of an individual; usually refers to physical manifestations of sexual development.

somite (so'mīt) One of paired, segmented blocks of epithelioid cells on either side of the neural tube of the embryo; they give rise to connective tissue, bone, muscle, and skin; the size of the

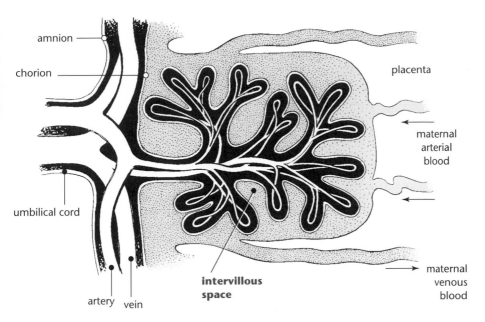

amnion

chorion

placenta

maternal arterial blood

umbilical cord

artery vein

intervillous space

maternal venous blood

embryo may be expressed in terms of the number of somites.

sonogram (so'no-gram) See ultrasonogram.

sonograph (so'no-graf) See ultrasonograph.

sonography (so-nog'ră-fe) See ultrasonography.

sonolucent (so-no-loo'sent) See anechoic.

sore (sor) **1.** Common term for any open skin lesion. **2.** Aching.

    hard s. See chancre.

    soft s. See chancroid.

souffle (soo'fl) A sound, heard on auscultation, which has a soft blowing quality.

    fetal s. A blowing, whistling sound synchronous with the fetal heartbeat, heard during late pregnancy; caused by blood flowing through the umbilical vessels when the cord is subject to torsion, tension, or pressure. Also called funic souffle; umbilical souffle.

    funic s. See fetal souffle.

    mammary s. A blowing murmur heard at the medial border of a breast during late pregnancy and lactation; attributed to a change of dynamics in blood flow through the internal thoracic (mammary) artery.

    placental s. See uterine souffle.

    umbilical s. See fetal souffle.

    uterine s. A sound heard over the uterus in late pregnancy, synchronous with the maternal heartbeat; caused by the blood flow through engorged uterine blood vessels; also may be heard in nonpregnant women with large myomatous tumors of the uterus or with enlarged ovaries. Also called placental souffle.

sound (sownd) A cylindrical, usually curved, instrument for exploring body cavities or for dilating a canal or tubular structure.

sounding (sownd'ing) Introduction of a sound into a cavity, canal, channel, or any tubular structure.

    uterine s. Introduction of a sound into the cavity of the uterus through the cervical canal.

space (spas) Any body area between specified boundaries; a delimited three-dimensional area.

    Douglas' s. See rectouterine pouch, under pouch.

    epidural s. The space between the dura mater of the spinal cord and the periosteum of the vertebral canal; it contains loose areolar and fibrous tissue, as well as a plexus of veins.

    intervillous s. The space in the placenta in which maternal blood bathes the chorionic villi, thus allowing exchange of materials between the fetal and maternal circulations; it is bounded by the chorionic plate on the fetal side and by the basal plate on the maternal side.

    paravesical s. One of two spaces bordered anteriorly by the pubic symphysis, posteriorly by the transverse cervical ligament, laterally by the internal obturator muscle, and medially by a medial umbilical ligament.

    presacral s. The area between the parietal peritoneum and the anterior aspect of the sacrum. It is continuous with the retrorectal space.

    prevesical s. See retropubic space.

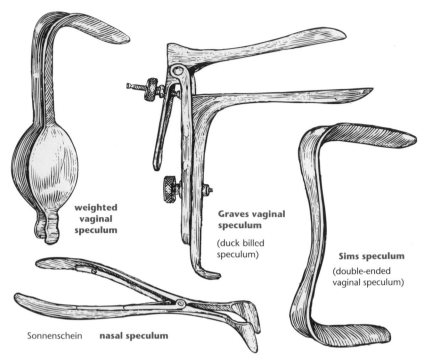

weighted vaginal speculum

Graves vaginal speculum

(duck billed speculum)

Sims speculum

(double-ended vaginal speculum)

Sonnenschein **nasal speculum**

rectouterine s. See rectouterine pouch, under pouch.

rectovaginal s. The space between the posterior wall of the vagina and the rectum, from the perineal body to the peritoneal fold forming the rectouterine pouch.

retromammary s. The area of loose connective tissue between the breast and the deep fascia covering the chest muscles. Also called submammary space.

retroperitoneal s. The space between the posterior parietal peritoneum and the muscles and bones of the posterior abdominal wall; it is occupied by the kidneys, adrenal glands, pancreas, ureters, duodenum, ascending and descending colon, and nerves and vessels.

retropubic s. The fat-filled area of loose connective tissue bordered anteriorly by the pubic bone and transversalis fascia and posteriorly by the anterior wall of the bladder and the umbilical prevesical fascia; it extends up to the umbilicus between the medial umbilical ligaments. Also called prevesical space; Retzius' space.

retrorectal s. The area between the anterior aspect of the sacrum and the rectum. It is continuous with the presacral space.

Retzius' s. See retropubic space.

submammary s. See retromammary space.

vesicovaginal s. The space between the

posterior wall of the bladder and the anterior wall of the vagina and extending down to the upper end of the urethra.

specific (spĕ-sif'ik) **1.** Relating to a single disease. **2.** A remedy intended for a particular disease. **3.** In immunology, a special affinity, such as that of an antibody for the corresponding antigen.

specificity (spes-ĭ-fis'ĭ-te) The state of being specific.

diagnostic s. Applied to a screening test: the proportion of individuals who are truly free of a disease in a screened population, and who are identified as such by the test (i.e., it is a measure of the probability that a disease-free person will be correctly identified by the screening test).

speculum (spek'u-lum), pl. specula Instrument for dilating and holding open the orifice of a body cavity or canal to facilitate inspection of its interior.

duckbill s. See Graves vaginal speculum.

Graves vaginal s. A two-valved speculum used in examination of the adult vagina; available in small, medium, and large sizes. Also called duckbill speculum.

Huffman-Graves s. A narrow variation of the Graves speculum, designed for use in a patient with a small vaginal opening such as seen in adolescents.

nasal s. A small, short-bladed speculum for

inspecting the cavity of the nose; also used to inspect a child's vagina.

Pederson's s. A speculum similar to the Huffman-Graves speculum and used for the same purposes.

Sims s. A double-ended, retractor-like vaginal speculum.

vaginal s. Any of several specula designed for inspection of the vagina.

weighted vaginal s. A single blade retractor-like vaginal speculum with a weighted element that frees both hands of the examiner or surgeon; frequently used on obese patients and patients that have borne many children.

sperm (sperm) See spermatozoon.

spermatic (sper-mat'ik) Relating to sperm.

spermatid (sper'mă-tid) One of the four cells resulting from the division of the spermatocyte; it develops into the spermatozoon without further division.

spermatoblast (sper'mă-to-blast) See spermatogonium.

spermatocide (sper-mat'ŏ-sīd) See spermicide.

spermatocyte (sper-mat'o-sīt) One of the spherical cells housed in the wall of a seminiferous tubule of the testis; it represents an early stage in the development of a spermatozoon.

primary s. A large cell in the outer wall of the seminiferous tubule resulting from the mitotic division of a type B spermatogonium (stem cell); it contains the full diploid number of chromosomes (46).

secondary s. A cell resulting from the meiotic division of the primary spermatocyte; it contains the haploid number of chromosomes (23) and represents the first reduction division, followed by the second reduction division (by mitosis) which results in two spermatids.

spermatocytogenesis (sper-mat-ŏ-si-tŏ-jen'ĕ-sis) The mitotic proliferation of the undifferentiated germ cell (spermatogonium) and development of first spermatocytes, then spermatids; first stage in the process of sperm differentiation in the testis.

spermatogenesis (sper-mat-ŏ-jen'e-sis) The whole process of formation of spermatozoa, including spermatocytogenesis and spermiogenesis, carried out in the seminiferous tubules of the testis.

spermatogenetic (sper-mat-ŏ-je-net'ik) See spermatogenic.

spermatogenic (sper-mat-ŏ-jen'ik) Sperm-producing. Also called spermatogenetic.

spermatogonium (sper-mat-ŏ-go'ne-um), pl.

spermatogonia An undifferentiated young cell located in the seminiferous tubules of the testis; it either gives rise to new spermatogonia (type A) or differentiates to a more developed primary spermatocyte (type B), which eventually becomes a spermatozoon. Also called spermatoblast.

spermatolysin (sper-mă-tol'ĭ-sin) A specific antibody to spermatozoa formed in the female following exposure to spermatozoa.

spermatolysis (sper-mă-tol'ĭ-sis) Destruction and dissolution of spermatozoa.

spermatolytic (sper-mă-to-lit'ik) Destructive to spermatozoa.

spermatozoa (sper-mă-to-zo'ă) Plural of spermatozoon.

spermatozoon (sper-mă-to-zo'on), pl. spermatozoa The mature male sex cell produced in the testes; in humans, it consists of an ovoid head (4 to 6 μm long) containing the nucleus, a short neck (0.3 μm), a middle section (4 μm) containing mitochondria, and a long motile tail (40 to 50 μm), containing circular fibers, by means of which the cell moves up through the female reproductive

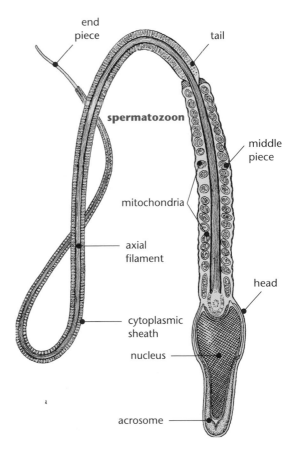

end piece

tail

spermatozoon

middle piece

mitochondria

axial filament

head

cytoplasmic sheath

nucleus

acrosome

tract to fertilize the ovum. Also called sperm; sperm cell.

spermicide (sper'mĭ-sīd) Any agent that kills spermatozoa. Also called spermatocide.

spermiogenesis (sper-me-o-jen'ĕ-sis) Second stage in the formation of spermatozoa (spermatogenesis) during which the immature round cell (spermatid) transforms morphologically and biochemically into the elongated testicular spermatozoon.

sphincter (sfingk'ter) **1.** Any circular muscle that normally maintains constriction of a natural body opening and that is capable of relaxing in order to permit passage of substances through the opening. **2.** A portion of a tubular structure that functions as a sphincter.

    anal s. *External anal s:* a flat, elliptical band of muscle fibers encircling the anal opening; consists of three parts: subcutaneous, superficial and deep; it closes the anal canal and anus. *Internal anal s:* a muscular ring formed from the thickened inner circular coat adjacent to the caudal end of the rectum, and surrounding about 2.5 cm of the anal canal; it is in contact with, but separate from, the external anal sphincter; it closes the anal canal and anus.

    artificial urethral s. A sphincter created by surgical procedures for the treatment of urinary incontinence; designed for patients for whom standard surgical procedures are contraindicated.

    s. of bladder A thickening of the middle, circular layer of muscle fibers of the bladder surrounding the internal urethral opening at the neck of the bladder; it is composed of nonstriated (smooth) muscle and is not under voluntary control. Along with the sphincter of the urethra, it controls the urine outflow from the bladder. Also called sphincter vesicae; vesicular sphincter.

    s. of urethra A flat muscle that closely surrounds the terminal part of the urethra in the female and the membranous portion of the urethra in the male; it is composed of striated muscle and is normally under voluntary control after early infancy. Along with the vesicular sphincter, it controls the urine outflow from the bladder by compressing the urethra. Also called sphincter urethrae.

    s. urethrae See sphincter of urethra.

    s. vesicae See sphincter of bladder.

    vesicular s. See sphincter of bladder.

sphingomyelin (sfing-go-mi'ĕ-lin) Any of a group of phospholipids present in large quantities in brain and nerve tissue.

spider (spi'der) **1.** Any arachnid with four pairs of legs, a body divided into a cephalothorax and an abdomen, a complex of spinnerets, and a cluster of up to eight eyes. **2.** A spider-shaped pattern.

    arterial s. See spider telangiectasia, under telangiectasia.

    vascular s. See spider telangiectasia, under telangiectasia.

spin- Combining form meaning spine.

spina (spi'na), pl. spinae **1.** The vertebral column. **2.** Any sharp bony projection.

    s. bifida Congenital defect of the vertebral column in which the posterior portion (vertebral arch) of one or several vertebrae fails to develop; the resulting gap allows spinal membranes, and sometimes the spinal cord and nerve roots, to protrude. Also called cleft spine.

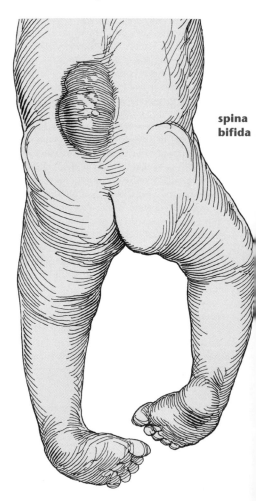

spina bifida

s. bifida occulta Spina bifida without protrusion of the spinal cord or its membranes.

spindle (spin'dl) Any spindle-shaped or fusiform anatomic structure.

    achromatic s. See mitotic spindle.

    central s. The middle mitotic spindle between the centrioles in a dividing cell.

    Krukenberg s.'s Spindle-shaped, brownish-red opacities on the inner (posterior) surface of the cornea; they occur with increased frequency in the pregnant state.

    mitotic s. The fusiform figure in the nucleus of a dividing cell; formed by fine, viscous microtubules extending between the two centrioles and connecting the chromosomes at their centromeres. Also called achromatic spindle; nuclear spindle.

    nuclear s. See mitotic spindle.

spine (spīn) 1. A sharp-pointed projection of bone. 2. The vertebral column; see under column. 3. A short projection.

    cleft s. See spina bifida, under spina.

    iliac s. Any of the four spines of the ilium (lateral part of the hipbone). *Anterior inferior iliac s.*, the blunt projection on the front border of the ilium just above the anterior part of the acetabulum; it provides attachment to the rectus muscle of the thigh (rectus femoris muscle) and to the iliofemoral ligament. *Anterior superior iliac s.*, the spine forming the front end of the crest of the ilium; it provides attachment to the lateral end of the inguinal ligament and, just below, to the sartorius muscle. *Posterior inferior iliac s.*, the wide projection at the lower end of the posterior border of the ilium, where it makes a sharp bend forward to form the upper border of the greater sciatic notch; it provides attachment to the piriform muscle. *Posterior superior iliac s.*, the spine forming the back end of the crest of the ilium; it provides attachment to the sacrotuberal ligament and the dorsal (posterior) sacroiliac ligament; the spine cannot usually be felt, but its position is indicated by a prominent dimple lateral to the second spinous tubercle of the sacrum.

    ischial s. A bony spine situated on the posterior aspect of the ischium (posterior part of the hipbone) near the posteroinferior border of the acetabulum; it provides attachment to the sacrospinal ligament. Also called sciatic spine.

    pubic s. See pubic tubercle, under tubercle.

    sciatic s. See ischial spine.

spinnbarkeit (spin'bar-kīt) A state of extreme stretchability of the cervical mucus, which, when spread on a glass slide, dries in a fernlike pattern; indicative of ovulation; it peaks on the 14th day of the menstrual cycle. Also spelled spinnbarkheit.

spironolactone (sper-o-no-lak'tōn) Diuretic drug that blocks the action of the adrenal hormone aldosterone on the kidney tubules, producing sodium loss with potassium retention. Also used in the treatment of androgen excess. Adverse effects may include numbness, weakness, nausea, and vomiting. It has a potential risk of causing antiandrogenic effects on the fetus when taken during pregnancy.

spondyloschisis (spon-dī-los'kī-sis) A congenital cleft in the vertebral arch of one or more vertebrae.

sponge (spunj) 1. The skeleton of some marine animals. 2. A piece of cotton, folded gauze, or rolled collagen.

    absorbable gelatin s. An absorbable, gelatin-based sponge used to control bleeding.

spot (spot) 1. A small, circumscribed area that differs in color from its surroundings. 2. To discharge a slight amount of blood through the vagina.

    blue s. (1) A bluish mark on the skin caused by the bite of a flea or lice. (2) See mongolian spot.

    mongolian s. A bluish or purplish area on the skin present at birth; a type of birthmark most commonly occurring on the lower back over the sacrum, but occasionally noted on the shoulders, back, and buttocks; usually fades over the years but traces may persist into adulthood. The lesion may be mistaken for a bruise, causing suspicion of child abuse. Also called blue spot.

    soft s. See fontanel.

spotting (spot'ing) Slight, unexpected vaginal bleeding; it may be insignificant (e.g., occurring as the fertilized ovum attaches to the uterine wall), or it may indicate an abnormal condition.

spread (spred) 1. To disseminate; applied to an infectious disease. 2. See metastasize.

squama (skwa'mă), pl. squamae 1. A thin plate of bone. 2. A scalelike structure.

squamous (skwa'mus) 1. Scaly. 2. Resembling scales.

stage (stāj) 1. A phase in any process, such as the course of a disease, the life cycle of an organism, a physiologic development, or a procedure. 2. The platform of a microscope on which the slide with the specimen is placed for viewing.

    incubative s. See incubation period, under period.

STAGING CRITERIA FOR CLASSIFICATION OF MELANOMAS

CLARK'S STAGING		BRESLOW'S STAGING	
Stage	**Invasion level**	**Stage**	**Tumor thickness**
I	Melanoma in situ: above basement membrane	I Ia Ib	0.75 mm or less 0.75 mm or less 0.75 mm to 1.5mm
II	Tumor passes through basement membrane; invades papillary dermis	II IIa IIb	 1.5 to 3.99 mm > 4.00 mm
III	Tumor extends through papillary dermis and touches on reticular dermis but does not penetrate it	III	Tumor has spread
IV	Tumor extends into the reticular dermis		
V	Tumor has invaded subcutaneous tissue		

indifferent gonad s. The stage during the fifth week of gestation (prior to gonad differentiation into ovaries or testes) in which the midportion of each urogenital ridge thickens with a condensed cell mass, forming the gonadal ridge, which morphologically is neither an ovary nor a testis; the stage lasts 7 to 10 days.

s.'s of labor. See labor.

latent s. See latent period (1), under period.

staging (stā'jing) A clinical method of providing an estimate of the gravity of a cancerous tumor, based on the size of the primary tumor and the extent of local and distant spread. Also called tumor staging.

Haagensen s. A four-stage clinical staging for cancer of the breast. *Stage A*, no skin edema, ulceration, or solid fixation to skin or chest wall; clinically negative axillary nodes. *Stage B*, no skin edema, ulceration, or solid fixation to skin or chest wall; nodes are palpable (but are not larger than 2.5 cm in transverse diameter). *Stage C*, presence of any five of the following grave signs: edema of skin (less than one-third of breast surface), skin ulceration, solid fixation to chest wall, massive size of axillary nodes (more than 2.5 cm in transverse diameter), fixation of axillary nodes

to skin or deep structures. *Stage D*, encompasses all advanced tumors, including any combination of two or more grave signs of stage C; extensive edema (more than one-third of breast surface), satellite skin nodules, inflammatory carcinoma; parasternal tumor of internal mammary nodes, edema of arm, distant metastasis.

TNM (tumor-node-metastasis) s. An international system for staging tumors, used as a basis for treating cancer; it measures three basic parameters: T for the size and local invasion of the primary tumor, N for the number of involved lymph nodes, M for the presence of metastasis; each letter is followed by a number, from 0 through 4, to indicate the extent of tissue involvement. Lower case letters are sometimes added as a means of providing additional information: aTNM (autopsy staging), cTNM (clinical-diagnostic staging), pTNM (post-surgical pathologic staging), rTNM (retreatment staging), sTNM (surgical-evaluation staging).

tumor s. See staging.

staining (stā'ning) **1.** The act of applying an artificial color. **2.** Modification of the natural color of a tissue or structure.

meconium s. A greenish-brown discoloration of the fetal membranes caused by the presence of meconium in the amniotic fluid; a frequent occurrence after 40 weeks of gestation.

stalk (stawk) An elongated connection resembling a stem; a pedicle.

    allantoic s. A narrow connection between the urogenital sinus of the embryo and the allantoic sac.

    body s. A precursor of the umbilical cord, composed of a mesenchymal mass of tissue connecting the ventral portion of the tail end of the embryo to the inner face of the chorionic vesicle.

    yolk s. The stalk connecting the yolk sac to the ventral aspect of a young embryo.

standard (stan'dard) A unit or specification established as a measure or model for comparison, uniformity, or control.

    s. of care A description of the conduct expected of an individual in a given situation regarding the care of a patient.

    minimum s. A standard of medical care based on the modes of treatment employed by the members of a medical specialty group in good standing.

staphylococci (staf-ĭ-lo-kok'si) Plural of staphylococcus.

Staphylococcus (staf-ĭ-lo-kok'us) Genus of Gram-positive, nonmotile bacteria (family Micrococcaceae) that tend to aggregate in grapelike clusters.

    S. aureus A species often carried in the nasal cavity; it is the causative agent of boils, carbuncles, abscesses, and other pus-forming infections.

    S. epidermidis A variety normally present on the skin, causing minor infections in skin wounds (e.g., stitch abscesses).

staphylococcus (staf-ĭ-lo-kok'us), pl. staphylococci Any microorganism of the genus *Staphylococcus.*

stasis (sta'sis) Reduction or stoppage of a flow (e.g., of blood or lymph).

    venous s. Impairment or cessation of blood flow in a vein. Also called hypostatic congestion.

stathmokinesis (stath-mo-kĭ-ne'sis) The arresting of mitosis (e.g., by a drug used in chemotherapy).

station (sta'shun) The position of the presenting part of the fetus in the birth canal, relative to the level of the maternal ischial spines; designated –3 to +3 (if the long axis of the birth canal is divided into thirds above and below the level of the spines), or –5 to +5 (depending on the number of centimeters the presenting part is above or below the spines).

status (sta'tus, stat'us) State; condition.

    Karnofsky performance s. A system that employs numbers from 100 to 0 to evaluate the degree of gravity of a patient with epithelial ovarian cancer: 100 (no complaints, no evidence of disease); 90 (able to conduct normal activities, minor signs or symptoms of disease); 80 (able to conduct normal activities with effort, some signs or symptoms of disease); 70 (able to care for self but unable to conduct normal activities or perform active work); 60 (needs occasional help but is able to care for personal needs); 50 (needs considerable assistance and frequent medical care); 40 (disabled, needs special care and assistance); 30 (severely disabled, hospitalization indicated); 20 (sick, needs hospitalization and active support treatment); 10 (near death and worsening rapidly); 0 (dead).

    Zubrod s. A system of numbers from 0 to 4 for evaluating the condition of a patient with epithelial ovarian cancer: 0 (no symptoms); 1 (symptoms present but patient is fully ambulatory); 2 (requires nursing help, is bedridden less than 50% of the day); 3 (bedridden more than 50% of the day); 4 (bedridden constantly).

stenion (sten'e-on) One of two craniometric points on the temporal areas of the skull, at each end of the shortest transverse diameter.

stenosis (stĕ-no'sis), pl. stenoses Abnormal constriction or narrowness of a channel or an opening.

    cervical s. Pathologic constriction of the internal opening of the cervix, causing scanty or absent menstruation and cyclic uterine pain; may result from injury to the tissues (e.g., during an abortion performed with minimal cervical dilatation).

stenotic (stĕ-not'ik) Affected with stenosis; abnormally narrowed.

stent (stent) A device used for support of a tubular structure during a surgical procedure (e.g., anastomosis), or of a body orifice or cavity during skin grafting. Also used in a blood vessel or ureter after correction of a blockage.

    urethral s. Device for keeping open the urethral channel (urethra) when compressed by an enlarged prostate.

stenting (stent'ing) The placing of a stent in a body structure.

sterile (ster'il) **1.** Incapable of reproducing. **2.** Free from living disease-causing microorganisms.

sterility (stĕ-ril'ĭ-te) **1.** Inability to produce offspring. In males, lack of sperm production; in females, inability to conceive. Sterility may or may not be reversible. Compare with infertility. **2.** The state of being free from living microorganisms.

sterilization (ster-ĭ-lĭ-za'shun) **1.** Destruction or elimination of living microorganisms by physical methods, chemical agents, or filtration. **2.** A treatment that deprives living organisms of the ability to reproduce.

  female s. See tubal sterilization.

  Irving s. See Irving's operation, under operation.

  Kroener s. See fimbriectomy.

  Madlener s. See Madlener's operation, under operation.

  male s. See vasectomy.

  Pomeroy s. See Pomeroy's operation, under operation.

  tubal s. Sterilization of the female by any of several surgical techniques performed on the fallopian (uterine) tubes; may be a tying (ligation) of the tubes, constriction of a small loop of the tubes with a tight band, insertion of a plastic or metal clip on each tube, electrocoagulation of tubal tissues, or cutting away a section of the tubes or their fimbriated ends. Also called female sterilization. See also tubal ligation, under ligation.

  Uchida s. See Uchida procedure, under procedure.

sternad (ster'nad) Toward or in the direction of the breastbone (sternum).

sternal (ster'nal) Relating to the breastbone (sternum).

sterno-, stern- Combining forms meaning sternum.

sternoclavicular (ster-no-klă-vik'u-lar) Relating to the breastbone (sternum) and the collarbone (clavicle). Also called sternocleidal.

sternum (ster'num) A long, flat bone forming the middle part of the anterior wall of the thoracic cage; composed of three parts: manubrium, body, and xiphoid process; it articulates with both clavicles and cartilages of the first seven pairs of ribs. Commonly called breastbone.

steroid (ste'roid) One of a large family of chemical substances that includes the adrenocortical hormones, the male and female sex hormones, and the D vitamins.

  anabolic s. Any of a group of drugs with protein-building properties that are synthetic derivatives of the male hormone testosterone; they help to strengthen bones and to accelerate muscle recovery after injury caused by strenuous exercise. Anabolic steroids have been abused by athletes, resulting in severe depression upon withdrawal; other adverse

effects of abuse include acne, baldness, liver and adrenal gland damage, infertility and impotence in men, and virilization in women; if taken in childhood, they may stunt growth.

steroid 17α-hydroxylase/17,20-lyse ($P450_{17\alpha}$) Enzyme that has a crucial role in the formation of androgen-like compounds such as testosterone, androstenedione, and dehydroepiandrosterone.

stimulation (stim-u-la'shun) **1.** The act of exciting the body or any of its parts to increased functional activity. **2.** The state of being stimulated.

  vibroacoustic s. A technique to assess the fetal condition. An artificial larynx is placed 1 cm above or on the maternal abdomen and is activated for several seconds. A normal response is considered to be a fetal heart rate acceleration of at least 15 beats per minute for at least 15 seconds of the stimulus. This is usually accompanied by prolonged fetal movements.

stimulator (stim'u-la-tor) **1.** See stimulant. **2.** Any device for delivering low voltage electrical stimuli to any part of the body.

  long-acting thyroid s. (LATS) A substance found in the blood of most patients with Graves' disease; it mimics the stimulating action of the hormone thyrotropin but its effect on the thyroid gland is more prolonged.

stone (stōn) An abnormal concretion in the body, usually in the lumen of ducts or hollow organs, formed by accumulation of mineral salts. Also called calculus.

  kidney s. Stone formed in the kidney, ranging in size from a tiny particle to a large concretion filling the renal pelvis; usually composed of calcium oxalate, calcium phosphate, and uric acid. Also called renal calculus; nephrolith.

  urinary s. Concretion formed anywhere within the urinary tract (kidney, ureter, bladder, urethra); frequently causing obstruction, bleeding, and pain. Also called urinary calculus; urolith.

  vesical s. Concretion formed or retained in the bladder. Also called cystolith; vesical calculus.

storm (storm) A sudden increase in the severity of an illness.

  thyroid s. See thyrotoxic crisis, under crisis.

strain (strān) In bacteriology, a group of microorganisms originating from a common ancestor and retaining the characteristics of the ancestor.

strait (strāt) A narrow space or passage.

inferior pelvic s. See pelvic plane of outlet, under plane.

superior pelvic s. See pelvic plane of inlet, under plane.

stratum (stra'tum), pl. strata Latin for layer, especially of differentiated tissue comprising one of several associated layers. See layer.

s. basale See basal layer, under layer.

s. compactum See compact layer, under layer.

s. functionale See functional layer, under layer.

s. spongiosum See spongy layer, under layer.

streptococcal (strep-to-kok'al) Relating to streptococcus.

streptococcemia (strep-to-kok-se'me-ă) The presence of streptococci in the blood.

streptococci (strep-to-kok'si) Plural of streptococcus.

Streptococcus (strep-to-kok'us) A genus of Gram-positive round or ovoid bacteria occurring in pairs or in chains held together by incomplete wall separation; some species occur harmlessly in the mouth, throat, or intestinal tract of humans; others can cause disease. They are classified according to their hemolytic activity on blood agar into alpha-, beta-, or gamma-streptococci and according to their antigenic composition into groups A through O.

streptococcus (strep-to-kok'us), pl. streptococci Any member of the genus *Streptococcus*.

group B s. A group frequently causing vaginal and rectal infections in women during pregnancy and the postpartum period; the organisms are the major cause of sepsis and meningitis in newborn infants, who acquire the infection just before or during passage through the mother's infected birth canal; they also cause urinary tract infection of nonpregnant women, especially those who have an underlying chronic condition (e.g., diabetes mellitus).

streptomycin (strep-to-mi'-sin) An antibiotic obtained from *Streptomyces griseus*, formerly used to treat a variety of infections, especially tuberculosis; excessive dosage may damage the vestibulocochlear (8th cranial) nerve, disturbing balance and causing ringing in the ears and hearing impairment. Intrauterine exposure causes similar damage to the fetus.

stress (stres) Any physical or psychological condition that tends to disrupt the normal functions of the body or mind.

stria (stri'ă), pl. striae A thin stripe or line on a tissue, especially one of several that are more or less parallel.

striae atrophicae A series of glistening white streaks in the skin of the abdomen, buttocks, thighs, and breasts caused by overstretching and weakening of elastic tissues; associated with pregnancy, obesity, rapid growth during puberty, and Cushing's syndrome. Also called gravidic lines; lineae albicantes; lineae atrophicae; lineae gravidarum; stretch marks; striae distensae; striae gravidarum.

striae distensae See striae atrophicae.

striae gravidarum See striae atrophicae.

Rohr s. Strands of fibrin occasionally present at the base of the intervillous space, where the invading trophoblast meets the decidua during early pregnancy.

striate, striated (stri'āt, stri'āt-ed) Having striae; striped.

stripe (strīp) A narrow layer or section differing in color or texture from adjacent parts.

endometrial s. The endometrium as it appears in ultrasonograms. Measurement of its thickness is useful in the management of abnormal uterine bleeding.

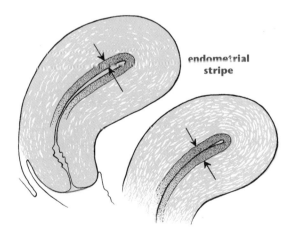

endometrial stripe

stroma (stro'ma) The supporting framework of an organ.

s. of ovary, s. ovarii The framework of the ovary composed of a dense network of reticular fibers and spindle-shaped cells in the superficial portion (cortex) of the ovary, and loose connective tissue with elastic fibers, nonstriated muscle cells, and abundant blood vessels (especially veins) in the inner portion (medulla).

stromal, stromic (stro'mal, stro'mik) Relating to

stroma.

stromatogenous (stro-mă-toj'ĕ-nus) Originating in the connective tissue of an organ.

struma (stroo'mă) Goiter.

>**Hashimoto's s.** See Hashimoto's thyroiditis, under thyroiditis.

>**s. lymphomatosa** See Hashimoto's thyroiditis, under thyroiditis.

>**s. ovarii** Benign tumor of the ovary composed entirely, or predominantly, of mature thyroid tissue; occasionally causes hyperthyroidism; may undergo malignant transformation.

>**Riedel's s.** See Riedel's thyroiditis, under thyroiditis.

stump (stump) The remaining portion of a partially resected structure (e.g., the remaining end of a limb after amputation).

>**cervical s.** The portion of the uterine cervix remaining after a subtotal hysterectomy.

stupor (stu'por) A state of semiconsciousness in which vigorous stimuli are needed to evoke a response.

sub- Prefix meaning under; secondary; less than completely.

subclavicular (sub-klă-vik'u-lar) Beneath the collarbone (clavicle).

subclinical (sub-klin'ĭ-kal) Without manifestation of symptoms; applied to a disease producing no symptoms because it is very mild or because it is at an early phase of its course.

subdural (sub-doo'ral) Located beneath or internal to the outer, fibrous covering of the brain and spinal cord (i.e., the dura mater).

subfertility (sub-fer-til'ĭ-te) Less than normal ability to reproduce.

subinvolution (sub-in-vo-lu'shun) Failure of an organ to return completely to its normal size, as when the uterus remains abnormally large after childbirth.

>**s. of placental site** Condition in which blood vessels at the implantation site of the placenta fail to obliterate completely following delivery, causing a persistent postpartum discharge (lochia) and bleeding.

substance (sub'stans) Matter; material of a specified constitution.

>**compact s. of bone** See compact bone, under bone.

>**cortical s. of bone** See compact bone, under bone.

>**mullerian-inhibiting s.** A glycoprotein produced by the Sertoli cells of the fetal testis; acting locally (unlike a hormone), it causes regression of the mullerian duct of the same side of its origin.

>**radiopaque s.** See contrast medium, under medium.

>**spongy s. of bone** See spongy bone, under bone.

suburethral (sub-u-re'thral) Beneath the urethra.

suction (suk'shun) Aspiration; sucking.

suctioning (suk'shun-ing) The act of aspirating or sucking (e.g., gas or fluid) by mechanical means.

>**nasopharyngeal s.** Suctioning of the nares, mouth, and pharynx of an infant at birth, as soon as the head is delivered.

sulfonamides (sul-fon'ă-mids) A group of synthetic antibacterial compounds effective against a wide range of Gram-positive and Gram-negative organisms; currently used only in specific circumstances. Commonly called sulfa drugs. When taken in pregnancy close to term, they may cause kernicterus in the newborn infant.

super- Prefix meaning above; excessive.

superfecundation (soo-per-fe-kun-da'shun) Fertilization of two ova within a short period of time (during the same ovulatory cycle) but not at the same sexual act and not necessarily by the same man.

superfetation (soo-per-fe-ta'shun) A theoretic situation in which two ova released at two consecutive cycles are fertilized, yielding two fetuses at one birth.

superovulation (soo-per-o-vu-la'shun) The production of a greater than normal number of ova, usually resulting from administration of gonadotropins (hormones) for assisted fertilization procedures.

supra- Prefix meaning above.

supraclavicular (soo-pră-klă-vik'u-lar) Above the collarbone (clavicle).

suprainguinal (soo-pră-in'gwi-nal) Above the groin.

suprapubic (soo-pră-pu'bik) Above the pubic arch.

suprasternal (soo-pră-ster'nal) Above the breastbone (sternum).

surfactant (sur-fak'tant) A surface-active lipoprotein, principally dipalmitoylphos-phatidylcholine, formed in pneumocytes that line the alveoli; it normally serves to decrease the surface tension of fluids within the alveoli; thus it permits lung tissues to expand during inspiration and prevents alveoli from collapsing and sticking together after each breath. In the fetus, it is produced after the 35th week of gestation; its appearance in the amniotic fluid is a marker for fetal lung maturity, and prevents respiratory

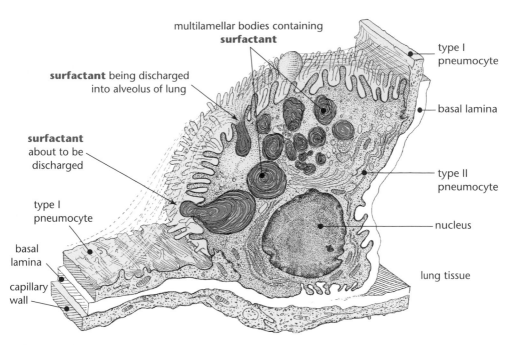

multilamellar bodies containing **surfactant**

surfactant being discharged into alveolus of lung

surfactant about to be discharged

type I pneumocyte

basal lamina

capillary wall

type I pneumocyte

basal lamina

type II pneumocyte

nucleus

lung tissue

distress syndrome from developing. Naturally-occurring and synthetic surfactants have been used for prophylaxis and rescue of newborns with respiratory distress syndrome.

surgery (sur'jer-e) Medical specialty concerned with the treatment of disease, injury, or deformity by means of manual and instrumental procedures.

　　ambulatory s. Operative procedures performed on an outpatient basis; may be performed in a physician's office, a surgical center, or a hospital. Also called outpatient surgery.

　　cytoreductive s. See debulking operation, under operation.

　　elective s. Surgery of a nonemergency nature; although recommended, it can be scheduled in advance without affecting the health of the patient or the expected result of the procedure.

　　exploratory s. Any operation performed to determine the extent of a disease or to establish a diagnosis.

　　outpatient s. See ambulatory surgery.

　　transexual s. A series of major operations on the genitourinary tract designed to change a person's anatomic gender. Procedures may include some or all of the following. *Male-to-female change:* breast implantation, removal of penile erectile tissue, repositioning of urethra, creation of a vaginal pouch, removal of testes, and creation of labia. *Female-to-male change:*

removal of breasts, uterus, and ovaries; formation of a penile graft, and reconstruction of a new urethra.

　　vaginal incontinence s. Any procedure for the surgical treatment of urinary stress incontinence in which the structures of concern (mainly the urethrovesical junction) are approached through the vagina, as opposed to an abdominal incision.

surveillance (sur-vāl'ans) **1.** Careful watching. **2.** An ongoing scrutiny of morbidity and mortality reports, identification of infectious agents, available vaccines, and other similar activities to detect changes in trend or distribution of a disease; the goal is to initiate control measures as soon as the need arises.

　　immunologic s. The concept that the immune system recognizes and destroys malignant cells as they arise.

survival (sur-vi'val) The act or process of remaining alive.

　　actuarial s. See life table, under table.

suture (soo'chur) **1.** Stitch or stitches used in surgery to unite two surfaces. **2.** To apply a surgical stitch. **3.** The material used in closing a wound with stitches. **4.** An immovable fibrous articulation uniting the bones of the cranium.

　　coronal s. The junction on top of the skull, between the posterior border of the frontal bone and the anterior borders of the two parietal bones.

frontal s. The suture between the two halves of the developing frontal bone, prior to complete ossification into one bone; ossification usually occurs from the second year of life to about the eighth year when the process is completed. Also called metopic suture.

lambdoid s. The junction between the occipital and parietal bones, at the back of the skull; it resembles the Greek letter lambda (λ). Also called parieto-occipital suture.

metopic s. See frontal suture.

parieto-occipital s. See lambdoid suture.

sagittal s. The median suture between the upper margins of the two parietal bones, at the top of the skull.

squamosoparietal s. See squamous suture.

squamous s. The suture on either side of the skull, between the squamous part of the temporal bone and the parietal bone.

swelling (swel'ing) **1.** A temporary enlargement that may or may not be inflammatory. **2.** In embryology, an elevation or protuberance indicating an early stage of development of certain structures.

genital s.'s In embryology, two pairs of swellings developed beside the opening of the urogenital sinus. In the female, they persist as the labia minora and majora; in the male, they undergo further development to form the scrotal pouch. Also called labioscrotal swellings.

labioscrotal s.'s See genital swellings.

sympathomimetic (sim-pă-tho-mĭ-met'ik) Producing effects similar to those of the sympathetic nervous system.

symphysial, symphyseal (sim-fiz'e-al) Relating to a symphysis.

symphysis (sim'fĭ-sis), pl. symphyses **1.** A type of articulation in which the two opposing bone surfaces are covered with a thin layer of hyaline cartilage and united by a plate of fibrocartilage. **2.** In pathology, the abnormal fusion of two surfaces.

pubic s. The symphysis between the pubic bones at the anterior plane of the pelvis; the bones are united by an interpubic disk of fibrocartilage, and by the superior pubic ligament above and the arcuate pubic ligament below.

synchondrosis (sin-kon-dro'sis), pl. synchondroses The union of two bones by cartilage; usually the cartilage is replaced by bone (e.g., the junction between skull bones or the pelvic bones of the newborn infant).

synclitism (sin'klit-izm) The attitude of the fetal

head in relation to the maternal pelvis as it descends into the pelvis; the head enters the pelvis with its sagittal suture in the transverse plane of the maternal pelvis, midway between the pubic bone and the sacrum. Also called obliquity.

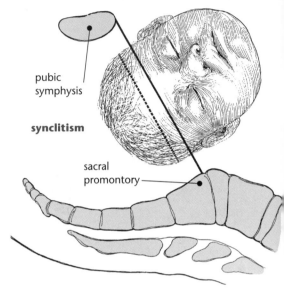

pubic symphysis

synclitism

sacral promontory

syncytiotrophoblast (sin-sit-e-o-trof'o-blast) In embryology, the peripheral part of the trophoblast; it penetrates maternal tissues to attach the blastocyst to the uterus and eventually enters into the formation of the placenta. Also called syntrophoblast.

syndrome (sin'drōm) A set of signs and/or symptoms that occur together with reasonable consistency.

acquired immune deficiency s. See AIDS.

adrenogenital s. General term for a group of syndromes characterized by masculinization of women, feminization of men, or precocious sexual development in children; caused by either hyperplasia or malignant tumors of the adrenal cortex.

amniotic band s. A fetal condition in which a band of amnion causes constriction and possible amputation of digits and limbs. Webbing of digits, clubfoot, and fusion deformities of the cranium and face may also be present.

anaphylactoid s. of pregnancy See amniotic fluid embolism, under embolism.

androgen insensitivity s.'s See complete testicular feminization and incomplete testicular feminization, under feminization.

aortic arch s. See Takayasu's arteritis, under

arteritis.

Argonz-DelCastillo s. See Forbes-Albright syndrome.

Asherman's s. See posttraumatic uterine adhesions, under adhesion.

Beckwith-Wiedemann s. Autosomal dominant inheritance characterized by enlarged tongue, umbilical hernia, and low blood sugar, associated with increased incidence of large-for-gestational age fetuses.

Behçet's s. A rare disorder of unknown cause characterized by recurrent oral and genital ulcerations.

Bernard-Soulier s. Autosomal recessive inheritance characterized by markedly reduced adhesion of platelets (due to deficiency or dysfunction of glycoprotein receptors) and extremely large size of platelets; consequent postpartum hemorrhage and reduced platelet numbers in the fetus have been reported.

binge-and-purge s. See bulimia.

Boerhaave's s. Spontaneous rupture of the lower esophagus; in pregnancy, it may be due to the increased pressure of retching and vomiting.

carpal tunnel s. A complex of symptoms caused by abnormal pressure upon the median nerve as it passes between the transverse carpal ligament and the wrist bones (carpus); may result from an injury to the wrist (e.g., a Colles' fracture), or from repetitive wrist and finger movements; symptoms include numbness of the thumb, index and middle fingers with pain in the wrist and the palm. May also occur during pregnancy as a self-limited condition with symptoms appearing usually at night, and abating within a few months after delivery.

cat's cry s. See cri-du-chat syndrome.

Chiari-Frommel s. (CFS) Prolonged milk secretion, absence of menstruation, and atrophy of the uterus after childbirth; generally associated with a benign tumor of the anterior lobe of the pituitary (adenohypophysis).

cold agglutinin s. The presence of circulating antibodies that can agglutinate red blood cells, especially at temperatures below 37°C.

complete androgen insensitivity s. See complete testicular feminization, under feminization.

congenital rubella s. Syndrome present at birth that includes one or more of the following symptoms: ocular abnormalities (cataracts, glaucoma, abnormally small size of one or both eyes), cardiac anomalies (patent ductus arteriosus, septal defects), deafness, abnormally small head, and growth retardation; may be associated with such conditions as reduced number of platelets in the blood, anemia, hepatitis, encephalitis, changes in long bones, and chromosomal abnormalities. Caused by transplacental fetal infection with the rubella virus during the first trimester of gestation as a result of maternal infection, which may or may not produce the typical rash.

congenital varicella s. Malformations of the cerebral cortex, eyes, kidneys, long bones, and skin; the result of maternal chickenpox in the first 12 weeks of pregnancy; the responsible microorganism (varicella-zoster virus) is transmitted to the fetus through the placenta. See also extended rubella syndrome.

Conn's s. See primary aldosteronism, under aldosteronism.

cri-du-chat s. Congenital disorder marked by severe mental retardation, a typical plaintive catlike cry in infancy, and anomalies of the heart; caused by a chromosomal defect in which chromosome 5 lacks part of its short arm. Also called cat's cry syndrome.

Cushing's s. The group of symptoms and physical characteristics of Cushing's disease, including a round face, central obesity, prominent fat pad on the upper back ('buffalo hump'), reddish complexion, abdominal striations, high blood pressure, and impaired carbohydrate tolerance; may be caused by long-term corticosteroid therapy, abnormalities of the pituitary or adrenal glands, or by ACTH-secreting nonpituitary tumors. When present in pregnancy (unusual) it causes an increased risk of spontaneous abortion, stillbirths and preterm labor; may also cause reduced function of the adrenal cortex in the newborn infant.

D s. See trisomy 13 syndrome.

Dandy-Walker s. Congenital hydrocephalus secondary to outlet obstruction of the fourth ventricle due to atresia of its median and lateral apertures (foramina of Magendi and Luschka); may be an autosomal dominant or recessive inheritance, or the result of major chromosomal alterations. Also called Dandy-Walker malformation.

defibrination s. Deficiency of blood platelets and blood clotting proteins (factors II,V, VIII, and X).

dead fetus s. See retained dead fetus

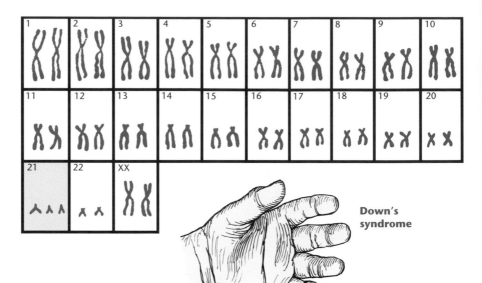

Down's syndrome

syndrome.

DelCastillo's s. See Forbes-Albright syndrome.

Down's s. The occurrence of various degrees of mental retardation and characteristic physical features such as posteriorly flattened skull, thickened tongue, broad hands and feet, and other anomalies; caused by the abnormal presence of three chromosomes (trisomy) instead of the normal two for the pair designated number 21. Also called trisomy 21 syndrome.

E s. See trisomy 18 syndrome.

Edwards' s. See trisomy 18 syndrome.

Eisenmenger's s. The presence of congenital heart disease, pulmonary hypertension, and a right-to-left shunt; in pregnancy, the syndrome is associated with a high incidence of both maternal and fetal death.

empty sella s. Congenital malformation at the base of the skull characterized by incomplete development of the sellar diaphragm, enlargement of the sella turcica (forming a fluid-filled extension of the subarachnoid space), and flattening of the pituitary (causing the pituitary fossa to appear empty in x-ray pictures). Secretion of pituitary hormones may be normal, deficient, or excessive.

extended rubella s. Generalized inflammation of the brain, with lesions of the white and gray matter, and type I diabetes mellitus, manifested during the second and third decades of life; caused by intrauterine infection with the virus causing chickenpox (varicella-zoster virus), acquired through the placenta from a maternal infection occurring usually after the first 16 weeks of pregnancy. See also congenital varicella syndrome.

familial adenomatous polyposis s. Autosomal dominant disorder secondary to a mutated gene of the long arm of chromosome 5 (5q21) in which patients develop thousands of polypoid adenomas in the large intestine, with a lesser number in the proximal small bowel. The chance of developing adenocarcinoma in at least one of these adenomas is 100%, especially in the descending colon.

fetal alcohol s. A syndrome that includes growth retardation, abnormally small head, characteristic facial features, mental retardation, and heart and kidney abnormalities; affects infants born to mothers who abuse alcohol intake during early pregnancy.

fetal cocaine s. Characteristic small size for gestational age, hyperirritability, anomalies of the genitourinary tract, prune belly, and abnormally small head; occurs in infants born to cocaine abusers.

fetal hydantoin s. Broad low nasal bridge, epicanthal folds, prominent ears, mental and growth deficiency, and a high incidence of absent fifth finger or toenail; caused by maternal ingestion of hydantoin analogs during pregnancy.

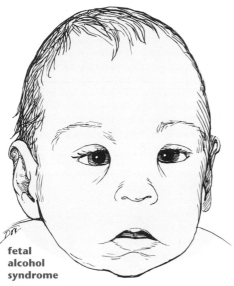

fetal alcohol syndrome

Forbes-Albright s. Combination of a profuse milky secretion from the nonlactating breast and absence of menstruation, unassociated with a recent pregnancy; thought to result from overproduction of pituitary prolactin stimulated by a benign tumor of the anterior lobe of the pituitary. Also called Argonz-DelCastillo syndrome; DelCastillo syndrome.

fragile X s. Inherited defect of the chromosome X causing mental retardation, large testicles, and big ears and chin in males, and mild mental retardation in females; may be associated with increased incidence of large-for-gestational age (LGA) infants.

gray baby s. A pale, bluish coloration of the skin, abdominal distention, collapse of blood vessels, and death.

hantavirus pulmonary s. A respiratory illness caused by a hantavirus and manifested as a pneumonitis that may progress to adult respiratory distress syndrome. Rodents are thought to act as vectors in its transmission.

HELLP s. Destruction of red blood cells (hemolysis), elevated liver enzymes, and low platelet count; may occur in pregnant women in association with severe preeclampsia and eclampsia in the last trimester of pregnancy.

hyperstimulation s. In assisted reproduction, ovarian enlargement, abdominal distention, and weight gain. Severe cases may include ascites, pleural effusion, electrolyte imbalance, and hypovolemia with low blood pressure and reduced urine output; in addition, the ovaries become greatly

enlarged, with many follicular cysts, stromal edema, and multiple corpora lutea.

immune deficiency s., immunologic deficiency s. A group of symptoms indicating impairment of one or more of the major functions of the immune system; may be primary, which is usually hereditary and evident between 6 months to 2 years of age, or secondary, which is the result of altered immune function by a variety of factors (e.g., infection, chemotherapy, radiation, immunosuppression, autoimmunity, etc.). See also AIDS.

incomplete androgen insensitivity s. See incomplete testicular feminization, under feminization.

Jervelle-Lange Neilsen s. An autosomal recessive condition characterized by a long QT interval and congenital deafness. It is associated with fainting episodes, ventricular tachycardia, and sudden death.

Kallman's s. Underdeveloped gonads with absence of secondary sexual characteristics occurring with absence or impairment of the sense of smell.

large edematous ovary s. Swollen condition of one ovary and masculinization of the patient.

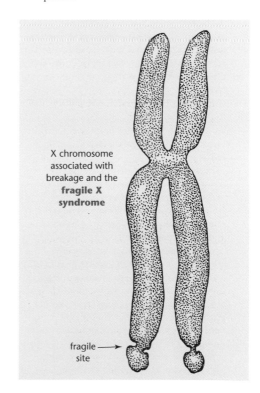

X chromosome associated with breakage and the **fragile X syndrome**

fragile → site

luteinized unruptured follicle s. (LUFS) Cyclical menstruation occurring in the absence of ovulation, with the ovum remaining within the ovary.

Mayer-Rokitansky-Küster-Hauser s. An absent vagina and a rudimentary uterus occurring with normal fallopian (uterine) tubes and ovaries; secondary sexual characteristics and growth are also normal. Also called Rokitansky-Küster-Hauser syndrome.

McCune-Albright s. The occurrence of multiple cystlike bone lesions (polyostotic fibrous dysplasia), dark- or light-brown skin patches with irregular edges, and precocious puberty. Cause is unknown.

meconium aspiration s. (MAS) An intense inflammatory reaction and air obstruction resulting in severe respiratory distress of the newborn; caused by fetal aspiration of meconium-stained amniotic fluid during intrauterine life or during the birth process.

meconium plug s. Total blockage of the lower intestinal tract (rectosigmoid) with a mass of hard meconium, associated with abdominal distention. Preterm infants, some infants of diabetic mothers, and maternal treatment with magnesium sulfate are risks for the development of the syndrome.

Meckel's s. An autosomal recessive inheritance characterized by sloping forehead, occipital protrusion of brain tissue and its covering membranes, and multiple cysts within the kidneys. Death usually occurs at the time of birth.

Meigs' s. The presence of noninflammatory fluid in the abdominal cavity (ascites) and around the lungs (hydrothorax) occurring in association with an ovarian tumor, usually a fibroma.

nephrotic s. (NS) A clinical symptom complex caused by a variety of kidney diseases in adults and children; characterized by generalized swelling with sodium and water retention, low plasma albumin concentration, and severe proteinuria.

new mother s. Condition frequently affecting new mothers in the first 2 weeks to few months after delivery; characterized by some or all of the following symptoms: fatigue, moodiness, tendency to weep easily, anxiety about baby care, anger at the baby and baby's father, and guilty feelings about having hostile thoughts.

Oglivie s. Massive abdominal distension with dilatation of the cecum, caused by decreased or absent propulsive activity of the colon; occurs sometimes after parturition. Rarely, the cecal wall may rupture.

ovarian hyperstimulation s. (OHSS) Massive enlargement of the ovaries, ascites, pleural effusion, and electrolyte and coagulation imbalances; occurs as a complication of hormonal therapy for *in vitro* fertilization.

ovarian resistance s. Condition in which ovarian follicles do not mature in response to follicle-stimulating hormone (FSH); caused by absence of FSH receptors or by a postreceptor defect. Also called resistant ovary syndrome; Savage syndrome.

Perrault s. The occurrence of deficient development of ovaries or testes and deafness.

Plummer-Vinson s. The combination of long-standing iron deficiency with formation of ledgelike webs of mucous membrane protruding into the lower pharynx; symptoms include difficult swallowing, dry mouth, and lesions in the mouth, pharynx, and esophagus. Seen most commonly in middle-aged women. Also called sideropenic dysphagia.

polycystic ovary (PCO) s. See polycystic ovary disease, under disease.

postconcussion s. See posttraumatic syndrome.

postmaturity s. The occurrence of prolonged gestation, an excessively large fetus,

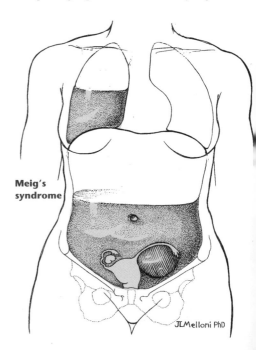

Meig's syndrome

JLMelloni PhD

and reduced placental capacity.

posttraumatic s. A group of symptoms following a head injury (with or without concussion) and persisting from weeks to a year or longer; they include persistent headache, irritability, giddiness, fatigue, difficulty in concentration, sleep disturbance, anxiety, and depression. Also called postconcussion syndrome.

posttraumatic stress s. See posttraumatic stress disorder (PTSD), under disorder.

Potter's s. Congenital absence of kidneys and skeletal deformities of the face, hip, and feet, associated with deficient amniotic fluid. The infant is small for its gestational age and dies shortly after birth.

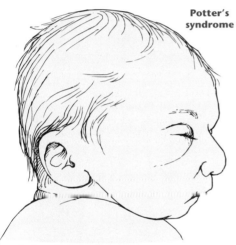

Potter's syndrome

features include:
epicanthal folds, low-set ears, receding chin, and wide-set eyes.

premenstrual s. (PMS) The occurrence of all or some of the following symptoms during the week preceding onset of the menstrual flow: lumbar and low abdominal pain, irritability, headache, tenderness of breasts, pelvic congestion, fluid retention, and weight gain. Also called premenstrual tension.

Reifenstein's s. An X-linked recessive inheritance; a form of male pseudohermaphroditism associated with hypospadias, small testes and sterility, absence of beard, short stature, and often enlarged breasts.

Reiter's s. (RS) Urethritis, conjunctivitis, arthritis, and sometimes mucocutaneous lesions; recurrences or chronicity occur in more than one-half of patients. Cause is unknown; usually develops after nonspecific urethritis or bacillary dysentery.

resistant ovary s. See ovarian resistance syndrome.

respiratory distress s. (RDS) of newborn Acute difficult breathing and bluish coloration of the skin most commonly occurring as a complication of premature birth; also seen in infants born to diabetic mothers and in those delivered by cesarean section; caused by deficient fetal production of surfactant, a substance that prevents the air sacs (alveoli) in the infant's lungs from collapsing and sticking together. An adequate level of surfactant is normally reached after the 35th week of gestation. Also called hyaline membrane disease of newborn.

retained dead fetus s. Symptom complex occurring when a dead fetus remains in the uterus; may include disseminated intravascular coagulation (DIC) and, after 5 weeks, abnormally low level of the plasma protein fibrinogen in the circulating blood; may cause excessive bleeding during delivery. Also called dead fetus syndrome.

Rokitansky-Küster-Hauser s. See Mayer-Rokitansky-Küster-Hauser syndrome.

Savage s. See ovarian resistance syndrome.

Sheehan's s. Syndrome usually caused by lack of blood supply to the anterior lobe of the pituitary (adenohypophysis), typically associated with hemorrhage and shock following childbirth; causes such symptoms as atrophy of sex organs, inability to lactate, hair loss, cold intolerance, and wrinkling of skin. The syndrome may also occur in men and nonpregnant women in association with sickle cell anemia, trauma, and disseminated intravascular coagulation (DIC). Also called postpartum necrosis of pituitary.

sicca s. See Sjögren's syndrome

Sjögren's s. Immunologic disorder marked by progressive destruction of lacrimal and salivary glands; characterized by dry eyes (keratoconjunctivitis sicca) and dry mouth (xerostomia); may occur in association with other diseases, such as rheumatoid arthritis, systemic lupus erythematosus (SLE), or scleroderma; usually seen in women 40–60 years of age. Also called sicca syndrome.

Swyer s. Absence of ovaries, underdeveloped genitalia, and normal female testosterone levels occurring in a female with an XY karyotype (an abnormal chromosome constitution for a female).

thoracic outlet s. A condition characterized by pain, paresthesias, numbness, or weakness in the neck or upper extremity resulting from compression of the brachial plexus, subclavian artery or subclavian vein at the thoracic outlet secondary to the presence of a cervical rib or fibromuscular bands.

TORCH s. Chronic nonbacterial infections occurring in the perinatal period (i.e., shortly before, during, or after birth) and causing similar clinical and laboratory findings. The term is an acronym: toxoplasma, other infections (e.g., syphilis, hepatitis B, coxsackie virus, Epstein-Barr virus, varicella-zoster, and human parvovirus), rubella, cytomegalovirus infection, and herpes simplex.

toxic shock s. (TSS) Sudden onset of high fever, muscle ache, vomiting, diarrhea, and a rash on the palms and soles, followed by low body temperature, low blood pressure, and shock; multiple organ dysfunction is common and may include kidneys, liver, and central nervous system; caused by infection with toxin-producing strains of *Staphylococcus aureus* or *Streptococcus pyogenes* (e.g., in the vagina in association with prolonged tampon use, contraceptive cap, or diaphragm; in surgical wounds, typically after the second day of surgery; and in focal tissue infections).

trisomy 18 s. Uncommon syndrome characterized by mental deficiency, skull deformities, abnormally small chin, low-set ears, webbed neck, deafness, heart defects, and Meckel's diverticulum; caused by the presence

of chromosome 18 in triplicate rather than the normal duplicate. Few children survive beyond the first year. Also called E syndrome; Edwards' syndrome; trisomy E syndrome.

trisomy 21 s. See Down's syndrome.

trisomy E s. See trisomy 18 syndrome.

Turner's s. Anomaly affecting females in which there are only 45 chromosomes instead of the normal 46, the missing chromosome being one of the X chromosomes; main features include rudimentary or absent ovaries, infantile genitalia, webbed neck, and short stature.

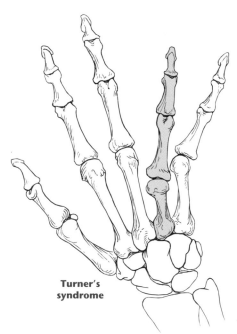

Turner's syndrome

trisomy 18 syndrome

medial deviation of second, fourth, and fifth fingers

rockerfoot deformity

twin–twin transfusion s. Syndrome diagnosed in identical (monozygotic) twins when there is a hemoglobin difference greater than 5 g/dl between the twins; it occurs when the fetuses share a single (monochorionic) placenta and there is a blood vessel communication between the two umbilical circulations, with a deep artery-to-vein flow from one twin to the other without a compensatory return flow. The donor twin tends to be pale, anemic, dehydrated, of low birth weight and decreased blood volume; it may die of heart failure. The recipient twin frequently has an abnormally large number of red blood cells, a high birth weight, increased organ mass, and an enlarged heart; although ruddy and apparently healthy, it may die of heart failure within 24 hours. Also called third circulation.

vulvar vestibulitis s. Tenderness to slight pressure on the vestibule of the vulva (e.g., upon touching with a Q-tip); severe pain, burning, and stinging sensations are experienced on attempts at vaginal entry; the pain may last for months or even years after intercourse. Cause is unknown.

syndromic (sin-drom'ik) Relating to a syndrome.

syngeneic (sin-je-ne'ik) Genetically identical or nearly identical; applied to identical (monozygous) twins or to animals so highly inbred that they have complete compatibility of genes. Also called isogenic; isologous; isoplastic.

syntrophoblast (sin-trof'o-blast) See syncytiotrophoblast.

syphilid (sif'ĭ-lid) Any of the infectious skin lesions of secondary syphilis; they may last weeks or months after onset and are rarely itchy although they resemble a variety of highly itchy skin rashes; some occur on the trunk and extremities and resemble the lesions of measles, others are brown macules and papules on the palms and soles, others resemble psoriasis around the hairline, others are pus-filled blisters at the nasolabial fold and the mouth.

syphilis (sif'ĭ-lis) An infectious disease caused by the bacterium *Treponema pallidum*, transmitted through sexual contact or any other primary contact; first symptoms develop after an incubation period of 12 to 30 days. The microorganisms can cross the placenta and infect the fetus.

congenital s. An infectious disease of the fetus acquired *in utero* through maternal transmission; it may be manifested by a number of abnormalities (including hepatosplenomegaly, osteochondritis, jaundice, anemia, skin lesions, rhinitis, and lymphadenopathy) with which the affected fetus may be born, or which may become manifest weeks or months later.

primary s. The first stage of the disease, characterized by the appearance of a small ulcer that develops into a chancre and heals 6 to 12 weeks later; it occurs either on the genitals, oral cavity, or near the anus.

secondary s. The second stage of syphilis, beginning after healing of the initial chancre and lasting indefinitely; characterized by variable infectious skin lesions, mucous patches, fever, and other constitutional symptoms.

tertiary s. The final, noninfectious stage of the disease, beginning after a lapse of several months or years; may take one or more of three forms: widespread development of masses of granulomatous tissue (gummas); involvement of the cardiovascular system (e.g., aneurysm in the ascending aorta, aortic valve incompetence); or involvement of the central nervous system.

syphiloid (sif'ĭ-loid) Resembling syphilis.

syringoma (sir-ing-go'mă) A tiny, subcutaneous, benign tumor of sweat glands, usually multiple, occurring most frequently about the lower eyelids and cheeks; found also on the vulva.

system (sis'tem) **1.** A functionally related group of parts or organs. **2.** An organized set of interrelated ideas, procedures, techniques, etc. **3.** A method of arrangement or classification.

APACHE scoring s. II Criteria developed to predict the survival of seriously ill patients based on the severity of their disease. The term APACHE is an acronym for acute physiology and chronic health evaluation.

autonomic nervous s. (ANS) The division of the nervous system that innervates the striated muscles of the heart and the smooth muscles and glands of the body; composed of two parts, the sympathetic nervous system and the parasympathetic nervous system.

Bethesda s. of classification, Bethesda s. See under classification.

cardiovascular s. (CVS) A closed system composed of the heart and blood vessels through which blood is pumped and circulated in the body.

central nervous s. (CNS) The portion of the nervous system consisting of the brain and spinal cord.

closed urinary drainage s. An indwelling urinary drainage system designed to reduce or eliminate the possibility of contamination and infection of the urinary tract; consists of an apparatus (packed under sterile conditions) that includes catheter, lubricant, gloves, drainage tube, and collection reservoir.

digestive s. The alimentary canal from the mouth to the anus and the associated glands; the organs associated with the ingestion, digestion, and absorption of food, and with the elimination of those constituents that are unabsorbed.

endocrine s. The system composed of ductless glands, including the pituitary (hypophysis), adrenal, thyroid, and parathyroid glands, the pineal body, pancreatic islets, interstitial cells of the testis, interstitial, follicular, and luteal cells of the ovary, the placenta, and certain specialized cells of the thymus, kidney, and lungs.

genitourinary s. The reproductive organs and the organs for the secretion and passage of urine. Also called urogenital system.

immune s. A complex system of cells (T lymphocytes) and protein molecules (major histocompatibility complex) acting together to protect the body from harmful organisms and substances; it normally distinguishes between foreign (nonself) proteins and the body's own (self) proteins.

lymphatic s. A closed system consisting of lymphoid tissue, lymph nodes, and lymph vessels; it forms an alternative route for the absorption of lymph and its return to the blood via the thoracic duct and right lymphatic duct.

lymphoid s. Specialized lymphoid tissues and organs considered collectively; they have in common the ability to produce substances, such as antibodies, that can inactivate foreign (nonself) matter; it includes the thymus, bone marrow, lymph nodes, spleen, and gut-associated lymphoid tissue; it operates in close association with the macrophage system.

macrophage s. The phagocytic cells present in the bone marrow, spleen, and liver, where they free the blood or lymph of foreign matter; it includes all major phagocytic cell types, except the polymorphonuclear leukocytes. Also called mononuclear phagocyte system.

mononuclear phagocyte s. See macrophage system.

musculoskeletal s. All the muscles and

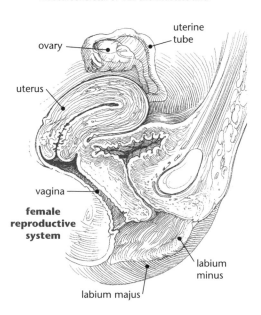

uterine tube

ovary

uterus

vagina

female reproductive system

labium minus

labium majus

bones of the body and their connecting structures considered collectively.

nervous s. The nervous tissues of the body; includes the brain and spinal cord (central nervous system), the cranial and spinal nerves (peripheral nervous system), and the sympathetic and parasympathetic nerves (autonomic nervous system).

parasympathetic nervous s. The smaller of the two divisions of the autonomic nervous system (ANS) that emerges from certain cranial and sacral spinal nerves (craniosacral outflow); some of the structures innervated include the ciliary muscles of the eye, the sphincter muscle of the pupil, salivary glands, heart, stomach, small intestine, cecum, appendix, colon, rectum, bladder, erectile tissue of penis/clitoris, testes, ovaries, fallopian (uterine) tubes, and the uterus. Physiologically, parasympathetic action is usually localized.

peripheral nervous s. (PNS) The nervous system that connects the central nervous system (CNS) to the rest of the body; composed of the 12 pairs of cranial nerves arising from the brain, the 31 pairs of spinal nerves arising from the spinal cord, and the sympathetic trunks and their ganglia and branches.

renin–angiotensin-aldosterone s. A biochemical feedback system important in the regulation of blood pressure, fluid volume, and sodium balance.

reproductive s. The organs and structures associated with reproduction and with the procreative act. Also called genital system. *Female reproductive s.*, the genital organs in the female, consisting of the ovaries, fallopian (uterine) tubes, uterus, vagina, and external genitalia. *Male reproductive s.*, the genital organs in the male, consisting of the testes, excretory ducts, seminal vesicles, prostate, and penis.

sympathetic nervous s. The larger of the two divisions of the autonomic nervous system (ANS), confined to the thoracolumbar region; some of the structures innervated include all sweat glands of the skin, arrector muscles of the hairs, muscular walls of blood vessels, heart, lungs, and abdominopelvic viscera. Physiologically, sympathetic action is systemic.

two-cell s. An explanation of the sequence of events involved in estrogen formation in the ovary, particularly in the maturing follicle, based on the cooperative participation of theca and granulosa cells.

urogenital s. See genitourinary system.

World Health Organization scoring s., WHO scoring s. A classification of gestational trophoblastic neoplasia that identifies nine prognostic factors with 29 variables (scores). The prognostic factors relate to metastatic disease (i.e., any spread of disease outside the uterus) and are grouped into: *good prognosis metastatic disease* (short duration, low pretreatment human chorionic gonadotropin [hCG] titer, no metastasis to brain or liver, no significant prior chemotherapy); and *poor prognosis metastatic disease* (long duration, high pretreatment hCG titer, brain or liver metastasis, significant prior chemotherapy, term pregnancy).

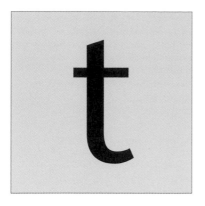

tabes (ta'bez) Progressive wasting away.

> **t. dorsalis** Manifestations of the tertiary stage of syphilis (neurosyphilis) resulting from damage to the sensory nerve roots and the posterior column of the spinal cord; characterized by loss of muscular coordination, shooting pains in the extremities, Charcot's joints, incontinence, and impotence.

tabetic (tă-bet'ik) Relating to tabes.

tabetiform (tă-bet'ĭ-form) Resembling tabes dorsalis.

tachy- Combining form meaning speed.

tachycardia (tak-ĭ-kar'de-ă) An abnormally fast heartbeat; usually applied to one exceeding 100 beats per minute. Also called tachyrhythmia.

> **atrial t.** See paroxysmal supraventricular tachycardia.

> **fetal t.** Tachycardia of the fetus in which the heart rate is 160 beats per minute or more (normal rate is 120–160 beats/minute); causes may include maternal or fetal infection, fetal oxygen deficiency (hypoxia), or maternal use of certain drugs.

> **paroxysmal supraventricular t.** (PSVT) Tachycardia of rapid onset and cessation, occurring abruptly and recurrently; characteristically seen in young individuals, including pregnant women, without evidence of heart disease. Formerly called atrial tachycardia.

> **sinus t.** (ST) Tachycardia of slow onset and cessation, occurring as a physiologic response to a variety of stresses that place a demand on the pumping action of the heart (e.g., exercise, anxiety, fever, low blood pressure, depletion of blood volume, congestive heart failure).

tachyphylaxis (tak-e-fĭ-lak'sis) Rapidly decreasing response to a pharmacologically or physiologically active substance after repetitive administration of the substance.

tachypnea (tak-ip-ne'ă) Abnormally rapid, shallow breathing.

> **transient t. of newborn** Benign condition of near-term or term babies who have respiratory distress shortly after delivery; usually lasts 3 to 5 days; thought to be caused by delayed resorption of fetal lung fluid. Popularly called wet lung.

tachyrhythmia (tak-e-rith'me-ă) See tachycardia.

tag (tag) **1.** A small outgrowth. **2.** To introduce or add an easily identifiable substance (e.g., a radioactive isotope) as a marker or label. **3.** The material so introduced or added.

> **anal skin t.** A polyp-like projection in the anus.

> **skin t.** A soft, flesh-colored or deeply pigmented appendage of the skin, usually occurring on the neck and upper chest.

tail (tāl) Any tapered extension of a structure.

> **axillary t.** Breast tissue extending from the superolateral part of the breast toward the axilla, along the lower border of the pectoralis major muscle; sometimes it passes through the deep fascia into the axilla, and lies in close proximity to the pectoral group of lymph nodes and vessels and the axillary blood vessels and nerves. Also called tail of Spence.

> **t. of Spence** See axillary tail.

talipes (tal'ĭ-pez) General term that denotes a deformity involving the talus (ankle bone) and the foot, which results in an abnormal shape and position.

> **t. equinovarus** Congenital deformity of the foot in which the ankle is plantar-flexed and the foot is inverted and adducted (i.e., directed toward the middle).

tamponade (tam-pon-ād') Application of external pressure (e.g., to stop bleeding).

tandem (tan'dem) **1.** An intracavitary applicator containing radioactive material used in local irradiation (e.g., of a gynecological cancer). **2.** Denoting an arrangement of two or more objects placed one behind the other.

tap (tap) **1.** To deliver a quick, gentle blow or blows (e.g., when eliciting a tendon reflex). **2.** To strike lightly but sharply and audibly. **3.** To withdraw fluid from a body cavity.

> **spinal t.** See lumbar puncture, under puncture.

Taxol (tak'sol) Trade name for a preparation of paclitaxel.

technetium 99m (tek-ne'she-um) (99mTc) Radioisotope of technetium, suitable as a radiotracer for scanning of many organs because of its readily detected gamma rays and relatively short half-life (6 hours). However, radioactivity has been reported to remain in the milk of lactating women from 15 hours to 3 days.

technique (tek-nēk') A systematic method of accomplishing a skillful task (e.g., a surgical operation, a scientific experiment, laboratory testing, natural childbirth, and the use of diagnostic and therapeutic devices).

Brandt-Andrews t. A method of expediting delivery of the placenta by elevating the uterus out of the abdomen while placing pressure just above the symphysis; simultaneously the placenta is expressed into the vagina.

breathing t.'s Techniques used in the Lamaze method of natural childbirth for coping with the labor process; consist of slow, deep breathing using the chest muscles, and rapid shallow breathing and panting just before full cervical dilatation; during the second stage of labor pushing efforts alternate with panting.

Irving's t. See Irving's operation, under operation.

Kerr t. A transverse rather than longitudinal incision through the lower uterine segment in the performance of cesarean section. It is the most common type of cesarean currently performed.

Madlener's t. See Madlener's operation, under operation.

McDonald's t. Measurement of the pregnant uterus by placing a centimeter tape on the abdomen and following the curvature of the abdominal surface from the pubic bone margin to the top of the uterine mass; useful for detecting fetal growth retardation, especially in the third trimester. Also called McDonald's maneuver.

moving strip t. A form of radiation therapy in which the area to be irradiated is divided into four contiguous segments (strips), each 2.5 cm wide; the treatment field is gradually increased, and then decreased, at the level of one strip at a time every 2 days for a total of 12 days.

Pastore t. A technique for delivery of the placenta; the uterine fundus is elevated with the fingers of the right hand placed on the patient's abdomen; the left hand is placed flat on the abdomen with the fingers superior to the pubic symphysis to prevent the fundus from entering the pelvis; when contractions occur and the placenta separates, the fundus is gently squeezed and pushed downward with the right hand; when the placenta is felt to pass into the cervix or vagina, the fundus is

elevated further; the placenta is then extracted by gentle cord traction.

Pomeroy's t. See Pomeroy's operation, under operation.

technology (tek-nol'o-je) The application of scientific knowledge to the practical purposes of any field, including methods, techniques, and instrumentation.

assisted reproductive t. (ART) The field of reproductive medicine involved with techniques used to increase fecundability by nonphysiologic methods that enhance the probability of fertilization, e.g., *in vitro* fertilization (IVF), gamete intrafallopian transfer (GIFT), zygote intrafallopian transfer (ZIFT), tubal embryo transfer (TET), peritoneal oocyte and sperm transfer (POST), subzonal insertion of sperm by microinjection (SUZI), and intracytoplasmic sperm injection (ICSI).

telangiectasia (tel-an-je-ek-ta'ze-ă) Abnormal dilatation of groups of tiny blood vessels in skin or mucous membranes.

hereditary hemorrhagic t. An autosomal dominant disease in which branched spider telangiectasias appear on the skin and mucous membranes, especially on the skin of the fingers, lips, and face, and on the oral and nasal mucosa. A frequent cause of nosebleed and gastrointestinal bleeding. Also called Osler-Weber-Rendu disease.

spider t. A group of minute focal dilated arterioles arranged in a radial pattern around a central core, typically seen above the waist; the presence of a small number of spider telangiectasias on the face, neck, upper chest, or arms is frequently associated with hyperestrogenic states, such as pregnancy and estrogen therapy (most disappear after delivery); they are also seen normally in children. The occurrence of a large number of spider telangiectasias usually indicates an underlying systemic disease (e.g., cirrhosis of the liver). Also called arterial spider; nevus araneus; spider angioma; spider nevus; vascular spider.

telangiectatic (tel-an-je-ek-tat'ik) Relating to telangiectasia.

tele-, telo- Combining forms meaning at a distance; end.

telogen (tel'o-jen) The resting phase of the hair growth cycle, following the growth phase (catagen).

temperature (tem'per-ă-tur) (t) **1.** Heat intensity as measured in any of several arbitrary scales. **2.** Popular term for fever.

neonate t. The range of normal temperatures in a term newborn infant. Skin temperature 36.0–36.5°C (96.9–97.7°F); core temperature, 36.5–37.5°C (97.7–99.5°F).

normal body t. The average oral temperature in healthy human adults (40 years or younger): 36.8°C (98.2°F), with upper limits ranging between an early morning temperature of 37.2°C (98.9°F) and an evening temperature of 37.7°C (99.9°F); other variables include exercise, eating and drinking, age and, in women, the time of the menstrual cycle.

template (tem'plāt) **1.** A gauge or pattern for checking locations, dimensions, or contours. **2.** In genetics, the macromolecular mold for the synthesis of complementary macromolecules, as in replication of DNA and the transcription of DNA to RNA.

Syed-Noblett t. A template for delivering interstitial radiation therapy for advanced carcinoma of the cervix when anatomic landmarks are obscured by tumor growth.

temporal (tem'pŏ-ral) Relating to the side of the head or temple (e.g., bones of the skull, lobes of the brain).

temporo-occipital (tem-pŏ-ro ok-sip'-ĭ-tal) Relating to the temporal and occipital bones of the skull.

temporoparietal (tem-pŏ-ro-pă-ri'e-tal) Relating to the temporal and the parietal bones, at the sides and upper part of the head.

tendon (ten'dun) Fibrous band attaching a muscle to a bone.

central t. of perineum See perineal body, under body.

conjoined t. The fused tendons of two abdominal muscles: the transverse muscle of the abdomen (transversus abdominis) and the internal oblique muscle of the abdomen (obliquus internus abdominis); it inserts onto the crest of the pubic bone and the pectineal line. Also called inguinal falx.

tent (tent) **1.** A covering of plastic or canvas placed over a patient's bed for inhalation of oxygen (oxygen tent) or steam (steam tent). **2.** An expandable, cylindrical plug for keeping an orifice open.

Laminaria t. A sterile tent made of dried stems of the seaweed *Laminaria digitata*, measuring 1 to 2 mm in diameter and 5 to 7 mm in length, with a cord attached to one end to facilitate removal. The tent is inserted in the cervical canal and left in place 6 to 12 hours for gradual, atraumatic expansion of the cervix; employed as a preoperative procedure in first trimester abortion by suction aspiration or D & C, or during second trimester abortion as a supplement to other procedures; also used to soften and dilate an 'unripe' cervix in preparation for induction of labor at or near term. See also *Laminaria digitata*.

terato- Combining form meaning developmental malformation.

teratogen (ter'ă-to-jen) Any environmental agent, microorganism, or drug that causes physical defects in the developing embryo or fetus.

teratogenesis (ter-ă-to-jen'ē-sis) The origin of fetal malformations.

teratogenic (ter-ă-to-jen'ik) Causing birth defects in the developing embryo.

teratoid (ter'ă-toid) Resembling a malformed fetus.

teratology (ter-ă-tol'ŏ-je) The subspecialty of developmental anatomy concerned with abnormal development in all its aspects.

teratoma (ter-ă-to'mă) Any of a group of tumors derived from cell types of the three germ layers (i.e., endoderm, mesoderm, and ectoderm); seen most commonly in the ovary and testis, also along the midline of the chest between the lungs; some are benign, others malignant; may occur at any age.

benign cystic t. See dermoid cyst, under cyst.

immature t. of ovary See malignant teratoma of ovary.

malignant t. of ovary An uncommon, bulky tumor, usually solid with areas of tissue degeneration and hemorrhage; it contains embryonic elements of all three germ layers (i.e., tissue elements differentiating toward cartilage, glands, muscle, bone, nerve); extraovarian spread depends on the

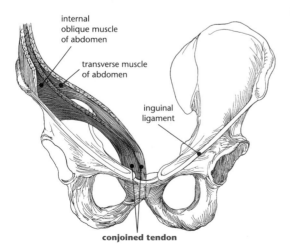

internal
oblique muscle
of abdomen

transverse muscle
of abdomen

inguinal
ligament

conjoined tendon

predominant cell type present and degree of tissue immaturity; occurs most commonly unilaterally in adolescent and young women. Also called immature teratoma of ovary; solid teratoma of ovary.

mature benign t. See dermoid cyst, under cyst.

sacrococcygeal t. Teratoma occurring usually as a large mass in the area of the sacrum and coccyx of newborn infants.

solid t. of ovary See malignant teratoma of ovary.

teratomatous (ter-ă-to'mă-tus) Of the nature of teratomas.

teratophobia (ter-ă-to-fo'be-ă) Abnormally exaggerated fear of giving birth to a malformed baby.

term (term) A definite time period; applied to a newborn infant at the end of a normal-length pregnancy (36 weeks to 42 weeks).

tertigravida (ter-tĭ-grav'ĭ-dă) A woman who is pregnant for the third time. Also called gravida III.

tertipara (ter-tip'ă-ră) A woman who has had three pregnancies reaching the period of viability. Also called para III.

test (test) **1.** An examination. **2.** A means of determining the presence, quality, constitution, or concentration of a substance. **3.** To perform such a function. **4.** A systematic procedure to assess the function of specific parts of the body. **5.** A substance used in a test.

agglutination inhibition t. for pregnancy See immunologic pregnancy test.

alpha-fetoprotein t., AFP t. A prenatal screening test based on detection of AFP (a fetal glycoprotein) in maternal serum; performed on pregnant women between 14 and 16 weeks of gestation, especially women over 35 years of age; abnormally high levels of AFP are usually associated with open neural-tube defects (e.g., spina bifida); abnormally low levels are usually indicative of Down's syndrome (trisomy 21). Positive results may be followed by amniocentesis to determine AFP levels in amniotic fluid and final diagnosis. See also alpha-fetoprotein.

Apt t. A test used to determine the presence of fetal hemoglobin. Addition of dilute sodium hydroxide to a fluid specimen will turn maternal blood brown while fetal blood remains red. Applications include testing maternal blood in cases of suspected abruptio placentae, and vaginal fluid in patients in whom vasa previa may be present.

Bonney's t. See Marshall's test.

bubble stability t. See foam stability test.

chorionic villus sampling t., CVS t. See chorionic villus sampling, under sampling.

clot retraction t. A bedside test that can provide qualitative evidence of hypofibrinogenemia. The inability of 2 ml of blood to clot and retract in a 5-ml glass test tube under observation over a period of time is a clinical measure of low sodium fibrinogen.

contraction stress t. (CST) A test for assessing a fetus at risk for compromised placental respiratory function (placental insufficiency). A monitoring device is placed on the maternal abdomen to continuously monitor the fetal heart rate and uterine contractions; contractions are induced by intermittent stimulation of the nipples, or by intravenous infusion of dilute oxytocin, until three (no more than five) contractions occur within 10 minutes; each contraction should last no longer than 40 to 60 seconds; uterine stimulation is then discontinued but the fetal heart rate is monitored until contractions have subsided. Interpretation of test results depends on the occurrence of late decelerations (i.e., when there is a fetal heart-rate decrease beginning at, or after, the peak of a uterine contraction and returning to baseline levels well after the contraction has ended). Results are interpreted as follows: *negative (normal),* no late decelerations occur, baseline fetal heart rate is normal; *positive (abnormal),* late decelerations occur with each three contractions in a 10-minute period; and *equivocal (suspicious),* intermittent or nonrepetitive late decelerations occur, observed in less than half of the contractions. When oxytocin is used to evoke the uterine contractions for the test, it is called oxytocin challenge test (OCT).

cotton-tipped applicator t., Q-tip t. A test for assessing the anatomic support of the urethra and bladder; a lubricated cotton-tipped applicator is introduced into the urethra with the tip at the urethrovesical junction; the resting position of the applicator is horizontal; with straining, the urethrovesical junction descends, causing the end of the applicator to rotate upward and form an angle which, when greater than 30 degrees, indicates poor urethral and bladder support.

t. of cure Reculturing after a course of therapy to be certain of the anticipated effect (e.g., after the use of certain penicillins for the treatment of gonorrhea).

do-it-yourself t. A health test usually

performed at home, using a test kit sold over the counter at drugstores (e.g., pregnancy test, blood-glucose monitoring test, hidden [occult] fecal blood test).

effort tolerance t. See exercise test.

exercise t., exercise tolerance t. A test to assess cardiovascular function usually through the use of exercise on a treadmill or pedaling a stationary bicycle (bicycle ergometer) while under continuous electrocardiographic monitoring; useful in detecting coronary artery disease. Also called stress test; effort tolerance test.

fern t., ferning t. A qualitative test used to detect ovulation; also used as an adjunctive test to confirm rupture of the membranes during pregnancy; a fernlike pattern or arborization appears on a dried specimen spread on a histologic slide; elevated estrogen secretion (e.g., during ovulation) is indicated when the pattern is present in a specimen of endocervical mucus; rupture of the membranes is indicated when the pattern occurs in a specimen of vaginal fluid. See also ferning.

fluorescent treponemal antibody absorption t. A confirmatory test for detecting antibody against *Treponema pallidum*, the syphilis-causing microorganism; the patient's serum (after removing nonspecific antibodies) is mixed on a glass slide with Nickol's strain of *Treponema pallidum* and incubated; syphilis is confirmed when specific antibodies attaching to the treponemal organisms are demonstrated with fluorescence-labeled antihuman globulin serum. Positive tests are seen in 80 to 90% of cases of primary syphilis, and practically all cases of secondary and late syphilis; minimally reactive tests may be indicative of systemic lupus erythematosus, pregnancy, or genital herpes; normal findings show no fluorescence. *Treponema pallidum* antibodies are not detected in the blood for 14 to 21 days after initial infection. The test is also used to screen for suspected false-positive results of Venereal Disease Research Laboratory (VDRL) tests. Also called FTA test; FTA-ABS test.

foam stability t. An amniotic fluid test to detect risk of respiratory distress syndrome (RDS) in the fetus; amniotic fluid from mature fetal lungs contains an essential surface-active substance (surfactant); for the test, amniotic fluid is placed in a test tube together with saline and ethanol and shaken vigorously for 15 seconds before being placed upright for 15 minutes; pulmonary maturity is indicated when the surfactant causes a ring of bubbles to form on the surface of the solution; if the bubbles fail to appear or are poorly formed, the test is negative and it indicates varying

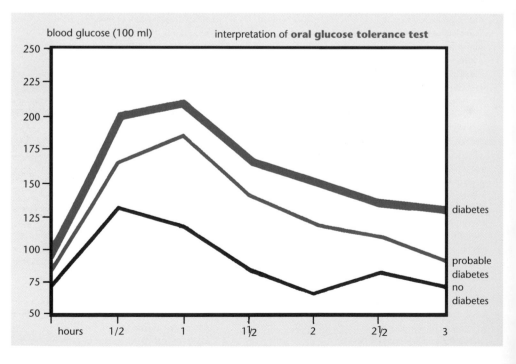

degrees of high risk of respiratory distress syndrome. Also called bubble stability test; shake test.

FTA t. See fluorescent treponemal antibody absorption test.

FTA-ABS t. See fluorescent treponemal antibody absorption test.

gestational diabetes t. A screening glucose tolerance test routinely administered between 24 and 28 weeks of pregnancy for the detection of abnormal carbohydrate metabolism; the patient drinks 50 g of glucose solution or equivalent, and a blood sample is drawn 1 hour later. Generally, a plasma value over 140 mg/dl is an indication for an extended glucose tolerance test. See also gestational diabetes, under diabetes.

glucose tolerance t. (GTT) A 3-hour metabolic test for the diagnosis of diabetes mellitus; it measures the ability of the liver to absorb and store excessive amounts of blood sugar (glucose) as glycogen. The patient ingests a high carbohydrate load for 3 days before the test (at least 150 g of carbohydrate per day); then, after an overnight fast of 10 to 12 hours, a fasting blood glucose level is obtained; levels are taken thereafter at 1, 2, and 3 hours. Usually, the fasting glucose level rises quickly and then falls to normal (below 140 mg/dl) within 2 hours; in a diabetic patient, the glucose level increase is greater and the time it takes to return to normal is prolonged (the 2-hour level is 140 mg/dl or above).

guaiac t. A chemical test for detection of occult blood; the specimen is mixed with glacial acetic acid and gum guaiac solution; blood is present if a blue tint appears upon the addition of hydrogen peroxide.

hamster egg t. See sperm penetration assay, under assay.

HIV infection t.'s Tests for detecting HIV infection. Two commonly used testing programs, ELISA (enzyme-linked immunosorbent assay) and Western blot analysis, aim to detect HIV-specific antibody, a protein produced by the infected person's immune system in response to the presence of the HIV virus. In current practice, all blood donors are ELISA-tested; in this test, the presence of antibody in a blood sample is indicated by a reaction-dependent color, which is then measured by spectrophotometry. Unlike ELISA, the Western blot analysis gives information about particular antibodies among the several that HIV antigens may elicit; it uses electrophoresis and is thus more expensive and demanding of expertise than the ELISA test. False-negative results cannot be totally disregarded because some sera contain too little anti-HIV antibody to be detected (e.g., sera from individuals who have been infected very recently, typically during the first 6 weeks of infection, or from individuals who form antibody very slowly). See also enzyme-linked immunosorbent assay (ELISA), under assay; Western blot analysis, under analysis.

home pregnancy t.'s Any do-it-yourself pregnancy test using commercial over-the-counter kits for detection of human chorionic gonadotropin (hCG) in a urine sample; detection of hCG in the sample indicates pregnancy since this hormone is not usually present in nonpregnant women.

t. for hydrocephalus See scinticisternography.

human chorionic gonadotropin pregnancy t. See immunologic pregnancy test.

immunologic pregnancy t. A test for detection and confirmation of pregnancy by means of immunologic techniques, based on the antigenic properties of the glycoprotein hormone hCG (human chorionic gonadotropin); by measuring urine levels of hCG, pregnancy can be detected as early as 10 days after a missed menstruation (measurable hCG is not normally found in the urine of nonpregnant women). The test is also used to aid in the diagnosis of hydatidiform mole, choriocarcinoma, and other hCG-secreting tumors. Also called agglutination inhibition test for pregnancy; human chorionic gonadotropin pregnancy test; pregnancy test.

latex t. See latex agglutination test.

latex agglutination t. A passive agglutination test in which minute spherical particles of latex in suspension are used as passive carriers of absorbed antigens; the particles clump together (agglutinate) in the presence of antibody specific for the absorbed antigen (e.g., when rheumatoid factor is present in the serum, agglutination of the latex particles occurs); frequently used as a test for rheumatoid arthritis, and for the detection of human chorionic gonadotropin (hCG) in urine when testing for pregnancy. Also called latex fixation test; latex particle agglutination test; latex test.

latex fixation t. See latex agglutination test.

latex particle agglutination t. See latex agglutination test.

Marshall's t. An adjunctive test to help in

the diagnosis of urinary stress incontinence, performed in addition to the physical examination of the urethrovesical angle; the anterior vaginal wall is digitally elevated in an anterior direction; the patient is asked to cough forcefully while in both the supine and upright positions; the digital pressure supposedly prevents leakage of urine by re-establishing the urethrovesical angle. Also called Bonney's test; Read's test.

microhemagglutination t. A version of the *Treponema pallidum* hemagglutination test.

nonstress t. (NST) A test for detecting oxygen deficiency in the fetus (fetal hypoxia); fetal movements are recorded and fetal heart rate changes are monitored by applying a recording system to the maternal abdomen. Normally, an increase of the fetal heart rate occurs in response to spontaneous fetal activity; decreased movements usually occur during fetal sleep; they can also occur with such situations as maternal intake of alcohol or drugs or chronic smoking. Test results are interpreted as follows: *reactive,* at least four fetal movements occur in a 20-minute period and the heart rate accelerates by at least 15 beats per minute during fetal movements, indicating well-being of the fetus; *nonreactive,* no fetal movement occurs in a 20-minute period, or no heart rate acceleration occurs with fetal movement, usually indicating fetal compromise and frequently associated with a poor outcome (deep fetal sleep lasting up to 45 minutes, resulting in absent fetal movement, may give a false nonreactive result); *uncertain reactivity,* fewer than four fetal movements occur in a 20-minute period, or the heart rate accelerates less than 15 beats per minute with fetal movements.

oxytocin challenge t. (OCT) See contraction stress test.

pad t. A clinical evaluation of urine loss wherein a patient wears a preweighed sanitary pad and performs activities which may result in urine incontinence; the pad is then reweighed to determine urine loss.

Pap smear t. See Pap test.

Pap t., Papanicolaou t. A microscopic examination of cells shed or scraped from the female genital tract for evidence of abnormal cells; used especially for early detection of cancer of the cervix. The same test may also be used to examine the respiratory, urinary, and gastrointestinal tracts, and to detect intracellular inclusions indicative of herpesvirus infection. Also called Pap smear test; Papanicolaou examination. See also Pap smear, under smear.

plain slide t. See saline slide test.

postcoital t. A test of questionable reliability for evaluating the adequacy of the ejaculate content and cervical environment to determine the cause of infertility; it is performed on the estimated date of ovulation, between 2 and 8 hours after intercourse; a specimen of cervical mucus is obtained and inspected for clarity, ferning, elasticity, and the number and activity of spermatozoa present.

potassium hydroxide slide t. A test for diagnosing a fungal vaginal infection; one drop of vaginal discharge is mixed with a 10% aqueous solution of potassium hydroxide on a histologic slide; the potassium hydroxide dissolves epithelial cells and other extraneous material, thereby facilitating visualization of the network of fungal filaments (mycelium) if present.

PPD t. See tuberculin test.

pregnancy t. See immunologic pregnancy test.

preimplantation t. A woman's unfertilized eggs (ova) are removed and fertilized in a Petri dish; some cells are later removed from each embryo and tested for genetic defects; only those embryos found to be disease-free are transferred to the uterus for implantation.

Q-tip t. See cotton-tipped applicator test.

Read's t. See Marshall's test.

rollover t. A clinical screening procedure performed at 28 to 32 weeks of gestation, predictive of asymptomatic women who may develop pregnancy-induced hypertension. The patient rests on her side for 15 to 20 minutes and her blood pressure is taken; she then rolls over to the supine position and her blood pressure is retaken. An increase in diastolic pressure of 20 mmHg or more is a positive test. Also called supine pressor response.

Rubin's t. See tubal insufflation test.

saline slide t. A test for demonstrating the presence of *Trichomonas vaginalis* in the vagina; a drop of vaginal discharge is mixed with a drop of normal saline solution on a histologic slide and warmed to body temperature; if present, motile organisms can be seen. Also called plain slide test.

Schiller's t. A test performed when cancer of the cervix or vaginal mucosa is suspected; the suspect area is painted with Lugol's or Schiller's iodine solution; a normal cervix stains dark brown; any portion of the epithelium that does not stain is considered either scar tissue or a neoplasm.

screening t. (1) A test applied to a group of apparently healthy people to separate some members of the group on the basis of established criteria. (2) A testing procedure designed to separate chemicals according to an established characteristic, such as carcinogenicity.

shake t. See foam stability test.

sniff t. See whiff test.

stress t. See exercise test.

tilt t. A rise in pulse or drop in blood pressure as a patient moves from the supine toward the upright position, indicating a loss of extracellular fluid (e.g., during hemorrhage or dehydration).

timed t. A test that is taken at a precise specified time interval (e.g., blood that is drawn each hour and tested for glucose levels in a glucose tolerance test).

TPHA t. See *Treponema pallidum* hemagglutination test.

TPI t. See Treponemal immobilization test.

Treponemal immobilization t. Test for syphilis; serum from a syphilitic patient will (in the presence of complement) immobilize the actively motile *Treponema pallidum* obtained from testes of a syphilitic rabbit. Also called TPI test.

***Treponema pallidum* hemagglutination t.** A serologic test for syphilis; tanned sheep red blood cells are coated with *Treponema pallidum* antigen, then combined with absorbed test serum; hemagglutination (positive reaction) occurs in the presence of specific anti-*Treponema pallidum* antibodies in the patient's serum. Also called TPHA test.

tubal insufflation t. A test to determine patency of the fallopian (uterine) tubes by transcervical introduction of carbon dioxide into the uterus; if the tubes are patent, the escape of gas into the abdominal cavity is heard on auscultation over the lower abdomen; the gas often accumulates under the diaphragm which can be demonstrated by x-ray film; it may be accompanied by discomfort or pain in the shoulder region. The test is generally administered as part of an evaluation of infertility. Also called Rubin's test.

tuberculin t. Any test for tuberculosis in which tuberculin or its purified protein derivative (PPD) is introduced into the skin either by means of an intradermal injection (Mantoux test), multiple punctures (tine test), or an adhesive patch (patch test). A delayed hypersensitivity reaction (manifested by a palpable and visible area of redness and induration larger than 5 mm in diameter within 48 to 72 hours) is indicative of a positive reaction. Also called PPD test.

urinary stress t. A test for urinary stress incontinence; a specified volume of fluid is instilled into the bladder; the patient stands with her feet separated shoulder-wide, then coughs or pushes forcefully; poor anatomic support of the bladder and urethra is suggested when urine leakage occurs during stress and stops shortly thereafter; a disorder of the bladder is suggested when leakage is delayed or continued.

urine concentration t. A test to assess the tubular function of the kidneys by measuring the relative density or osmolality of urine after a period of restricted fluids and controlled diet; the specific gravity of normal urine should measure 1.02 or more after several hours without fluids.

VDRL t. A nonspecific serologic test for diagnosing syphilis, using heat-activated serum and cardiolipin-lecithin-cholesterol antigen, as developed by the Venereal Disease Research Laboratory (VDRL) of the U.S. Public Health Service; a positive reaction is determined when flaky masses (flocculation) appear in the test.

Western blot t. See Western blot analysis, under analysis.

whiff t. A clinical observation that vaginal discharge secondary to either bacterial vaginosis or trichomonas vaginitis will emit a fishy odor after the addition of 10% potassium hydroxide. Also called sniff test.

testis (tes'tis). pl. **testes** One of two glands that produce spermatozoa and hormones (testosterone and small quantities of estrogenic hormones), normally suspended in the scrotum; the left testis often hangs 1 cm lower than the right one.

ectopic t. Abnormal condition in which a testis has strayed from its normal path of descent into the scrotum. Most common location is superficial to and over the inguinal canal; other (rare) locations are: just in front of the anus (perineal), over the femoral vessels (femoral or crural), under the skin at the root of the penis (penile), within the pelvic cavity (pelvic), and both testes in the same inguinal canal (transverse).

testosterone (tes-tos'tĕ-rōn) The most potent of the naturally produced male hormones (androgens), responsible for the development and maintenance of secondary sexual characteristics; produced in the testes by the

Leydig's cells under the control of luteinizing hormone of the pituitary.

tetanus (tet'ă-nus) An infectious, bacterial disease caused by the toxin of *Clostridium tetani*; initial symptoms include pain and stiffness in jaw, abdomen, and back muscles, progressing to rigidity (trismus) and reflex spasm; may follow any penetrating wound.

    t. neonatorum Tetanus of the newborn due to infection of the umbilical stump.

tetra- Prefix meaning four.

tetracycline (tet-ră-si'klēn) Any of a group of broad-spectrum antibiotic drugs prescribed to treat a variety of infections; possible side-effects include nausea, vomiting, and diarrhea; may discolor developing teeth or worsen the blood level of protein metabolites when kidney function is diminished; taken during pregnancy may cause such adverse effects as inhibition of bone growth, bone deformity, webbing or fusion of fingers or toes, and maternal liver toxicity.

tetralogy (te-tral'ŏ-je) A combination of four related entities.

    t. of Fallot Cyanotic congenital heart disease produced by coexistence of the following four abnormalities: narrowed valve of pulmonary artery (pulmonary stenosis), displaced aorta (dextro-position of aorta), hole in the muscular wall separating the ventricles (ventricular septal defect), and thickened wall of the right ventricle (right ventricular hypertrophy).

thalassemia (thal-ă-se'me-ă) A group of hereditary disorders characterized by deficient or absent production of one of the polypeptide chains of hemoglobin (the oxygen-carrying pigment of red blood cells).

    alpha t., α t. Disorder characterized by reduced formation of alpha-globin chains in precursors of red blood cells in bone marrow, caused by deletion of one or more of the four alpha-globin genes normally present in each cell. The number of deletions determines the severity of the disorder; lack of a single gene produces a silent carrier state, which has little or no effect on the blood and is completely asymptomatic; a lack of all four genes (hemoglobin Bart disease) is incompatible with life. The condition caused by lack of three alpha-globin genes was formerly called hemoglobin H disease.

    beta t., β t. Disorder characterized by a reduced quantity of hemoglobin in red blood cells due to diminished formation of the beta-globin chains in hemoglobin.

    beta t. major A generally severe form of

thalassemia, usually the result of inheritance of genes for beta thalassemia from both parents (homozygous state); characterized by severe anemia, bone abnormalities, growth retardation, enlargement of spleen and liver, and jaundice. Clinical manifestations usually appear after 4 to 6 months of age; death usually occurs before puberty; those females who survive are usually unable to conceive. Also called Cooley's anemia.

    beta t. minor Mild thalassemia rarely associated with significant clinical manifestations; may produce symptoms resembling those of iron deficiency anemia. Also called beta-thalassemia trait.

thalidomide (thă-lid'o-mīd) A sedative-hypnotic drug; it produces fetal deformities of the limbs and other defects when taken by pregnant women.

theca (the'kă), pl. thecae A sheath or capsule enveloping a structure.

    t. folliculi The envelope surrounding the vesicular ovarian follicle, composed of an external, fibrous layer (theca externa) and an internal, vascular, secretory layer (theca interna).

thecoma (the-ko'mă) A firm, yellow-to-orange, benign tumor of the ovary; composed of theca cells with varying degrees of lipid content; found most commonly in the fifth to seventh decades of life; it has estrogenic activity.

thecomatosis (the-ko-mă-to'sis) See hyperthecosis.

thelarche (the-lar'ke) The beginning of breast development in girls.

    premature t. The isolated development of breast tissue before 8 years of age, usually between 1 and 3 years; may develop unilaterally or bilaterally.

theleplasty (the'le-plas-te) See mammilaplasty.

thelerethism (thě-ler'ě-thizm) Erection of a nipple.

thelitis (the-li'tis) Inflammation of a nipple.

thelium (the'le-um) A nipple or nipple-like structure.

thelo-, thel- Combining forms meaning nipple.

thelorrhagia (the-lo-ra'je) Bleeding from the nipple.

theory (the'o-re) A hypothetical concept formulated to provide a coherent basis for investigation or to account for observed phenomena.

    'two hit' t. A proposal to explain the development of malignancies in genetically susceptible individuals. It states that there is an underlying genetic deficiency in growth-

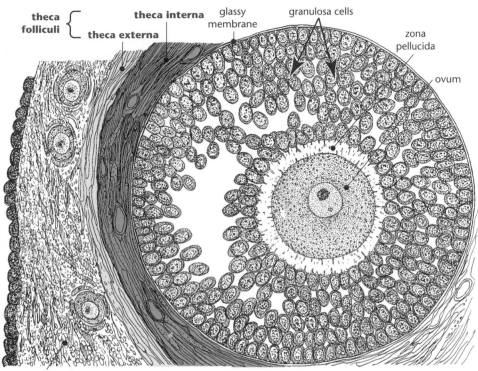

theca folliculi { theca interna · theca externa · glassy membrane · granulosa cells · zona pellucida · ovum

tunica albuginea

secondary vesicular follicle of ovary

controlling factors (the first 'hit'); the deficiency is then intensified by the loss (mutation, deletion) of additional genetic material required to maintain normal growth (the second 'hit').

therapy (ther'ă-pe) Treatment of disease, especially as undertaken in accordance with specific modalities.

    adjuvant t. Treatment used in addition to the primary therapy (e.g., radiation therapy in addition to surgery).

    combination antimicrobial t. The simultaneous administration of two or more antimicrobial drugs, rather than a single one.

    estrogen replacement t. Administration of estrogen, usually with progestin, to those women who have signs and symptoms of estrogen deficiency (e.g., some postmenopausal women and those who have had both ovaries removed).

    internal radiation t. See brachytherapy.

    maintenance drug t. In chemotherapy, administration of drugs at a dose level sufficient to forestall aggravation of the condition.

    pseudomenopause t. Temporary administration of drugs (e.g., danazol, GnRH

agonists), which suppress ovarian function; usually given as medical treatment of endometriosis.

    radiation t. Treatment of disease with high-energy rays or subatomic particles, such as x-rays, alpha and beta particles, gamma rays; radioactive materials include cobalt, radium, cesium, and iridium.

thermography (ther-mog'ră-fe) The technique of recording, in the form of an image, temperature patterns on the surface of the skin; used to provide clues to the presence of diseases or abnormalities that alter skin temperature (e.g., circulation problems, inflammation, tumors). Further investigation is usually necessary to confirm a diagnosis.

thermoregulation (ther-mo-reg-u-la'shun) Regulation of body core temperature, controlled by a special region of the hypothalamus in the brain.

thickness (thik'nes) The smallest measurement between two of an object's surfaces.

    nuchal t. One of several ultrasound measurements useful in identifying fetuses with Down's syndrome; usually performed in midtrimester. A nuchal thickness equal to, or greater than, 5 mm is considered a positive finding.

thioguanine (thi-o-gwa'nĕn) Antitumor drug used in the treatment of acute nonlymphocytic leukemia. Intrauterine exposure may cause fetal malformations and chromosomal abnormalities.

thoracopagus (tho-ră-ko'pă-gus) Conjoined twins united anteriorly, at the chest.

threadworm (thred'werm) See pinworm.

three-day blues See postpartum depression, under depression.

thrombo-, thromb- Combining forms meaning blood clot.

thrombocythemia (throm-bo-si-the'me-ă) See thrombocytosis.

thrombocytopenia (throm-bo-si-to-pe'ne-ă) Decreased number of platelets in blood (less than 150,000 per μl) Also called thrombopenia.

  isoimmune t. Thrombocytopenia caused by development of antiplatelet antibodies and consequent platelet destruction.

  neonatal t. Thrombocytopenia occurring in a newborn baby; may originate from the mother (e.g., infections, drug therapy, or maternal–fetal platelet incompatibility) or from the infant (e.g., disorders causing platelet destruction or dysfunction).

thrombocytosis (throm-bo-si-to'sis) An abnormally high number of platelets in the blood. Also called thrombocythemia.

thrombogenesis (throm-bo-jen'ĕ-sis) The formation of blood clots.

thrombopenia (throm-bo-pe'ne-ă) See thrombocytopenia.

thrombophilia (throm-bo-fil'e-ă) A hypercoagulable state secondary to a deficiency of natural inhibitors of coagulation (e.g., antithrombin II, protein C, and protein S).

thrombophlebitis (throm-bo-flĕ-bi'tis) Inflammation of the wall of a vein occurring in association with blood clot formation.

  deep t. Thrombophlebitis involving a deep vein, especially of the calf and thigh, causing pain and swelling of the limb; when a venous segment of the iliofemoral area is affected, symptoms become severe; may occur as an extension superficial thrombophlebitis.

  migratory t. Inflammation appearing first in one site, then another; associated with cancer, especially of internal organs.

  puerperal t. Thrombophlebitis occurring in a deep vein of the iliofemoral area during late pregnancy and after delivery; characterized by extreme swelling of the leg, with severe pain, tenderness, and elevated temperature; caused by compression of the vein by the pregnant uterus and the enhanced coagulability of

blood during pregnancy; usually considerable arterial spasm occurs causing the leg to become pale and cold with diminished pulses. Also called milk leg; painful white leg; phlegmasia alba dolens.

  septic pelvic t. Clotting in the veins of the pelvis, due to bacterial invasion of the vessel walls (usually by *Staphylococcus aureus*), causing chills, persistent high fever, elevated pulse and respiratory rates, and (rarely) pus formation. May occur after childbirth; predisposing factors include cesarean section after prolonged labor, premature rupture of the membranes, difficult delivery, existing systemic disease, anemia, and malnourishment.

  superficial t. The most common form of thrombophlebitis associated with pregnancy, usually involving a varicose superficial vein, particularly the long saphenous vein and its tributaries; characterized by a painful, palpable, cordlike induration of the affected vein and redness of the overlying skin; usually, there is no significant swelling of the limb as a whole.

thromboplastin (throm-bo-plas'tin) Protein complex that initiates the clotting of blood. Also called factor III.

thrombosis (throm-bo'sis) Formation of blood clots (thrombi) within an intact blood vessel.

  deep venous t. (DVT) Clotting of blood inside deep-seated veins, especially of the legs, often causing pain and tenderness in the thigh or calf; seen most commonly in people immobilized for long periods, those with chronic debilitating diseases, surgical patients, and those with cancer. The condition is a common source of embolism, especially pulmonary embolism.

thrombus (throm'bus), pl. thrombi A blood clot; a solid or semisolid mass formed inside an intact blood vessel (distinct from one formed to seal a cut or injured vessel); it is composed of the constituents of blood, primarily platelets and fibrin.

thrush (thrush) Infection of the mouth with the fungus *Candida albicans*, which forms white patches in the mucous membrane; seen most frequently in infants and in patients with a suppressed or deficient immune system, especially after a course of antibiotic

thyroiditis (thi-roi-di'tis) Inflammation of the thyroid gland.

  Hashimoto's t. Autoimmune inflammatory disorder responsible for most cases of primary hypothyroidism; characterized by progressive, painless enlargement of the thyroid gland, which becomes firm and rubbery and then slowly diminishes in size, eventually becoming atrophic and fibrous; seen most commonly in women between 30 and 50 years old. Affected pregnant women may be at a higher risk of miscarriage. Also called Hashimoto's struma; struma lymphomatosa.

postpartum t. Transient thyroiditis of autoimmune origin; characterized by hyperthyroidism, occurring 1 to 4 months after delivery, followed by hypothyroidism 4 to 8 months later; symptoms include depression, fatigue, and palpitations; the condition may recur in subsequent pregnancies.

Riedel's t. Uncommon condition in which the thyroid gland is replaced by fibrous tissue, which extends to contiguous neck structures. Also called Riedel's struma.

thyrotropin (thi-ro-tro'pin) Hormone of the anterior lobe of the pituitary (adenohypophysis) that stimulates the growth and function of the thyroid gland. Also called thyroid-stimulating hormone.

thyrotoxicosis (thi-ro-tok-sĭ-ko'sis) Toxic condition reflecting the response of tissues to an excess of thyroid hormone. Pregnancy outcomes depend on whether metabolic control is achieved.

thyroxine (thi-rok'sin) (T_4) Iodine-containing hormone, produced by the thyroid gland; its chief function is to aid in regulating the body's metabolism. Synthetic preparations are used in replacement therapy for deficiency states (e.g., hypothyroidism, cretinism, myxedema).

time (tīm) The duration of something such as an event or a process.

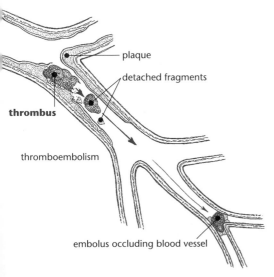

plaque

detached fragments

thrombus

thromboembolism

embolus occluding blood vessel

activated partial thromboplastin t. (APTT) Time required for plasma to form a fibrin clot subsequent to adding calcium and a phospholipid reagent.

clotting t. See coagulation time.

coagulation t. Time required for blood to clot in a test tube. Also called clotting time.

prothrombin t. (PT) Time required for a clot to form after calcium has been added to plasma in the presence of tissue thromboplastin.

tinea (tin'e-ă) Fungus infection of the skin, nails, or scalp usually caused by fungi belonging to the genera *Trichophyton, Microsporum,* and *Epydermophyton.* Popularly called ringworm.

t. cruris A reddened, intensely itchy area spreading from the genitals to the groin, perianal area, and inner thighs; usually caused by *Trichophyton rubrum* or *Epydermophyton floccosum.* Also called jock itch; ringworm of groin; tinea of groin.

t. of groin See tinea cruris.

t. versicolor Patches of dark and light scales on the skin, occurring most commonly on the trunk but occasionally involving the skin of the vulva; caused by a yeastlike fungus, *Malassezia furfur.*

tissue (tish'oo) A mass of similar cells and the substance that surrounds them, united to perform a particular function.

erectile t. Tissue containing an abundance of vascular spaces which, when engorged with blood, render the part firm (e.g., the penis and clitoris).

lymphatic t., lymphoid t. A lattice of reticular cells and fibers with interspaces containing predominantly masses of developing and mature lymphocytes; might also include some macrophages or other cells, as seen in lymph nodes, adenoids, spleen, tonsils, etc.

target t. (1) In immunology, the tissue against which antibodies are formed. (2) Tissue that responds to a specific hormone.

tobacco (to-bak'o) The dried, prepared leaves of the tobacco plant *(Nicotiana tabacum)* containing the alkaloid nicotine; tobacco smoke is a health hazard for smokers and exposed nonsmokers including the fetus, causing dose-related risk of low birth weight, reduced placental blood flow, reduced fetal breathing movements, stillbirth, and death of the newborn..

toco- Combining form meaning childbirth.

tocodynamometer (to-ko-di-nă-mom'ĕ-ter) A pressure sensor placed on the abdomen of a woman in labor to determine the frequency, duration, and strength of uterine contractions. It does not measure accurately the intensity of contractions or the resting tone of the uterus. Also called tocometer.

tocolysis (to-kol'ĭ-sis) Inhibition of uterine contractions.

tocometer (to-kom'ĕ-ter) See tocodynamometer.

Togaviridae (to-gă-vir'ĭ-de) Family of viruses that contain single-stranded RNA and replicate in cytoplasm; it includes the virus causing German measles (rubella).

togavirus (to-gă-vi'rus) Any member of the family Togaviridae.

tolerance (tol'er-ans) **1.** The body's ability to endure an insult (e.g., physiologic, chemical, or mechanical) without showing unfavorable effects. **2.** Tendency toward a reduced degree of response to repeated exposure to a stimulus.

> **drug t.** A condition of decreased responsiveness to a drug acquired by repeated intake of the drug; characterized by the necessity to increase the size of successive doses in order to produce effects of equal magnitude or duration. Compare with drug resistance, under resistance.

> **immunologic t.** The nonreactivity, or a lessened reactivity, to a particular antigen by an otherwise immunocompetent individual, acquired by previous exposure to that antigen.

> **impaired glucose t.** Abnormal result of an oral glucose tolerance test although the abnormality is not sufficient to be diagnostic of diabetes mellitus. Also called latent diabetes mellitus, preclinical diabetes mellitus, subclinical diabetes mellitus.

tomography (to-mog'ră-fe) Any imaging procedure that sequentially produces a clear image of one selected plane of internal body structures while all background and foreground planes appear blurred. Also called sectional roentgenography; body-section roentgenography.

> **computed t.** (CT) The combined use of x-ray transmission and a computer to construct cross-sectional (axial) images of a body part. Also called computed axial tomography.

> **computed axial t.** (CAT) See computed tomography.

-tomy Combining form meaning surgical cutting (e.g., thyroidotomy).

tone (tōn) The tension of a muscle at rest.

TORCH See TORCH syndrome, under syndrome.

torsade de pointes (tor-sahd dĕ pwant') In cardiology, a form of ventricular tachycardia in which the QRS complexes of the electrocardiogram are of changing amplitude and appear to twist around an electrically neutral

(isoelectric) point; hence the name ('twisting of the points').

torsion (tor'shun) A turning or twisting along a long axis.

> **t. of umbilical cord** Twisting of the umbilical cord usually occurring counterclockwise and which, if extreme, results in asphyxiation of the fetus.

tort (tort) An act that causes harm to another person (or the person's property) for which the injured party is seeking monetary compensation from the wrongdoer (tortfeasor).

> **intentional t.** In medical malpractice, a treatment involving body contact for which the patient gave neither actual nor implied consent; frequently refers to surgical procedures performed on a body structure for which the patient's consent was not previously obtained (e.g., removing both ovaries when consent was obtained for one only, or tying uterine tubes in addition to performing the cesarean section for which consent was obtained). See also informed consent, under consent.

> **negligent t.** In medical malpractice, the most common of medical professional liability actions; basically, it involves a claim that the physician violated a standard of care. See also standard of care, under standard; negligence.

torulopsosis (tor-u-lop'so-sis) Yeast infection usually involving the respiratory or genitourinary tracts; caused by *Torulopsis glabrata* (a species of the genus *Torulopsis*); seen usually as an opportunistic disease in severely debilitated persons, in those undergoing immunosuppressive therapy, or those with immune deficiency (e.g., AIDS).

tourniquet (toor'nĭ-ket) Device used in compressing blood vessels to reduce circulation to and from a part, usually an extremity.

> **scalp t.** Tourniquet applied to a patient's scalp during administration of anticancer drugs; reported to prevent associated hair loss.

toxemia (tok-se'me-ă) The presence of bacterial toxins in the bloodstream.

> **t. of pregnancy** See preeclampsia.

toxo-, toxico-, toxi- Combining forms meaning poison, toxin.

toxoplasmosis (tok-so-plaz-mo'sis) Disease caused by infection with the protozoan *Toxoplasma gondii*; it may resemble a mild cold or infectious mononucleosis in adults; a disseminated form may lead to inflammation of the liver, lungs, heart muscle, or brain and spinal cord and their membranes; another form of the disease involves the eyes; an infected pregnant woman can spread the disease to her unborn child, causing eye or brain damage or even death; the most common way of acquiring the disease is by eating raw or undercooked meat from infected animals and through contact with infected cat feces.

trachelectomy (tra-ke-lek'to-me) See cervicectomy.

trachelitis (tra-ke-li'tis) See cervicitis.

trachelo-, trachel- Combining forms meaning neck.

trachelorrhaphy (tra-ke-lor'ă-fe) Reparative operation on the 'neck' of the uterus (uterine cervix).

tract (trakt) **1.** A series of structures constituting a body system that performs a specialized function (e.g., the respiratory tract). **2.** A collection of nerve fibers possessing the same origin, termination, and function. **3.** A path.

> **genitourinary t.** See urogenital apparatus, under apparatus.

> **urinary t.** The passageway for the excretion of urine; it extends from the pelvis of the kidney, downward to the ureter, bladder, and urethra, ending at the external urethral orifice.

> **urogenital t.** See urogenital apparatus, under apparatus.

trait (trāt) **1.** In genetics, any inherited gene-determined characteristic; applied to a normal variation or to a disease. **2.** A distinguishing attribute or characteristic. **3.** A distinctive pattern of behavior.

> **beta-thalassemia t.** See beta thalassemia minor, under thalassemia.

trans- **1.** Prefix meaning through, across, beyond. **2.** In genetics, the position of two genes on opposite chromosomes of a homologous pair.

transcervical (trans-ser'vĭ-kal) Through the opening of the uterine cervix.

transcriptase (trans-krip'tās) Any enzyme that promotes transcription of genetic information. See also transcription.

> **reverse t.** An enzyme found in RNA tumor viruses (retroviruses of the family Retroviridae) that functions in transferring genetic code information back from RNA into DNA, that is, in reverse order from the usual DNA-to-RNA transcription. Used in genetic engineering.

transcription (trans-krip'shun) The transfer of genetic code information from various parts of the DNA molecule to new strands of messenger RNA (mRNA), which then carry this information from the cell nucleus to the cytoplasm.

transcutaneous (trans-ku-ta'ne-us) See transdermal.

transdermal (trans-der'mal) Applied on or entering through the skin, such as an electric nerve stimulation, or certain prolonged-release pharmaceuticals (e.g., estrogen patches in replacement therapy). Also called transcutaneous.

transfer (trans'fer) A passage from one place to another.

> **gamete intrafallopian t.** (GIFT) The placement of ova and spermatozoa together in the distal end of one or both fallopian (uterine) tubes. The procedure is performed with a laparoscope through the abdominal wall.

> **embryo t.** (ET) Procedure in which an embryo at the blastocyst stage (acquired through *in vitro* or *in vivo* fertilization) is transferred to the recipient's uterus through the vagina. The embryo may also be transferred to the recipient's fallopian (uterine) tubes via an abdominal incision.

> ***in vitro* fertilization and embryo t.** (IVF-ET) Fertilization by placing ova and spermatozoa together in a Petri dish and then placing the embryos within the recipient's uterus.

> **passive t.** The conveying of specific immunity to a nonimmune individual by introducing preformed antibody or immune cells from an immune or sensitized individual (e.g., the transfer of antibodies from a mother to her suckling newborn via colostrum and breast milk).

> **peritoneal oocyte and sperm t.** (POST) Procedure in which oocytes and spermatozoa are transvaginally injected into the rectouterine pouch under ultrasound guidance.

> **tubal embryo t.** (TET) The placement of 2- to 8-cell (cleaving) embryos in the fallopian (uterine) tubes.

> **zygote intrafallopian t.** (ZIFT) Procedure in which oocytes are fertilized *in vitro* and transferred into the fallopian (uterine) tube 24 hours later.

transferrin (trans-fer'rin) Iron-binding beta globulin; it facilitates blood transportation of iron to bone marrow and tissue storage areas.

transformation (trans-for-ma'shun) **1.** The conversion of a cell from a normal state to a malignant state due either to infection with a cancer-producing virus or to environmental factors. **2.** In molecular biology, genetic changes incurred by a cell through incorporation of DNA from another species.

> **neoplastic cell t.** Abnormal cell changes

including increased growth potential, changes in cell surface, biochemical deviations, and other attributes that invest the cell with the potential ability to invade, metastasize, and kill.

transfusion (trans-fu´zhun) Introduction of a fluid (e.g., blood, plasma) into the bloodstream.

    autologous blood t. Transfusion of the patient's own blood, retrieved and antiseptically prepared, to maintain circulating blood volume subsequent to blood loss at surgery.

    exchange t. Removal of blood containing a toxic substance and replacing it with donor blood, as performed in newborn infants with Rh-incompatibility isoimmune hemolytic anemia. Also called substitution transfusion.

    intrauterine t. Exchange transfusion of the fetus in the uterus by umbilical vein catheterization performed through the mother's abdominal wall under ultrasound guidance; conducted to maintain an effective red blood cell mass within the fetal circulation and to maintain the pregnancy.

    substitution t. See exchange transfusion.

translation (trans-la´shun) The decoding of genetic information contained in the messenger RNA (mRNA) molecule and conversion of this information into a protein of a particular amino acid sequence, as directed by the mRNA.

translocation (trans-lo-ka´shun) An error occurring during replication of chromosomes whereby a chromosome, or a fragment of it, becomes attached to another chromosome.

transluminal (trans-lu´mĭ-nal) Through a lumen (e.g., of a blood vessel).

transmembrane (trans-mem´brān) Through a membrane.

transmission (trans-mish´un) **1.** Transfer, as of disease or genetic information, from one individual to another. **2.** Conveyance (e.g., of nerve impulses).

    iatrogenic t. Transmission of infectious microorganisms through medical or dental interference (e.g., by contaminated instruments or equipment).

    vertical t. Direct, prenatal passage of an infective agent or genetic characteristic from mother to child.

transmural (trans-mu´ral) Across the wall of an organ or cyst.

transperitoneal (trans-per-ĭ-to-ne´al) Through the membrane (peritoneum) lining the abdominopelvic cavity.

transplacental (trans-plă-sen´tal) Through the placenta.

transplantation (trans-plan-ta´shun) The transfer

of living tissues or organs from one site to another in the same individual, between individuals of the same species, or between individuals of different species.

    allogeneic bone marrow t. The transplantation of bone marrow tissue from one individual to another of the same species but of a different genetic make-up (genotype).

    autologous bone marrow t. (ABMT) Treatment modality for patients with recurrent

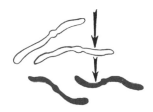

injury to a chromosome

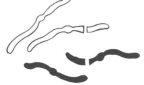

breakage of a chromosome

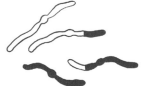

reciprocal **translocation** between non-homologous chromosomes

malignant disease and when an appropriate donor cannot be found; bone marrow tissue is obtained from the patient, is freed of leukemic cells, and reinfused after the patient has received large levels of chemotherapy and irradiation. The procedure is performed at a time when the patient is in remission.

    bone marrow t. Transplantation of bone marrow tissue from the iliac crest of the donor's hipbone; used in the treatment of blood malignancies, aplastic anemia, or immunodeficiency states.

    stem cell t. Transplantation of stem cells, which may be autologous or allogeneic, for the treatment of certain disorders (e.g., sickle cell anemia, thalassemias, leukemias, and various immunodeficiencies).

transport (trans'port) Movement of substances in the body, especially across cell membranes.

    active placental t. The selective transport of specific nutrients to the fetus, accomplished by enzymatic mechanisms in the placenta.

transposition (trans-po-zish'un) **1.** The presence of an organ or structure on the wrong side of the body. **2.** The state of being reversed. **3.** In genetics, the DNA-mediated movement of genetic material from one site to another in the chromosomes. **4.** The surgical movement of tissues or structures from one place to another.

    t. of great vessels, t. of great arteries Developmental malformation in which the aorta and pulmonary trunk arise from abnormal, opposite sites in the heart (i.e., the aorta originates from the right ventricle, the pulmonary trunk from the left ventricle); in essence, two independent blood circulations are formed, without exchange of oxygenated and deoxygenated blood. The affected infant survives when some anatomic communication exists between the two systems; this occurs when holes (septal defects) in the walls separating the right and left atria or ventricles are formed during fetal life or when the ductus arteriosus (which normally closes after birth) remains open; symptoms include bluish coloration of the skin and shortness of breath. The transposition occurs most frequently in children of diabetic mothers, especially sons. If not corrected surgically, the infant dies within 1 year.

transrectal (trans-rek'tal) Through the rectum, as in certain procedures (e.g., prostatic biopsy, ultrasonic evaluation of the genitourinary system).

transsexual (trans-seks'u-al) **1.** Relating to the surgical or hormonal intervention to alter an individual's external characteristics so that they resemble those of the opposite sex. **2.** Relating to transsexualism.

transsexualism (trans-seks'u-a-lizm) The overpowering desire to be of the opposite sex and desiring corrective surgery, usually from an early age.

transurethral (trans-u-re'thral) Through the urethra.

transvaginal (trans-vaj'ĭ-nal) Through the vagina.

transvestism (trans-ves'tizm) The persistent desire and practice of dressing in clothing of the opposite sex; especially by a male and usually for sexual gratification. Also called cross-dressing.

transvestite (trans-ves'tĭt) A person who practices transvestism.

treatment (trēt'ment) Any course of action or program adopted to restore health, prevent disease, or relieve symptoms.

    breast conservation t. See segmental mastectomy, under mastectomy.

    conservative t. Management of disease with the least aggressive of therapeutic options. Sometimes the term is used to mean medical as opposed to surgical.

    maintenance t. Treatment aimed at stabilizing the patient's condition, especially when no cure is available.

    palliative t. Treatment aimed at mitigating symptoms rather than curing the disease.

    preventive t., prophylactic t. Treatment given to prevent a person from acquiring a disease after exposure to the disease, or when expected to be exposed.

treatment port (trēt'ment port) In radiation therapy, the spot on the body at which the radiation beam is directed.

Treponema (trep-o-ne'mă) A genus of spiral bacteria (family Treponemataceae); several species cause disease in humans.

    T. pallidum Species causing syphilis in humans.

treponemicidal (trep-o-ne-mĭ-si'dal) Destructive to microorganisms of the genus *Treponema*. Also called antitreponemal.

triad (tri'ad) A group of closely related signs, symptoms, or anatomic structures.

    Virchow's t. The notion that there is a predisposition for thromboembolism consisting of circulatory stasis (i.e., impaired blood circulation), vascular damage, and hypercoagulability (i.e., abnormally high tendency to form clots).

triangle (tri'ang-gl) A three-cornered area.

    anal t. A triangular space with the angles placed at both ischial tuberosities and at the tip of the coccyx; the posterior part of the perineum containing the anus.

    t. of bladder See trigone of bladder, under trigone.

    femoral t. The area just below the fold of the groin, at the upper and inner part of the thigh; it is bounded above by the inguinal ligament, laterally by the medial border of the sartorius muscle, and medially by the medial border of the long adductor muscle; the femoral vessels divide the triangle into two parts. Also called Scarpa's triangle; femoral trigone.

    Hesselbach's t. See inguinal triangle.

inguinal t. Area of the anterior abdominal wall bounded below by the medial half of the inguinal ligament, medially by the lower edge of the straight muscle of the abdomen (rectus abdominus muscle), and laterally by a line from the middle of the inguinal ligament to the navel; an important area relating to direct and indirect inguinal hernias. Also called Hesselbach's triangle.

    Scarpa's t. See femoral triangle.

    umbilicomammillary t. A triangular area formed by a line joining the nipples of the breast with its apex at the navel.

    urogenital t. A triangular space with the angles placed at both ischial tuberosities and at the pubic symphysis; it contains the external urogenital organs.

    vesical t. See trigone of bladder, under trigone.

trichomonad (tri-kom'o-nad) Any member of the genus *Trichomonas*.

Trichomonas (trik-o-mo'nas) Genus of parasitic protozoan flagellates (family Trichomonadidae).

    T. vaginalis A pear-shaped, highly motile organism that infects the lower genital tract of females and the urethra and prostate of males. See also trichomoniasis.

trichomoniasis (trik-o-mo-ni'ă-sis) Infection of the genital tract with *Trichomonas vaginalis* almost always acquired through sexual intercourse; in females, it usually causes varying degrees of vulvar and vaginal irritation and itching, a profuse vaginal discharge, and inflammation of the vaginal epithelium; in pregnant women, the infection may cause low-birthweight infants or premature birth. Infected males are usually asymptomatic, serving mostly as vectors for transmission through sexual intercourse; a few experience inflammation of the urethra; the organism can be detected in the urine following prostatic massage.

tricyclic (tri-si'klik) Term used to describe a class of antidepressant drugs having three rings in their molecular structure.

trigone (tri'gōn) Triangle; a triangular space, eminence, or fossa.

    t. of bladder A small triangular, smooth area at the lower-posterior part of the bladder, between the two slit-like openings of the ureters and the internal orifice of the urethra; in this area the mucosa is closely adhered to the muscular layer of the bladder wall. Also called vesical triangle; vesical trigone; triangle of bladder.

    femoral t. See femoral triangle, under triangle.

    vesical t. See trigone of bladder.

trigonitis (trig-o-ni'tis) Inflammation of the lower portion (trigone) of the bladder.

trigonocephaly (tri-go-no-sef'ă-le) Early closure of the frontal suture, sometimes occurring during intrauterine life, and resulting in a keel-shape deformity of the skull.

triiodothyronine (tri-i-o-do-thi'ro-nēn) (TITh, T_3) One of the two principal hormones secreted by the thyroid gland (the other being thyroxine); it aids in regulating the body's metabolism.

    reverse t., reverse T_3 (rT_3) A product of the peripheral degradation of thyroxine; present in elevated levels in certain disease states; useful as an aid for diagnosis of fetal and infantile hypothyroidism.

trimethadione (tri-meth-ă-di'ōn) Drug with anticonvulsant properties; may cause abnormalities or death of the fetus when taken by a pregnant woman; abnormalities may include intrauterine growth retardation, mental retardation, impaired hearing, heart defects, and urogenital malformations.

trimester (tri-mes'ter) A period of 3 months.

    first t. The period of pregnancy from the first day of the last menstrual period before conception to the 98th day; the first 14 weeks of gestation.

    second t. The period of pregnancy from the 15th to the 28th weeks of gestation.

    third t. The period of pregnancy from the 29th to the 42nd weeks of gestation.

triplet (trip'let) **1.** One of three individuals born at one birth. **2.** In molecular biology, a unit of three successive bases in DNA or RNA that code for a specific amino acid in a protein molecule.

trisomy (tri'so-me) An abnormality in which an additional chromosome is present in the cells (i.e., 47 instead of 46); the extra chromosome is a copy of one of an existing pair, so that one particular chromosome is present in triplicate. The consequences of trisomy can range from early fetal death and spontaneous abortion to numerous abnormalities in the live-born child. See also trisomy 13 syndrome, trisomy 18 syndrome, and Down's syndrome, under syndrome.

tropho-, troph- Combining forms meaning nutrition.

trophoblast (trof'o-blast) The outer layer of cells forming the wall of the blastocyst; it plays an important role in attaching this early embryo to the uterine wall and in the eventual formation of the placenta.

trophoblastoma (trof-o-blas-to'mă) See choriocarcinoma.

truncus (trun'kus) Latin for trunk.

t. arteriosus The main arterial trunk of the embryonic heart; it gives rise to the aorta and the pulmonary trunk.

persistent t. arteriosus Congenital cardiovascular defect due to failure of the pulmonary trunk and aorta to normally separate during embryonic development; it results in a single blood vessel that takes origin astride a ventricular septal defect, receiving blood from both right and left ventricles.

trunk (trungk) **1.** The human body excluding the head and the extremities. Also called torso. **2.** The main stem of a nerve, vessel, or duct before it divides into branches.

costocervical t. A short arterial trunk arising from the back of each subclavian artery; in the vicinity of the neck of the first rib, it divides into the deep cervical and highest intercostal branches.

lumbar lymphatic t.'s Two large collecting lymphatic vessels, right and left, that drain lymph upward from the lumbar lymph nodes to the cisterna chyli.

lumbosacral t. A large nerve formed by the union of the lower part of the ventral division of the fourth lumbar nerve and the entire ventral branch of the fifth lumbar nerve; it enters into the formation of the sacral plexus.

lymphatic t.'s Large vessels that convey lymph to the thoracic duct, right lymphatic duct, or to the cisterna chyli.

sympathetic t.'s Two long chains of sympathetic ganglia extending on either side of the vertebral column, from the base of the skull to the coccyx; the two chains meet in front of the coccyx in an unpaired terminal ganglion (ganglion impar).

tube (tūb) **1.** An anatomic channel or canal. **2.** A hollow cylinder designed to function as a passage.

fallopian t. See uterine tube.

neural t. The epithelial tube of the early embryo formed by the closure of the neural groove; it develops into the brain and spinal cord.

uterine t. One of the two slender tubes extending from each superior angle of the uterus to the ovary and varying from 7 to 14 cm in length; may be divided into: *isthmus*, the narrow portion with its proximal segment

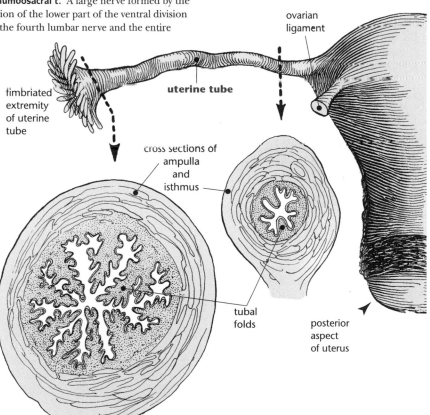

ovarian ligament

fimbriated extremity of uterine tube

uterine tube

cross sections of ampulla and isthmus

tubal folds

posterior aspect of uterus

embedded in the muscular wall of the uterus and communicating with the uterine cavity through an opening, the uterine ostium, which is about 1 mm in diameter; *ampulla,* the slightly wider and tortuous portion; *infundibulum,* the widest, funnel-shaped portion terminating near the ovary in communication with the abdominal cavity through an opening, the abdominal ostium, which is about 3 mm in diameter; the margin of the infundibulum is divided into numerous projections (fimbriae); one projection, the fimbria ovarica, is much longer than the others and forms a sort of gutter in contact with the ovary. The uterine tube is the channel through which ova gain access to the uterine cavity and the site where fertilization usually occurs. Also called fallopian tube; oviduct.

tubectomy (too-bek'to-me) See salpingectomy.

tubercle (too'ber-kl) **1.** A rounded elevation on a structure, such as a bone. **2.** The specific grayish lesion of tuberculosis. **3.** A nodule on the skin.

    areolar t.'s The numerous nodules just beneath the skin of the areola of the breast representing the enlarged condition of areolar sebaceous glands, a characteristic change normally occurring during pregnancy and lactation; the increased oily secretion provides lubrication for the nipple and areola during breast feeding.

    t. of iliac crest A prominence on the outer lip of the iliac crest of the hipbone, approximately 5 cm above and behind the anterior superior iliac spine.

    Müller's t., mullerian t. The first indication of the embryonic uterus and vagina; a median protrusion into the urogenital sinus, formed from the fused caudal ends of the paramesonephric ducts. Also called sinus tubercle.

    pubic t. A small tubercle at the lateral end of the pubic crest, on either side, about 2 cm from the pubic symphysis; it provides attachment to the tendons of the straight muscle of the abdomen (rectus abdominis muscle) and the pyramidal muscle. Also called pubic spine.

    t. of Rokitansky The solid elements that arise, and are contained, in a protrusion or nipple in the cyst wall of a benign cystic teratoma.

    sinus t. See Müller's tubercle.

tuberculosis (too-ber-ku-lo'sis) (TB, tb, TBC) A chronic, communicable disease caused by the bacterium *Mycobacterium tuberculosis,* which causes a distinctive ulcerating lesion in the tissues

affected; human infections are most commonly caused by *Mycobacterium hominis* and *bovis,* acquired by inhaling airborne droplets of the coughing and sneezing from infected persons and, only rarely, by drinking infected milk; people most at risk are those with debilitating or immunosuppressive conditions, including malnutrition, alcoholism, diabetes, chronic lung disease, extensive corticosteroid use, and AIDS.

    disseminated t. See miliary tuberculosis.

    miliary t. A form in which the bloodstream has carried the organisms to several organs, causing simultaneous development of numerous, minute foci of infection. Also called disseminated tuberculosis.

    pelvic t. Tuberculosis of the female genital tract usually involving the endometrium, fallopian (uterine) tubes, and ovaries; it occurs as a spread, via the bloodstream, from a primary infection; manifestations include dense adhesions without occlusion of the tube openings, and dilatation of tubal segments.

tubocornual (too-bo-kor'nu-al) Relating to a fallopian (uterine) tube and one of the upper elongated portions (cornua) of the uterus.

tuboscopy (too-bos'cŏ-pe) See falloposcopy.

tubo-ovarian (too'bo o-va're-an) Relating to a fallopian (uterine) tube and an ovary.

tubo-ovariectomy (too'bo o-va-re-ek'to-me) See salpingo-oophorectomy.

tubo-ovaritis (too'bo o-vă-ri'tis) See salpingo-oophoritis.

tuboperitoneal (too-bo-per-ĭ-to-ne'al) Relating to the fallopian (uterine) tubes and the lining (peritoneum) of the abdominopelvic cavity.

tuboplasty (too'bo-plas-te) See salpingoplasty.

tumor (too'mor) An overgrowth of tissue; a neoplasm.

    benign t. A tumor that does not spread to other areas of the body, does not infiltrate adjacent structures, and is unlikely to recur once removed.

    Brenner's t. A yellowish-brown solid tumor of the ovary; it is typically benign but (rarely) may undergo malignant transformation; usually occurs unilaterally in postmenopausal women.

    collision t. Synchronous squamous cell carcinomas and adenocarcinomas that infiltrate each other.

    desmoid t. See desmoid.

    embryonal t. General term for any tumor (usually malignant) believed to be derived from embryonic tissues. Also called embryoma.

    endodermal sinus t. (EST) See yolk-sac

tumor of ovary.

endometrioid t. of ovary Malignant tumor composed of a combination of solid and cystic masses, microscopically resembling endometrial adenocarcinoma; may occur bilaterally (40%) or unilaterally.

Ewing's t. See Ewing's sarcoma, under sarcoma.

fibroid t. See leiomyoma.

germ-cell t. of ovary Any of a group of ovarian tumors derived from cell types of the endoderm, mesoderm, or ectoderm (i.e., the germ layers); they include dermoids, dysgerminomas, malignant teratomas, and yolk-sac tumors.

gonadal stromal t. Any of various ovarian tumors that contain theca cells, granulosa cells, stromal fibroblasts of gonadal stromal origin, Sertoli cells, and Leydig cells.

granular cell t. A predominantly benign tumor of uncertain origin; it may occur anywhere in the body, most commonly seen in the tongue and subcutaneous tissue of the trunk (especially of the breast), and upper extremities. Formerly called granular cell myoblastoma.

granulosa cell t. An uncommon, benign (potentially malignant) tumor of the ovary that typically secretes large amounts of estrogen; it is usually confined to one ovary and may occur in any age group, causing vaginal bleeding in postmenopausal women; when occurring in young girls, it is commonly associated with pseudoprecocious puberty. Also called granulosa-theca cell tumor; folliculoma.

granulosa-theca cell t. See granulosa cell tumor.

Grawitz' t. See renal adenocarcinoma, under adenocarcinoma.

malignant t. A tumor that spreads from its original location to affect other parts of the body (i.e., forms metastases), may recur after removal, and eventually causes death if not treated early and appropriately. Often called cancer.

mixed t. Tumor composed of more than one tissue or cell type.

papillary t. See papilloma.

phyllodes t. A bulky, slow-growing, usually benign tumor of the breast, most commonly seen in premenopausal women, although it may occur at any age; it is composed chiefly of proliferative ducts and supportive tissues (stroma) of the breast; some have malignant potential; those that become malignant

metastasize to the lungs via the bloodstream. Formerly called cystosarcoma phyllodes.

Sertoli-Leydig t. An uncommon benign tumor of the testis or the ovary, composed of Sertoli cells or a mixture of Leydig and Sertoli cells in varying proportions and degrees of differentiation; on rare occasions, it may turn malignant. Also called androblastoma.

sex cord-stromal t.'s A group of ovarian tumors derived either from the sex cords of the embryonic gonad or from the supporting tissues (stroma) of the ovary (e.g., fibromas, granulosa-theca cell tumors, Sertoli-Leydig cell tumors).

yolk-sac t. of ovary A highly malignant tumor that grows rapidly and aggressively; it affects only one ovary and occurs mainly in young women (under 20 years of age) and children; microscopically, it consists of primitive cells and cystic spaces into which protrude tufts of blood vessels enveloped by immature epithelium. Most secrete alpha-fetoprotein (AFP). Also called endodermal sinus tumor.

tumorigenic (too-mor-ĭ-jen'ik) Causing tumors.

tumor sanctuary (too'mor sank'chŭ-wĕ-re) Sites in the body where tumor cells remain unaffected by anticancer drugs, permitting unimpeded growth of a tumor that has been successfully eliminated from the rest of the body by the drugs.

tunica (too'ni-kă), pl. tunicae A coat of condensed connective tissue covering an organ or lining a space. Also called tunic.

t. albuginea of ovary A delicate collagenous covering of the ovary situated between the outer germinal epithelium and the cortex of the ovary; it increases in density with passing age.

t. mucosa of uterus The endometrium.

t. mucosa of vagina The mucous membrane of the vagina.

twin (twin) One of two children born at one birth.

conjoined t.'s Twins with a varying degree of connection or fusion with each other. Also called Siamese twins.

dizygotic t.'s See fraternal twins.

fraternal t.'s Twins developed from two separate eggs fertilized at the same time; they may or may not be of the same sex. Also called dizygotic twins; heterozygous twins.

heterozygous t.'s See fraternal twins.

identical t.'s Twins resulting from a single egg that splits at an early stage of development; they are always of the same sex, have the same genetic constitution, and have pronounced resemblance to each other. Also called monozygotic twins; uniovular twins.

locked t.'s Twins whose heads become simultaneously impacted in the pelvis during delivery; while one twin descends through the birth canal in a breech presentation, the other follows in a vertex presentation, and the chin of the first locks in the neck and chin of the second.

monozygotic t.'s See identical twins.

Siamese t.'s See conjoined twins.

uniovular t.'s See identical twins.

vanishing t. Colloquial term for the spontaneous release of amniotic fluid occurring in the first trimester of pregnancy, with the pregnancy usually continuing normally to term; cause is unknown; believed to be due to a twin pregnancy in which the second fetus and its amniotic sac (membrane) are liquefied by enzymatic action (probably from the second fetus itself) early in the pregnancy, with consequent release of the amniotic fluid.

typing (tī p'ing) Determination of the type category to which any entity belongs.

blood t. See blood grouping.

DNA t. Test on a nucleated cell (e.g., of semen, blood, hair roots) to detect characteristics in genetic structure that are as unique to an individual as fingerprints.

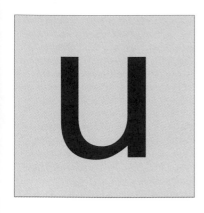

ulcer (ul′ser) Loss of tissue on the skin or mucous membrane, extending into the subcutaneous or submucosal tissues, frequently accompanied by inflammation.

gummatous u. An ulcer on the skin appearing in the late stage of syphilis.

soft u. See chancroid.

venereal u. See chancroid.

ultrasonic (ul-tră-son′ik) Relating to sound waves above 30,000 cycles per second, not perceptible by the human ear.

ultrasonogram (ul-tră-son′o-gram) A record made by ultrasonography. Also called echogram; sonogram.

ultrasonograph (ul-tră-son′o-graf) The apparatus used in ultrasonography. Also called echograph; sonograph.

ultrasonography (ul trǎ-son-ŏg′ra-fe) (US) Visualization of internal body structures by bouncing high-frequency sound waves off body tissues and converting the echoes (reflected pulses) of those waves into a pictorial display on a screen; used widely as a diagnostic procedure, a monitoring technique, and as an adjunct to certain surgical procedures. Also called sonography.

Doppler u. Diagnostic technique for recording and analyzing changes in the frequency of a continuous ultrasound wave, indicative of changes in a moving target (e.g., blood flow within vessels).

prenatal u. Transabdominal ultrasonography performed during pregnancy; may be applied to the maternal or the fetal condition.

real-time u. The production of serial ultrasound images displaying actual motion (e.g., of the fetus and the heart).

transabdominal u. Ultrasonography in which the transducer is placed on the skin of the abdomen, interfaced with a water-soluble

gel. Clinical applications include identification of intrauterine pregnancy, identification and location of the placenta, measurement of the fetus to estimate gestational age and weight, determination of amniotic fluid volume, detection of fetal anomalies and intrauterine growth retardation (IUGR), determination of fetal death, identification of uterine tumors, and detection of a foreign body (e.g., an intrauterine device).

transvaginal u. (TVUS) Ultrasonography in which the ultrasound probe is introduced into the vagina to examine the reproductive tract; usually performed to evaluate abnormal masses (e.g., of the ovaries or uterine tubes), to diagnose ectopic and molar pregnancies, and to examine the fetus for detection of abnormalities.

ultrasound (ul′tra-sound) Sound waves of frequency higher than the range audible to the human ear, especially in the 1 to 10 MHz range; the waves are propagated at a speed determined by the physical properties of the medium through which they travel; used in medicine for diagnostic purposes. See also ultrasonography.

umbilical (um-bil′ĭ-kal) Relating to the umbilicus. Also called omphalic.

umbilicus (um-bil′ĭ-kus) The depressed area on the abdominal wall where the umbilical cord was attached to the fetus. Popularly called navel; belly button.

Unasyn (ū na-sin) Trademark for an antibiotic combination of ampicillin and sulbactam.

uncinariasis (un-sin-ă-ri′ă-sis) See hookworm disease, under disease.

uniparental (u-nī-pă-ren′tal) Relating to one parent only.

unit (u′nit) (u) An entity regarded as an elementary constituent of a larger whole.

Alexandria u. The product of the average intensity of uterine contractions multiplied by the average duration of contractions and their frequency in a 10-minute interval.

Montevideo u. The product of the average intensity of uterine contractions (i.e., increased pressure above the baseline resting pressure) multiplied by the number of contractions in a 10-minute interval; used for measuring uterine activity.

up-regulation (up reg-u-la′shun) An increase in the number of active receptors on the cell surface in response to deficiency of a homologous hormone or neurotransmitter.

urachal (u′ră-kal) Relating to the urachus.

urachus (u′ră-kus) A canal present in the fetus between the navel and the apex of the bladder; it obliterates early during intrauterine life, becoming a thick fibrous cord known after birth as the median umbilical ligament. Occasionally the fetal structure remains completely or partly patent, forming a congenital anomaly (either a fistula, a cyst, or a sinus).

    patent u. See urachal fistula, under fistula.

uracil (u'ră-sil) A pyrimidine present in nucleic acid.

Ureaplasma (u-re-ă- plaz'mă) A genus of Gram-negative bacteria (family Mycoplasmataceae) which lack a cell wall and hydrolize urea with production of ammonia.

    U. urealyticum A sexually transmitted species causing disease of the genitourinary system; implicated in causing infertility in both males and females.

ureter (u-rē'ter) A long, slender musculai tube conveying urine from the pelvis of the kidney into the base of the bladder; in the adult, it measures from 25 to 30 cm in length and is slightly constricted in three places.

ureteral (u-re'ter-al) Relating to the ureter. Also called ureteric.

ureteric (u-rĕ-ter'ik) See ureteral.

ureterocystostomy (u-rĕ-ter-o-sis-tos'to-me) See ureteroneocystostomy.

ureteroneocystostomy (u-rĕ-ter-o-ne-o-sis-tos'tŏ-me) Transplantation of the distal end of a ureter to a site in the bladder other than the normal one. Also called ureterocystostomy.

ureteropelvic (u-re-ter-o-pel'vik) Relating to a ureter and the adjoining renal pelvis.

ureterostomy (u-re-ter-os'tŏ-me) Attachment of the distal end of a divided ureter to the skin of the lower abdomen and creation of an external opening through which urine may be discharged when the bladder has been removed.

ureterotomy (u-re-ter-ot'ŏ-me) Surgical division of a ureter.

ureterovaginal (u-re-ter-o-vaj'ĭ-nal) Relating to a ureter and the vagina.

ureterovesical (u-re-ter-o-ves'ĭ-kal) Relating to a ureter and the bladder.

ureterovesicostomy (u-re-ter-o-ves-ĭ-kos'to-me) Surgical procedure in which a divided ureter is implanted into a new site in the bladder.

urethra (u-re'thră) The canal conveying urine from the bladder to the exterior of the body.

    female u. The channel extending from the neck of the bladder to the urinary opening inferior and posterior to the clitoris.

    male u. The channel extending from the neck of the bladder to the opening at the tip of the glans penis; it conveys seminal secretions as well as urine. Designated *anterior*

urethra, the portion extending from the bulb of the penis to the tip of the glans penis (subdivided into bulbous, pendulous, and glandular parts), and *posterior urethra*, the portion extending from the neck of the bladder to the bulb of the penis (subdivided into prostatic and membranous parts).

urethral (u-re'thral) Relating to the urethra.

urethralgia (u-rĕ-thral'je-ă) Pain in the urethra.

urethratresia (u-re-thră-tre'ze-ă) Congenital imperforation or occlusion of the urethra.

urethrectomy (u-rĕ-threk'tŏ-me) Removal of the urethra, or a portion of it.

urethrism, urethrismus (u're-thrizm, u-re-thriz'mus) Irritability or chronic spasm of the urethra, usually associated with inflammation that may also involve the lower portion of the bladder. Also called urethrospasm.

urethritis (u-rĕ-thri'tis) Inflammation of the urethra; most common symptom is a burning sensation when passing urine; usually caused by infections (e.g., by sexually transmitted diseases and catheters left in place to drain the bladder); less frequently may be caused by chemical irritation (e.g., by antiseptics and spermicides).

    chlamydial u. Sexually transmitted disease caused by the bacterium *Chlamydia trachomatis*. See also nongonococcal urethritis.

    gonococcal u. Urethritis caused by gonococci; a form of gonorrhea; appears 2 to 7 days after sexual intercourse with an individual afflicted with gonorrhea.

    nongonococcal u. (NGU) A sexually transmitted disease caused by a variety of microorganisms, most commonly *Chlamydia trachomatis*; routine bacterial cultures often do not reveal the organisms. In males, the infection usually produces a mild burning sensation on urination and a slight grayish discharge, especially apparent before the first urination of the day; in females, it is usually asymptomatic. A pregnant woman may infect her newborn infant with serious consequences for the child. Also called nonspecific urethritis.

    nonspecific u. (NSU) See nongonococcal urethritis.

urethro-, urethr- Combining forms meaning urethra.

urethrocele (u-re'thro-sēl) A prolapse or sagging of the posterior wall of the female urethra into the vagina, commonly associated with a cystocele; often associated with (not the cause of) urinary incontinence.

urethrocystitis (u-re-thro-sis-ti'tis) Inflammation of the urethra and bladder.

urethrocystopexy (u-re-thro-sis'to-pek-se) An

operation for the treatment of genuine stress urinary incontinence (SUI). The concept of this procedure is to enhance continence of urine by surgically elevating the bladder neck (urethrovesical junction) to its normal anatomic position. Also called colpourethropexy; cystourethropexy.

> **Burch suprapubic u.** Procedure in which the bladder neck is sewn to the Cooper's (pectineal) ligaments in the space of Retzius (retropubic space).

> **Marshall-Marchetti-Krantz u.** Procedure in which the bladder neck is sewn to the periostium of the symphysis pubis in the space of Retzius (retropubic space).

urethrophyma (u-re-thro-fiˈmă) Any circumscribed growth of the urethra.

urethroplasty (u-reˈthro-plas-te) Surgical repair of an injury or defect of the urethra.

urethrorectal (u-re-thro-rekˈtal) Relating to the urethra and rectum.

urethrorrhagia (u-re-thro-raˈje-ă) Bleeding from the urethra.

urethrorrhea (u-re-thro-reˈa) Abnormal discharge from the urethra.

urethrospasm (u-reˈthro-spazm) See urethrism.

urethrostenosis (u-re-thro-ste-noˈsis) Abnormal constriction of the urethra.

urethrostomy (u-re-throsˈtŏ-me) Surgical construction of an opening into the urethra for temporary or permanent diversion of urine.

urethrovaginal (u-re-thro-vajˈĭ-nal) Relating to the urethra and the vagina.

urethrovesical (u-re-thro-vesˈĭ-kal) Relating to the urethra and bladder.

-uretic Combining form meaning urine (e.g., diuretic).

-uria Combining form meaning the presence of a particular substance in the urine (e.g., proteinuria).

urinalysis (ur-ĭ-nalˈĭ-sis) Analysis of urine.

urinary (uˈri-năr-e) Relating to urine.

urinary urgency (uˈrĭ-năr-e urˈjen-se) A strong urge to urinate.

urinate (urˈĭ-nāt) To micturate; to void.

urination (u-rĭ-naˈshun) The passing of urine. Also called micturition.

urine (uˈrin) The fluid excreted by the kidneys, normally stored in the bladder, and discharged through the urethra; composed of approximately 96% water and 4% solid matter (chiefly urea and sodium chloride), including many metabolic wastes.

> **residual u.** (RU) The urine left in the bladder after urination.

uriniferous (u-rĭ-nifˈer-us) Conveying urine.

urino-, urin- Combining forms meaning urine.

urinogenous (u-rĭ-nojˈĕ-nus) Producing urine.

urocystic (u-ro-sisˈtik) Relating to the urinary bladder.

urodynamics (u-ro-di-namˈĭks) The study of the activities of the urinary bladder, urethral sphincter muscle, and pelvic musculature by means of various pressure devices.

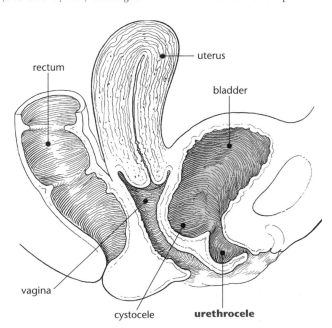

rectum
uterus
bladder
vagina
cystocele
urethrocele

urodynia (u-ro-din'e-ă) Pain or discomfort experienced during urination.

urogenital (u-ro-jen'ĭ-tal) See genitourinary.

urography (u-rog'ră-fe) X-ray examination of any part of the urinary tract.

> **excretory u.** See intravenous pyelography, under pyelography.

> **retrograde u.** Urography following introduction of a radiopaque substance into the bladder or ureters.

urogynecology (u-ro-gi-nĕ-kol'ŏ-je) The study, diagnosis, and treatment of diseases of the female urinary tract.

urokinase (u-ro-ki'nās) A protease used as a thrombolytic agent (i.e., to dissolve blood clots); not known to cause developmental anomalies in laboratory animals.

urolith (u'ro-lith) See urinary stone, under stone.

urologist (u-rol'ŏ-jist) A specialist in urology.

urology (u-rol'ŏ-je) The branch of medicine concerned with the study, diagnosis, and treatment (especially by surgical techniques) of diseases of the urinary tract of both male and female, and of the genital organs of the male.

> **gynecologic u.** Urology of the female reproductive system and lower urinary tract.

ursodeoxycholic acid (ur-so-de-ok-se-ko'lik as'id) A bile acid useful in the treatment of intrahepatic cholestasis of pregnancy.

uterine (u'ter-in) Relating to the uterus.

utero-, uter- Combining forms meaning uterus.

uteroglobin (u-ter-o-glob'in) A protein present in epithelial cells of the endometrium.

utero-ovarian (u'ter-o o-va're-an) Relating to the uterus and an ovary.

uteroplacental (u-ter-o-plă-sen'tal) Relating to the uterus and the placenta.

uteroplasty (u'ter-o-plas-te) Reparative surgery of the uterus.

uterosacral (u-ter-o-sa'kral) Relating to the uterus and the sacrum.

uterotomy (u-ter-ot'ŏ-me) See hysterotomy.

uterotonic (u-ter-o-ton'ik) **1.** Overcoming relaxation of the uterine wall. **2.** Any agent producing such an effect.

uterotonin (u-ter-o-ton'in) General term for any substance that increases the tone, or induces contraction, of uterine smooth muscle (e.g., oxytocin, prostaglandins, endothelin 1).

uterotropic (u-ter-o-trop'ik) Denoting a substance that has an affinity for the uterus.

uterotropin (u-ter-o-tro'pin) Any substance that activates the functional elements of the uterus in preparation for labor (i.e., by facilitating contractile effectiveness of the myometrium and softening of the cervix).

uterotubal (u-ter-o-too'bal) Relating to the uterus and a fallopian (uterine) tube.

uterovaginal (u-ter-o-vaj'ĭ-nal) Relating to the uterus and vagina.

uterovesical (u-ter-o-ves'ĭ-kal) Relating to the uterus and bladder.

uterus (u'ter-us) A hollow muscular organ of the female mammal situated in the pelvis between the bladder and rectum; its function is the nourishment of the developing young prior to birth; the mature human uterus is pear-shaped, thick walled, and approximately 76 mm long, reaching adult size by 15 years and diminishing after the menopause; it consists of a main portion (the corpus or body), an upper rounded portion (the fundus) into which opens on either side a fallopian (uterine) tube, and a lower portion (the cervix or neck) that opens into the vagina. Popularly called womb.

> **anomalous u.** A malformed uterus.

> **bicornuate u., u. bicornis** A uterus characterized by the presence of a vascular, fibromuscular partition that indents the fundus and may extend down into the uterine body, forming two distinct horns.

> **Couvelaire u.** A purplish hard uterus that has lost a great deal of its contractile power; caused by blood infiltration from a partially detached placenta; specifically, the center of the placenta detaches from the uterine wall while its margins remain attached, resulting in extensive bleeding into the myometrium and consequent disruption of muscle bundles. Also called uteroplacental apoplexy.

> **u. didelphys** A uterus separated throughout its length by a fibrous partition, which may extend through the vagina; each side has one separate uterine horn with a corresponding fallopian (uterine) tube; it may or may not have a double vagina. Also called double uterus.

> **double u.** See uterus didelphys.

> **gravid u.** A pregnant uterus.

> **inverted u.** A uterus that is, in effect, turned inside out, with its fundus prolapsed toward or through the cervix into the vagina. See uterine inversion, under inversion.

> **pubescent u.** An underdeveloped adult uterus.

> **septate u., u. septus** A uterus in which the uterine cavity is completely divided by a partition (septum).

> **subseptate u., u. subseptus** A uterus in which the uterine cavity is partly divided by a partition (septum) extending down from the fundus.

tipped u. A retrodisplaced uterus (i.e., one that is tilted in a backward direction).

unicornuate u., u. unicornis A uterus with one normal horn on one side and a rudimentary horn on the opposite side; the lumen of the rudimentary horn may or may not be continuous with the uterine cavity.

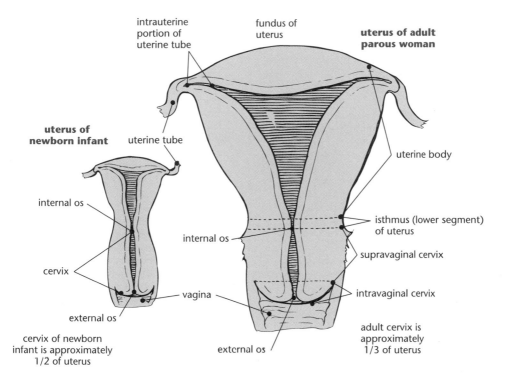

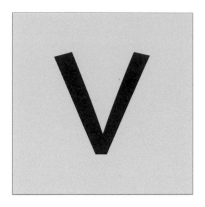

vaccine (vak'sēn) A preparation of dead or attenuated live viruses or bacteria for use in the prevention of infectious diseases by inducing active immunity.

attenuated v. See live vaccine.

hepatitis B v. Vaccine containing a formalin-inactivated hepatitis B surface antigen obtained from plasma of human carriers of the virus, or a genetically engineered (recombinant) subunit of the virus.

inactivated v. Any vaccine in which the nucleic acid components in the core of the infectious microorganism have been destroyed by chemical or physical means (e.g. formaldehyde or gamma radiation) without affecting the immunogenicity of the outer coat proteins.

live v. A vaccine prepared from living microorganisms that have been made to undergo physical changes by submission either to radiation or unfavorable temperatures, or to serial passage in laboratory animals or infected tissue/cell cultures; the result is a living avirulent, mutant strain capable of inducing protective immunity against the original organisms. Live vaccines are contraindicated in febrile or immunosuppressed patients and in pregnant women. Also called attenuated vaccine.

measles v. A vaccine containing the live attenuated measles virus, used for immunization against measles. It should not be given during pregnancy because it has deleterious effects on the fetus. Pregnancy should be avoided for 3 months following immunization. Because some viruses may be secreted in the mother's milk, caution should be exercised for use during lactation. See also live vaccine.

MMR v. A combination of live measles, mumps, and rubella vaccines.

MR v. A combination of live measles and rubella vaccines.

mumps v. Vaccine containing a suspension of the live attenuated mumps virus, used for immunization against mumps. It has a deleterious effect on the fetus. Pregnancy should be avoided for 3 months after vaccination. Because some viruses may be secreted in human milk and transmitted to the breast-fed infant, caution should be exercised for use during lactation. See also live vaccine.

rubella v. A live attenuated vaccine containing a strain of the rubella virus, used to induce immunity to rubella (German measles). It has substantive fetal risk, therefore it should not be given to pregnant women; pregnancy should be avoided for 3 months following vaccination. Lactating women immunized with the rubella vaccine secrete the virus in the milk and thereby transmit it to their breast-fed infants. See also live vaccine.

varicella virus v. A live attenuated vaccine containing the varicella virus, used to induce immunity to varicella (chickenpox). Pregnancy should be avoided for 3 months after vaccination. It should not be given to pregnant women. Because some viruses are secreted in human milk, caution should be exercised for use during lactation. See also live vaccine.

vagina (vă-ji'nă) 1. The musculomembranous structure of a female extending from the uterine cervix to the vulva. 2. Any sheathlike structure.

vaginal (vaj'ĭ-nal) 1. Relating to the vagina. 2. Relating to any sheath.

vaginectomy (vaj-i-nek'tŏ-me) Partial or total removal of the vagina.

vaginismus (vaj-ĭ-niz'mus) Painful spasmodic contractions of the vaginal wall; designated *global*, when precipitated by any attempt at vaginal penetration (e.g. with a tampon, penis, finger, or speculum), or *situational*, if tampons and pelvic examinations are tolerated, occurring only when vaginal sexual intercourse is attempted. Also called colpospasm.

vaginitis (vaj-ĭ-ni'tis) Inflammation of the vagina.

atrophic v. Thinning and dryness of the vaginal mucosa and loss of vaginal rugae, due to estrogen deficiency, causing painful sexual intercourse (coitus) and postcoital bleeding; seen commonly in women undergoing menopause, either occurring naturally or after surgical removal of the ovaries.

candidal v. Vaginitis caused by a candida species belonging to the family Cryptococcaceae. Symptoms include vulvar

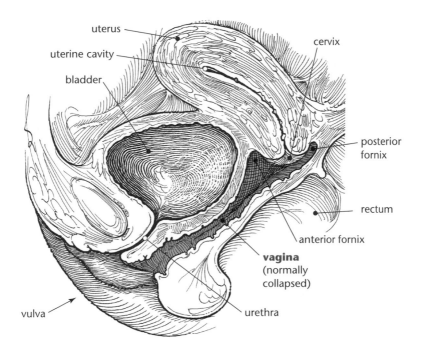

uterus

uterine cavity

bladder

cervix

posterior fornix

rectum

anterior fornix

vagina (normally collapsed)

vulva

urethra

pruritis and irritation, intensified by sexual intercourse; usually manifested by a thick 'cottage cheese'-like discharge with a pH of 4.0 to 5.0. Conditions that predispose to its occurrence include pregnancy, poorly controlled diabetes mellitus, or systemic antibiotic treatment. Also called candidiasis.

desquamative inflammatory v. Diffuse vaginitis occurring in the absence of estrogen deficiency; characterized by a profuse vaginal discharge containing pus and epithelial cells and vulvovaginal burning or irritation; may occur in association with superficial hemorrhagic spots in the upper vagina; the pH of vaginal secretions is higher than 4.5.

emphysematous v. Vaginitis accompanied by formation of gas-filled cysts within the upper vaginal tissues and adjacent cervix.

Gardnerella v. See bacterial vaginosis, under vaginosis.

nonspecific v. See bacterial vaginosis, under vaginosis.

senile v. See atrophic vaginitis.

trichomonas v. Vaginitis caused by the flagellated parasite *Trichomonas vaginalis*, a sexually transmitted organism; symptoms include a profuse discharge of abnormal odor, itchiness of the vulva, and a pH of vaginal secretions higher than 5.0; it often coexists with bacterial vaginosis. See also vaginosis.

vaginodynia (vaj-ĭ-no-din'e-ă) Pain in the vagina.

Also called colpodynia.

vaginofixation (vaj-ĭ-no-fik-sa'shun) See vaginopexy.

vaginohysterectomy (vaj-ĭ-no-his-ter-ek'tŏ-me) See vaginal hysterectomy, under hysterectomy.

vaginolabial (vaj-ĭ-no-la'be-al) Relating to the vagina and the labia.

vaginomycosis (vaj-ĭ-no-mi-ko'sis) Any fungal infection of the vagina.

vaginopathy (vaj-ĭ-nop'ă-the) Any vaginal disorder.

vaginoperineal (vaj-ĭ-no-per-ĭ-ne'al) Relating to the vagina and perineum.

vaginoperineorrhaphy (vaj-ĭ-no-per-ĭ-ne-or'ă-fe) See colpoperineorrhaphy.

vaginopexy (vaj'ĭ-no-pek-se) Suturing a prolapsed vaginal wall in an elevated normal position. Also called vaginofixation.

vaginoplasty (vaj'ĭ-no-plas-te) Reparative surgery of the vagina. Also called colpoplasty.

vaginoscopy (vaj-ĭ-nos'kŏ-pe) Visual examination of the vagina, usually with the aid of an instrument (vaginoscope).

vaginosis (vaj-ĭ-no'sis) Disease of the vagina.

bacterial v. (BV) Infection with multiple anaerobic and aerobic bacteria, usually causing a vaginal discharge that is grayish-white, homogeneous, and slightly viscous, and frequently coats the entire vaginal mucosa; the pH of the vagina is in the range 5.0 to 6.0. About half of infected women are asymptomatic. The condition has been implicated as a risk factor for acute inflammation and perinatal complications. Formerly called nonspecific vaginitis; *Gardnerella* vaginitis.

vaginotomy (vaj-ĭ-not'ŏ-me) See colpotomy.

vaginovesical (vaj-ĭ-no-ves'ĭ-kal) Relating to the vagina and bladder.

vaginovulvar (vaj-ĭ-no-vul'var) See vulvovaginal.

vagitus uterinus (va-ji'tus u-ter-i'nus) Crying of a fetus while still in the uterus; a rare phenomenon thought to occur when the fetus inspires air entering the amniotic cavity after the membranes rupture.

valproic acid (val-pro'ik as'id) An anticonvulsant used in the treatment of seizure disorders. Intrauterine exposure during the first trimester of pregnancy places the fetus at risk of developing spina bifida and other fetal malformations.

valve (valv) A fold of the lining membrane within a tubular structure or hollow organ, so placed as to permit passage of a body fluid in one direction only.

> **anterior urethral v.** A crescenteric valve in the male urethra, near the junction of the scrotum and penis.

> **aortic v.** The valve situated at the opening of the ascending aorta as it leaves the left ventricle; consists of three cusps designated according to their location in the fetus as posterior, left, and right (in the adult, a more accurate description is anterior, right posterior, and left posterior).

> **left atrioventricular v.** The valve between the left atrium and the left ventricle of the heart; composed of two cusps. Also called mitral valve.

> **mitral v.** See left atrioventricular valve.

> **posterior urethral v.'s** Abnormal congenital folds of mucous membrane found in the distal prostatic urethra; they constitute the most common obstructive lesions in the urethra of male newborns and older infants.

> **v. of pulmonary trunk** Valve situated at the opening of the pulmonary trunk as it leaves the right ventricle; composed of three semilunar cusps designated right, left, and anterior according to their location in the fetus (in the adult, a more accurate description is right anterior, left anterior, and posterior cusps).

> **right atrioventricular v.** The valve between the right atrium and the right ventricle of the heart; composed of three cusps (anterior, posterior, and septal). Also called tricuspid valve.

> **tricuspid v.** See right atrioventricular valve.

vancomycin (van-ko-mi'sin) An antibiotic effective against most Gram-positive organisms, particularly staphylococcus. It is given parenterally and is indicated in the treatment of serious infections or enterococcal endocarditis. Rapid infusion may result in diffuse hyperemia (red man syndrome).

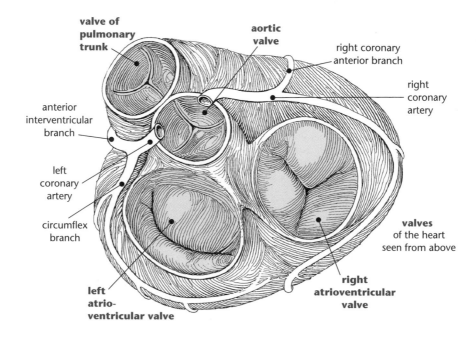

valve of pulmonary trunk

aortic valve

right coronary anterior branch

right coronary artery

anterior interventricular branch

left coronary artery

circumflex branch

valves of the heart seen from above

left atrio-ventricular valve

right atrioventricular valve

Congenital defects attributable to vancomycin have not been located. It is secreted in breast milk in small amounts, and may interfere with bowel flora or interfere with the interpretation of laboratory results.

vanillylmandelic acid (vă-nil-il-man-del'ik as'id) (VMA) A compound that is the major breakdown product of catecholamines (e.g. epinephrine and norepinephrine); it is excreted in the urine at a normal range of 2 to 10 mg per day; elevated levels of excretion suggest the presence of a pheochromocytoma (tumor of the adrenal gland).

variceal (var-ĭ-se'al) Relating to a varix.

varicella (var-ĭ-sel'ă) See chickenpox.

varicelliform (var-ĭ-sel'ĭ-form) Resembling chickenpox.

varices (var'ĭ-sēz) Plural of varix.

variciform (var-is'ĭ-form) Resembling a varix.

varicocele (var'ĭ-ko-sēl) A mass of dilated, tortuous veins just above and posterior to the testis, sometimes extending up to the groin, with the left side most commonly involved. The condition is a frequent finding in infertile men.

varicocelectomy (var-ĭ-ko-sĕ-lek'tŏ-me) Ligation and removal of the enlarged veins forming a varicocele.

varicose (var'ĭ-kōs) Abnormally dilated and tortuous; applied to lymphatic vessels, arteries, and especially veins.

Varivax (var'ĭ-vaks) A live attenuated strain of varicella virus used for human immunization. Presently, there is no data to ensure the safety of its administration during pregnancy. Pregnancy should be avoided for the 3 months after vaccination. There are no data about its secretion in breast milk.

varix (var'iks), pl. varices A dilated tortuous vessel, especially a vein.

vas (vas), pl. vasa A channel conveying body fluids such as blood, lymph, chyle, or semen; a vessel.

    v. deferens See deferent duct, under duct.

    vasa previa A configuration of fetal vessels that traverse the membranes and appear across the internal os ahead of the presenting part. It is associated with velamentous insertion of the umbilical cord and is clinically important because when membranes rupture, rupture of a fetal vessel may occur resulting in fetal exsanguination. See also velamentous insertion of the umbilical cord, under insertion.

vasectomy (vă-sek'tŏ-me) Removal of a section of both deferent ducts as a method of male sterilization. Also called deferentectomy; male sterilization.

vasoactive (vas-o-ak'tiv) Having an effect on blood vessels.

vasopressin (vas-o-pres'in) (VP) A hormone produced by the posterior lobe of the pituitary (neurohypophysis) and also prepared synthetically; it has a constrictive action on blood circulation of the viscera, including the uterus.

vault (vawlt) Any arched anatomic structure resembling a dome.

    vaginal v. The uppermost portion of the vagina. See also fornix.

vector (vek'tor) **1.** An organism (e.g. tick, rat, dog) that transmits pathologic microorganisms from one host to another. **2.** A DNA molecule into which a gene of interest is cloned and which is capable of replicating itself in a particular host.

veil (vāl) See caul.

vein (vān) (v) **1.** A vessel carrying blood toward the heart. **2.** A vessel in the heart wall carrying blood to the right atrium.

    appendicular v. *Location:* along the mesentery of the vermiform appendix. *Drains:* appendix. *Tributaries:* none. *Empties into:* ileocolic vein.

    axillary v. *Location:* from the lower border of the teres major muscle to the lateral border of the first rib. *Drains:* arm, axilla, superolateral chest wall. *Tributaries:* basilic, brachial, cephalic, subscapular, thoracoacromial, highest thoracic and lateral thoracic veins, posterior humeral circumflex vein, and anterior humeral circumflex vein. *Empties into:* subclavian vein.

    brachial v.'s *Location:* from the neck of the radius, they course upward to the lower border of the teres major muscle. *Drain:* forearm, elbow joint, arm, humerus. *Tributaries:* deep brachial vein, nutrient vein of humerus, superior and inferior ulnar collateral veins, radial veins, ulnar veins. *Empty into:* axillary vein.

    brachiocephalic v., left *Location:* from behind the medial end of the left clavicle, it courses downward and obliquely to the cartilage of the first rib. *Drains:* head and left arm. *Tributaries:* internal jugular, left subclavian, thymic, and left vertebral veins. *Empties into:* superior vena cava.

    brachiocephalilc v., right *Location:* from behind the medial end of the right clavicle, it courses downward toward the cartilage of the first rib. *Drains:* head and right arm. *Tributaries:* internal jugular and right subclavian veins. *Empties into:* superior vena cava.

    v. of bulb of vestibule *Location:* vestibule of the vagina. *Drains:* bulb of vestibule. *Tributaries:* none. *Empties into:* internal pudendal vein.

circumflex iliac v., deep *Location:* lower abdomen. *Drains:* internal oblique, transversus abdominis, iliac, psoas, and sartorius muscles. *Tributaries:* ascending branch. *Empties into:* external iliac vein (about 2 cm above level of inguinal ligament).

circumflex iliac v., superficial *Location:* from the ilium, it courses downward and obliquely to the level of the inguinal ligament. *Drains:* superficial inguinal lymph nodes, skin of groin. *Tributaries:* none. *Empties into:* great saphenous vein or femoral vein.

colic v., left *Location:* along the medial side of the descending colon and the left colic (splenic) flexure. *Drains:* descending colon and left flexure. *Tributaries:* ascending and descending branches, marginal veins. *Empties into:* inferior mesenteric vein.

dorsal v. of clitoris, deep *Location:* on the dorsum of the clitoris, deep to the fascia; it passes under the pubic symphysis. *Drains:* glans clitoris, corpus cavernosum (right and left). *Tributaries:* small branches from clitoris. *Empties into:* vesical venous plexus.

dorsal v.'s of clitoris, superficial *Location:* two veins on the dorsum of the clitoris. *Drain:* prepuce and mucosa of clitoris and surrounding area. *Tributaries:* small branches from mucosa of clitoris and surrounding area. *Empty into:* external pudendal veins or femoral veins.

epigastric v., inferior *Location:* from the rectus muscle of the abdominal wall, it descends to a level just above the inguinal ligament. *Drains:* rectus abdominis muscle, cremaster muscle, skin. *Tributaries:* superior epigastric veins, vein of round ligament, muscular and cutaneous branches. *Empties into:* external iliac vein.

epigastric v., superficial *Location:* lower anterior abdominal wall. *Drains:* lower anterior abdominal wall and overlying skin. *Tributaries:* thoracoepigastric vein. *Empties into:* great saphenous vein or femoral vein.

epigastric v.'s, superior *Location:* upper anterior abdominal wall to costal cartilages. *Drain:* upper anterior abdominal wall. *Tributaries:* subcutaneous abdominal veins. *Empty into:* internal thoracic veins.

femoral circumflex v.'s, lateral *Location:* posterolateral thigh. *Drain:* head and neck of femur, thigh muscles. *Tributaries:* ascending, descending, transverse branches. *Empty into:* femoral vein or deep femoral vein.

femoral circumflex v.'s, medial *Location:* posteromedial thigh. *Drain:* hip joint, adductor muscles of thigh. *Tributaries:* deep, ascending transverse acetabular branches. *Empty into:* femoral vein or deep femoral vein.

iliac v., common *Location:* from the front of the sacroiliac joint, it courses obliquely and upward to the level of the fourth lumbar vertebra. *Drains:* gluteal region, perineum, lower limb, lower abdominal wall. *Tributaries:* external iliac, internal iliac, iliolumbar, lateral sacral, middle sacral, and ascending lumbar veins. *Empties into:* inferior vena cava.

iliac v., external *Location:* from behind the inguinal ligament, it ascends to the front of the sacroiliac joint. *Drains:* abdominal wall, external genitalia, cremaster muscle, lower limb. *Tributaries:* femoral, inferior epigastric, and deep circumflex iliac. *Empties into:* common iliac vein.

iliac v., internal *Location:* from the greater sciatic notch to the brim of the pelvis. *Drains:* pelvic viscera, perineum, external genitalia, buttock, medial side of thigh. *Tributaries:* superior and inferior gluteal, internal pudendal, obturator, lateral sacral, vesical, uterine, lateral sacral, and iliolumbar veins. *Empties into:* common iliac vein.

intercostal v.'s anterior *Location:* upper nine intercostal spaces. *Drain:* intercostal spaces, pectoralis major and minor muscles, breast, skin of chest. *Tributaries:* costoaxillary veins, perforating veins. *Empty into:* internal thoracic veins, musculophrenic veins.

intercostal v., highest *Location:* first intercostal space. *Drains:* first intercostal space. *Tributaries:* none. *Empties into:* brachiocephalic vein.

intervertebral v.'s *Location:* intervertebral foramen. *Drain:* vertebral foramen. *Tributaries:* veins from spinal cord, internal and external vertebral venous plexuses. *Empty into:* vertebral vein (in neck), posterior intercostal vein (in thorax), lumbar veins (in abdomen), lateral sacral veins (in pelvis).

labial v.'s, anterior *Location:* vulva. *Drain:* anterior portion of labia majora, mons pubis. *Tributaries:* none. *Empty into:* external pudendal veins.

labial v.'s, posterior *Location:* vulva. *Drain:* posterior portion of labia majora, vestibule, labia minora. *Tributaries:* none. *Empty into:* internal pudendal vein.

lumbar v.'s *Location:* posterior wall of abdomen. *Drain:* muscles and skin of loins, posterior body wall. *Tributaries:* vertebral plexuses, dorsal and abdominal branches. *Empty into:* ascending lumbar vein, inferior vena cava.

lumbar v., ascending *Location:* ventral to transverse process of lumbar vertebrae. *Drains:* lumbar plexus, back muscles, spinal cord. *Tributaries:* lateral sacral veins, lumbar veins. *Empties into:* azygos vein (right side); hemiazygos vein (left side).

mesenteric v., inferior *Location:* from the area of the upper rectum, it ascends to the level of the body of the pancreas. *Drains:* upper rectum, sigmoid, descending colon. *Tributaries:* superior rectal, sigmoid, left colic, and rectosigmoid veins. *Empties into:* splenic vein or junction of splenic and superior mesenteric veins.

obturator v. *Location:* from high in the thigh, it enters the pelvis through the obturator canal. *Drains:* adductor region of thigh, hip joint, ilium, pelvic muscles. *Tributaries:* anterior and posterior branches, pubic and vesical veins, acetabular branch, medial circumflex femoral, iliac, and iliolumbar veins. *Empties into:* internal iliac vein, sometimes the inferior epigastric or common iliac vein.

ovarian v.'s *Location:* in the broad ligament near the ovary and uterine tube. *Drain:* ovary,

uterine tube, uterus, ureter. *Tributaries:* uterine plexus, pampiniform plexus, ureteric vein. *Empty into:* inferior vena cava (right vein), left renal vein (left vein).

paraumbilical v.'s *Location:* from the umbilicus, they course along the round ligament of the liver and the median umbilical ligament of the bladder. *Drain:* umbilicus. *Tributaries:* superior and inferior epigastric, superior vesical, lateral thoracic, and superficial epigastric veins. *Empty into:* portal vein.

pectoral v.'s *Location:* pectoral muscles. *Drain:* pectoral region. *Tributaries:* none. *Empty into:* subclavian vein.

pudendal v.'s, external *Location:* external genitalia, lower and medial part of abdomen. *Drain:* skin of lower part of abdomen, external genitalia. *Tributaries:* superficial dorsal vein of clitoris, anterior labial veins. *Empty into:* great saphenous vein or femoral vein.

pudendal v., internal *Location:* from the region of the ischial tuberosity, it passes to the pelvis through the greater sciatic foramen. *Drains:* perineum and genitalia. *Tributaries:* deep dorsal vein of clitoris, vesical venous plexus, labial and inferior rectal veins, and

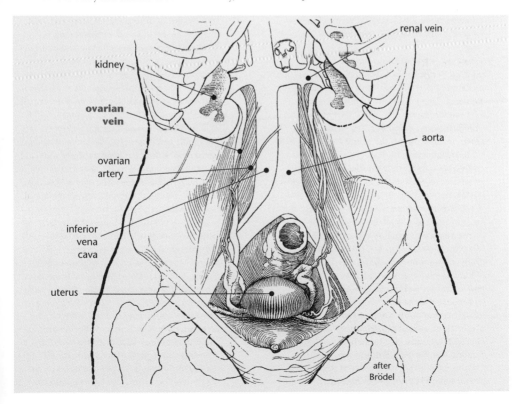

kidney

renal vein

ovarian vein

ovarian artery

aorta

inferior vena cava

uterus

after Brödel

veins from bulb of vestibule. *Empty into:* internal iliac vein.

pulmonary v.'s *Location:* from the lungs to the heart. *Drain:* lungs. *Tributaries:* veins from inferior and superior lobes of left lung and from superior, middle, and inferior lobes of right lung. *Empty into:* left atrium of heart.

rectal v.'s inferior *Location:* anal region. *Drain:* lower part of anal canal. *Tributaries:* external rectal plexus. *Empty into:* internal pudendal vein.

rectal v.'s middle *Location:* middle of the rectum in the lesser pelvis. *Drain:* muscular wall of middle of rectum and surrounding organs. *Tributaries:* lower part of perimuscular rectal plexus, middle part of external rectal plexus, veins from bladder. *Empty into:* internal iliac vein or inferior gluteal vein.

rectal v.'s superior *Location:* upper rectum to the brim of the pelvis. *Drain:* upper rectum. *Tributaries:* upper part of perimuscular rectal plexus, internal and external rectal plexuses. *Empty into:* inferior mesenteric veins.

sacral v.'s, lateral *Location:* from the dorsum of the sacrum and the coccyx, they course through the sacral foramina to the upper part of the pelvis. *Drain:* sacrum, skin and muscles of dorsum of sacrum and coccyx. *Tributaries:* spinal veins, sacral venous plexus. *Empty into:* superior gluteal or internal iliac veins.

sacral v., middle *Location:* front of the sacrum. *Drains:* sacrum, rectum. *Tributaries:* rectal and small lumbar veins. *Empties into:* left common iliac vein or junction of two common iliac veins.

saphenous v., accessory *Location:* posteromedial part of the thigh. *Drains:* posteromedial part of thigh. *Tributaries:* small saphenous vein, numerous small veins from posterior and medial thigh. *Empties into:* great saphenous veins.

saphenous v., great *Location:* from medial marginal vein of foot, it courses medially up the leg to about 4 cm below the pubic tubercle. *Drains:* thigh, sole of foot, leg, lower part of abdominal wall. *Tributaries:* medial marginal vein of foot, plus accessory saphenous, medial superficial, anterior femoral cutaneous, superficial epigastric, superficial circumflex iliac, external pudendal, small saphenous, and perforating veins. *Empties into:* femoral vein.

spinal v.'s *Location:* two median (anterior and posterior), two anterolateral, and two posterolateral veins in the pia mater of the spinal cord, forming a tortuous plexus. *Drain:* spinal cord. *Tributaries:* none. *Empty into:* internal vertebral venous plexus.

subclavian v. *Location:* from the lateral border of the first rib to the medial end of the clavicle. *Drains:* arm, neck, thoracic wall. *Tributaries:* axillary, external jugular, dorsal scapular, and pectoral veins, anterior jugular vein (occasionally) and vertebral vein (occasionally). *Empties into:* brachiocephalic vein.

subcostal v. *Location:* beneath the twelfth rib. *Drains:* upper abdominal wall below the twelfth rib, spinal cord. *Tributaries:* dorsal and spinal branches, intervertebral vein. *Empties into:* right side: azygos vein; left side: hemiazygos vein.

suprascapular v. *Location:* from the supraspinous and infraspinous fossae of the scapula, it courses upward and medially across the anterior scalene muscle. *Drains:* clavicle, scapula, skin of chest, muscles of scapular region, acromioclavicular and shoulder joints. *Tributaries:* suprasternal, articular, and acromial branches, nutrient veins of clavicle and scapula. *Empties into:* external jugular vein.

thoracic v.'s, internal *Location:* from the chest, they course upward just beyond the level of the clavicle. *Drain:* anterior thoracic wall, mediastinal lymph nodes, diaphragm. *Tributaries:* pericardiacophrenic, mediastinal, anterior intercostal, musculophrenic, superior epigastric, thymic, abdominal subcutaneous veins. *Empty into:* brachiocephalic vein.

thoracic v., lateral *Location:* lateral thoracic wall. *Drains:* chest muscles, mammary gland, axillary lymph nodes. *Tributaries:* lateral mammary vein, thoracoepigastric, intercostal veins. *Empties into:* axillary vein.

thoracoacromial v.'s *Location:* top of shoulder. *Drain:* pectoralis major and minor, subclavius and deltoid muscles, sternoclavicular joint, acromion. *Tributaries:* pectoral, acromial, deltoid, and clavicular branches. *Empty into:* axillary vein, subclavian vein (occasionally).

umbilical v *Location:* within umbilical cord. *Drains:* placenta. *Tributaries:* joined by fetal portal vein. *Empties into:* ductus venosus of the fetus.

uterine v.'s *Location:* lateral aspect of the uterus. *Drain:* uterus, upper part of vagina, round ligament of uterus, cervix, uterine tube. *Tributaries:* uterine venous plexus, ovarian vein, vaginal and tubal branches. *Empty into:* internal iliac vein.

vaginal v.'s *Location:* lateral aspect of vagina. *Drain:* vagina, fundus of urinary bladder, rectum. *Tributaries:* none. *Empty into:* internal iliac vein, uterine vein (occasionally).

varicose v.'s Abnormally dilated tortuous veins, resulting from prolonged increased pressure within the vessels; occur most commonly in the superficial veins of the legs; contributing factors include hereditary defects in the venous walls, obesity, compression by tumors, and prolonged dependent position of the legs.

vesical v.'s *Location:* urinary bladder. *Drain:* urinary bladder and adjacent structures.

Tributaries: vesical venous plexus. *Empty into:* internal iliac vein.

vitelline v.'s Veins returning blood from the yolk sac of an early embryo; they form a network around the duodenum and liver and empty directly into the primitive heart.

velamentous (vel-ă-men'tus) Resembling a curtain or veil; applied to certain body structures and membranes. See also velamentous insertion of umbilical cord, under insertion.

vellus (vel'us) Fine, soft, nonpigmented downy hair that replaces the lanugo hair (primary hair) of the neonate; it begins to appear in the early months of post-natal life. Also called vellus hair;

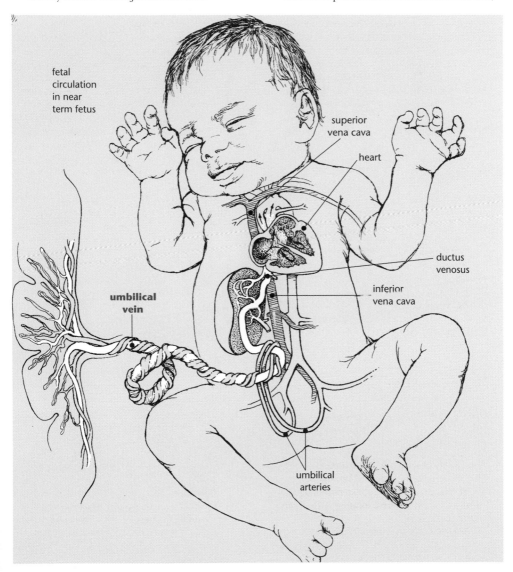

fetal circulation in near term fetus

superior vena cava

heart

ductus venosus

inferior vena cava

umbilical vein

umbilical arteries

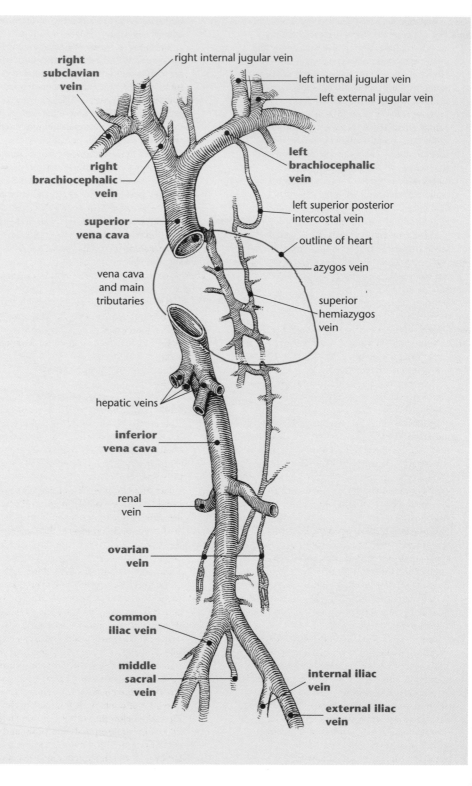

secondary hair.

vena (ve'nă), pl. venae Latin for vein.

    v. cava The largest vein in the body; designated *inferior v. cava*, the portion extending upward from the level of the fifth lumbar vertebra, along the vertebral column, to the right side of the heart; it drains the common iliac, lumbar, renal, testicular (male), ovarian (female), suprarenal, inferior phrenic, and hepatic veins; it empties into the lower portion of the right atrium of the heart; *superior v. cava*, the portion extending downward behind the breastbone (sternum) to the right side of the heart; it drains both brachiocephalic veins and empties into the upper portion of the right atrium of the heart.

    venae comitantes Veins (usually two) accompanying a corresponding artery.

venereal (vě-ne're-al) Relating to or resulting from sexual contact (e.g. a sexually transmitted disease).

venereology (vě-nēr-e-ol'ō-je) The study of venereal disease.

veno-, veni- Combining forms meaning veins.

ventilation (ven-tĭ-la'shun) The physiologic process through which air in the lungs is exchanged with atmospheric air.

    alveolar v. (V_A) The amount of inspired gas per minute entering the tiny air sacs in the lungs.

    artificial v. The maintenance of respiratory movements by manual or mechanical means. Also called artificial respiration.

    assisted v. Respiration in which the patient's own breathing effort initiates the cycle but the volume of air entering the lungs is increased by mechanical means. Also called assisted respiration.

    continuous positive pressure v. (CPPV) Administration of air or a mixture of gases to the lungs under continuously positive pressure applied by a ventilator. The pressure in the airways fluctuates to allow air or gases to flow in and out of the lungs. Also called continuous positive pressure breathing; positive pressure respiration.

    controlled v. Artificial ventilation requiring no effort from the patient; each inspiration is initiated by a timing mechanism of the respirator. Also called controlled respiration.

    controlled mechanical v. (CMV) (1) See continuous positive pressure ventilation. (2) See intermittent positive pressure ventilation.

    high-frequency v. A variety of ventilatory methods and devices designed to provide ventilation at rapid rates and low tidal volumes, hence reducing the risk of causing injury by pressure changes (barotrauma).

    intermittent mandatory v. (IMV) Delivery of a positive-pressure breath by the ventilator at preset intervals while the patient breathes spontaneously between mechanical breaths.

    intermittent positive pressure v. (IPPV) Administration of air or a mixture of gases to the lungs under intermittent positive pressure applied by a ventilator during each inspiration. Also called intermittent positive pressure breathing; positive pressure respiration.

    maximum voluntary v. (MVV) The maximum volume of air that a person can voluntarily breathe as deeply and as quickly as possible in a given period of time (e.g. 12 seconds). Also called maximum breathing capacity (MBC).

    mechanical v. Ventilation accomplished by automatically cycling devices.

ventilator (ven-tĭ-la'tor) Any device used to provide ventilation.

    babybird v. A ventilator for infants (one of the earliest) that requires an adjunct monitor and an alarm system.

ventouse (ven-tus') See vacuum extractor, under extractor.

ventricle (ven'trĭ-kl) A cavity, especially within the heart or the brain.

    fourth v. of brain A cavity filled with cerebrospinal fluid (CSF), located within the brain, in front of the cerebellum and behind the pons and upper half of the medulla oblongata; it communicates with the third ventricle above and with the central canal of the spinal cord below.

    lateral v.'s of brain Two relatively large, irregular cavities contained within the frontal, occipital, and temporal lobes of the brain; they are filled with cerebrospinal fluid (CSF) and each communicates with the third ventricle below.

    left v. The cavity within the lower left side of the heart; it receives blood from the left atrium through the left atrioventricular valve and, by contracting its walls, pumps blood into the systemic circulation via the aorta.

    right v. The cavity within the lower right side of the heart; it receives blood from the right atrium through the right atrioventricular valve and, by contracting its walls, pumps blood into the lungs via the pulmonary trunk.

    third v. of brain A narrow median cleft in the brain, below the corpus callosum; it is filled with cerebrospinal fluid (CSF) and communicates with the two lateral ventricles above, and with the fourth ventricle below.

ventriculomegaly (ven-trĭ-ku-lo-meg'ă-le) An abnormally expanded state of a cerebral ventricle, as seen in hydrocephalus.

verapamil (ver-ap'ă-mil) A calcium channel-blocking agent used in the treatment of cardiac arrhythmias and hypertension; it may decrease uterine blood flow. It is not known to cause developmental anomalies.

verruca (vě-roo'kă), pl. verrucae A wart.

    v. acuminata See condyloma acuminatum, under condyloma.

verruciform (vě-roo'sĭ-form) In the shape of a wart.

verrucosis (ver-oo-ko'sis) The condition of having multiple warts.

verrucous, verrucose (ver'oo-kus, ver'oo-kōs) Having a wartlike roughness.

versicolor (ver-sĭ-kol'or) Turning or changing color.

version (ver'zhun) The manual turning of a fetus in the uterus to alter its position to one more favorable for delivery.

    bimanual v., bipolar v. A maneuver for turning the fetus by using two hands; may be external or combined.

    Braxton Hicks v. A seldom-used procedure in which the forefinger and/or middle finger of one hand are introduced through the vagina into the uterus to displace the presenting part of the fetus (often the shoulder) while the head is guided toward the birth canal by the operator's other (external) hand placed on the abdomen.

    cephalic v. Version performed in modern obstetrics only by external manipulations and before 38 weeks of gestation, usually with the aid of ultrasonographic scanning; the procedure is used to turn the fetal presenting part from breech to cephalic presentation. The operator's hands are placed on the patient's abdomen and each pole of the fetus is located by palpation; then gently but firmly the breech is displaced upward and laterally while moving the fetal head downward toward the birth canal (like a forward somersault).

    combined v. Version in which one hand is introduced into the uterus and the other is placed on the patient's abdomen.

    external v. Version conducted entirely by placing the hands on the patient's abdomen for application of force.

    external cephalic v. See cephalic version.

    internal v. Direct turning of the fetus by introducing a hand into the uterus.

    internal podalic v. See podalic version.

    podalic v. Internal version performed only

rarely (e.g. for a second twin with fetal distress or for a small dead fetus in a transverse lie); a hand is introduced into the uterus through the fully dilated cervix; the fetus is turned by seizing both feet and drawn through the cervix; a total breech extraction is then performed.

    spontaneous v. Version accomplished by contractions of the uterus alone.

vertebra (ver'tě-bră), pl. vertebrae One of the 33 bones forming the spinal (vertebral) column; they are divided into seven cervical, 12 thoracic, five lumbar, five sacral, and four coccygeal vertebrae.

vertex (ver'teks) **1.** The highest point at the vault of the skull. **2.** The crown of the fetal head.

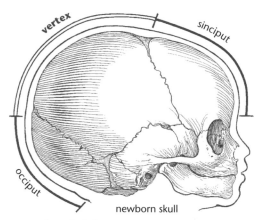

newborn skull

vesica (vě-sĭ'kă) Latin for bladder; blister.

vesical (ves'ĭ-kal) Relating to a bladder, usually the urinary bladder.

vesicle (ves'ĭ-kl) **1.** A small fluid-filled blister on the skin. **2.** Any small saclike structure.

    blastodermic v. See blastocyst.

    seminal v. One of two sac-like glandular structures situated behind the bladder in the male; its secretion is one of the components of semen.

vesico-, vesic- Combining forms meaning bladder; vesicle.

vesicocervical (ves-ĭ-ko-ser'vĭ-kal) Relating to the bladder and the cervix.

vesicocele (ves'ĭ-ko-sēl) See cystocele.

vesicolithiasis (ves-ĭ-ko-lĭ-thi'ă-sis) See cystolithiasis.

vesicolithotomy (ves-ĭ-ko-lĭ-thot'ŏ-me) See cystolithotomy.

vesicopubic (ves-ĭ-ko-pu'bic) Relating to the bladder and pubic bone.

vesicorectal (ves-ĭ-ko-rek'tal) Relating to the bladder and the rectum.

vesicostomy (ves-ĭ-kos'tŏ-me) See cystostomy.

vesicotomy (ves-ĭ-kot'ŏ-me) See cystotomy.

vesicoureteral (ves-ĭ-ko-u-re'ter-al) Relating to the bladder and ureters.

vesicourethral (ves-ĭ-ko-u-re'thral) Relating to the bladder and urethra.

vesicouterine (ves-ĭ-ko-u'ter-in) Relating to the bladder and uterus.

vesicouterovaginal (ves-ĭ-ko-u-ter-o-vaj'ĭ-nal) Relating to the bladder, uterus, and vagina.

vesicovaginal (ves-ĭ-ko-vaj'ĭ-nal) Relating to the bladder and vagina.

vesicovaginorectal (ves-ĭ-ko-vaj-ĭ-no-rek'tal) Relating to the bladder, vagina, and rectum.

vesiculopapular (vĕ-sik-u-lo-pap'u-lar) Relating to superficial blisters (vesicles) and small, solid elevations (papules).

vesiculopustular (vĕ-sik-u-lo-pus'tu-lar) Relating to superficial blisters (vesicles) and small accumulations of pus (pustules).

vessel (ves'el) Tubular structure conveying a body fluid.

　　chorionic v.'s Branches of the umbilical blood vessels that fan out throughout the connective tissue layer of the chorionic plate (placental tissues on the fetal side). Also called placental surface vessels.

　　great v.'s The aorta and vena cava.

　　lymph v. A vessel conveying lymph.

　　placental surface v.'s See chorionic vessels.

vestibule (ves'tĭ-būl) A small cavity or chamber at the entrance of a canal.

　　v. of vagina The space between the labia minora into which open the vagina, urethra, and the ducts of the greater and lesser vestibular glands. Also called vestibule of vulva.

　　v. of vulva See vestibule of vagina.

vestibulitis (ves-tĭ-bu-li'tis) Inflammation of a vestibule.

　　vulvar v. Condition marked by redness and irritation in the vestibule of the vagina, with small red patches in the vulvar region; causes are varied; may arise from abrasions from sexual intercourse, using tampons, bike riding, or wearing tight-fitting pants; may also be caused by recurrent yeast infection or trauma (e.g. from caustic chemicals or laser surgery used to treat vulvar genital warts); often the cause is unknown.

vestibulo- Combining form meaning a vestibule.

vestibulourethral (ves-tib-u-lo-u-re'thral) Relating to the vestibule of the vagina and the urethra.

viability (vi-ă-bil'ĭ-te) The condition of being viable.

viable (vi'ă-bl) Capable of living (e.g. a fetus that has developed sufficiently to be able to live outside of the uterus).

vibroacoustic (vi-bro-ă-koōs'tik) Having both vibratory and acoustic components. See also vibroacoustic stimulation, under stimulation.

villi (vil'i) Plural of villus.

villitis (vil-i'tis) The presence of inflammatory lesions in the placental villi associated with unfavorable pregnancy outcomes; the condition is usually chronic, with a tendency to recur in subsequent pregnancies; cause is unknown.

villoma (vi-lo'mă) See papilloma.

villositis (vil-o-si'tis) Inflammation of the villous portion of the placenta.

villosity (vi-los'ĭ-te) The presence of villi.

villous (vil'us) Covered with minute hairlike projections (villi).

villus (vil'us), pl. villi A minute, vascular, hairlike projection from the free surface of a membrane.

　　chorionic villi The slender vascular projections of the chorion that enter into the formation of the placenta and through which all substances are exchanged between maternal and fetal circulations.

vinblastine (vin-blas'tēn) The sulfate salt of a vinca alkaloid extracted from *Vinca rosea*, used primarily in the treatment of breast cancer and germ cell tumors of the ovary.

vincristine (vin-kris'tēn) The sulfate salt of a vinca alkaloid extracted from *Vinca rosea*, used primarily in the treatment of cervical carcinoma and genital tract sarcomas.

virile (vir'il) 1. Relating to male sexual functions. 2. Having male characteristics.

virilism (vir'ĭ-lizm) The occurrence of secondary male characteristics in the female or prepubescent males, usually caused by excessive amounts of androgenic hormone.

virilization (vir-ĭ-lĭ-za'shun) The abnormal appearance of secondary male characteristics, especially in the female. Also called masculinization.

virus (vi'rus), pl. viruses An infectious parasite thriving and replicating only within living cells; usually composed of a protein shell enclosing a nucleic acid, either DNA or RNA (not both); viruses range in size from 30 to 300 nm, are visible under the electron microscope, and are spherical, polyhedral, or rod-shaped.

　　DNA v.'s A class of viruses having an inner core of DNA and multiplying chiefly in the nuclei of cells; included are those causing herpes simplex, herpes zoster, chickenpox, smallpox, warts, and certain malignant tumors.

　　Epstein-Barr v., EB v. (EBV) See human herpesvirus 4, under herpesvirus.

hepatitis A v. (HAV) A 27-nm RNA virus (genus *Enterovirus*, family Picornaviridae) causing hepatitis A; spread by contaminated food and water. Formerly called infectious hepatitis virus.

hepatitis B v. (HBV) A 42-nm DNA virus (family Hepadnoviridae) causing hepatitis B; found in body fluids, including saliva; spreads via transfusion, needle-stick accidents, shared needles, the sexual route, or in childbirth. Formerly called serum hepatitis virus.

hepatitis C v. (HCV) A 50-nm RNA virus (family Flaviviridae), the cause of hepatitis C; spreads chiefly through transfusion and shared needles. Formerly classified as a non-A, non-B virus.

hepatitis Delta v. (HDV) A 37-nm RNA virus that requires the presence of the HBV (coinfection) to survive; spreads by infected blood or sexual contact. Also called delta agent.

hepatitis E v. (HEV) A 30-nm RNA virus (family Caliciviridae) causing hepatitis E, mainly spread by contaminated water, via the gastrointestinal tract. Formerly classified as a non-A, non-B virus.

herpes v. See herpesvirus.

human immunodeficiency v. (HIV) A virus (subfamily Lentivirinae, family Retroviridae) causing acquired immune deficiency syndrome (AIDS); two types are known (HIV-1, HIV-2); the two types produce identical symptoms but HIV-2 can linger in the body much longer than HIV-1 before causing symptoms.

human papilloma v. (HPV) See human papillomavirus under papillomavirus. See also *Papillomavirus.*

human T-cell lymphotropic v. (HTLV) A virus (subfamily Oncovirinae, family Retroviridae) causing T-cell leukemia or lymphoma; two types are known (HTLV-1, HTLV-2).

infectious hepatitis v. Former name for hepatitis A virus.

measles v. A virus of the genus *Morbillivirus* (family Paramyxoviridae) that causes measles.

oncogenic v. Any of a variety of DNA and RNA viruses that are known to cause cancer in animals and others that have been implicated in causing cancer in humans, including the human papilloma virus (HPV), Epstein-Barr virus (EBV), hepatitis B virus (HBV), and human T-cell leukemia virus (HTLV). Also called tumor virus.

RNA v.'s A large class of viruses having an inner core of RNA and multiplying chiefly in the cytoplasm of cells; included are those causing poliomyelitis, meningitis, yellow fever, encephalitis, mumps, measles, rabies, German measles, and the common cold.

rubella v. A virus of the genus *Rubivirus* (family Togaviridae) causing German measles (rubella).

serum hepatitis v. Former name for hepatitis B virus.

tumor v. See oncogenic virus.

visceral (vis'er-al) Relating to the internal organs (viscera).

viscid (vis'id) Thick and sticky.

viscous (vis'kus) Characterized by a relatively high resistance to flow.

voiding (void'ing) The act of discharging a body waste, especially urine.

double v. Popular term used to describe the act of urinating a second time several minutes after the first; a method of fully emptying the bladder practiced by patients with a large cystocele.

volume (vol'ūm) (V) A measure of the space occupied by matter in any state or form.

closing v. (CV) Lung volume at which airways at the bases of the lungs begin to close during expiration and airflow from the lungs is mainly from the upper portions.

expiratory reserve v. (ERV) The quantity of air that can be expelled from the lungs after a normal expiration.

forced expiratory v. (FEV) Maximal volume of air exhaled from the lungs during a particular time interval, starting from maximal inspiration.

inspiratory reserve v. (IRV) The quantity of air that can be inspired after a normal inspiration.

lung v.'s The following four volumes: expiratory reserve, inspiratory reserve, residual, and tidal volumes.

mean corpuscular v., mean cell v. (MCV) The average volume of red blood cells; calculated by multiplying the hematocrit by 1000, divided by the red cell count.

minute v. The total amount of air expelled from the lungs in 1 minute.

plasma v. The total volume of blood plasma.

residual v. (RV) (1) The amount of air remaining in the lungs after a maximum expiration. Also called residual capacity. (2) In urogynecology, the amount of urine remaining in the urinary bladder after micturition.

tidal v. (V_T) The amount of air expired or inspired in one breath in normal breathing.

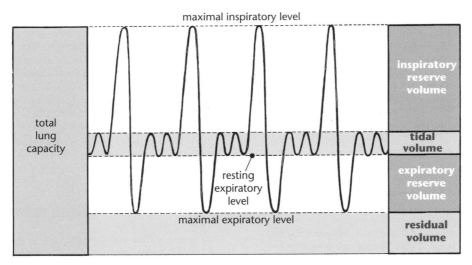

vomiting (vom'it-ing) The forceful expulsion of stomach contents through the mouth.

    pernicious v. Persistent, uncontrollable vomiting.

    v. of pregnancy Vomiting occurring during pregnancy, usually at 2 to 12 weeks of gestation, especially in the morning but may occur at any time.

VP 16 See etoposide.

vulva (vul'vă) The external female genitalia; consists of the prominence over the pubic bone (mons pubis), the labia majora and minora, clitoris, vestibule of the vagina, bulb of the vestibule, greater and lesser vestibular glands, and the vaginal orifice.

vulvar (vul'var) Relating to the vulva.

vulvectomy (vul-vek'tŏ-me) Partial or complete removal of the vulva.

    radical v. An operation for the treatment of invasive vulvar cancer consisting of *en bloc* removal of the skin of the vulva and the subcutaneous tissue to the depth of the urogenital diaphragm, with wide margins around the cancer being taken. Areas of primary lymphatic drainage are concurrently eliminated by bilateral removal of inguinal and femoral lymph nodes. The extent of the surgery can often be tailored to the location of the lesion.

    skinning v. Removal of the skin of the vulva, including the epidermis and dermis, usually as a treatment of multifocal vulvar *in situ* disease (i.e., vulvar intraepithelial neoplasia [VIN]). The purpose of the surgery is to maximize a functional and cosmetic result since VIN is a disease of young women.

vulvitis (vul-vi'tis) Inflammation of the vulva.

    atrophic v. See lichen sclerosus of vulva,

under lichen.

    diabetic v. Vulvitis associated with diabetes mellitus; caused by a chronic vulvovaginal infection by the yeastlike fungus *Candida albicans*; it may respond poorly to treatment if the diabetes is not controlled.

    gonorrheal v. Vulvitis caused by infection of the glandular structures of the vulva by the bacterium *Neisseria gonorrhoeae*.

    leukoplakic v. See lichen sclerosus of vulva, under lichen.

vulvo- Combining form meaning vulva.

vulvocrural (vul-vo-kroo'ral) Relating to the vulva and the thigh.

vulvodynia (vul-vo-din'e-ă) Chronic pain or burning sensations of the vulva without evidence of disease or abnormalities, usually causing sexual dysfunction; thought to be a form of peripheral neuralgia. It is a diagnosis of exclusion.

    dysesthetic v. A pain syndrome usually found in women in the sixth decade of life or older, marked by a burning or rawness that is limited to the vulvar vestibule and is usually not accompanied by redness (erythema) or even sensitivity to a cotton-tipped applicator.

vulvouterine (vul-vo-u'ter-in) Relating to the vulva and uterus.

vulvovaginal (vul-vo-vaj'ĭ-nal) Relating to the vulva and vagina. Also called vaginovulvar.

vulvovaginitis (vul-vo-vaj-ĭ-ni'tis) Inflammation of the vulva and vagina.

vulvovaginoplasty (vul-vo-vaj-ĭ-no-plas'ty) Reparative or reconstructive surgery of the vulva and vagina.

    Williams' v. Surgical construction of an artificial vagina using the labia majora to form the vaginal pouch.

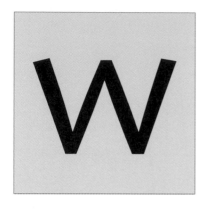

wall (wawl) In anatomy, a structure serving to enclose, divide, or protect a body cavity or part.

warfarin (war'fă-rin) Compound used in the prevention and treatment of abnormal blood clotting. Administration at any time during pregnancy can cause birth defects or abortion. Maternal ingestion of warfarin during the first trimester may result in a syndrome characterized by incomplete or defective development of nasal structures and stippled epiphyseal calcifications resembling chondrodysplasia punctata (a congenital bone abnormality).

wart (wort) A small, horny outgrowth on the skin or mucous membrane, usually of viral origin. Also called verruca.

    anorectal w. See condyloma acuminatum.

    common w. A wart with an irregular upper surface, usually ranging in size from 1 mm to 2 cm in diameter; seen most commonly on the back (dorsum) of the hand. Also called verruca vulgaris.

    fig w. See condyloma acuminatum.

    genital w. See condyloma acuminatum.

    moist w. See condyloma acuminatum.

    pointed w. See condyloma acuminatum.

    telangiectatic w. See angiokeratoma.

    venereal w. See condyloma acuminatum.

washing (wosh'ing) The removal of soluble material (e.g., from cells).

    sperm w. An adjunct to intrauterine insemination in which the semen sample is diluted and centrifuged prior to introduction into the uterus.

watchful waiting (wach'ful wāt'ing) An option consisting of closely monitoring a disease process and its progress instead of intervening (or changing therapy).

water-on-the-brain Colloquialism for hydrocephalus.

water, waters (wah'ter, s) Colloquial terms for amniotic fluid.

wave (wāv) A periodic increase and subsidence, as an oscillation propagated from point to point in a medium, characterized by alternate elevations and depressions.

    sine w. A wave characterized by a rise from zero to maximum positive potential, then descending back to zero and to maximum negative potential.

    ultrasonic w. A high-frequency sound wave, greater than 20,000 Hz; it cannot be heard by humans; used therapeutically and in diagnostic imaging.

wave-form (wāv-form) The graphic shape of a wave (i.e., on a chart).

weight (wāt) The product of the pull of gravity upon a body.

    birth w. The weight of a term infant at birth, usually ranging from 3000 to 3600 g.

    fetal w. The weight of a developing offspring from the ages of 16 to 40 gestational weeks; approximately 110 g at 16 weeks, 1100 g at 28 weeks, and 3400 g at 40 weeks.

    fetal w. calculation, Johnson's See Johnson's calculation of fetal weight, under calculation.

    low birth w. A newborn weight that is 2500 g or less.

    very low birth w. A newborn weight that is 1500 g or less.

whipworm (hwip'werm) Common term for a minute whiplike roundworm, *Trichuris trichiura*, parasitic in human intestines; transmitted by direct hand-to-mouth contact or by ingesting contaminated food or water.

whites (hwīts) Popular term for leukorrhea.

window (win'do) **1.** In anatomy, an opening in any partition-like structure or membrane. **2.** In radiology, a clear (radiolucent) area in an x-ray picture. **3.** In pharmacology, a range of drug concentration in the blood. **4.** A time interval (e.g., between ingestion of a poison and the production of irreversible organ damage).

    implantation w. The time period during which the uterine wall will allow implantation of the fertilized ovum; its length in humans has been estimated to be between 1 and 4 days.

womb (woom) Popular term for uterus.

    falling of w. See prolapse of uterus, under prolapse.

    neck of w. See uterine cervix, under cervix.

worm (werm) Common name for any of the elongated soft-bodied invertebrates of the phyla Annelida (segmented worms), Nematoda (roundworms), and Platyhelminthes (flatworms).

    seat w. See pinworm.

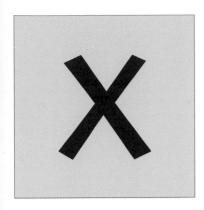

xenon (ze'non) An odorless gaseous element; symbol Xe, atomic number 54, atomic weight 131.3; present in minute proportions in the atmosphere.

xenon 133 (^{133}Xe) A gamma-emitting radioactive inert gas with a half-life of 5.27 days; a radioisotope of xenon; used to measure blood flow and regional pulmonary ventilation.

xeromenia (zēr-o-me'ne-ă) The occurrence of the usual symptoms of menstruation but without a menstrual blood flow.

xerotocia (zēr-o-to'se-ă) See dry labor, under labor.

Xg blood group Erythrocyte antigen controlled by a gene located on the X chromosome.

xiphopagus (zĭ-fop'ă-gus) Conjoined twins fused in the area of the xiphoid process of the breastbone.

X-linked (eks'linkt) Determined by a gene located on the X chromosome.

x-ray The common term for roentgenogram. See roentgenogram.

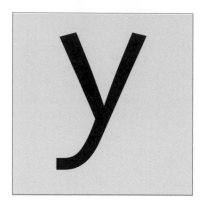

yaws (yawz) A bacterial skin infection characterized by eruptions of papules on the face, hands, feet, and around the external genitalia; caused by a spirochete, *Treponema pertenue*. Also called frambesia.

yolk (yōk) The nutrient portion of an ovum.

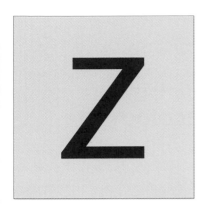

zidovudine (zi-do'vu-dēn) A drug used in the management of immune deficiency syndrome (AIDS); adverse effects include anemia and gastrointestinal symptoms. Formerly called azidothymidine (AZT).

zona (zo'nă), pl. zonae A zone, especially an encircling region distinguished from adjacent parts by some distinctive characteristic.

> **z. dermatica** An area of thick elevated skin surrounding the protrusion of a meningocele.

> **z. pellucida** A gel-like glycoprotein layer surrounding a developing ovum in the ovarian follicle; it plays a role in fertilization as it is penetrated by the sperm; it persists while the zygote undergoes cell divisions up to the blastocyst stage, when it degenerates and

disappears just prior to implantation into the uterine wall.

> **z. reaction** See under reaction.

zone (zōn) (z) Any area or space with differentiating characteristics; a region.

> **basal z.** See basal layer, under layer.

> **compact z.** See compact layer, under layer.

> **functional z.** See functional layer, under layer.

> **spongy z.** See spongy layer, under layer.

> **erogenous z., erotogenic z.** Any area of the body that, when appropriately stimulated, produces sexual sensations.

zygo-, zyg- Combining forms meaning a joining.

zygosity (zi-gos'ĭ-te) A state relating to the fertilized egg (zygote); often used as a word termination. Relating to twin pregnancies, development from one zygote (monozygosity) or from two zygotes (dizygosity). Relating to the genetic characteristic, whether they are identical (homozygosity) or different (heterozygosity).

zygote (zi'gōt) The single fertilized cell formed by the union of the male and female reproductive cells (gamete); a fertilized ovum or egg.

zygotene (zi'go-tēn) In meiosis, the second stage of prophase (following leptotene) in which homologous chromosomes approach each other and pair off point for point, forming a bivalent structure. See also diplotene; leptotene; pachytene.

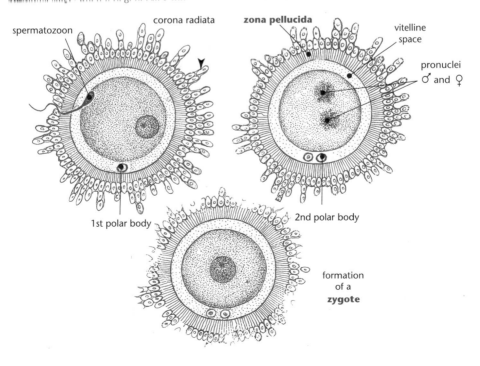

formation of a **zygote**

Selected abbreviations used in obstetrics and gynecology

A	age; area; atrium; auricle; blood type A+, A–; dominant allele	**ADH**	alcohol dehydrogenase; antidiuretic hormone
a	recessive allele	**ADL**	activities of daily living
AAA	abdominal aortic aneurysm; acute anxiety attack	**adm.**	admission
		ADR	adverse drug reaction
AAL	anterior axillary line	**ADS**	anonymous donor's sperm
AASH	adrenal androgen-stimulating hormone	**ADT**	admission–discharge transfer; anterior drawer test
Ab	abortion; antibody		
ABMT	autologous bone marrow transplant	**AE**	above elbow (said of amputations and prostheses); adverse event
ABO	blood groups A, B, AB, and O		
ABP	androgen-binding protein; arterial blood pressure	**AF**	amniotic fluid; anterior fontanel; atrial fibrillation; atrial flutter
ABVD	adriamycin (doxorubicin), bleomycin, vinblastine, dacarbazine (a chemotherapeutic regimen for treating cancer)	**AFAFP**	amniotic fluid alpha-fetoprotein
		AFE	amniotic fluid embolism
		AFI	amniotic fluid index
		AFP	alpha-fetoprotein
ABX	antibiotics	**Ag**	antigen; silver
aC	arabinosylcytosine	**AGA**	appropriate for gestational age (infant)
AC	acromioclavicular (joint); adrenal cortex; adriamycin, cyclophosphamide; air conduction; alternating current; anticoagulant	**AH**	abdominal hysterectomy; arterial hypertension; artificial heart
		AHF	acute heart failure; antihemophilic factor
ac	acromioclavicular (joint); acute; adrenal cortex; air conduction; alternating current; anchored catheter	**AI**	aortic insufficiency; artificial insemination; artificial intelligence
ACA	anterior cerebral artery; anticardiolipin antibody	**AID**	acute infectious disease; anti-inflammatory drug; artificial insemination by donor; automatic implantable defibrillator
ACE	angiotensin-converting enzyme; adrenocortical extract		
ACEI	angiotensin-converting enzyme inhibitor	**AIDS**	acquired immune deficiency syndrome
ACh	acetylcholine	**AIH**	artificial insemination by husband (homologous insemination)
AChE	acetylcholinesterase		
ACI	after-care instructions	**AIS**	adenocarcinoma *in situ*
ACLS	advanced cardiac life support	**ALEC**	artificial lung-expanding compound
ACOG	American College of Obstetricians and Gynecologists	**ALL**	acute lymphoblastic leukemia
		ALS	advanced life support; amyotrophic lateral sclerosis; antilymphocyte serum
ACPS	acrocephalopolysyndactyly		
ACTH	adrenocorticotropic hormone	**AMH**	antimullerian hormone
ACV	acyclovir	**AMI**	acute myocardial infarction
AD	addict; adenovirus; Alzheimer's disease; analgesic dose; autosomal dominant	**AMP**	adenosine monophosphate
		AN	anesthesia; aneurysm; anorexia nervosa
		ANA	antinuclear antibody
AdC	adrenal cortex	**AND**	anterior nasal discharge
ADCC	antibody-dependent-cell-mediated cytotoxicity	**anes.**	anesthesia
		ANP	atrial natriuretic peptide

ANS	anterior nasal spine; autonomic nervous system		AWS	alcohol withdrawal syndrome
AOC	area of concern		AZT	azidothymidine (zidovudine)
AP	acid phosphatase; alkaline phosphatase; angina pectoris; antepartum; anterior pituitary; anteroposterior (view); appendix; arterial pressure		B	bacillus; blood type B+, B–; bicuspid; boron
			BA	backache; bile acid; blood alcohol; bone age; boric acid; bronchial asthma
A & P	anterior and posterior; auscultation and palpation; auscultation and percussion		BB	blood bank; breast biopsy
APC	acetylsalicylic acid, phenacetin, and caffeine; antigen-presenting cell; atrial premature contraction		BBA	born before arrival (of physician or midwife)
			BBB	blood–brain barrier; bundle-branch block
APH	antepartum hemorrhage; anterior pituitary hormone		BBT	basal body temperature
			BC	birth control; blood culture; bone conduction; bronchial carcinoma
APO	apolipoprotein			
app.	apparent; appendix		BCC	basal cell cancer; basal cell carcinoma; benign cellular changes
appr.	approximate			
appx	appendix		BCG	bacillus Calmette-Guerin (vaccine); ballistocardiograph
appy	appendectomy			
APTS	acid phosphatase test for semen		BCP	birth control pill
APTT	activated partial thromboplastin time		BD	below diaphragm; bile duct; birth defect; Bowen's disease; brain dead
AR	alarm reaction; aortic regurgitation; artificial respiration; attributable risk; autosomal recessive		BE	barium enema; breast examination
			BFPR	biologic false-positive reaction
Ar	argon		BG	blood glucose; bone graft
A & R	advised and released		BID	brought in dead
ARBD	alcohol-related birth defects		bil.	bilirubin
ARC	AIDS-related complex; American Red Cross		blad.	bladder
			Bld	blood
ARD	acute respiratory disease; acute respiratory distress		Bld Bk	blood bank
			BLS	basic life support; blind loop syndrome
ARDS	acute respiratory distress syndrome; adult respiratory distress syndrome		BM	basal metabolism; basement membrane; bone marrow; bone mass; bowel movement
ARF	acute renal failure; acute respiratory failure; acute rheumatic fever			
			BMD	bone mineral density
ARM	artificial rupture of membranes		BMI	body mass index
ARP	at-risk period		bmk	birthmark
ART	acid reflux test; acoustic reflex test; assisted reproductive technology		BMR	basal metabolic rate
			BMT	bone marrow transplant
AS	anal sphincter; aortic stenosis; arteriosclerosis; artificial sweetner; atherosclerosis		BO	bowel obstruction
			BOA	born on arrival
			BOW	bag of waters
ASA	acetylsalicylic acid (aspirin); antisperm antibody		BP	blood pressure; bypass
			BPD	biparietal diameter; bronchopulmonary dysplasia
ASAP	as soon as possible			
ASCUS	atypical squamous cells of undetermined significance		BPM	beats per minute; breaths per minute
			BPP	biophysical profile
ASD	atrial septal defect		BPS	binge-and-purge syndrome
ASIS	anterosuperior iliac spine		Bq	becquerel
ASX	asymptomatic		B.R.	bed rest
ATB	antibiotic		BRBPR	bright red blood per rectum
ATN	acute tubular necrosis		BRM	biologic response modifier
AUDS	atypia of undetermined significance		BS	blood sugar; breath sounds; bowel sounds
AVH	acute viral hepatitis			
AVM	arteriovenous malformation		BSE	breast self examination
AVP	arginine vasopressin		BSL	blood sugar level

BSO	bilateral salpingo-oophorectomy	**CCF**	congestive cardiac failure
BT	bedtime; benzidine test; biuret test; blind test; blood transfusion; body temperature	**CCMS**	clean-catch midstream (urine specimen)
		Ccr	creatinine clearance
		CCRU	critical care recovery unit
BTC	basal temperature chart	**CD**	cadaver donor; cardiac disease; cesarean delivery; cluster designation; cluster determinant; cluster of differentiation (system); communicable disease; consanguineous donor; contact dermatitis; curative dose
BTL	bilateral tubal ligation		
BUN	bleeding of unknown origin; blood urea nitrogen		
BV	bacterial vaginosis; blood vessel; blood volume		
BW	birth weight; body weight	**CD3**	antigenic marker on T cell associated with T cell receptor
BX, Bx	biopsy		
		CD4	antigenic marker of helper/inducer T cells
C	calculus; carbohydrate; carbon; cathode; Celsius; Centigrade; cervical (spinal nerves, vertebrae); cesarean; complement; concentration; contraction; coulomb; large calorie		
		CD8	antigenic marker of suppressor/cytotoxic T cells
		CDI	color Doppler imaging
		CEA	carcinoembryonic antigen
CA	cancer; cardiac arrest; chronological age	**CE & R**	central episiotomy and repair
		cerv.	cervical; cervix
Ca	calcium; cancer; carotid artery; cathode; cerebral aqueduct; chronological age	**CES**	cauda equina syndrome
		CF	cancer-free; cardiac failure; complement fixation; complement-fixing (antibody); coupling factor; cystic fibrosis
ca	cancer		
CAD	computer-assisted diagnosis; coronary artery disease		
		CFS	Chiari-Frommel syndrome
CAF	cyclophosphamide, adriamycin, 5-FU	**CG**	cholecystogram; chorionic gonadotropin; chronic glomerulonephritis
CAH	chronic active hepatitis; congenital adrenal hyperplasia		
CALLA	common acute lymphoblastic leukemia antigen	**C–H**	crown–heel (applied to the length of a fetus)
cAMP	cyclic adenosine monophosphate	**CHAP**	cyclophosphamide, hexamethylmelamine, doxorubicin, cisplatin (chemotherapeutic regimen for ovarian cancer)
CAN	cord (umbilical) around neck		
CASA	computer-assisted semen analysis		
CASH	cancer and sex hormone		
CAT	cataract; computerized axial tomography	**CHD**	congenital heart disease; congenital hip dislocation; coronary heart disease
cath.	catheter; catheterize	**chemo**	chemotherapy
CATSCAN	computer-assisted tomography scanner	**CHF**	congestive heart failure
		CHN	congenital hairy nevus
CB	catheterized bladder; cesarean birth; chronic bronchitis; code blue	**CI**	cervical incompetence; color index; confidence interval
CBC	complete blood count	**CIA**	chemiluminescent immunoassay
CBD	common bile duct; closed bladder drainage	**CID**	cytomegalovirus inclusion disease
		Cin	insulin clearance
CBE	clinical breast examination	**CIN**	cervical intraepithelial neoplasia
CBG	capillary blood gases; corticosteroid-binding globulin	**CIN I**	cervical intraepithelial neoplasia (with mild dysplasia)
CBR	complete bed rest	**CIN II**	cervical intraepithelial neoplasia (with moderate dysplasia)
CC	cardiac catheterization; cardiac cycle; cerebral concussion; chief complaint; chronic complainer; (umbilical) cord compression; creatinine clearance; critical care		
		CIN III	cervical intraepithelial neoplasia (with severe dysplasia)
		CIS	carcinoma *in situ*; Cancer Information Service
cc	cubic centimeter	**CL**	corpus luteum; critical list
CCB	calcium channel blocker	**clav.**	clavicle

CMI	cell-mediated immunity
CMID	cytomegalic inclusion disease
CMN	cystic medial necrosis
CMV	controlled mechanical ventilation; cytomegalovirus
CNS	central nervous system
coc	coccygeal
COD	cause of death
COLD	chronic obstructive lung disease
COMT	catechol-O-methyl transferase
C-ONC	cellular oncogene
COP	colloid osmotic pressure
COPD	chronic obstructive pulmonary disease
cor.	coronary
CORD	chronic obstructive respiratory disease
CP	cerebral palsy; chemically pure; chest pain; chronic pain; cleft palate; cor pulmonale; creatine phosphate
C & P	cystoscopy and pyelography
CPAP	continuous positive air pressure; continuous positive airway pressure
C-parvum	*Corynebacterium parvum*
CPD	cephalopelvic disproportion; comparison point decision; compound
CPID	chronic pelvic inflammatory disease
CPP	chronic pelvic pain
CPPB	continuous positive pressure breathing
CPPV	continuous positive pressure ventilation
CPR	cardiac pulmonary reserve; cardiopulmonary resuscitation
CPX	complete physical examination
CR	cardiorespiratory; cellular receptor; chest roentgenogram; clinical record; code red; colon resection; complete remission; conditioned reflex; conditioned response; creatinine
C–R	crown–rump (applied to length of fetus)
CRC	colorectal cancer
CRH	corticotropin-releasing hormone
CRL	crown–rump length (of fetus)
CRS	Chinese restaurant syndrome; colorectal surgery
CS	cardiogenic shock; carotid sinus; cesarean section; cigarette smoke; cigarette smoker; conditioned stimulus; congenital syphilis
CSF	cerebrospinal fluid; colony-stimulating factor
CSP	criminal sexual psychopath
CST	contraction stress test
CT	calcitonin; carotid tracing; carpal tunnel; cerebral thrombosis; clotting time; coagulation time; computed tomography; connective tissue; corneal transplant
ct	count

CTB	ceased to breathe
CTL	cytotoxic T lymphocyte; cytotoxic lymphocyte
CU	cause unknown; clinical unit; convalescent unit
CUSA	cavitron ultrasonic surgical aspirator
CV	cardiovascular; closing volume (of lung); coefficient of variation
CVA	cardiovascular accident; cerebrovascular accident; costovertebral angle
CVD	cardiovascular disease
CVP	central venous pressure
CVS	cardiovascular system; chorionic villus sampling
CVST	chorionic villus sampling test
CWP	childbirth without pain
Cx	cervix; convex
CXR	chest x-ray
cyc	cycle
CYS	cystoscopy
D	day; deceased; deuterium; dexter; diagnosis; diopter; donor; dorsal; dose; drug
d	day; deceased; density; deuteron; died
DA	delayed action; developmental age; drug addict; ductus arteriosus
DAD	dispense as directed
DB	date of birth; disability
Db	diabetic
dbl	double
DBW	desirable body weight
DC	dendritic cells; diagonal conjugate; diagnostic center; discharge; discontinue
D & C	dilatation and curettage
DC & B	dilatation, curettage, and biopsy
DCIS	ductal carcinoma *in situ*
DD	dangerous drug; degenerative disease; differential diagnosis
DDAVP	deamino D-arginine vasopressin (desmopressin acetate)
ddC	dideoxycytidine
DDH	developmental dysplasia of hip
ddl	dideoxyinosine
D & E	dilatation and evacuation
def.	defecation
dehyd.	dehydration
DES	diethylstilbestrol
DESI	direct egg sperm injection
DFS	dead fetus syndrome
DFU	dead fetus *in utero*
DGI	disseminated gonococcal infection
DHA	dehydroepiandrosterone
DHEA	dehydroepiandrosterone
DHEAS	dehydroepiandrosterone sulfate

DHT	dihydrotestosterone	**EBV**	Epstein-Barr virus
diag.	diagnosis	**ECC**	emergency cardiac care; endocervical curettage
diam.	diameter		
DIC	disseminated intravascular coagulation	**ECF**	eosinophil chemotactic factor; extended care facility; extracellular fluid
DIE	died in emergency room		
dilat.	dilatation; dilated		
DIPI	direct intraperitoneal insemination	**ECG**	echocardiogram; electrocardiogram; electrocardiograph; electrocardiography
disch.	discharge		
DKA	diabetic ketoacidosis		
DL	danger list; diffuse lymphoma	**ECHO**	echocardiogram; echoencephalogram; Enteric Cytopathogenic Human Orphan (virus)
DLE	dialyzable leukocyte extract; discoid lupus erythematosus; disseminated lupus erythematosus		
		ECMO	extracorporeal membrane oxygenation
DLMP	date of last menstrual period	**E. coli**	*Escherichia coli*
DM	diabetes mellitus; diabetic mother; diastolic murmur; dopamine	**ECS**	electrocerebral silence; electroconvulsive shock
DMOOC	diabetes mellitus out of control	**EDC**	estimated date of confinement
DNA	does not apply; deoxyribonucleic acid	**EDD**	effective drug duration; expected date of delivery
DND	died a natural death		
DNI	do not intubate	**EDRF**	endothelium-derived relaxing factor
DNR	do not resuscitate (order)	**EFM**	electronic fetal monitoring
DOA	date of admission; dead on arrival	**EGF**	epidermal growth factor
DOB	date of birth	**EKG**	electrocardiogram; electrocardiograph; electrocardiography
DOC	deoxycholate; deoxycorticosterone		
DOC-SO 4	deoxycorticosterone sulfate	**ELISA**	enzyme-linked immunosorbent assay
DOD	date of death	**EM**	electron micrograph; electron microscope; electron microscopy; emergency medicine; emotionally disturbed; erythema migrans; external monitor
DOE	date of examination; dyspnea on exertion		
DOM	dominance		
DOPA	dopamine		
DORx	date of treatment		
DOS	date of surgery	**EMB**	endometrial biopsy
DOT	died on (operating room) table	**EMC**	emergency medical care; endometrial curettage
DPA	dual-photon absorptiometry		
DPPC	dipalmitoylphosphatidylcholine	**EMS**	early morning specimen; emergency medical service
DR	delivery room; diabetic retinopathy		
DRE	digital rectal examination	**En.**	enema
DRG	diagnosis-related group	**ENDO**	endoscopy
dRVVT	dilute Russel viper venom time	**enz**	enzyme
DS	discharge summary; donor's serum; double strength; Down's syndrome	**EP**	ectopic pregnancy; electrophoresis; emergency procedure; erythropoietin
DSM	Diagnostic and Statistical Manual	**EPF**	early pregnancy factor
DU	decubitus ulcer; diagnosis undetermined; duodenal ulcer	**epis**	episiotomy
		epith	epithelium
DUB	dysfunctional uterine bleeding	**EPM**	electronic fetal monitoring; electronic pacemaker
DVT	deep vein thrombosis		
D & X	dilatation and extraction	**ER**	emergency room; endoplasmic reticulum; estrogen receptor
Dx	diagnosis		
DXA	dual-energy x-ray absorptiometry	**ERA**	endometrial resection and ablation
DZ	disease; dizygotic (twins); dizziness	**ERCP**	endoscopic retrograde cholangiopancreatography
		ERPF	effective renal plasma flow
EACP	epsilon-aminocaproic (acid)	**ERT**	estrogen replacement therapy
EB	epidermolysis bullosa; Epstein-Barr (virus)	**ERV**	expiratory reserve volume
		ESR	electron spin resonance; erythrocyte sedimentation rate
EBF	erythroblastosis fetalis		
EBL	estimated blood loss		
EBM	expressed breast milk	**ESRD-DM**	end stage renal disease – diabetes

mellitus

ESS	endometrial stromal sarcoma
EST	electroshock therapy; electroshock treatment; endodermal sinus tumor
Est	estrogen
ET	embryo transfer; endotracheal; endotracheal tube; etiology; exercise test; expiratory time
ETC	estimated time of conception
EU	excretory urography
EUS	external urethral sphincter
Ex	excision
exog.	exogenous
EXP	exploration
F	factor; Fahrenheit; failure; fasting; female; fertility; fetal; flow; fluorine; foramen; force; formula
F1	first filial generation
F2	second filial generation
f	fluid; focal length; frequency
FA	false aneurysm; fatty acid; femoral artery; fetal age; fluorescent antibody; folic acid; frontanterior (position)
FAE	fetal alcohol effects
FAS	fetal alcohol syndrome
FB	feedback; foreign body
FBP	femoral blood pressure
FBS	fasting blood sugar; fetal blood sample
FCD	fibrocystic disease
FCM	flow cytometry
FCS	fetal cocaine syndrome
FD	fatal dose; forceps delivery
FDIU	fetal death *in utero*
FDLMP	first day of last menstrual period
FECG	fetal electrocardiogram
FEV	forced expiratory volume
FFA	free fatty acids
FFI	free from infection
FGF	fibroblast growth factor
FGT	female genital tract
FH	family history
FHCM	familial hypertrophic cardiomyopathy
FHH	fetal heart heard
FHNH	fetal heart not heard
FHR	fetal heart rate
FHT	fetal heart tone
FHx	family history
FICU	fetal intensive care unit
FIGO	International Federation of Gynecology and Obstetrics
FISH	fluorescence *in situ* hybridization
fist.	fistula
FIUO	for internal use only
fl.	fluid
FM	face mask; fetal monitor; fetal

movements; forensic medicine

FMC	fetal movement counting
FMF	familial Mediterranean fever; fetal movement felt
FMP	first menstrual period
FN	false-negative
FNA	fine needle aspiration
FNAB	fine-needle aspiration biopsy
FOB	fecal occult blood; fiberoptic bronchoscopy
FOD	free of disease
FP	false-positive; family physician; family planning; frontoposterior (fetal position); frozen plasma
FRC	functional residual capacity
FSH	follicle-stimulating hormone
FSH-LH	follicle-stimulating hormone–luteinizing hormone
FSH-RH	follicle-stimulating hormone-releasing hormone
FT	family therapy; frontotransverse (fetal position); full term
FTA	fluorescent titer antibody (test)
FTA-ABS	fluorescent treponemal antibody absorption (test)
FTAAT	fluorescent treponemal antibody absorption test
FTND	full term normal delivery
FTP	failure to progress (labor)
FTT	failure to thrive
FU	fluorouracil; follow up
FUE	fever of undetermined etiology
FUO	fever of undetermined origin; fever of unknown origin
FVC	forced vital capacity
Fx	fracture
FXS	fragile X syndrome
G	gas; gauge; gauss; glucose; glycine; glycogen; gram; guanosine
g	gender; gram; gravitational constant; gravity; grou
GA	gastric analysis; general anesthesia; gestational age
GABA	gamma-aminobutyric acid
GBG	gonadal steroid-binding globulin
GBS	group B streptococcus
GC	gas chromatography; gonococcus; gonorrheal cervicitis
GDM	gestational diabetes mellitus
GEN	gender; generic; genetics; genital
GEPH	gestational edema with proteinuria and hypertension
GER	gastroesophageal reflux; geriatrics
GF	gastric fluid; germ-free; growth factor
GFR	glomerular filtration rate

GH	growth hormone; general hospital	**HBs**	hepatitis B surface
GHD	growth hormone deficiency	**HBsAb**	antibody to the hepatitis B surface antigen
GH-RF	growth hormone-releasing factor		
GH-RH, GHRH		**HBsAg**	hepatitis B surface antigen
	growth hormone-releasing hormone	**HBV**	hepatitis B virus
GIFT	gamete intrafallopian transfer	**HBW**	high birth weight
GIH	growth hormone-inhibiting hormone (somatostatin)	**HC**	head circumference; (fetal) head compression; home care; hydrocortisone; hydroxycorticoid
gl.	gland		
GLUT	glucose transport (protein)	**HCC**	hepatocellular carcinoma
GN	glomerulonephritis; Gram-negative	**hCG**	human chorionic gonadotropin
Gn	gonadotropin	**HCM**	hypertrophic cardiomyopathy
Gn-RH	gonadotropin-releasing hormone	**hCS**	human chorionic somatomammotropin
GnRHa	gonadotropin-releasing hormone analog; gonadotropin-releasing hormone agonist	**Hct**	hematocrit
		HCV	hepatitis C virus
		HDL	high-density lipoprotein
GOG	Gynecologic Oncology Group	**HDN**	hemolytic disease of newborn; high-density nebulizer
G6PD	glucose-6-phosphate dehydrogenase		
grav.	gravid	**HDR**	high-dose rate (brachytherapy)
GSH	growth-stimulating hormone	**HDV**	hepatitis D (Delta) virus
GST	genetic screening test	**HE**	heterologous
GTD	gestational trophoblastic disease	**HELLP**	hemolysis, elevated liver enzymes, low platelet count
GTN	gestational trophoblastic neoplasia		
GTT	glucose tolerance test	**hem.**	hemorrhage; hemorrhoid
GU	gastric ulcer; genitourinary	**hep**	heparin; hepatitis
GUS	genitourinary system	**HEV**	hepatitis E virus; high endothelial venules
GVHD	graft-versus-host disease	**HF**	heart failure
GYN	gynecology	**HFD**	high forceps delivery
		HG	herpes genitalis
H	head; heart; hemisphere; hernia; heroin; hydrogen; hypodermic	**Hg**	mercury
		Hgb	hemoglobin
h	height; horizontal; hour; hundred	**hG**	human gonadotropin
HA	headache; hemolytic anemia; hepatitis A; hospital admission	**hGH**	human growth hormone
		hgt	height
HAA	hepatitis-associated antigen	**HHV**	human herpesvirus
HAAg	hepatitis A antigen	**HIV**	human immunodeficiency virus
HAI	hospital-acquired infection	**HIV-1**	human immunodeficiency virus type 1
HAMA	human anti-murine antibody	**HIV-2**	human immunodeficiency virus type 2
HAP	hospital-acquired pneumonia	**HLA**	human leukocyte antigen
HAV	hepatitis A virus	**hLH**	human luteinizing hormone
HB	bundle of His; heart block; hepatitis B; hospital bed	**HM**	heart murmur; human milk; hydatidiform mole
Hb	hemoglobin	**HMD**	hyaline membrane disease
HBAb	hepatitis B antibody	**HMG**	high mobility group
HBAg	hepatitis B antigen	**hMG**	human menopausal gonadotropin
HBc	hepatitis B core	**HMM**	hexamethylmelamine
HBcAb	antibody to hepatitis B core antigen	**HO**	homologous
HBcAg	hepatitis B core antigen	**H & P**	history and physical (examination)
HBe	hepatitis B e	**HPA**	hypothalamic-pituitary-adrenal (axis)
HBeAb	antibody to hepatitis B e antigen	**HPF**	high-power field
HBeAg	hepatitis B e antigen	**HPI**	history of present illness
HbF	fetal hemoglobin; hemoglobin F	**hPL**	human placental lactogen
HbH	hemoglobin H	**HPV**	human papillomavirus
HBIG	hepatitis B immune globulin	**H & R**	hysterectomy and radiation
HBO	hyperbaric oxygen	**HRCT**	high-resolution computed tomography
HBP	high blood pressure	**HRT**	hormone replacement therapy;

	hyperparathyroidism
HS	half-strength; hazardous substance; heart sounds; hereditary spherocytosis; herpes simplex; house surgeon
HSG	hysterosalpingogram
HSIL	high-grade squamous intraepithelial lesion
HSV	herpes simplex virus
HT	Hashimoto's thyroiditis; height; high temperature; hypertension
Ht	heart; height
HUAM	home uterine activity monitoring
HTN	hypertension
hTSS	human toxic shock syndrome
HV	has voided; herpes virus; hyperventilation
HVGR	host-versus-graft reaction
hyst.	hysterectomy
HZI	hemizona assay index
IAS	interatrial septum
IASD	interatrial septal defect
IAT	impedance audiometry test; intraoperative autologous transfusion
IB	inclusion body; infectious bronchitis
IBD	inflammatory bowel disease
IBI	intermittent bladder irrigation
IBC	iron-binding capacity
IC	immune complex; indwelling catheter; inspiratory capacity; intensive care; intermittent catheterization; intracranial; irritable colon
ICA	internal carotid artery; intracranial aneurysm; islet cell antibody
ICAO	internal carotid artery occlusion
ICD	immune complex disease; International Classification of Diseases; intrauterine contraceptive device
ICF	intermediate care facility; intracellular fluid
ICH	intracranial hemorrhage
ICN	intensive care nursery
ICP	intracranial pressure
ICS	intercostal space
ICSH	interstitial cell-stimulating hormone
ICSI	intracytoplasmic sperm injection
IDAM	infant of drug-abusing mother; infant of drug-addicted mother
IDDM	insulin-dependent diabetes mellitus
IDM	infant of diabetic mother
IDP	intraductal papilloma
IE	infective endocarditis
Ig	immunoglobulin
IgA	immunoglobulin A (gamma A globulin)
IgD	immunoglobulin D (gamma D globulin)

IGDM	infant of gestational diabetic mother
IgE	immunoglobulin E (gamma E globulin)
IGF	insulin-like growth factor
IgG	immunoglobulin G (gamma G globulin)
IgM	immunoglobulin M (gamma M globulin)
IGT	impaired glucose tolerance
IGTT	intravenous glucose tolerance test
IHD	ischemic heart disease
IICU	infant intensive care unit
IL	interleukin
IM	infectious mononucleosis; intramuscular
IMB	intermenstrual bleeding
IMR	individual medical record; infant mortality rate
IMV	intermittent mandatory ventilation
INC	incontinence
IND	investigational new drug
INF	infant; interferon; intravenous nutritional feeding
inop.	inoperable
INPT	inpatient
int. obst.	intestinal obstruction
IODAM	infant of drug-addicted mother
IODM	infant of diabetic mother
IP	incubation period; inpatient; intraperitoneal
IPCD	infantile polycystic disease
IPD	inflammatory pelvic disease; intermittent peritoneal dialysis
IPG	impedance plethysmography
IPP	inflatable penile prosthesis; intermittent positive pressure
IPPB	intermittent positive pressure breathing
IPPV	intermittent positive pressure ventilation
IPT	immunologic pregnancy test
IR	immune response; insulin reaction; insulin resistance; insulin resistant
IRC	inspiratory reserve capacity
IRDS	infant respiratory distress syndrome
IRMA	immunoradiometric assay
IRV	inspiratory reserve volume
IS	immunosuppressive; inguinal syndrome; intercostal space
ISSVD	International Society for the Study of Vulvar Disease
IU	immunizing unit; International Units; intrauterine
IUCD	intrauterine contraceptive device
IUD	intrauterine device
IUGR	intrauterine growth retardation
IUI	intrauterine insemination
IV	interventricular; intravenous
i.v.	*in vitro* [Latin] in glass; *in vivo* [Latin]

	within a living body
IVC	inferior vena cava; inspiratory vital capacity
IVDA	intravenous drug abuse; intravenous drug abuser
IVF	*in vitro* fertilization
IVF-ET	*in vitro* fertilization and embryo transfer
IVH	intraventricular hemorrhage
IVP	intravenous pyelogram; intravenous pyelography; increased vascular permeability
IVT	intravenous transfusion
IVU	intravenous urography
JCV	JC virus
JD	juvenile delinquent; juvenile diabetes
JDM	juvenile-onset diabetes mellitus
JOD	juvenile-onset diabetes
JPS	juvenile polyposis syndrome
JRA	juvenile rheumatoid arthritis
KA	ketoacidosis
KB	ketone bodies
KDA	known drug allergies
KI	karyotype index
KS	Kaposi's sarcoma; ketosteroid
17-KS	17-ketosteroids
KS/OI	Kaposi's sarcoma and opportunistic infections
KT	kidney transplant
KUB	kidney, ureter, and bladder
L	lumbar (spinal nerves, vertebrae)
LA	left arm; left atrium; left auricle; local anesthesia; long acting; lupus anticoagulant
La	labial; lanthanum
LAC	laceration; lupus anticoagulant
LAE	left atrial enlargement
LAH	left atrial hypertrophy
LAK	lymphokine-activated killer (cell)
LAL	left axillary line
LASER	light amplification by stimulated emission of radiation
LATS	long-acting thyroid stimulator
LAVH	laparoscopically assisted vaginal hysterectomy
LB	large bowel; left breast; left buttock; live birth
LBB	left breast biopsy
LBO	large bowel obstruction
LBP	low back pain; low blood pressure
LBR	labor room
LBW	low birth weight (infant)
LC	lethal concentration; living child; living children

LCCS	low cervical cesarean section
LD	lethal dose; levodopa; living donor; loading dose; low dosage; Lyme disease
L & D	labor and delivery
LDH	lactate dehydrogenase
LDL	low-density lipoprotein; loudness discomfort level
L-dopa	levodopa
LDR	labor, delivery, and recovery (room); low-dose rate (brachytherapy)
LE	lower extremity; lupus erythematosus
LEEP	loop electrosurgical excision procedure
leio.	leiomyoma
LF	low forceps; low frequency
LFA	left femoral artery; left frontoanterior (fetal position); low friction arthroplasty; lymphocyte functional antigen
LFH	left femoral hernia
LFP	left frontoposterior (fetal position)
LFT	left frontotransverse (fetal position)
LGA	large for gestational age (infant)
LGV	lymphogranuloma venereum
LH	luteinizing hormone
LHF	left heart failure; luteinizing hormone-releasing factor
LH-RF	luteinizing hormone-releasing factor
LH-RH	luteinizing hormone-releasing hormone
Li	labeling index; lithium
LIC	left iliac crest
LIP	lymphocytic interstitial pneumonia
LLQ	left lower quadrant (of abdomen)
LM	licentiate in midwifery
LMA	left mentoanterior (fetal position)
LME	left mediolateral episiotomy
LMP	last menstrual period; left mentoposterior (fetal position); low malignancy potential; lumbar puncture
LMS	leiomyosarcoma
LMT	left mentotransverse (fetal position)
LN	lymph node
LNB	lymph node biopsy
LNMP	last normal menstrual period
LOA	left occipitoanterior (fetal position)
LOP	left occipitoposterior (fetal position)
LOT	left occipitotransverse (fetal position)
LP	lichen planus; light perception; lipoprotein; lumbar puncture
Lp(a)	lipoprotein (a)
LPS	last Papanicolaou smear; lipopolysaccharide
LR	labor room; light reaction
LRH	luteinizing hormone-releasing hormone
LS	lichen sclerosis; lumbosacral

L/S	lecithin/sphingomyelin (ratio)
LSA	left sacroanterior (fetal position)
LSCS	lower segment cesarean section
LSD	life-sustaining device; lysergic acid diethylamide
LSH	lutein-stimulating hormone
LSIL	low-grade squamous intraepithelial lesion
LSP	left sacroposterior (fetal position)
LST	left sacrotransverse (fetal position)
LT	left; leukotriene; long term; low temperature; lymphotoxin
LTA	lymphocyte-transforming activity
LTCS	low transverse cesarean section
LUFS	luteinizing unruptured follicle syndrome
lum	lumbar
LUQ	left upper quadrant (of abdomen)
LV	left ventricle; leukemia virus; live vaccine; lung volume
LVEDP	left ventricular end-diastolic pressure
LX	local irradiation
Lys	lysine
M	male; malignant; mass; maximum; median; meter; minimum; mol; molar; mother; murmur; muscle
MA	medical authorization; menstrual age; mentoanterior (fetal position); moderately advanced
MAC	membrane-attack complex; minimum alveolar (anesthetic) concentration; methotrexate, dactinomycin (actinomycin D), and chlorambucil; *Mycobacterium avium* complex;
MAF	macrophage-activating factor
MAI	*Mycobacterium avium-intracellulare*
MAIDS	murine acquired immune deficiency syndrome
MAL	midaxillary line
malig.	malignant
mammo.	mammogram
MAP	mean airway pressure; mean arterial pressure; muscle action potential
MAS	meconium aspiration syndrome; milk-alkali syndrome
MBC	maximum breathing capacity
MBL	menstrual blood loss
MBM	mother's breast milk
MC	mast cell; maximum concentration; metacarpal; miscarriage
MCA	middle carotid artery; middle cerebral artery; multiple congenital abnormalities
MCC	midstream clean-catch (urine sample)
MCHC	mean corpuscular hemoglobin concentration; mean cell hemoglobin concentration
MCL	maximum contamination level; midclavicular line
MCV	mean corpuscular volume; mean cell volume
MDR-TB	multiple drug-resistant tuberculosis
ME	medial episiotomy; mediastinal emphysema
mec.	meconium
MENS	multiple endocrine neoplasia syndrome
MESA	microsurgical epididymal sperm aspiration
MET	metastasis
MeV	megavolt; megavoltage; million electron volts
M & F	male and female; mother and father
MFD	mid-forceps delivery; minimum fatal dose
MG	mammary gland; myasthenia gravis
MH	medical history; menstrual history; mental health
MHA	major histocompatibility antigen; microhemagglutinin
MHA-TP	microhemagglutination for *Treponema pallidum*
MHC	major histocompatibility complex; mental health clinic
MHx	medical history
MI	maturation index; mitotic index; mitral insufficiency; myocardial infarction
MID	minimal infecting dose; minimal inhibiting dose
MIF	migration-inhibiting factor; mullerian-inhibiting factor
misc	miscarriage; miscellaneous
MLE	midline episiotomy
MMMT	malignant mixed mesodermal tumor
MMR	measles–mumps–rubella (vaccine)
MMS	mixed mesodermal sarcoma
MODY	maturity-onset diabetes of youth
MOPD	multiple oocytes per disk
MP	mean pressure; menstrual period; mentoanterior (fetal position); multiparous
MPC	mucopurulent cervicitis
MPD	maximal permissible dose; multiple personality disorder
MPS	meconium plug syndrome; mononuclear phagocyte system; mucopolysaccharide; mucopolysaccharidosis
MR	may repeat; measles–rubella (vaccine); medical record; medical resident; mental retardation; mitral regurgitation; Moro's reflex

MRI	magnetic resonance imaging		osteochondritis dissecans
MS	mitral stenosis; morphine sulfate;	OCT	oxytocin challenge test
	multiple sclerosis; musculoskeletal	ODA	overall disease assessment
MSAFP	maternal serum alpha-fetoprotein	OGTT	oral glucose tolerance test
MSH	melanocyte-stimulating hormone	OFA	oncofetal antigen
MSL	midsternal line	OFC	occipitofrontal circumference
MT	mammary tumor; mentotransverse	OHSS	ovarian hyperstimulation syndrome
	(fetal position); muscles and tendons	OM	osteomalacia; osteomyelitis
multip	multiparous	OMI	oocyte maturation inhibitor
MVC	maximum vital capacity	ONCO	oncology
MVV	maximum voluntary ventilation	OP	occipitoposterior (fetal position);
			operative procedure; osteoporosis
Narco	narcolepsy	OT	occipitotransverse (fetal position); oral
NB	needle biopsy; newborn		temperature; oxytocin
NBM	no bowel movement; nothing by mouth	OTC	ornithine transcarbamoylase; over the
NBW	normal birth weight		counter (drugs)
ND	natural death; neonatal death;	OV	office visit; ovary; ovum
	neoplastic disease; new drug; no	Ov	ovary; ovum
	disease; normal delivery; not diagnosed;	OXT	oxytocin
	notifiable disease		
NDA	new drug approval	P450c21	21-hydroxylase
NE	nerve ending; neurologic examination;	PAS	periodic acid–Schiff (stain)
	no effect; norepinephrine	PAL	posterior axillary line
NEC	necrotizing enterocolitis	Palp	palpable; palpate; palpated
NEEP	negative end-expiratory pressure	PAP	Papanicolaou (test); peroxidase anti-
NEO	neonatology		peroxidase (complex); prostatic acid
ng	nanogram		phosphatase; pulmorary artery pressure
NGF	nerve growth factor	PAPP	pregnancy-associated plasma protein
NGU	nongonococcal urethritis	Pap smear	Papanicolaou smear
NI	neonatal isoerythrolysis; no	Pap test	Papanicolaou test
	improvement	PBA	partial-birth abortion
NICC	neonatal intensive care center	PBD	proliferative breast disease
NICU	neonatal intensive care unit	PBG	porphobilinogen
NIDDM	non-insulin-dependent diabetes mellitus	PBI	protein-bound iodine
NK	natural killer (cells); no ketones	PBP	penicillin-binding protein
NMP	normal menstrual period	PC	phosphatidylcholine; platelet count;
NMR	nuclear magnetic resonance		postcoital; premature contraction
NNACS	neonatal neurologic and adaptive	PCA	patient care aide; patient-controlled
	capacity score		anesthesia; posterior cerebral artery
NP	nasopharynx; no pain; not pregnant	PCAN	potential child abuse and neglect
NPH	neutral protamine Hagedorn (insulin);	PCB	polychlorinated biphenyl; postcoital
	no previous history; normal-pressure		bleeding
	hydrocephalus	PCC	pericardiocentesis; positional
n-RNP	anti-ribonucleic protein (antibody)		contraceptive
NST	nonstress test	PCG	phonocardiogram
NSU	nonspecific urethritis	PCL	persistent corpus luteum; posterior
NTD	neural tube defect		cruciate ligament
		P_{CO_2}	partial pressure of carbon dioxide
OA	occipitoanterior (fetal position)	PCOD	polycystic ovary disease
OB	obstetrics; occult bleeding	PCOS	polycystic ovary syndrome
OB/GYN	obstetrics and gynecology	PCP	phencyclidine pill (phencyclidine
OBN	occult blood negative		hydrochloride); *Pneumocystis carinii*
OBP	occult blood positive		pneumonia
OBS	organic brain syndrome	PCR	polymerase chain reaction; protein
OCCC	oocyte–cumulus–corona complex		catabolic rate
OCD	obsessive–compulsive disorder;	PCT	porphyria cutanea tarda; postcoital test;

	proximal convoluted tubule
PCTA	percutaneous transluminal angioplasty
PCU	pain control unit
PCWP	pulmonary capillary wedge pressure
PDA	patent ductus arteriosus
PDR	Physicians' Desk Reference
PE	physical examination; pleural effusion; probable error; pulmonary edema; pulmonary embolism
PEEP	positive end-expiratory pressure
PEG	pneumoencephalogram; pregnancy-associated endometrial globulin
PEP	primer extension pre-amplification
PET	positron emission tomography; pre-eclamptic toxemia
PFC	pelvic flexion contracture; persistent fetal circulation; plaque-forming cell
PFO	patent foramen ovale
PG	pregnant; prostaglandin
PGDH	prostaglandin dehydrogenase
PGI	prostacyclin
PGU	postgonococcal urethritis
pH	hydrogen-ion concentration
PI	periodontal index; physician intervention; ponderal index; pregnancy induced; present illness; pulmonary infarction; pulmonary insufficiency
PICU	pediatric intensive care unit
PID	pelvic inflammatory disease; prolapsed intervertebral disk
PIE	pulmonary interstitial edema; pulmonary interstitial emphysema
PIF	preimplantation factor; prolactin-inhibiting factor
PIH	pregnancy-induced hypertension; prolactin-inhibiting hormone
PLISSIT	permission, limited information, structured suggestions, intensive therapy
PLM	percent-labeled mitosis
PMB	postmenopausal bleeding
PMN	polymorphonuclear neutrophil
PMO	postmenopausal osteoporosis
PMPO	palpable postmenopausal ovary
PMS	passive maternal smoking; premenstrual syndrome
PMT	premenstrual tension
PNC	prenatal care
PND	pelvic node dissection
PNS	peripheral nervous system
Po2	partial pressure of oxygen
POF	premature ovarian failure
POL	premature onset of labor
POMC	pro-opiomelanocortin
POS	polycystic ovary syndrome
POST	peritoneal oocyte and sperm transfer
post op	postoperative

PPD	purified protein derivative (TB skin test); postpartum day
PPH	primary pulmonary hypertension
PPHN	persistent pulmonary hypertension of newborn
PPV	positive predictive value
PR	partial remission; peer review; proctologist; progesterone receptor; prosthion
PRF	prolactin-releasing factor
PRH	prolactin-releasing hormone
primip.	primiparous
PRL	prolactin
PROG	progesterone
PROM	premature rupture of membranes
PROST	pronuclear stage transfer
prox.	proximal
PSIS	posterosuperior iliac spine
PSTT	placental-site trophoblastic tumor
PSVT	paroxysmal supraventricular tachycardia
PT	parathyroid; paroxysmal tachycardia; prothrombin time
PTB	patellar-tendon-bearing (base or prosthesis); prior to birth
PTH	parathyroid hormone; posttransfusion hepatitis
PTH-rP	parathyroid hormone-related protein
PTSD	posttraumatic stress disorder
PTT	partial thromboplastin time; patellar tendon transfer
PTU	propylthiouracil
PUB	cisplatin, vinblastine, bleomycin
PUBS	percutaneous umbilical blood sampling
PUPPP	pruritic urticarial papules and plaques of pregnancy
PUVA	psoralen (plus) ultraviolet A
PV	peripheral vessels; polycythemia vera; portal vein
PWA	person with AIDS
PWM	pokeweed mitogen
Px	physical examination; pneumothorax; prognosis
PZD	partial zona dissection
Q	coulomb; quadrant; quotient; volume of blood
QCT	quantitative computed tomography
R	rate; reaction; rectum; respiration; roentgen
r	oxidation–reduction potential; respiration; roentgen
RA	radioactive; radium; ragweed antigen; residual air; rheumatoid arthritis; right atrium
RADIUS	routine antenatal diagnostic imaging

	with ultrasound		rate
RAP	recurrent abdominal pain	rRNA	ribosomal ribonucleic acid
RBB	right breast biopsy	RS	rectal sinus; Reiter's syndrome;
RBC	red blood cell; red blood count;		rheumatoid spondylitis; right side; right
	retinoblastoma		sacral
rbc	red blood cell	RSA	right sacroanterior (fetal position)
RBF	renal blood flow	RSP	right sacroposterior (fetal position)
RBOW	ruptured bag of waters	RST	right sacrotransverse (fetal position)
RBP	resting blood pressure; retinoid-binding	RSV	respiratory syncytial virus; Rous sarcoma
	protein		virus
RC	red cell; retention catheter	RT	radiation therapy; rectal temperature;
RCC	rape crisis center; red cell count; renal		renal transplant; reverse transcriptase;
	cell carcinoma		rubella titer
R/CS	repeat cesarean section	RTA	renal tubular acidosis
RCT	randomized control trial	RTx	radiation therapy
rDNA	recombinant deoxyribonucleic acid	RU	residual urine; roentgen unit
RDS	respiratory distress syndrome	RUQ	right upper quadrant (of abdomen)
RDVT	recurrent deep vein thrombosis	RV	residual volume; right ventricle; rubella
rem	roentgen-equivalent-man		vaccine; rubella virus
RF	renal failure; respiratory failure;	RVF	recto-vaginal fistula
	rheumatoid factor; risk factor	RVU	retroversion of uterus
RFA	right frontoanterior (fetal position)		
RFB	retained foreign body (in surgery)	S	heart sound; sacral (spinal nerves;
RFLP	restriction fragment length		vertebrae); saline; section; sedimentation
	polymorphism		coefficient; septum; serum; suction
RFP	right frontoposterior (fetal position)	s	second
RFT	right frontotransverse (fetal position)	SA	sacroanterior (fetal position); sarcoma;
RHD	rheumatic heart disease		semen analysis; serum albumin; surface
RhIg	Rh immunoglobulin		antigen
RI	radiation intensity; radioisotope;	SAB	spontaneous abortion
	regional ileitis; regular insulin	SB	shortness of breath; spina bifida;
RIA	radioimmunoassay		stillbirth; stillborn
RICS	right intercostal space	SBE	self breast examination; subacute
RM	radical mastectomy; repetition		bacterial endocarditis
	maximum; right mental	SCAN	scintiscan; suspected child abuse or
Rm	remission		neglect
RMA	right mentoanterior (fetal position)	SCC	squamous cell carcinoma; squamous
RMP	right mentoposterior (fetal position)		cell cancer
RMS	rhabdomyosarcoma	SCD	sudden cardiac death
RMT	right mentotransverse (fetal position)	SCID	severe combined immunodeficiency
RNA	ribonucleic acid	SD	septal defect; skin dose; standard
RO	right occipital		deviation; sterile dressing;
R/O	rule out		streptodornase; sudden death
ROA	right occipitoanterior (fetal position)	SDS	same-day surgery
ROC	receiver-operating-characteristic (curve)	sem.	semen
ROI	region of interest	SF	seminal fluid; spinal fusion; symptom-
ROM	range of motion (of a joint); rupture of		free; synovial fluid
	membranes	SGA	small for gestational age (infant)
ROP	retinopathy of prematurity; right	SGH	subgaleal hemorrhage
	occipitoposterior (fetal position)	SGO	Society of Gynecologic Oncology
ROT	right occipitotransverse (fetal position)	SHBG	sex hormone-binding globulin
RPF	relaxed pelvic floor; renal plasma flow	SI	International System of Units; sacroiliac
	(rate)		(joint); stress incontinence
RPLND	retroperitoneal lymph node dissection	SIFT	sperm intrafallopian transfer
RPR	rapid plasma reagin (test)	SIG	sigmoidoscopy
RR	recovery room; relative risk; respiratory	sigmo	sigmoidoscopy

SIJ	sacroiliac joint
SIL	squamous intraepithelial lesion
SIMV	spontaneous intermittent mandatory ventilation; synchronized intermittent mandatory ventilation
SIN	salpingitis isthmica nodosa
SLE	systemic lupus erythematosus
SM	sadomasochism; self-monitoring; simple mastectomy; small; smoker; smooth muscle; synovial membrane; systolic murmur
SMS	sperm motility study
SNS	sacral nerve stimulation
Sod.	sodomy
SP	sacroposterior (fetal position)
SPA	single-photon absorptiometry; spermatozoa penetration assay; suprapubic aspiration
SPBT	suprapubic bladder tap
sp. cd.	spinal cord
sp. fl.	spinal fluid
SPROM	spontaneous premature rupture of membranes
sp. tap	spinal tap
SR	sarcoplasmic reticulum; sedimentation rate; sinus rhythm; stomach rumble; suture removed; systems review
SRIF	somatotropin release-inhibiting factor
SRM	sexual maturity rating
SRY	sex-determining region of Y (chromosome)
ST	sacrotransverse (fetal position); scar tissue; smokeless tobacco; survival time
staph.	*Staphylococcus* (usually implies *Staphylococcus aureus*)
STB	stillborn
STD	sexually transmitted disease; standard test dose
STS	serologic test for syphilis
SUI	stress urinary incontinence
SUZI	subzonal insertion (of sperm)
SVD	sudden vaginal delivery
T	thoracic (nerves, vertebrae)
T_3	triiodothyronine
T_4	thyroxine
TA	toxin-antitoxin; transplantation antigen; tricuspid atresia; truncus arteriosus; tumor antigen
TAA	thoracic aortic aneurysm; tumor-associated antigen
TAE	total abdominal eventration
TAF	tumor-angiogenesis factor
TAH	total abdominal hysterectomy
TAH/BSO	total abdominal hysterectomy/ bilateral salpingo-oophorectomy

TAUS	transabdominal ultrasonography
TB	tracheobronchitis; tuberculin; tuberculosis
TBG	thyroid-binding globulin; thyroxine-binding globulin
TBLC	term birth, living child
TBW	total body water
TBS	The Bethesda System
TCA	terminal cancer; transluminal coronary angioplasty; trichloroacetic acid
TCT	thrombin-clotting time; total cholesterol test
TDF	testis-determining factor
TDI	toluene diisocyanate; therapeutic donor insemination
TE	thromboembolism; total ejaculate
TEBG	testosterone-estradiol-binding globulin
TEE	transesophageal echocardiography
TEST	tubal embryo stage transfer
TET	treadmill exercise test; tubal embryo transfer
TF	tetralogy of Fallot; tracheal fistula; transfer factor; tube feeding; tuning fork
TG	tendon graft; thyroglobulin; triglyceride
TH	thyroid hormone; total hysterectomy
TIBC	total iron-binding capacity
TID	therapeutic insemination, donor
TIH	therapeutic insemination, husband
TIL	tumor-infiltrating lymphocyte
TIS	tumor *in situ*
TIT	tubal insufflation test
TL	time lapse; tubal ligation
TLC	thin-layer chromatography; total lung capacity; total lymphocyte count
TNF	tumor necrosis factor
TNI	total nodal irradiation
TNM	tumor–node–metastasis (staging)
TO	target organ
TOA	time of arrival; tubo-ovarian abscess
TOF	tetralogy of Fallot
tomo	tomogram
TOP	termination of pregnancy
TORCH	toxoplasmosis, other infections, rubella, cytomegalovirus infection, and herpes (simplex)
TORCHS	toxoplasmosis, other infections, rubella, cytomegalovirus infection, herpes (simplex), and syphilis
TP	tubal pregnancy
tPA	tissue plasminogen activator
TPH	transplacental (fetal) hemorrhage
TPHA	*Treponema pallidum* hemagglutination assay
TPI	*Treponema pallidum* immobilization (test)
TPN	total parenteral nutrition
TPR	temperature, pulse, and respiration; testosterone production rate; total

	peripheral resistance
TRAP	twin-reversed-arterial perfusion
TRH	thyrotropin-releasing hormone
TRUS	transrectal ultrasonography
TS	toxic substance; transsexual; tricuspid stenosis
TSA	tumor-specific antigen
TSH	thyroid-stimulating hormone
TSI	thyroid-stimulating immunoglobulin
TT	tendon transfer; thrombin time; tilt table; total time
TTE	transthoracic echocardiogram
TTN	transient tachypnea of the newborn
TTP	thrombotic thrombocytopenic purpura
TTTS	twin–twin transfusion syndrome
TURP	transurethral resection of prostate
TV	total volume; transvestite; tricuspid valve
TVC	total vital capacity
TV-GIFT	transvaginal gamete intrafallopian transfer
TVH	total vaginal hysterectomy
TVS	transvaginal sonography
TV-TEST	transvaginal tubal embryo stage transfer
TVUS	transvaginal ultrasonography
TWAR	Taiwan acute respiratory (organism)
Tyr	tyrosine
U	unit; uracil; uranium; uridine; urine; urology
u	unit
UA	unstable angina; uric acid; urinalysis
U/A	urinalysis
UAC	umbilical artery catheterization
UC	ulcerative colitis; unsatisfactory condition; urea clearance; urine culture; uterine contraction
UCO	urinary catheter out
UG	urogenital
UGF	urinary gonadotropin factor
UI	unidentified; urinary incontinence
umb.	umbilical; umbilicus
UO	under observation; urinary output
UPI	uteroplacental insufficiency
UQ	upper quadrant
US	ultrasonography; ultrasound
USI	urinary stress incontinence
UT	urinary tract; uterus
UTI	urinary tract infection
UTV	unable to void
UVC	umbilical vein catheterization
V	volume
V_A	alveolar ventilation
V_T	tidal volume
v	valve; ventilation; ventral; ventricular; volt; volume; vomiting

Vag.	vagina
VAIN	vaginal intraepithelial neoplasia
VB	vertebral body; viable birth
VBAC	vaginal birth after (previous) cesarean section
VBL	vertex–breech length; vinblastine
VC	vasoconstriction; vena cava; vital capacity
VCE	vagina, cervix, endocervix
VCF	vaginal contraceptive film
VCR	vincristine
VD	vasodilator; venereal disease; viral diarrhea; voided
VDAC	vaginal delivery after cesarean
VDG	venereal disease-gonorrhea
VDRL	Venereal Disease Research Laboratory
VDS	venereal disease-syphilis; vindesine
VE	vaginal examination
VH	vaginal hysterectomy; ventricular hypertrophy; viral hepatitis
VHDL	very-high-density lipoprotein
VI	vaginal irritation
VIN	vulvar intraepithelial neoplasia
VIN I	vulvar intraepithelial neoplasia, mild (with mild dysplasia)
VIN II	vulvar intraepithelial neoplasia, moderate (with moderate dysplasia)
VIN III	vulvar intraepithelial neoplasia, severe (with severe dysplasia)
VIP	vasoactive intestinal peptide; vasoactive intestinal polypeptide; voluntary interruption of pregnancy
VIS	vaginal irrigation smear
VLBW	very low birth weight (infant)
VLDL	very-low-density lipoprotein
VMA	vanillylmandelic acid
V-ONC	viral oncogene
VP	variegate porphyria; vasopressin; venipuncture; venous pressure
VRL	vinorelbine
VS	vital sign; volumetric solution; voluntary sterilization
VSD	ventricular septal defect; virtual safe dose
VV	varicose veins; vesicovaginal
VVC	vulvovaginal candidiasis
VVF	vesicovaginal fistula
VP	vasopressin
VZ	varicella zoster
VZIG	varicella-zoster immune globulin
VZV	varicella zoster virus
WBC	white blood cell; white blood count
WBCT	whole blood clotting time
WHO	World Health Organization
Xe	xenon
XU	excretory urogram

46XX	normal number of female chromosomes
46XY	normal number of male chromosomes
Y	yellow; yttrium
YAC	yeast artificial chromosomes
ZEEP	zero end-expiratory pressure
ZIFT	zygote intrafallopian transfer
ZFY	zinc finger protein on Y (chromosome)